Peripheral Nerve Issues after Orthopedic Surgery

Preface

Anatomy is power. For surgeons, there is no greater truth. A thorough knowledge of anatomy is required to deliver thoughtful and effective care, particularly when evaluating and treating patients with peripheral nerve injuries. In this book, we have made every effort to provide a comprehensive, image-rich resource of peripheral nerve anatomy for both practicing surgeons and trainees.

Many times, peripheral nerve injuries occur within the context of recent surgery. These unexpected events disrupt the patient's expected recovery and are stressful to both the patient and surgeon. As peripheral nerve surgeons, we are often asked to assist our colleagues in the evaluation and care of these patients. To capture the collaborative spirit of this relationship, we have paired subspecialty surgeons with peripheral nerve experts for the various anatomic locations throughout the body. These pairings allow the sharing of multiple perspectives on the prevention, evaluation, prognosis, and management of peripheral nerve issues after commonly performed surgeries in the upper and lower extremities.

We hope that this book and its many anatomic illustrations will be a useful resource that enriches your knowledge and empowers you during the care of your patients.

The Editors

St. Louis, MO, USA — Christopher J. Dy
St. Louis, MO, USA — David M. Brogan
Atlanta, GA, USA — Eric R. Wagner

Contents

Contributors

Eduard Alentorn, MD, MSc, PhD, FEBOT.2-4 Instituto Cugat, Hospital Quirónsalud Barcelona, Barcelona, Spain

Mutualidad Española de Futbolistas, Delegación Cataluña, Federación Española de Fútbol, Barcelona, Spain

Fundación García-Cugat, Barcelona, Spain

John M. Apostolakos, MD, MPH Department of Orthopaedic Surgery, Hospital for Special Surgery, New York, NY, USA

Heather Baltzer, MSc, MD, FRCSC, FACS Department of Plastic and Reconstructive Surgery, University of Toronto, Toronto, ON, Canada

Laura E. Bashour, MS Dell Medical School at the University of Texas at Austin, Austin, TX, USA

Marschall B. Berkes, MD Department of Orthopedic Surgery, Washington University School of Medicine, St. Louis, MO, USA

Jared Bookman, MD Department of Orthopedic Surgery, New York University School of Medicine, New York, NY, USA

Jay T. Bridgeman, MD, DDS Division Chief Hand and Microvascular Surgery, Department of Orthopedic Surgery, University of Missouri, Columbia, MO, USA

David M. Brogan, MD, MSc Department of Orthopedic Surgery, Washington University, St. Louis, MO, USA

Robert C. Bucelli, MD, PhD Department of Neurological Surgery, Washington University School of Medicine, Saint Louis, MO, USA

Department of Neurology, Washington University School of Medicine, Saint Louis, MO, USA

Charles A. Daly, MD Division of Upper Extremity Surgery, Department of Orthopedic Surgery, Emory University, Atlanta, GA, USA

Mihir Desai, MD, MS Division of Hand and Upper Extremity, Department of Orthopaedic Surgery at Vanderbilt University Medical Center, Nashville, TN, USA

Christopher F. Dibble, MD, PhD Department of Neurological Surgery, Washington University School of Medicine, Saint Louis, MO, USA

Department of Neurology, Washington University School of Medicine, Saint Louis, MO, USA

Christopher J. Dy, MD, MPH, FACS Department of Orthopedic Surgery, Washington University, St. Louis, MO, USA

Matthew Florczynski, MSc, MD Department of Orthopaedic Surgery, University of Toronto, Toronto, ON, Canada

Paige M. Fox, MD PhD Chase Hand and Upper Limb Center, Division of Plastic and Reconstructive Surgery, Stanford University School of Medicine, Stanford, CA, USA

Jared M. Gopman, MD Division of Plastic and Reconstructive Surgery, Department of Surgery, Icahn School of Medicine at Mount Sinai Hospital, New York, NY, USA

Michael B. Gottschalk, MD Division of Upper Extremity Surgery, Department of Orthopedic Surgery, Emory University, Atlanta, GA, USA

Jacob K. Greenberg, MD Department of Neurological Surgery, Washington University School of Medicine, Saint Louis, MO, USA

Department of Neurology, Washington University School of Medicine, Saint Louis, MO, USA

Jacques Hacquebord, MD Department of Orthopedic Surgery, Hansjörg Wyss Department of Plastic Surgery, New York University School of Medicine, New York, NY, USA

Hand Surgery Service, Bellevue Hospital Center, New York, NY, USA

Steven L. Henry, MD Institute of Reconstructive Plastic Surgery, Dell Medical School at the University of Texas at Austin, Austin, TX, USA

J. Ryan Hill, MD Department of Orthopedic Surgery, Washington University School of Medicine, St. Louis, MO, USA

Callie Jewett, MD Department of Orthopaedic Surgery at Vanderbilt University Medical Center, Nashville, TN, USA

Robin N. Kamal, MD Chase Hand and Upper Limb Center, Department of Orthopaedic Surgery, Stanford University School of Medicine, Stanford, CA, USA

Steve Key, MA FRCS Joint Replacement Unit, Royal National Orthopaedic Hospital, Stanmore, UK

Steven T. Lanier, MD NorthShore University Health System, Evanston, IL, USA

Kenneth M. Lin, MD Department of Orthopaedic Surgery, Hospital for Special Surgery, New York, NY, USA

Milton T. Little, MD Cedars-Sinai Medical Center, Los Angeles, CA, USA

Andrés A. Maldonado, MD, PhD Department of Plastic, Hand and Reconstructive Surgery, BG Trauma Center Frankfurt am Main, Academic Hospital of the Goethe University Frankfurt am Main, Frankfurt am Main, Germany

Department of Plastic Surgery, University Hospital Getafe, Madrid, Spain

Benjamin A. McArthur, MD Dell Medical School at the University of Texas at Austin, Austin, TX, USA

Moira M. McCarthy, MD Department of Orthopaedic Surgery, Hospital for Special Surgery, New York, NY, USA

Eitan Melamed, MD Division of Plastic and Reconstructive Surgery, Department of Surgery, Icahn School of Medicine at Mount Sinai Hospital, New York, NY, USA

Elmhurst Hospital Center, Elmhurst, NY, USA

Travis J. Miller, MD Division of Plastic and Reconstructive Surgery, Stanford University, Stanford, CA, USA

Mitchel R. Obey, MD Department of Orthopedic Surgery, Washington University School of Medicine, St. Louis, MO, USA

Daniel A. Osei, MD, MSc Department of Orthopaedic Surgery, Hospital for Special Surgery, New York, NY, USA

Ryan Paul, MD, FRCSC Department of Orthopaedic Surgery, University of Toronto, Toronto, ON, Canada

Department of Plastic and Reconstructive Surgery, University of Toronto, Toronto, ON, Canada

Lukas Pindur, MD Department of Plastic, Hand and Reconstructive Surgery, BG Trauma Center Frankfurt am Main, Academic Hospital of the Goethe University Frankfurt am Main, Frankfurt am Main, Germany

Bridget P. Pulos, MD Department of Anesthesiology, Mayo Clinic, Rochester, MN, USA

Nicholas Pulos, MD Department of Orthopedic Surgery, Mayo Clinic, Rochester, MN, USA

Tom Quick, MA MD(res) FRCS Peripheral Nerve Injury Unit, Royal National Orthopaedic Hospital, Stanmore, UK

Centre for Nerve Engineering, University College London, London, UK

Anil S. Ranawat, MD Department of Orthopaedic Surgery, Hospital for Special Surgery, New York, NY, USA

Wilson Z. Ray, MD Department of Neurological Surgery, Washington University School of Medicine, Saint Louis, MO, USA

Department of Neurology, Washington University School of Medicine, Saint Louis, MO, USA

Alexander Rothy, MD Joseph M. Abell Arthroplasty and Value-Based Health Care Delivery Fellow, Dell Medical School at the University of Texas at Austin, Austin, TX, USA

Kyle Schweser, MD Division Chief Foot and Ankle Surgery, Department of Orthopedic Surgery, University of Missouri, Columbia, MO, USA

Maksim A. Shlykov, MD, MS Department of Orthopedic Surgery, Washington University School of Medicine, St. Louis, MO, USA

John Skinner, FRCS Joint Replacement Unit, Royal National Orthopaedic Hospital, Stanmore, UK

Katherine M. Velicki, BA Washington University School of Medicine, St. Louis, MO, USA

Steven Weinfeld, MD, FAAOS Summit Medical Group, NJ, Berkeley, NJ, USA

Kitty Wu, MD Department of Plastic and Reconstructive Surgery, Western University, London, ON, Canada

Part I

Overview and Evaluation of Nerve Injuries after Orthopedic Surgery

1 Nerve Compression, Nerve Injury, and Nerve Regeneration: An Overview

Steven T. Lanier and David M. Brogan

1.1 Peripheral Nerve Anatomy and Physiology

The architecture of a peripheral nerve includes axons and perineural Schwann cells enveloped within a connective tissue matrix. Axons can be myelinated or unmyelinated and are somatotopically grouped within a peripheral nerve into units called fascicles [1]. The connective tissue framework of the nerve includes endoneurium that surrounds individual axon fibers within fascicles, a perineurium surrounding individual fascicles, and an epineurium which encircles groups of fascicles and forms the external sheath of a nerve. Within this connective tissue framework is a vascular supply that nourishes the nerve. A detailed understanding of neural anatomy and physiology provides the basis for our understanding of various mechanisms and patterns of nerve injury as well as potential for recovery. Figure 1.1 provides an overview of this architecture; each individual component is discussed in greater detail below.

S. T. Lanier (✉)
NorthShore University Health System, Evanston, IL, USA
e-mail: SLanier@northshore.org

D. M. Brogan
Department of Orthopedic Surgery, Washington University, St. Louis, MO, USA
e-mail: brogand@wustl.edu

1.1.1 Axon

The axon is the basic functional unit of a nerve, and a peripheral nerve can be conceptualized as a cable of axon fibers. Most major peripheral nerves contain a combination of motor, sensory, and autonomic axons. Neuronal cell bodies of motor axons are found in the ventral horn of the spinal cord, whereas sensory and autonomic cell bodies are found adjacent to the spinal cord in dorsal root ganglia and autonomic ganglia, respectively (Fig. 1.2).

Axons are long, thin processes that extend peripherally from neuron cell bodies and transmit information that is encoded in the form of bursts of electrical activity known as action potentials. The axon itself consists of an axolemmal cell membrane that houses a fluid axoplasm, a network of neurofibrils used for axoplasmic transport, and other cellular organelles. Motor axons carry efferent information from the central nervous system (CNS) to end effectors such as skeletal muscles, and sensory axons carry afferent information from sensory end organs back to the CNS. Anterograde and retrograde axoplasmic transport are energy-requiring processes that are responsible for the shuttling of materials to and from the cell body, which can be disrupted with axonal injury. An important component of this includes anterograde transport of neurotransmitter filled vesicles to the neuromuscular junction.

C. J. Dy et al. (eds.), *Peripheral Nerve Issues after Orthopedic Surgery*,
https://doi.org/10.1007/978-3-030-84428-8_1

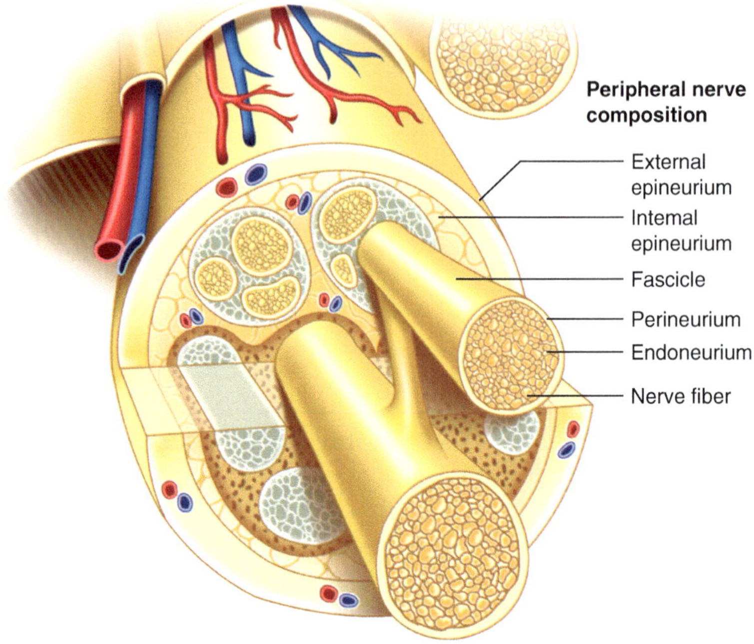

Fig. 1.1 Peripheral nerve architecture. Myelinated and unmyelinated axon fibers are surrounded by endoneurium and grouped together into fascicles by perineurium. Fascicles within the nerve are surrounded by an inner epineurium, and the entire nerve is enveloped by the outer epineurium. Longitudinal extrinsic blood vessels on the epineurial surface communicate with an intrinsic vascular plexus within the inner connective tissue framework of the nerve

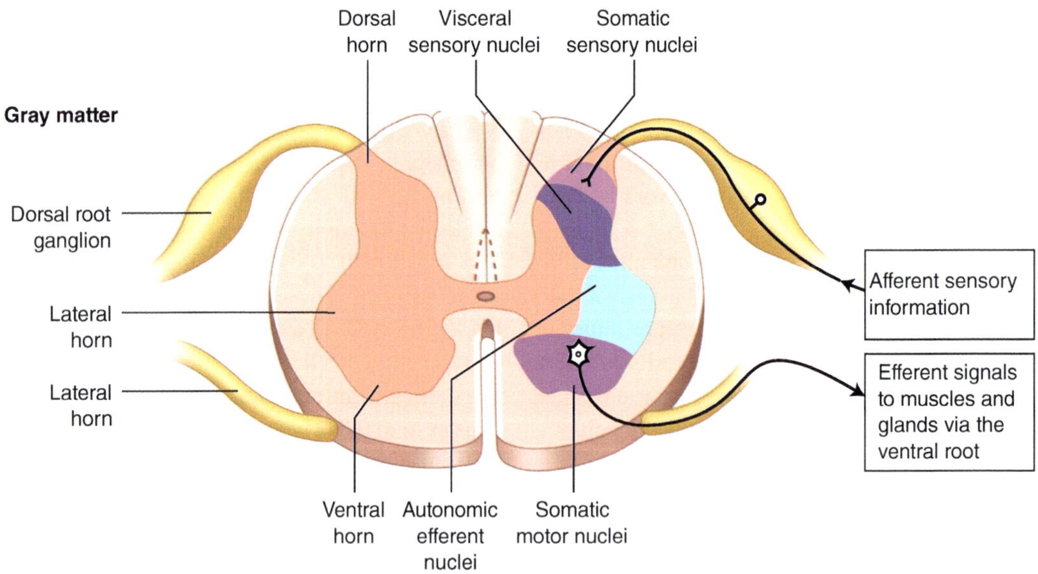

Fig. 1.2 Cross-sectional anatomy of the spinal cord. Motor cell bodies are located in the ventral horn of the spinal cord and send efferent motor axons distally. Afferent sensory information is carried from end organs proximally to bipolar sensory nerve cell bodies located in dorsal root ganglia, adjacent to the spinal cord. These bipolar sensory axons form a second synapse with sensory cell bodies in the dorsal horn of the spinal cord. Distal to the dorsal root ganglia, the motor efferent fibers and sensory afferent fibers join together into spinal nerves. Spinal nerves then branch into dorsal and ventral rami

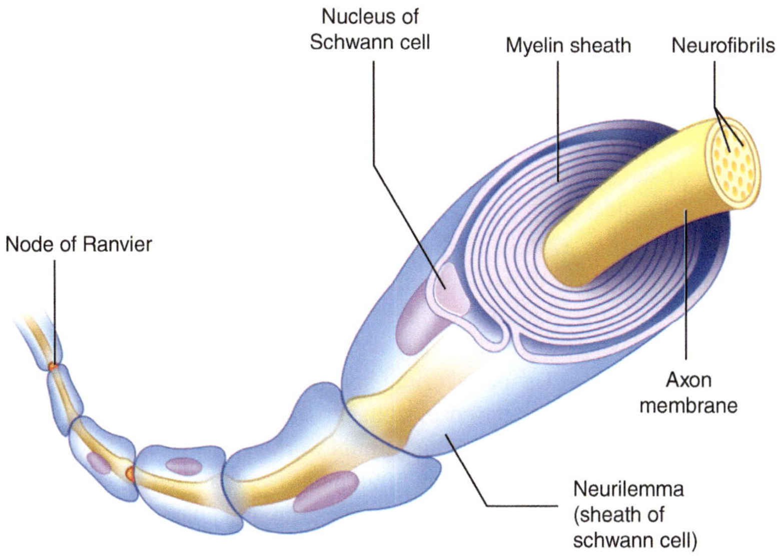

Fig. 1.3 Myelinated axon. Myelinated axon fibers are enveloped by concentric rings of myelin produced by a single Schwann cell. Myelin sheaths from adjacent Schwann cells are arranged in parallel and separated by spaces called Nodes of Ranvier. Myelin serves to insulate nerve impulses and results in "saltatory conduction," by which impulses travel quickly across myelinated sections to the Nodes of Ranvier

Axon fibers vary in diameter and in whether or not they are encased in a myelin sheath. The speed with which electric impulses are transmitted down an axon increases with fiber diameter and with myelination. Myelinated fibers are larger in diameter and are surrounded by concentric rings of myelin produced by a single Schwann cell (Fig. 1.3). Unmyelinated fibers are relatively small in comparison, averaging on the order of 1 micron. Based on these characteristics, axon fibers are classified into three broad types according to their size and speed: Groups A (motor, light touch, and proprioception fibers), B (sympathetic preganglionic motor fibers), and C (pain and temperature fibers). Group A has multiple subtypes, ranging in speed from 10 m/s (sharp pain) to 100 m/s (large motor), depending on their specific function [2].

Myelin forms a multilaminar sheath around the axon fiber composed of proteins and phospholipids produced by a single Schwann cell. Sodium channels cluster in the interspaces between Schwann cells along the length of the axon known as Nodes of Ranvier, and the electrical impulse is transmitted quickly across insulated segments between these nodes in a process referred to as saltatory conduction. In this way, myelination speeds up axon potential propagation by several fold. The conduction velocity of unmyelinated axons range from 0.5 to 10 meters per second, while myelination results in a 15 fold increase to speeds of up to 150 meters per second [3].

1.1.2 Connective Tissue Framework

The connective tissue of a peripheral nerve can be thought of as a series of tubes within larger tubes. The endoneurium immediately surrounds both myelinated and unmyelinated axons within a fascicle. It forms a continuous sheath composed of an outer layer of collagen that runs the entire length of the axon from cell body to end organ. Within this endoneurial tube, the axon is bathed in a low-protein endoneurial fluid that is analogous to cerebrospinal fluid in the CNS [4]. Fibroblasts produce collagen fibers and glycosaminoglycans within the endoneurial space and are seen to hypertrophy when a nerve is recovering from injury. Endoneurial blood vessels provide nutrient flow. The non-fenestrated endothelial cells of these endoneurial vessels are connected by tight junctions that control free diffusion of molecules into the endoneurium, thus forming a blood–nerve barrier. Endoneurial pericytes play a role in modulating this barrier, which is often disrupted after nerve injury.

Axons, with their surrounding endoneurium, are grouped together into fascicles by the perineurium. The perineurium is a lamellar structure of elongated, flat perineurial cells connected to each other by tight junctions and serves as the main diffusion barrier between the endoneurium and external environment [5]. The perineurial barrier allows selective transport and vesicular transport of substances into and out of the endoneurial environment, while limiting passive diffusion. The number of perineurial cell layers increases with the size and number of axons within a fascicle, generally thinning as fascicles branch peripherally. The perineurium houses an extracellular matrix composed of collagen and fibronectin that provide a structural framework to modulate compressive forces and endoneurial pressure, thus maintaining endoneurial homeostasis.

Fascicles are themselves grouped together by the epineurium. An inner epineurium immediately surrounds the fascicles, while an outer epineurium composed of collagen and elastin fibers forms the outer layer of the peripheral nerve itself. The ratio of connective tissue to neural tissue in a peripheral nerve varies along the course of the nerve, with a greater degree of connective tissue usually found in areas where the nerve is subject to strain, such as across joints [6].

1.1.3 Vascular Supply

Peripheral nerves have a rich extrinsic and intrinsic blood supply that are interconnected [7, 8]. Extrinsic blood vessels travel longitudinally along the course of the nerve on the outer surface of the epineurium. Smith describes these extrinsic, longitudinal vessels as being located within a loose, areolar connective tissue network around the nerve called the mesoneurium. Anastomotic channels called vasa nervorum connect extrinsic vessels to a rich, longitudinal vascular plexus located in the perineurium between fascicles, thus feeding the intrinsic blood supply. Further oblique branches from this perineurial plexus anastomose with the intrinsic endoneurial vasculature. Extrinsic vessels feed the intrinsic system at various points along the nerve, though the robustness of this intrinsic circulation allows long segments of a peripheral nerve to be dissected free of the extrinsic mesoneurium without the nerve becoming ischemic, such as is required for an ulnar nerve transposition at the elbow.

1.1.4 Fascicular Anatomy

Axons within the peripheral nerve are grouped together into fascicles which vary in size between nerves and along the longitudinal axis of a given peripheral nerve. Somatotopy refers to the functional clustering of nerve fibers within a fascicle [1]. Distally, peripheral nerves have a high degree of somatotopic organization with fascicles containing groups of axons destined to innervate a specific muscle or carrying sensory information from a very specific region of the skin. These fascicles can often be dissected for several centimeters proximal to their end target. As one moves proximally along the peripheral nerve, the internal topography of the nerve becomes less cable like and more plexiform, with increasing interconnections between fascicles. Despite increasing fascicular interconnections proximally, recent experimental evidence using tracer technology and advanced imaging techniques indicates that the somatotopic organization of axons is largely maintained throughout the course of the peripheral nerve [1]. This fascicular organization of the peripheral nerve can have important implications for nerve repair.

1.2 Classification of Nerve Injuries and Implications for Prognosis

Iatrogenic injury accounts for almost 20% of peripheral nerve traumatic injuries, and orthopedic surgeons are at the highest risk of causing such injuries [9]. Knowledge of the normal anatomic structure of peripheral nerves is a prerequisite to understand the pathophysiology of nerve injury, as function follows structure. Clinically, nerve injuries may present as anything from a mild sensory impairment (resolving within days to weeks) to a more profound loss of motor function. Prognostic information may be gleaned from accurate classification of the degree of nerve injury; therefore, Seddon devised a classification system dividing injured nerves into one of three broad categories: neurapraxia, axonotmesis, and neurotmesis [10]. While this may be an intuitive system, it belies important distinctions regarding the degree of nerve injury and potential for recovery. Recognizing these limitations, a more specific classification was devised by Sunderland to better correlate the differing degrees of injury with the underlying pathology. Ranging from Grade 1, a temporary alteration in nerve function, to Grade 5, complete severance of the nerve, Sunderland's classification correlates increasing degrees of dysfunction with increasing damage to the internal architecture of the nerve (Table 1.1). Knowledge of this classification system is important for the nerve surgeon faced with treatment of a postoperative complication, as accurate characterization can provide prognostic information for the affected patient. Ninety seven per cent of patients with Grade 1 injuries (neurapraxia) regain normal function and 83% of those with Grade 5 injuries (complete transection of the nerve) achieve little or no functional recovery [11]. However, accurate determination of the degree of nerve injury is at times best determined in retrospect, based on the ultimate recovery of the patient.

1.2.1 Nerve Injury

As described above, the presence of Wallerian degeneration is an important distinction between a transient conduction block and a more severe injury requiring axonal regrowth. Mechanisms of possible nerve injury include compressive neuropathies, traction injuries, or some form of traumatic transection. The molecular processes and subsequent changes in neuronal physiology can vary based on the degree and duration of nerve injury.

Table 1.1 Sunderland Classification of Nerve Injury [12]

Grade	Neural Elements Injured	Clinical Manifestations
1	Axonal conduction alone is interrupted, without significant derangement to the surrounding neural architecture	Rapid recovery of transient sensory deficits, with or without temporary muscle paresis or paralysis
2	Disruption of axonal continuity resulting in Wallerian degeneration in the affected axons, with maintained endoneurial tubes	Partial or complete loss of sensation or motor function. Recovery of function follows described innervation patterns of muscle with complete or near complete restoration of function
3	Disruption of endoneurial tubes and their contents	Longer period of recovery compared to second degree injuries, with incomplete recovery due to intraneural fibrosis and misdirection of regenerating axons due to loss of endoneurial tubes
4	Disruption of a larger percentage of the nerve (fascicular disruption) affecting the perineurium	Severe loss of sensory or motor function with minimal spontaneous regeneration may often result in a neuroma in continuity
5	Transection of the nerve, with disruption of the epineurium	Complete loss of all function with no spontaneous regeneration, requires repair

1.2.2 Compression Injuries

Compression of a nerve decreases venous return within the nerve and leads to increased edema that correlates with the degree of compression [13]. The degree of global nerve injury depends in part on the severity of compression – 30 mmHg has demonstrated breakdown of myelin, with 80 mmHg applied over 2 hours resulting in axonal loss in a rat sciatic nerve model [13]. Similar pressure thresholds in a rabbit tibial nerve model have demonstrated venous disruption at 20 mmHg, impairment of capillary flow at 40–50 mmHg, and cessation of intraneural blood flow at 60–80 mmHg [14]. Two hours of severe compression at 400 mmHg resulted in persistent alterations in blood flow at 3 and 7 days post-injury.

Animal studies of acute compression have shed light on the lasting physiologic effects of isolated neural trauma. Sustained acute compressive injuries, similar to that described above, have served as the basis of several early investigations in the field. Rydevik applied increasing amounts of pressure to a rabbit vagus nerve for 2 hours and found that 50 mmHg resulted in a reversible blockage of axonal transport, while 200 and 400 mmHg resulted in sustained blockage for up to 1 and 3 days. While these pressures did not induce Wallerian degeneration, the authors note that smaller unmyelinated fibers such as the vagal nerve are more resistant to injury than larger myelinated fibers [15]. A similar experiment conducted on rabbit tibial nerves showed minimal effect on nerve conduction velocity at 50 mm Hg compression. However, 200 and 400 mm Hg resulted in reduction of conduction velocity that persisted for at least 2 weeks, with evidence of axonal injury and demyelination [16]. Prior studies demonstrated that a traumatic compression of 50 mmHg for 2 hours resulted in alterations of epineurial vessels, while prolonged trauma or increased pressure resulted in endoneurial damage [17]. A clinical corollary for the surgeon is that even minor pressure or retraction to a nerve applied for a long duration during a case can result in alterations in axonal transport or even axonal damage from acute compression. The degree of dysfunction should be related to the magnitude and duration of the compressive injury.

These changes found in the epineurial and endoneurial vessels after prolonged compression help to explain the pathophysiology of chronic compression as well. The first manifestation of compressive nerve injury is edema with subsequent fibrosis of the perineurium and epineurium. Persistent intraneural pressure elevation leads to loss of myelin around the axons (Fig. 1.4) with a resultant increase in latency detectable on nerve

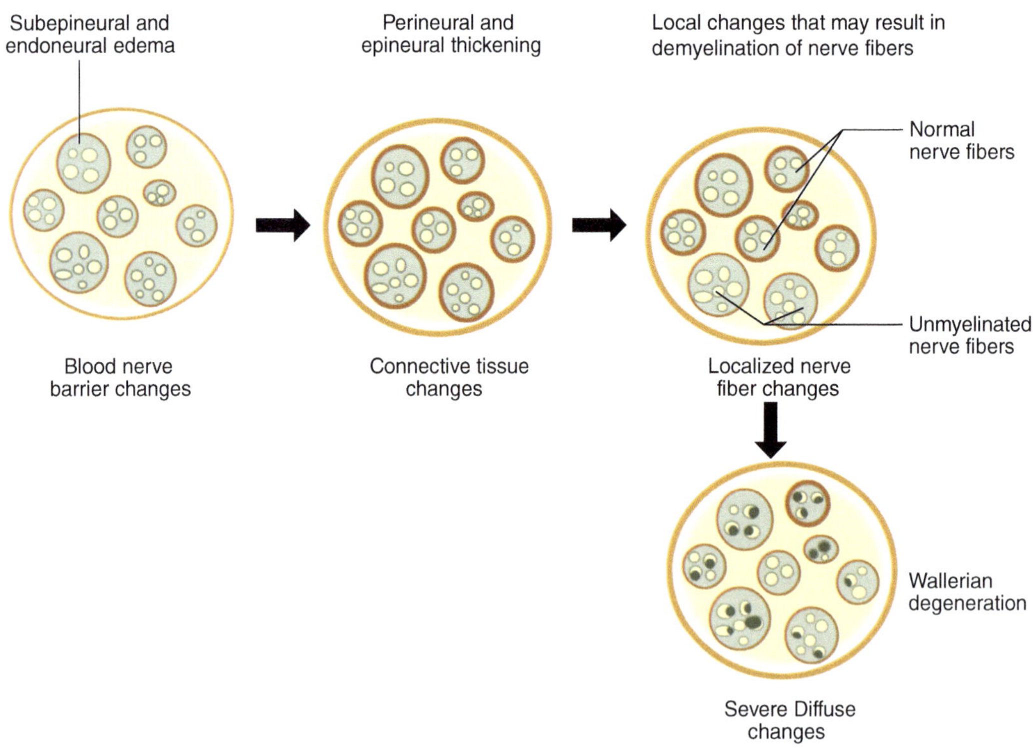

Fig. 1.4 Sequelae of nerve compression. Progressive ischemic changes occur in the peripheral nerve in response to compression, resulting ultimately in fibrosis

conduction studies (NCS). As the injury progresses, endoneurial ischemia develops, with subsequent axonal degeneration, venous congestion, and inflammation [18]. Initial treatment strategies of compressive neuropathy rely on decreasing pressure experienced by the nerve. In the most common compressive neuropathy, carpal tunnel syndrome [19] is accomplished with splints to alter wrist position or steroid injections to reduce swelling and decrease pressure in the carpal tunnel. Surgical release can substantially improve nocturnal symptoms and results in more than 80% patient satisfaction, but persistent slowing in nerve conduction studies is present in almost 80% of patients at 1 year [20].

The increased edema seen with chronic compressive neuropathies and the discomfort accompanying electrodiagnostic testing has given rise to interest in the use of ultrasound (US) to diagnose peripheral entrapment neuropathies. The overall cross-sectional area of the median nerve on ultrasound has been found to correlate with severity of carpal tunnel syndrome [21]. Beyond morphologic changes, intraneural blood flow has been identified as a possible predictor of median nerve entrapment at the wrist. A critical review of studies using Doppler sonography to identify carpal tunnel syndrome reported a median sensitivity of 72% and a median specificity of 88% [22]. A meta-analysis performed by Fowler et al. evaluating ultrasound findings of structural changes yielded similar findings, with a diagnostic sensitivity of 77.6% and specificity of 86.8% [23].

While the electrophysiologic changes associated with carpal tunnel release are well studied [24], less is known about the natural history of the above morphologic changes to the nerve. Li et al. examined the changes in median nerve cross-sectional area and total length of nerve edema before and after carpal tunnel release. They found that a significant improvement in cross-sectional area and nerve diameter was seen between 4 and 12 weeks postoperatively; however, a return to normal nerve diameter was not seen until 1 year after surgery. Even at 1 year follow-up, cross-sectional area was marginally increased compared to healthy controls [25].

1.2.3 Stretch Injury

Uninjured peripheral nerves have the capacity to glide within the extremities – this has been measured at almost 20 mm for the median nerve at the wrist [26]. Animal studies have shown acute changes in nerve conduction with increasing stretch of nerves – Wall demonstrated a transient 70% decline in conduction amplitude after a 6% strain on a rabbit tibial nerve for 20 minutes. When the strain was increased to 12%, a complete conduction block was found, with only a 40% recovery at 2 hours post-injury [27]. Kwan further investigated the ex vivo mechanical properties of rabbit tibial nerve, as well as in vivo responses to stress and strain in the rabbit tibial and sciatic nerve. Ex vivo testing of the tibial nerve resulted in a stress/strain curve demonstrating significant intrinsic strain in vivo with minimal stress. The viscoelastic behavior of the nerve allowed stress relaxation under mild strains, but failure of the nerve under high tension occurred due to perineurial disruption, beginning at a 27% increase beyond in situ strain. Nerve conduction velocity was maintained at 60% of normal amplitude after an hour of 6% strain, but dropped to 40% of normal within 20 minutes of application of a 12% strain [28].

Laser Doppler flowmetry has been used to better characterize the physiologic mechanisms contributing to decreased neural function under stress and strain. Peak conduction velocity and blood flow were measured under conditions of increasing strain in a rabbit tibial nerve. While an 8% and 16% strain both resulted in similar reductions in blood flow, only the 16% strain caused a drop in peak conduction velocity, leading the authors to conclude that ischemia alone cannot explain changes in nerve function due to significant strain [29].

1.2.4 Nerve Transection/Severe Axonotmetic Injury

While the peripheral nervous system has a capacity for axonal regeneration, particularly in compressive neuropathies or mild stretch injuries, the repair of a transected nerve yields inferior outcomes compared to the native state. This is likely due to derangement of the internal architecture and resultant misdirection of recovering axons. Maximal return of motor strength may not occur for up to 4 years [30] as collateral sprouting occurs and the nerve must regenerate to its target from the site of injury. Recovery of nerve function and growth is estimated as 1 mm/day or 1 inch per month in humans and typically regarded as 2–3.5 mm/day after transection in rats and rabbits [31]. Therefore, nerve injuries occurring near the shoulder may take more than a year to reach target muscles in the hand. This poor return of function and lengthy time to achieve some recovery has profound consequences on the emotional and financial well-being of the patient. Indirect costs alone from lost wages after traumatic brachial plexus injuries of the upper extremity have been estimated at more than $1.1 million [32]. Therefore, maximizing functional recovery by early and accurate diagnosis and subsequent intervention is paramount for the treating surgeon. A basic understanding of the pathophysiologic processes of nerve injury, degeneration, and repair by nerve surgeons is therefore critical to help inform clinical decision making.

1.2.5 NAD+ Homeostasis Is Critical to Preserving Distal Axonal Integrity

Upon transection or severe injury of a nerve, a complex interplay of irreversible changes occurs, beginning within 6 hours of injury. Initial extracellular calcium levels rise in the proximal and distal stumps, which leads to a series of molecular events that consume nicotinamide adenine dinucleotide (NAD+), increase levels of nicotinamide mononucleotide (NMN), and reduce levels of ATP [33]. In uninjured nerves, NAD^+ is present in higher concentrations than NMN. NAD^+ is generated by nicotinamide mononucleotide adenyltransferase 1 (Nmnat1) utilizing NMN as a precursor. The loss of ATP from the axons leads to dysfunction of its normal energy balance, resulting in mitochondrial destabilization and release of intracellular calcium from mitochondrial stores [33]. This second release of calcium appears to be critical for axonal degradation and initiation of Wallerian degeneration, resulting in destabilization of microtubules as well as fragmentation of axons, with their subsequent clearance by glial cells.

The onset of Wallerian degeneration stimulates Schwann cell transdifferentiation from a pro-myelinating phenotype into a regenerative phenotype critical to the process of neuronal regrowth. This Schwann cell transdifferentiation occurs due to upregulation of the transcriptional factor c-Jun [34] after nerve injury, due to increased intracellular Ca^{2+} levels [35]. C-Jun is critical to the formation of Bands of Bungner and promotion of axonal regeneration across the repair site [36]. Macrophages also appear to have a role in the regulation of Schwann cell response to nerve injury, assisting in proliferation of mature Schwann cells from a regenerative phenotype to a remyelination phenotype (transdifferentiation), likely via Gas6 [37], as part of the overall inflammatory process leading from nerve injury to nerve repair. The transcription factor Krox-20 functions to inhibit c-Jun activation, serving as a negative control to promote differentiation of Schwann cells back into the myelinating phenotype [38].

SARM-1 has been identified as the central executioner of Wallerian degeneration by cleavage of NAD^+ through the intrinsic NADase activity housed in its Toll/Interleukin-1 Receptor [39] (TIR) domain, which results in an imbalance of NMN vs NAD+. The importance of the relative balance of NMN and NAD+ to neuronal homeostasis has been underscored by the finding that the Wld^s protein prevents or delay axonal degeneration, through synthesis of NAD^+ with its nicotinamide mononucleotide adenyltransferase 1 (Nmnat1) enzymatic domain [40]. Animals with this phenotype demonstrate delayed Wallerian degeneration after nerve injury, supporting the concept that loss of NAD^+ and subsequent ATP loss is critical to initiation of Wallerian degeneration. However, the exact mechanism by which SARM-1 is activated after injury is still unclear, although some reports suggest that it is related to the intrinsic neuronal immune response to injury [41]. Loss of SARM-1 prevents consumption of NAD+ after axonal injury, resulting in conserved levels of ATP [42] and ultimately preventing calcium influx as well as Wallerian degeneration [43].

1.2.6 Assessment of Nerve Injury

Imaging can play a role in the evaluation of peripheral nerve dysfunction after surgery. No clear consensus exists on the ideal imaging method, but both ultrasound (US) and magnetic resonance imaging (MRI) have proven to be effective. MRI relies on detecting the difference in proton concentrations between tissues – therefore, pathologic conditions that result in increased edema or proton shifts may be amenable to evaluation with MRI. Increased T2 signal within a rat sciatic nerve after axonotmetic injury has been correlated with nerve conduction changes and muscle strength. An increase in signal distal to the site of the injury was visualized immediately, and this signal persisted until 2 weeks prior to complete restoration of compound motor action potentials (CMAP) in the foot. A proximal to distal resolution of the edema correlated well with functional recovery at the affected level [44]. Cudlip demonstrated similar increases in T2 signal intensity after a crush injury with a forceps, as well as a transient increase in sham-operated controls [45]. A more recent retrospective clinical series correlated intraoperative findings of a neuroma with preoperative MRI findings. All 20 neuromas in this series showed indistinct margins, and the portion of the nerve distal to the injury was larger in diameter than the more proximal nerve [46].

Traditional MRI has given way in recent years to magnetic resonance neurography, a specific technique utilizing MRI but focused on visualization of peripheral nerves. The precise spatial resolution of MR neurography (0.3–0.5 mm) allows detection of changes in a myriad of nerve properties to more precisely identify and characterize peripheral nerve pathology [47]. The characteristics that can be evaluated include changes in nerve diameter, contour, fascicular arrangement, continuity, signal intensity, and fat planes. This precision is helpful in the diagnosis of peripheral nerve injuries and the distinction between neurapraxic, axonotmetic, and neurotmetic injuries, which may influence clinical decision making (Table 1.2).

Enthusiasm for the wealth of information available from MR neurography is tempered by its potential cost and lack of availability in certain centers. A less expensive and more readily accessible alternative to evaluate peripheral nerve pathology is ultrasound (Fig. 1.5). The feasibility of ultrasound in detecting peripheral nerve injuries has been demonstrated in a cadaver study of 12 arms [48]. A sonographer blinded to the location of the nerve injuries was able to accurately detect nerve transection with a sensitivity of 89% and a specificity of 95%. Small case series have shown the potential of localization of iatrogenic injuries using ultrasound by examining for diffuse axonal swelling, nerve discontinuity, and compression of nerves by overlying plates [49].

Ultrasound also allows evaluation of the surrounding tissue to assess for hematoma or scar tissue. Karabay [50] examined clinical applications of ultrasound in the diagnosis of nine patients with iatrogenic upper extremity peripheral nerve injuries over a period of 3 years. All but one of the injuries involved the radial or posterior interosseous nerve (PIN), and five of the nine were indicated for exploration of the nerve based on the ultrasound findings. In one of the patients, the nerve could not be visualized due to body habitus. The authors used the following criteria as ultrasound evidence of a nerve injury:

1. Complete lack of nerve continuity
2. Formation of a neuroma or general fusiform swelling of the nerve at the suspected site of injury
3. Loss of fascicular pattern, or in partial injuries, evidence of intact epineurium on one side and disruption of the epineurium on the other side of the nerve
4. Hypoechoic texture of the nerve on ultrasound or generalized swelling of the nerve (possible stretch or contusion injury)

Table 1.2 Nerve injury classification (grading) based on Seddon's and Sunderland's classifications, electrophysiology, and magnetic resonance neurography (MRN) findings [47]

Sunderland class of nerve injury	Seddon class of nerve injury	Myelin	Axon	Endoneurium	Perineurium	Epineurium	Electrophysiology			MRN findings
							SNAP	CMAP	EMG	
I	*Neurapraxia*	Abnormal	Normal	Normal	Normal	Normal	Normal	Normal or CB	Normal but IP Decreased	Hyperintense nerve
II	*Axonotmesis*	Abnormal	Abnormal	Normal	Normal	Normal	Ampl Decreased	Ampl Decreased	SA and IP Decreased	Hyperintense and thickened nerve with/without prominent fascicles
III		Abnormal	Abnormal	Abnormal	Normal	Normal				
IV		Abnormal	Abnormal	Abnormal	Abnormal	Normal			0	Heterogeneous nerve signal with lateral or fusiform neuroma in continuity
V	*Neurotmesis*	Abnormal	Abnormal	Abnormal	Abnormal	Abnormal	Absent	Absent	No MUPS	Complete nerve gap

Please note muscle denervation change is typically absent in class I injury and full recovery is expected in class I/II injuries. In class III–V injuries, prognosis is guarded
SNAP sensory nerve action potential, *Ampl* amplitude, *CMAP* compound motor action potential, *EMG* electromyography, *CB* conduction block, *IP* interference pattern, *MUPS* motor unit potentials, *SA* spontaneous activity

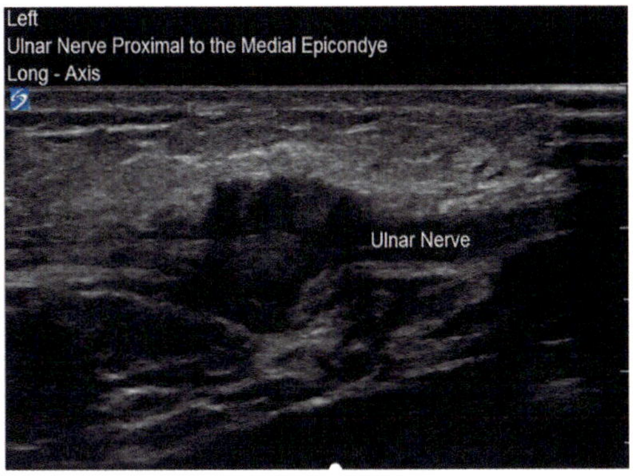

Fig. 1.5 Ultrasound of a neuroma. An ulnar nerve neuroma is imaged just proximal to the medial epicondyle – note the large bulbous structure consistent with a neuroma continuous with the normal caliber of the ulnar nerve proximally

A retrospective review comparing the sensitivity and specificity of ultrasound and MRI in identifying peripheral nerve pathology demonstrated a higher rate of true positives found in ultrasound, with a similar rate of true negatives between the modalities. Ultrasound was accurate and MRI was inaccurate in the diagnosis of 25% of patients [51]. The inaccuracy of MRI in fully identifying the peripheral nerve lesion was attributed to a more limited field of view with MRI, resulting in missed pathology outside of this field of view. The authors suggest that ultrasound is the preferred imaging modality for peripheral nerve pathology when the anatomic location is suitable for ultrasonography of nerves.

1.2.7 EMG/NCS

Despite advances in peripheral nerve imaging, nerve conduction studies and EMG remain the gold standard for diagnosis of peripheral nerve pathology. As the validity of the studies can be operator dependent, it is important for a peripheral nerve surgeon to develop a relationship with a trained electrophysiologist whom they trust to perform meticulous and accurate testing. Two types of electrophysiology tests are commonly employed – nerve conduction studies (NCS) and electromyography (EMG). NCS evaluates the health of the nerve itself, specifically the ability of the axons and myelin to propagate an electrical signal. However, NCS and EMG are only useful predictors of nerve function at a minimum of 2–3 weeks post-injury. After injury, nerves will undergo Wallerian degeneration, thus the true extent of the lesion will not be evident until this process has finished – earlier tests may give inaccurate diagnoses.

The treating nerve surgeon should have a basic understanding of the terminology and principles used in interpreting nerve conduction studies. In nerve conduction studies, stimulating electrodes are utilized to impart an electrical stimulus to the target nerve. In assessing sensory conduction, stimulating electrodes are placed over the area of sensory innervation and recording electrodes are placed proximally over the nerve to be assessed. This represents an orthodromic study, as it mimics the typical direction of a sensory nerve action potential (SNAP) propagation. Several parameters of a SNAP are of interest in identifying nerve pathology (Figs. 1.6 and 1.7). The latency of a signal refers to the elapsed time between the stimulus and the onset (or peak) of the sensory action potential. Nerve conduction velocity can be calculated by determining the latency at different locations and measuring the distance between these locations. Latency increases at further distances from the spinal cord, and changes in latency and conduction velocity reflect alterations in myelination [52]. In addition to latency, the amplitude of a signal gives critical information about the SNAP. Amplitude is a general measure of the strength of the conducted signal, which correlates to the number of axons that are functioning. In axonotmetic injuries, conduction may be possible, but with reduced amplitudes, reflecting the severity of the injury [52]. Similar to sensory nerve conduction studies, motor nerve conduction studies can be performed by placing a stimulating electrode proximally over the nerve of interest and recording the compound motor action potential (CMAP) generated by the muscle distally. CMAP latency and amplitude are measured in a method analogous to that used for SNAP latency and amplitude.

A commonly discussed phenomenon in brachial plexus injuries is that of a patient with a

Waveforms:

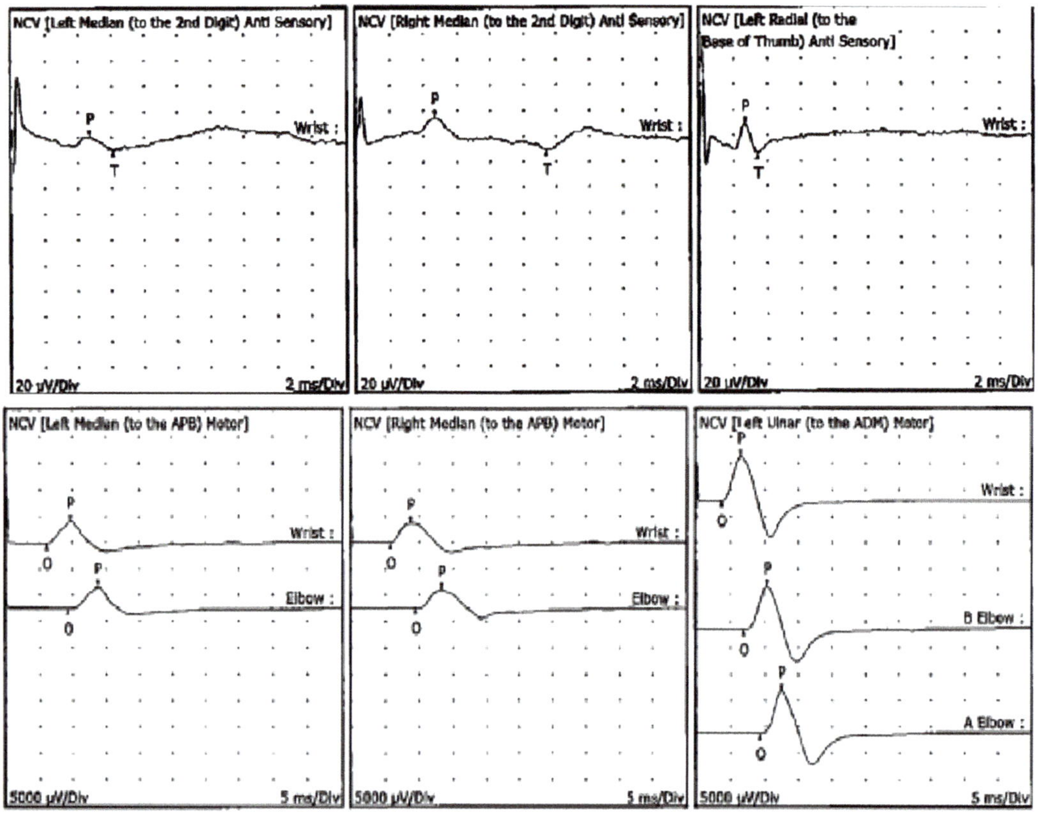

Fig. 1.6 Sensory and motor nerve conduction study waveforms. Example of sensory and motor nerve conduction studies in a patient with moderate bilateral carpal tunnel syndrome. Note the comparison of median SNAP to the radial nerve SNAP on the far right (top row). The amplitude in the left SNAP is severely reduced, latency is also increased as seen in the delay from the stimulus artifact on the far left of the waveform to the peak of the action potential. CMAP is also demonstrated for bilateral median nerves and the left ulnar nerve (bottom row) – note the reduction in CMAP amplitude on the right side compared to the left, and the increased latency of both compared to the normal ulnar nerve

severe preganglionic lesion, anesthesia throughout the extremity, no motor function, and a normal SNAP on nerve conduction tests. This constellation of signs and symptoms occurs when the connection of the sensory nerve is maintained to the dorsal root ganglion (DRG), but the spinal connection more proximally is disrupted. The SNAP appears normal as the conduction to the sensory cell body in the DRG is maintained, but this data is not transmitted to the brain. Similarly, the connection to the anterior horn cells controlling motor function is disrupted, resulting in muscle paralysis.

Electromyographic studies are commonly performed as a complement to the nerve conduction studies described above (Fig. 1.7). The focus of the electromyography is on the muscle itself by utilizing small needles placed within the muscle. A denervated muscle will display signs of electrical instability, manifesting as spontaneous fibrillation potentials, positive sharp waves, or fasciculations. These spontaneous activities begin at 2–6 weeks post-injury and continue until complete degeneration of the muscle fiber or reinnervation occurs [53]. Fasciculations are another type of increased insertional activity that

Summary													
			Insertional	Spontaneous				MUAP					Comments
Muscle	Nerve	Roots	Activity	Fib	PSW	Fasc	Other	Dur	Amp	Poly	Recruit	Activate	Comments
R. Deltoid (middle)	Axillary	C5-C6	Increased	2+	3+	None	-				None	None	-
R. Biceps brachii (long head)	Musculocutaneous	C5-C6	Increased	2+	3+	None	-				None	None	-
R. Triceps brachii	Radial	C6-C8	Increased	2+	3+	None	-				None	None	-
R. Flexor carpi ulnaris	Ulnar	C7-T1	Increased	3+	3+	None	-				None	None	-
R. Extrnsor indicis proprius	Radial	C7-C8	Increased	3+	3+	None	-				None	None	-
R. Flexor carpi radialis	Median	C6-C7	Increased	3+	3+	None	-				None	None	-
R. First dorsal interosseous	Ulnar	C8-T1	Increased	3+	3+	None	-				None	Poor	-
R. Abductor pollicis brevis	Median	C8-T1	Increased	3+	3+	None	-				None	None	-
R. Supraspinatus	Suprascapular	C5-C6	Increased	3+	3+	None	-				None	None	-

Fig. 1.7 EMG after nerve injury. EMG results from a patient with a multiple root preganglionic avulsion injury to the brachial plexus 6 weeks prior to the nerve study are displayed. Note the fibrillations and sharp waves seen throughout the right upper extremity consistent with acute denervation and resulting electrical instability of the muscle. No evidence of polyphasic motor units is identified given the severity of the injury and lack of recovery

can be present in neuropathic and myelopathic disorders – they stem from spontaneous discharge of the entire muscle unit and can be found in anterior horn cell disease, myelopathy, and radiculopathy [54]. After nerve injury, polyphasic potentials may be found and can be categorized into either nascent potentials or long duration motor units from collateral sprouting. The presence of these long duration units will help to quantify the injury as subacute, as this sprouting does not occur immediately. Nascent potentials, which are usually shorter in duration, represent true axonal recovery and must be distinguished from polyphasic potentials from sprouting for prognostic purposes [55].

1.2.8 Injury Recognition and Time to Surgery

The importance of timely recognition and accurate diagnosis of peripheral nerve injuries is underscored by the fact that early repair of nerves may result in improved outcomes compared to delayed repair [56]. Atrophic changes within denervated muscles and histologic changes around the motor end plates result in worse functional outcomes after long periods of denervation [57], due in part to the need for the nerve to create new functional end plates in the atrophied muscle. Some surgeons have found the time to surgery to have such a dramatic effect on functional recovery that they have advocated for urgent brachial plexus exploration and repair within 7 days of the injury [58]. Earlier surgery could lead to earlier muscle reinnervation to minimize motor fiber changes, as well as better pain relief. In a series of 148 patients with brachial plexus injuries and at least one nerve root avulsion, Kato et al. demonstrated improved pain relief in patients undergoing surgery within 1 month of injury [59].

While the timing of surgery for brachial plexus injuries is controversial, most experts would suggest that the standard of care within the United States is to proceed with observation and surgery within 3–6 months of the injury or sooner if a plateau in recovery is evident [60, 61]. For iatrogenic nerve injuries after operation, consideration could be given to immediate re-operation if there is a high index of suspicion for any injury beyond Grade 1 or 2. When nerve injuries are recognized intraoperatively, they should be repaired primarily or within 3–4 weeks if the zone of injury is uncertain. Similarly, if postoperative US or MRI demonstrates evidence of transection or neuroma in continuity, surgery should be performed without a significant delay [62]. Timing may be delayed secondary to limited access to peripheral nerve surgeons, as has been demonstrated in brachial plexus injuries [63]. This, coupled with failure to diagnose the nerve injury or failure to refer the patient to an experienced surgeon, can lead to unacceptable delays in a majority of patients. Ideally, peripheral nerve injuries, particularly iatrogenic injuries, are operated on within 3–4 months [62]. Despite these recommendations, only about 1/3 of patients are seen and treated within 6 months of their injury [9].

1.2.9 Nerve Repair and Regeneration

In the most severe injury, neurotmesis, nerve repair is required to approximate damaged nerve ends. An ideal nerve repair will have minimal gapping, minimal tension, appropriate fascicular alignment, and no evidence of fascicles extruded from the periphery of the repair [64]. Approximation of the nerve ends with minimal gap is critical to facilitate axonal bridging from the healthy proximal nerve to the distal degenerative nerve. Transdifferentiation of the Schwann cells into a pro-regenerative phenotype is an important component of neuronal regeneration. A growth cone consisting of filopodia responds to neurotrophic and neurite promoting factors to cross the nerve gap between the repaired ends and initiate regeneration within the distal segment [65], as shown in Fig. 1.8.

The regenerating fibers must then regrow the length of the axonal segment to the target organ at a speed of 1 mm/day [67]. Therefore, nerve transections far from the target muscles result in significant delays in recovery, accompanied by muscle wasting of 60–80% of volume 4 months after injury [65, 67].

1.3 Downstream Effects of Nerve Injury on Muscle

Distinct changes in the neuromuscular junction and muscle itself begin to occur shortly after a traumatic nerve transection. Muscle fibers begin to atrophy early after denervation, with a 70% reduction in muscle cross-sectional area by 2 months after injury [67]. This is accompanied by muscle fibrosis, characterized histologically by fibroblast proliferation and collagen deposition within the muscle. Dropout of motor fibers begins to occur between 6 and 12 months after denervation [67]. Histologic studies from both animal models and biopsies of human denervated muscle show a time-dependent condensation of motor end plates with loss of normal morphology and a significant reduction in surface area and volume [68]. Postsynaptic acetylcholine receptors on the neuromuscular junction begin to redistribute and over time are lost [69]. After 6 months of denervation, the possibility of full muscle recovery with innervation begins to decrease. By 12–18 months after denervation, the above changes in the neuromuscular junction and progressive muscle fibrosis are permanent and preclude reinnervation by regenerating axons and recovery of motor function [70].

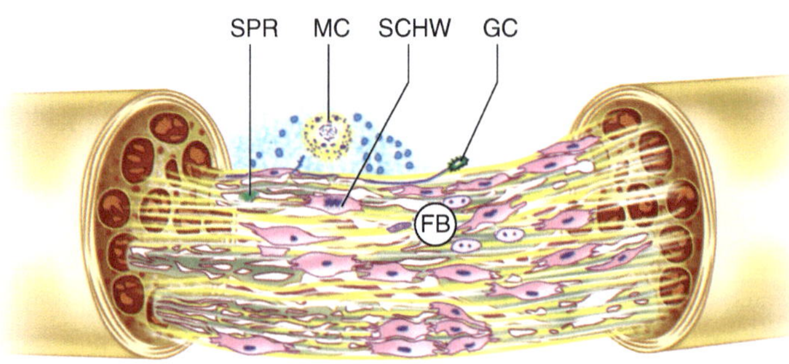

Fig. 1.8 Nerve regeneration after repair. A growth cone from the proximal nerve stump guided by neurotrophic factors bridges the gap between repaired nerve ends (SPR: Sprouts; MC: Mast Cell; SCHW: Schwann Cell; GC: Growth Cone; FB: Fibroblast). [66]

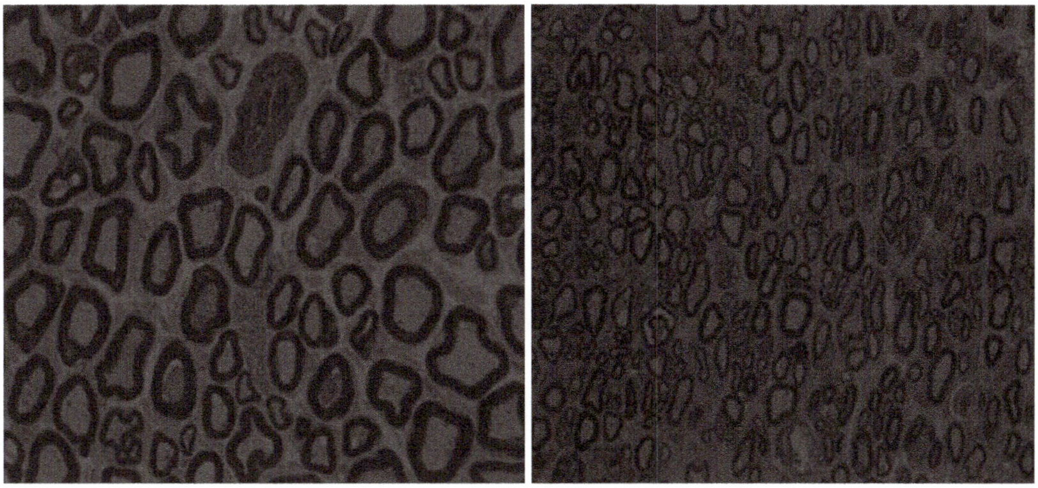

Fig. 1.9 Histology of a recovering nerve. Histologic section demonstrating normal nerve (left) and recovering nerve after transection and repair (right). Note smaller, disorganized axons and thinner myelin sheaths

Due to the downstream cascade of pathologic events, clinical results of nerve repairs are not encouraging – primary repairs of major peripheral nerves generally result in useful function (classified as good or excellent results) in less than half of patients [71] and up to a third of patients may have little or no recovery whatsoever [72], in part due to the disorganized nature of axonal recovery (Fig. 1.9). Return of normal function is almost never achieved and should not be expected; one series of iatrogenic nerve injuries showed improvement after surgery in only 70% of cases [9]. This is likely due to a combination of the delay in reinnervation due to the length of regeneration required and inefficient healing of the nerve across the transected ends. Clinically, this manifests as patients waiting for months to years to achieve any form of recovery of their paralyzed muscles, with modest success at best.

1.4 Nerve Repair Techniques

The goal of peripheral nerve repair is a tension-free coaptation that aligns fascicular topography. A great deal of work over the past 50 years has elucidated technical factors that play an important role in the success of a nerve repair. Nerve regeneration following repair is influenced by intrinsic characteristics of the injured nerve, the surrounding environment the injured nerve is placed in, and the technique with which the nerve is repaired. The surgeon must pay attention to all of these aspects of the nerve repair in order to give an injured nerve the best chance of recovery.

1.4.1 End-to-End Coaptation

The first step in performing a nerve repair is to assess the soft tissue wound bed and coverage. If needed, a flap reconstruction can be performed to provide a well-vascularized bed and coverage for the regenerating nerve. Once the wound bed is optimized, the next step is to determine the health of the injured nerve segments. Successful nerve regeneration requires unimpeded axonal sprouting from the proximal segment of a cut nerve. A severe crush injury, scar, or fibrosis of the end of the proximal nerve stump impairs axonal sprouting; therefore, scarred segments of the proximal stump must be resected prior to coaptation [73]. Evaluation of the nerve stump is primarily clinical and subjective. The nerve end is inspected for visible fascicles and is palpated. A healthy nerve is soft to the touch and compressible; in contrast, a damaged fibrotic nerve may be firm and incompressible. Bleeding from epineurial vessels is another sign of nerve health, and

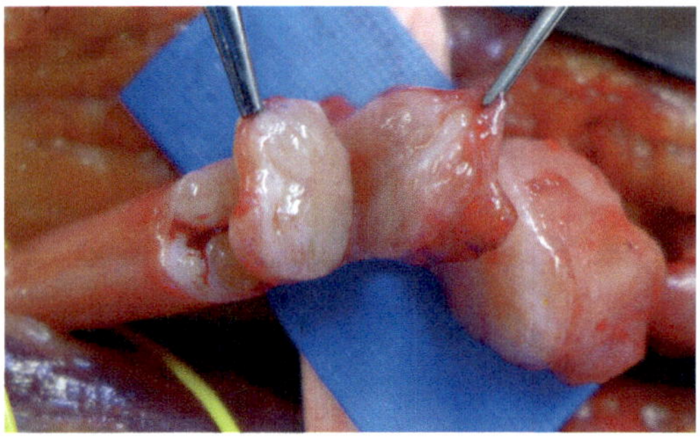

Fig. 1.10 Zone of transition within a neuroma that has been serially sectioned to reveal areas of fibrosis with increasingly healthy nerve tissue proximal to the zone of injury. Image copyright the authors and used with permission

resection of the proximal nerve stump to such a healthy level takes precedence over attempts to preserve length (Fig. 1.10). Similar considerations guide preparation of the distal nerve stump.

Once the nerve is prepared, attention must be paid to aligning fascicular groups to the extent possible. In sharp lacerations or injuries without extensive soft tissue destruction and loss, the position of the nerve stumps within their tissue bed provides insight into the correct orientation of the proximal and distal stumps with respect to each other. The surgeon should note this orientation and can place marking sutures in the epineurium on the superficial surface of the nerve prior to performing a neurolysis and mobilizing the nerve segments. Visual cues such as the alignment of large epineurial blood vessels commonly encountered on major peripheral nerves provide an additional tool to ensure fascicular alignment. While in theory a grouped fascicular repair could most accurately realign fascicles, it may not be a practical option for several reasons. In traumatic nerve injuries, the fascicular anatomy may be distorted to the extent that accurate identification is not possible. Additionally, a grouped fascicular repair necessitates increased intraneural dissection as well as the placement of intraneural sutures, both of which may lead to scarring within the nerve that could impair regeneration. Given these considerations, the vast majority of nerve surgeons perform an epineurial repair. Gently coapting the edges of the nerve together can allow space for mismatched fascicles to find their appropriate distal target with the help of neurotrophic and chemotactic factors, taking advantage of the intrinsic properties of neurotropism.

A tension-free nerve coaptation is critical for successful axon growth across the repair site. Tension creates two fundamental problems. First, a repair under significant tension is at risk of pulling apart and forming a critical gap across which sprouting axons cannot reliably regenerate.

Second, tension itself has physiologic effects on the repaired nerve. Above a certain threshold, strain on a nerve begins to decrease intraneural circulation. In a rabbit tibial nerve model, Lundborg and colleagues showed that between 8% and 15% strain there is a precipitous drop in intraneural circulation [74]. Below 8%, nerve elongation blood flow was not affected; however, at 8% strain, a detectable decrease in the flow of epineural and perineurial venules occurred, though intra-fascicular and capillary flow remained unaffected. Above 8% strain they observed a gradual and continuous decrease in arterial blood flow until blood intra-fascicular capillary and arteriole flow ceased at 15% strain. This strain-dependent decrease in intraneural blood flow is presumably a result of tension-induced increases in intra-fascicular pressures when the nerve is placed on stretch. Above the critical 15% strain level, nutrition to an already injured and regenerating nerve is impaired. Furthermore, tension on a nerve has been shown to negatively affect nerve conduction independently of nerve ischemia. Rabbit sciatic nerves placed at 16% strain for a 1 hour period showed an irreversible 30% drop in conduction velocity that was independent of recovery of blood flow following relaxation [29]. Similar effects on conduction velocity with stretched repairs were reported by Terzis et al., and tension-induced connective tissue proliferation may provide an obstructive barrier to axonal bridging across the coaptation site.

The resistance to stretch of a peripheral nerve will vary by the ratio of connective tissue to axons and the degree of elasticity of the connective tissue of the nerve. As mentioned above, anatomic regions where nerves are physiologically subjected to strain, such as across joints, display a higher percentage of connective tissue surrounding and within fascicles. Like other connective tissues, nerves exhibit time-dependent mechanical creep stress relaxation, which allows them to accommodate to a low level of tension placed on a repair [75]. A safe baseline would be to keep the degree of strain on both the proximal and distal nerve segments to less than 10% [76].

In clinical practice, surgeon judgment is used to make the determination of how much tension is too much tension for a primary nerve repair. A useful heuristic to help make this determination is the breaking or pullout strength of a single epineurial suture. Experimental data from a cadaveric study evaluating median nerve repair indicates that an epineurial repair with a single 9-0 nylon suture will reliably fail by suture breakage at a strain of between 5% and 8% [77]. The 8-0 nylon and prolene sutures tended to fail by pullout rather than breakage, and strain at failure exceeded 9% in some specimens. Thus, if a single 9-0 nylon is able to bring together the two ends of a nerve coaptation without the suture breaking, this indicates that the level of strain is likely below what would be deleterious to nerve regeneration. An epineurial repair is performed with as few 9-0 nylon sutures as necessary to align the two nerve ends and provide sufficient strength to resist gapping when the nerve is placed on gentle stretch. Many surgeons reinforce their suture repair with a fibrin glue sealant to decrease the chances of gapping.

Flexion of joints and positioning can at times aid to take tension off of the nerve coaptation. Postoperative splints can be used to gently flex joints that are then gradually extended in the postoperative period. However, it is of paramount importance to avoid reliance on joint positioning to the extent that a contracture is induced. The repair should be checked for gapping through a full range of motion of adjacent joints prior to wound closure to help guide the positioning of postoperative immobilization.

1.4.1.1 Nerve Grafting

When a tension-free primary nerve coaptation cannot be achieved, the nerve gap must be bridged by an interposition graft. The graft serves as a scaffold for sprouting axons to grow from the proximal to distal nerve stump en route to reinnervating their end target. Currently available options for bridging a nerve gap include autologous nerve graft, processed nerve allograft, and synthetic nerve conduits.

1.4.2 Autologous Nerve Grafting

Autologous nerve graft, or autograft, is still held by most peripheral nerve surgeons to be the "gold standard" for nerve grafting and the go-to choice for grafting of motor nerves and longer gaps in critical sensory nerves. The sural nerve is the most commonly used donor nerve given the length of available graft and well-tolerated resultant sensory deficit. The sural nerve can be used as a single nerve graft or several grafts together in parallel (a "cable graft") in order to provide a better size match for larger, poly-fascicular nerve repairs (Fig. 1.11). However, a number of additional donor options exist, including the anterior interosseous nerve (AIN), posterior interosseous nerve (PIN), lateral antebrachial cutaneous nerve (LABCN), medial antebrachial cutaneous nerve (MABCN), among others [78]. Each of these nerves has different cross-sectional areas and fascicular numbers, which can be taken into account to choose the optimal donor graft for a particular nerve reconstruction [79].

Some authors have reported the use of expendable motor nerves, such as the obturator nerve, for autograft reconstruction of motor and mixed peripheral nerves [80]. The authors cite an advantage of avoiding the sensory deficit in the donor distribution and the chance for neuroma formation or neuropathic pain at the donor site. The rationale for use of a motor nerve graft comes from animal research that has suggested that the internal architecture and neurotrophic factors unique to motor nerves may make them better suited to guide regeneration of a mixed periph-

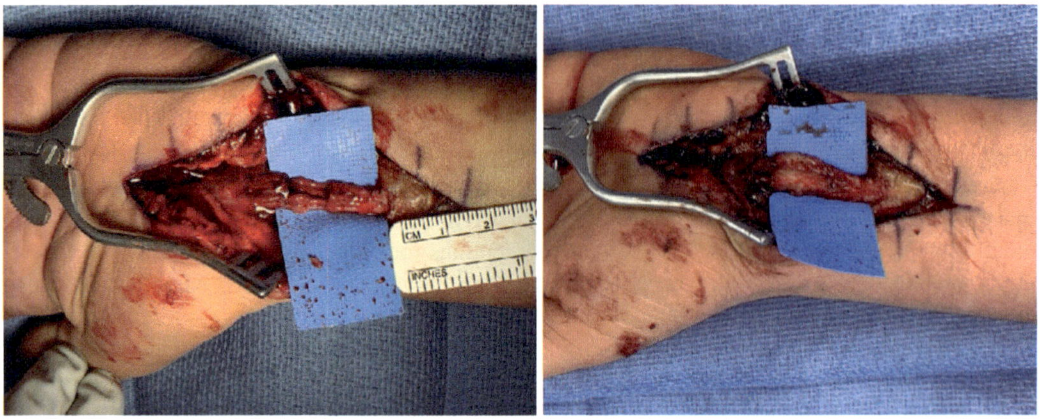

Fig. 1.11 Resection of neuroma in continuity from the median nerve (left) with subsequent sural nerve grouped fascicular repair using sural nerve autograft (right)

eral nerve defect due to so-called "modality-specific regeneration" [81]. Experiments by Mackinnon and colleagues have shown that the enhanced regeneration with use of a motor nerve graft is not seen with grafting of a pure motor nerve, only with grafting of a mixed sensory and motor nerve [82]. They hypothesize that the larger endoneurial tubes in a pure motor nerve may provide a better environment to permit directional sprouting when both motor and sensory axons are attempting to regenerate down the same graft. While these considerations merit further investigation, there is currently no clinical evidence to support the routine use of an autologous motor nerve donor for grafting of peripheral nerve defects.

Outcomes of nerve autografting have been reported in a number of retrospective case series and comparative studies, many of these in the upper extremity. However, interpretation of these results is challenging due to the heterogeneity of injury types and concomitant soft tissue damage, patient ages, delay to surgery, and technical details of repair – all of which have been shown to influence nerve regeneration. Sensory recovery following autologous nerve grafting is length dependent. For example, in a large series of over 100 digital nerve repairs with autograft, the vast majority of patients with gaps 2 cm or less demonstrated S3 or better sensation, while only two-thirds of patients with gaps 2–5 cm and very few with gaps >5 cm achieved this level of recovery [83]. A recent meta-analysis affirms excellent results for autograft repair of digital nerve gaps between 2 and 3 cm in length, with approximately 50% of patients achieving S4 recovery and 88% achieving S3+ or better. Over 50% of patients repaired with autograft achieved <6 mm static 2PD [84]. With respect to motor and mixed nerves, Ruijs et al. performed a meta-analysis of 23 studies and 623 median and ulnar nerve repairs using autograft and showed that 47% of patients recovered M4 strength and 40% of patients recovered at least a sensory recovery of pain and touch sensation without hyperalgesia (S3+) [85]. These numbers are useful as a rough estimate, though gap width and level of injury data were incomplete which precluded a more granular stratification of outcomes based on these variables.

Despite a proven track record, there are a number of disadvantages to nerve autografting. The main disadvantage is that an autograft results in donor site morbidity, has a finite length, and carries a risk of complications at a second surgical site, including increased operative time, wound healing problems, scar sensitivity, neuroma, or neuropathic pain. As a result, much effort over the past 30 years has been devoted to the development of alternatives to the use of autologous nerve grafts.

1.4.3 Nerve Conduits

A nerve conduit is a hollow tube that provides a relatively closed environment for axonal sprouting and regeneration from the proximal to distal segments of a cut nerve. The idea is that when the two ends of the nerve cannot be directly coapted, the conduit serves as a channel to permit the diffusion of neurotrophic growth factors and provide a mechanical barrier to the loss of axonal sprouts in order to increase the efficiency of regeneration. Extruded fluid trapped within the conduit forms a fibrin matrix that serves as a structural framework to guide axonal regeneration across the gap. The cross-sectional area of the fibrin bridge between nerve ends within a conduit decreases as the length of nerve gap is increased, limiting axonal bridging [86].

Modern conduits are fabricated from biocompatible, absorbable synthetic materials such as type I collagen, polyglycolic acid (PGA), and polylactide-caprolactone. Excellent results have been reported for the use of PGA conduits for short sensory nerve gaps, and it has compared favorably to both direct repair across a small gap and use of nerve autograft. A prospective, multicenter study comparing digital nerve repairs with PGA conduits to either direct repair or nerve autograft showed a higher proportion of excellent results and lower mean two-point discrimination for repairs utilizing the PGA conduit for both short nerve gaps and nerve gaps greater than 8 mm, ranging up to 25 mm [87]. Another large series on use of PGA conduits for sensory gaps less than 25 mm reported 94% meaningful recovery with an average static two-point discrimination of 8 mm [88]. In this study, patients were prospectively randomized to either PGA conduit or autologous vein conduit; no difference was found in sensory recovery, with the cost of the conduit offset by the cost of the additional surgical time need to harvest the vein. Similar outcomes have been reported with collagen conduits [89, 90]. While polycaprolactone has also shown some success in short sensory nerve gaps, high reported complications, including nerve irritation, extrusion, and fistulization with wound formation, have limited widespread adoption [91, 92].

Based on the accumulated body of evidence on the use of nerve conduits since their introduction in the 1980s, conduit use is limited to reconstruction of short sensory nerve gaps, <3 cm in length. Studies on the use of conduit for mixed and motor nerve defects yielded disappointing results, with the majority demonstrating minimal meaningful motor recovery, even for short nerve defects [93, 94]. A recent comprehensive review of conduit use confirmed that there is insufficient high-quality evidence to support the use of nerve conduits in larger gap motor or mixed motor/sensory nerves [95].

1.4.4 Processed Nerve Allograft

Processed nerve allograft is a commercially available product prepared from cadaveric nerves through a process of chemical decellularization to remove myelin and Schwann cells, leaving behind the endoneurial basement membrane architecture, extracellular matrix proteins and glycosaminoglycans, and neurotrophic factors to guide axonal regeneration. Revascularization of the allograft occurs via epineurial vessels at the proximal and distal coaptation sites [96]. Allograft has supported the regeneration of myelinated axons across gaps as long as 4–6 cm in animal models – longer regeneration is limited by the inability of Schwann cells to migrate further along a processed nerve allograft [97, 98]. Avance nerve graft by AxoGen is currently the only commercially available processed nerve allograft on the market and is available in diameters up to 5 mm and lengths of 10, 30, 50, or 70 mm.

Support for the use of allografts has been bolstered by the RANGER study (Registry Study of Avance Nerve Graft Evaluating Recovery Outcomes), an ongoing, multicenter, prospective longitudinal study to assess outcomes using processed nerve allograft for sensory, mixed sensory/motor, and pure motor peripheral nerve gaps. A number of studies from the RANGER cohort have established efficacy of Avance nerve graft for short sensory nerve repairs, <3 cm. Cho et al. reported meaningful recovery for 89% of digital nerve repairs, as defined as S3 or S4 recovery, with a mean gap length of 2.3 cm and range up to 3.5 cm. Mean static two-point discrimination for these patients was 8 mm [99]. More recent follow-up data from this same cohort looking at larger digital nerve gaps, averaging 3.5 cm and ranging up to 5 cm, showed similar outcomes with the majority achieving S3+ recovery [100]. A meta-analysis of the literature to date on use of processed nerve allograft for digital nerve gaps less than 2.5 cm showed equivalent results to autograft for sensory recovery [84].

Safa et al. recently reported on outcomes of mixed and motor nerve reconstructions from the RANGER cohort with a mean follow-up of more than 2 years [101]. Outcomes included nerve-specific functional testing for British Medical Research Council grade, as well as pinch and grip strength. Twenty-two patients with a mean age of 38 years met inclusion criteria. Mean gap length was 33 mm, ranging from 10 to 70 mm, and all repairs were acute, averaging 9 days after injury. Overall, 73% of patients achieved meaningful motor recovery (defined as M3 or greater), while 50% of patients achieved a higher threshold of recovery (defined as M4 or greater). Outcomes were stratified by gap length, with findings of 80% meaningful motor recovery (defined as M3 or greater) for a gap of 10–25 mm, 62% for a gap of 26–49 mm, and 76% for a gap of 50–70 mm. Median nerve repairs performed better than ulnar nerve repairs, though the study was not powered for this comparison. This study was limited by a small sample size, though it does provide some support for the use of processed nerve allograft for mixed and motor nerve defects up to 7 cm in length. While these results are encouraging, data from the RANGER cohort to date is still not considered sufficient by most peripheral nerve surgeons to indicate the routine use of processed nerve allograft in lieu of autograft for critical motor and mixed nerve gaps when sufficient donor nerve is available [95].

1.4.5 Future Directions in Nerve Recovery and Repair

The use of immune modulation by administration of tacrolimus (FK506) has garnered attention in the literature as a technique for improving peripheral nerve regeneration, as it has shown some tendency to improve results of immediate nerve repair when given at the time of nerve transection in a rat model. The mechanism by which FK506 improves regeneration is unclear, but possible mechanisms include a generalized decrease in inflammation, faster restoration of the blood–nerve barrier, effects on calcium levels, and modification of signaling pathways [102]. FK506 treatment has been shown to result in a transient increase in ED2-positive macrophages compared to controls, but not ED1-positive macrophages [103]. Local administration of FK-506 has shown better functional results than systemic administration in a rat model [104] and better axonal regeneration when applied topically in low doses [105]. The effects of a delay in administration of FK-506 are less clear, with one study showing diminished effects on axonal regeneration, particularly when repair is also delayed [106].

Polyethylene glycol (PEG) fusion is another technique that has gained attention in recent years for its ability to rapidly restore nerve continuity and function. Mammalian nerves have the capability to perform plasmalemmal sealing after transection to help mitigate further damage. More recently, polyethylene glycol, in conjunction with methylene blue, has been utilized to promote fusion of the transected fascicles after close approximation with sutures [107]. The cut ends must be washed with calcium-free hypotonic saline and treated with an antioxidant (methylene blue), followed by polyethylene glycol [108]. This results in return of nerve action potential minutes after repair and more rapid recovery of function over the course of days to weeks [109–111]. Clinical implementation of this technique may be limited due to the need to perform membrane fusion prior to the release of the mitochondrial calcium, the critical event that destabilizes the axonal membrane and triggers Wallerian degeneration. While PEG fusion has been successfully performed up to 24 hours after injury [112], it seems unlikely the window for intervention will extend beyond 1 day, due to the inevitable initiation of Wallerian degeneration. This will pose a formidable challenge in successful adaptation of this technique to clinical practice, but early findings give hope that future research may identify additional ways to prevent Wallerian degeneration and improve outcomes after nerve injury.

References

1. Stewart JD. Peripheral nerve fascicles: anatomy and clinical relevance. Muscle Nerve. 2003;28(5):525–41.
2. Swenson R. Clinical and functional neuroscience. Dartmouth Medical School; 2006.
3. Purves D. Neuroscience. 4th ed. Sunderland, MA, Sinauer; 2008. xvii, 857, G-16, IC-7, I-29 p.
4. Mizisin AP, Weerasuriya A. Homeostatic regulation of the endoneurial microenvironment during development, aging and in response to trauma, disease and toxic insult. Acta Neuropathol. 2011;121(3):291–312.
5. Peltonen S, Alanne M, Peltonen J. Barriers of the peripheral nerve. Tissue Barriers. 2013;1(3):e24956.
6. Millesi H, Zoch G, Reihsner R. Mechanical properties of peripheral nerves. Clin Orthop Relat Res. 1995;314:76–83.
7. Smith JW. Factors influencing nerve repair. I. Blood supply of peripheral nerves. Arch Surg. 1966;93(2):335–41.
8. Smith JW. Factors influencing nerve repair. II. Collateral circulation of peripheral nerves. Arch Surg. 1966;93(3):433–7.
9. Kretschmer T, et al. Evaluation of iatrogenic lesions in 722 surgically treated cases of peripheral nerve trauma. J Neurosurg. 2001;94(6):905–12.
10. Seddon H. A classification of nerve injuries. Br Med J. 1942;2(4260):237.
11. Noble J, et al. Analysis of upper and lower extremity peripheral nerve injuries in a population of patients with multiple injuries. J Trauma Acute Care Surg. 1998;45(1):116–22.
12. Sunderland S. A classification of peripheral nerve injuries producing loss of function. Brain. 1951;74(4):491–516.
13. Powell H, Myers R. Pathology of experimental nerve compression. Lab Investig. 1986;55(1):91–100.
14. Rydevik B, Lundborg G, Bagge U. Effects of graded compression on intraneural blood flow: an in vivo study on rabbit tibial nerve. J Hand Surg. 1981;6(1):3–12.
15. Rydevik B, et al. Blockage of axonal transport induced by acute, graded compression of the rabbit vagus nerve. J Neurol Neurosurg Psychiatry. 1980;43(8):690–8.
16. Rydevik B, Nordborg C. Changes in nerve function and nerve fibre structure induced by acute, graded compression. J Neurol Neurosurg Psychiatry. 1980;43(12):1070–82.
17. Rydevik B, Lundborg G. Permeability of intraneural microvessels and perineurium following acute, graded experimental nerve compression. Scand J Plast Reconstr Surg. 1977;11(3):179–87.
18. Ibrahim I, et al. Suppl 1: carpal tunnel syndrome: a review of the recent literature. Open Orthop J. 2012;6:69.
19. Somaiah A, Roy A, Spence. Carpal tunnel syndrome. Ulster Med J. 2008;77(1):6–17.
20. Prick J, et al. Results of carpal tunnel release. Eur J Neurol. 2003;10(6):733–6.
21. Zuniga AF, et al. Blood flow velocity but not tendon mechanics relates to nerve function in carpal tunnel syndrome patients. J Neurol Sci. 2020:116694.
22. Vanderschueren GA, Meys VE, Beekman R. Doppler sonography for the diagnosis of carpal tunnel syndrome: a critical review. Muscle Nerve. 2014;50(2):159–63.
23. Fowler JR, Gaughan JP, Ilyas AM. The sensitivity and specificity of ultrasound for the diagnosis of carpal tunnel syndrome: a meta-analysis. Clin Orthop Relat Res. 2011;469(4):1089–94.
24. Rotman MB, et al. Time course and predictors of median nerve conduction after carpal tunnel release. J Hand Surg Am. 2004;29(3):367–72.
25. Li M, et al. Sonographic follow-up after endoscopic carpal tunnel release for severe carpal tunnel syndrome: a one-year neuroanatomical prospective observational study. BMC Musculoskelet Disord. 2019;20(1):157.
26. Wright TW, et al. Excursion and strain of the median nerve. JBJS. 1996;78(12):1897–903.
27. Wall EJ, et al. Stress relaxation of a peripheral nerve. J Hand Surg Am. 1991;16(5):859–63.
28. Kwan MK, et al. Strain, stress and stretch of peripheral nerve rabbit experiments in vitro and in vivo. Acta Orthop Scand. 1992;63(3):267–72.
29. Driscoll PJ, Glasby MA, Lawson GM. An in vivo study of peripheral nerves in continuity: biomechanical and physiological responses to elongation. J Orthop Res. 2002;20(2):370–5.
30. Rosén LBD, Lundborg G, Birgitta B. Assessment of functional outcome after nerve repair in a longitudinal cohort. Scand J Plast Reconstr Surg Hand Surg. 2000;34(1):71–8.
31. Geuna S, et al. Histology of the peripheral nerve and changes occurring during nerve regeneration. Int Rev Neurobiol. 2009;87:27–46.
32. Hong T, et al. Indirect cost of traumatic brachial plexus injuries in the United States: level 4 evidence. J Hand Surg. 2018;43(9):S55–6.

33. Llobet Rosell A, Neukomm LJ. Axon death signalling in Wallerian degeneration among species and in disease. Open Biol. 2019;9(8):190118.
34. Parkinson DB, et al. c-Jun is a negative regulator of myelination. J Cell Biol. 2008;181(4):625–37.
35. Gonzalez S, et al. Blocking mitochondrial calcium release in Schwann cells prevents demyelinating neuropathies. J Clin Invest. 2016;126(3):1023–38.
36. Arthur-Farraj PJ, et al. c-Jun reprograms Schwann cells of injured nerves to generate a repair cell essential for regeneration. Neuron. 2012;75(4):633–47.
37. Stratton JA, et al. Macrophages regulate Schwann cell maturation after nerve injury. Cell reports. 2018;24(10):2561–2572.e6.
38. Parkinson DB, et al. Krox-20 inhibits Jun-NH2-terminal kinase/c-Jun to control Schwann cell proliferation and death. J Cell Biol. 2004;164(3):385–94.
39. Essuman K, et al. The SARM1 toll/interleukin-1 receptor domain possesses intrinsic NAD+ cleavage activity that promotes pathological axonal degeneration. Neuron. 2017;93(6):1334–1343.e5.
40. Coleman MP, et al. An 85-kb tandem triplication in the slow Wallerian degeneration (Wlds) mouse. Proc Natl Acad Sci. 1998;95(17):9985–90.
41. Wang Q, et al. Sarm1/Myd88-5 regulates neuronal intrinsic immune response to traumatic axonal injuries. Cell Rep. 2018;23(3):716–24.
42. Gerdts J, et al. SARM1 activation triggers axon degeneration locally via NAD+ destruction. Science. 2015;348(6233):453–7.
43. Lopez-Schier H, et al. Systemic loss of Sarm1 is glioprotective after neurotrauma. bioRxiv. 2018:493163.
44. Bendszus M, et al. MRI of peripheral nerve degeneration and regeneration: correlation with electrophysiology and histology. Exp Neurol. 2004;188(1):171–7.
45. Cudlip SA, et al. Magnetic resonance neurography of peripheral nerve following experimental crush injury, and correlation with functional deficit. J Neurosurg. 2002;96(4):755–9.
46. Ahlawat S, et al. MRI features of peripheral traumatic neuromas. Eur Radiol. 2016;26(4):1204–12.
47. Chhabra A, Madhuranthakam AJ, Andreisek G. Magnetic resonance neurography: current perspectives and literature review. Eur Radiol. 2018;28(2):698–707.
48. Cartwright MS, et al. Diagnostic ultrasound for nerve transection. Muscle Nerve. 2007;35(6): 796–9.
49. Peer S, et al. Examination of postoperative peripheral nerve lesions with high-resolution sonography. Am J Roentgenol. 2001;177(2):415–9.
50. Karabay N, et al. Ultrasonographic evaluation of the iatrogenic peripheral nerve injuries in upper extremity. Eur J Radiol. 2010;73(2):234–40.
51. Zaidman CM, et al. Detection of peripheral nerve pathology: comparison of ultrasound and MRI. Neurology. 2013;80(18):1634–40.
52. Mallik A, Weir A. Nerve conduction studies: essentials and pitfalls in practice. J Neurol Neurosurg Psychiatry. 2005;76(suppl 2):ii23–31.
53. Quan D, Bird SJ. Nerve conduction studies and electromyography in the evaluation of peripheral nerve injuries. Univ Pa Orthop J. 1999;12:45–51.
54. Lee DH, Claussen GC, Oh S. Clinical nerve conduction and needle electromyography studies. J Am Acad Orthop Surg. 2004;12(4):276–87.
55. Feinberg J. EMG: myths and facts. HSS J. 2006;2(1):19–21.
56. Mohseni M-A, Pour JS, Pour JG. Primary and delayed repair and nerve grafting for treatment of cut median and ulnar nerves. Pak J Biol Sci. 2010;13(6):287.
57. Gutmann E, Young JZ. The re-innervation of muscle after various periods of atrophy. J Anat. 1944;78(Pt 1–2):15.
58. Birch R. Timing of surgical reconstruction for closed traumatic injury to the supraclavicular brachial plexus. J Hand Surg (European Volume). 2015;40(6):562–7.
59. Kato N, et al. The effects of operative delay on the relief of neuropathic pain after injury to the brachial plexus: a review of 148 cases. J Bone Joint Surg. British volume. 2006;88(6):756–9.
60. Giuffre JL, et al. Current concepts of the treatment of adult brachial plexus injuries. J Hand Surg Am. 2010;35(4):678–88.
61. Hems T. Timing of surgical reconstruction for closed traumatic injury to the supraclavicular brachial plexus. J Hand Surg (European Volume). 2015;40(6):568–72.
62. Antoniadis G, et al. Iatrogenic nerve injuries: prevalence, diagnosis and treatment. Dtsch Arztebl Int. 2014;111(16):273.
63. Dy CJ, et al. A population-based analysis of time to surgery and travel distances for brachial plexus surgery. J Hand Surg. 2016;41(9):903–909.e3.
64. Isaacs J, et al. Technical assessment of connector-assisted nerve repair. J Hand Surg Am. 2016;41(7):760–6.
65. Lee SK, Wolfe SW. Peripheral nerve injury and repair. J Am Acad Orthop Surg. 2000;8(4):243–52.
66. Lundborg G. A 25-year perspective of peripheral nerve surgery: evolving neuroscientific concepts and clinical significance. J Hand Surg Am. 2000;25(3):391–414.
67. Burnett MG, Zager EL. Pathophysiology of peripheral nerve injury: a brief review. Neurosurg Focus. 2004;16(5):1–7.
68. Chan JP, et al. Examination of the human motor endplate after brachial plexus injury with two-photon microscopy. Muscle Nerve. 2019;
69. Kang H, et al. Terminal Schwann cells participate in neuromuscular synapse remodeling during reinnervation following nerve injury. J Neurosci. 2014;34(18):6323–33.
70. Sakuma M, et al. Lack of motor recovery after prolonged denervation of the neuromuscular junction

is not due to regenerative failure. Eur J Neurosci. 2016;43(3):451–62.
71. Kallio P, Vastamäki M. An analysis of the results of late reconstruction of 132 median nerves. J Hand Surg. 1993;18(1):97–105.
72. Vastamäki M, Kallio P, Solonen K. The results of secondary microsurgical repair of ulnar nerve injury. J Hand Surg. 1993;18(3):323–6.
73. Millesi H. Factors affecting the outcome of peripheral nerve surgery. Microsurgery. 2006;26(4):295–302.
74. Lundborg G, Rydevik B. Effects of stretching the tibial nerve of the rabbit. A preliminary study of the intraneural circulation and the barrier function of the perineurium. J Bone Joint Surg Br. 1973;55(2):390–401.
75. Kendall JP, et al. Tension and creep phenomena in peripheral nerve. Acta Orthop Scand. 1979;50(6 Pt 2):721–5.
76. Trumble TE, McCallister WV. Repair of peripheral nerve defects in the upper extremity. Hand Clin. 2000;16(1):37–52.
77. Smetana BS, et al. Testing of direct neurorrhaphy strain. J Hand Surg Am. 2019;44(7):615 e1–6.
78. Poppler LH, et al. Alternatives to sural nerve grafts in the upper extremity. Hand (N Y). 2015;10(1):68–75.
79. Higgins JP, et al. Assessment of nerve graft donor sites used for reconstruction of traumatic digital nerve defects. J Hand Surg Am. 2002;27(2):286–92.
80. Iorio ML, Felder JM 3rd, Ducic I. Anterior branch of the obturator nerve: a novel motor autograft for complex peripheral nerve reconstruction. Ann Plast Surg. 2011;67(3):260–2.
81. Brenner MJ, et al. Repair of motor nerve gaps with sensory nerve inhibits regeneration in rats. Laryngoscope. 2006;116(9):1685–92.
82. Kawamura DH, et al. Matching of motor-sensory modality in the rodent femoral nerve model shows no enhanced effect on peripheral nerve regeneration. Exp Neurol. 2010;223(2):496–504.
83. Kallio PK. The results of secondary repair of 254 digital nerves. J Hand Surg Br. 1993;18(3):327–30.
84. Mauch JT, et al. A systematic review of sensory outcomes of digital nerve gap reconstruction with autograft, allograft, and conduit. Ann Plast Surg. 2019;82(4S Suppl 3):S247–55.
85. Ruijs AC, et al. Median and ulnar nerve injuries: a meta-analysis of predictors of motor and sensory recovery after modern microsurgical nerve repair. Plast Reconstr Surg. 2005;116(2):484–94; discussion 495–6.
86. Safa B, Buncke G. Autograft substitutes: conduits and processed nerve allografts. Hand Clin. 2016;32(2):127–40.
87. Weber RA, et al. A randomized prospective study of polyglycolic acid conduits for digital nerve reconstruction in humans. Plast Reconstr Surg. 2000;106(5):1036–45; discussion 1046–8.
88. Rinker B, Liau JY. A prospective randomized study comparing woven polyglycolic acid and autogenous vein conduits for reconstruction of digital nerve gaps. J Hand Surg Am. 2011;36(5):775–81.
89. Wangensteen KJ, Kalliainen LK. Collagen tube conduits in peripheral nerve repair: a retrospective analysis. Hand (N Y). 2010;5(3):273–7.
90. Lohmeyer JA, et al. The clinical use of artificial nerve conduits for digital nerve repair: a prospective cohort study and literature review. J Reconstr Microsurg. 2009;25(1):55–61.
91. Chiriac S, et al. Experience of using the bioresorbable copolyester poly(DL-lactide-epsilon-caprolactone) nerve conduit guide Neurolac for nerve repair in peripheral nerve defects: report on a series of 28 lesions. J Hand Surg Eur Vol. 2012;37(4):342–9.
92. Bertleff MJ, Meek MF, Nicolai JP. A prospective clinical evaluation of biodegradable neurolac nerve guides for sensory nerve repair in the hand. J Hand Surg Am. 2005;30(3):513–8.
93. Moore AM, et al. Limitations of conduits in peripheral nerve repairs. Hand (N Y). 2009;4(2):180–6.
94. Liodaki E, et al. Removal of collagen nerve conduits (NeuraGen) after unsuccessful implantation: focus on histological findings. J Reconstr Microsurg. 2013;29(8):517–22.
95. Rbia N, Shin AY. The role of nerve graft substitutes in motor and mixed motor/sensory peripheral nerve injuries. J Hand Surg Am. 2017;42(5):367–77.
96. Best TJ, et al. Revascularization of peripheral nerve autografts and allografts. Plast Reconstr Surg. 1999;104(1):152–60.
97. Saheb-Al-Zamani M, et al. Limited regeneration in long acellular nerve allografts is associated with increased Schwann cell senescence. Exp Neurol. 2013;247:165–77.
98. Poppler LH, et al. Axonal growth arrests after an increased accumulation of Schwann cells expressing senescence markers and stromal cells in acellular nerve allografts. Tissue Eng Part A. 2016;22(13–14):949–61.
99. Cho MS, et al. Functional outcome following nerve repair in the upper extremity using processed nerve allograft. J Hand Surg Am. 2012;37(11):2340–9.
100. Rinker B, et al. Use of processed nerve allografts to repair nerve injuries greater than 25 mm in the hand. Ann Plast Surg. 2017;78(6S Suppl 5):S292–5.
101. Safa B, et al. Recovery of motor function after mixed and motor nerve repair with processed nerve allograft. Plast Reconstr Surg Glob Open. 2019;7(3):e2163.
102. Konofaos P, Terzis JK. FK506 and nerve regeneration: past, present, and future. J Reconstr Microsurg. 2013;29(03):141–8.
103. Kvist M, Danielsen N, Dahlin LB. Effects of FK506 on regeneration and macrophages in injured rat sciatic nerve. J Peripher Nerv Syst. 2003;8(4):251–9.
104. Goldani E, et al. Locally applied FK506 improves functional recovery in rats after sciatic nerve transection. Int J Innov Res Med Sci. 2017:**2**(06).

105. Davis B, et al. Local FK506 delivery at the direct nerve repair site improves nerve regeneration. Muscle Nerve. 2019;60(5):613–20.
106. Brenner MJ, et al. Delayed nerve repair is associated with diminished neuroenhancement by FK506. Laryngoscope. 2004;114(3):570–6.
107. Bittner GD, et al. The curious ability of polyethylene glycol fusion technologies to restore lost behaviors after nerve severance. J Neurosci Res. 2016;94(3):207–30.
108. Bittner G, et al. Rapid, effective, and long-lasting behavioral recovery produced by microsutures, methylene blue, and polyethylene glycol after completely cutting rat sciatic nerves. J Neurosci Res. 2012;90(5):967–80.
109. Ghergherehchi CL, et al. Behavioral recovery and spinal motoneuron remodeling after polyethylene glycol fusion repair of singly cut and ablated sciatic nerves. PLoS One. 2019;14(10):e0223443.
110. Bamba R, et al. A novel technique using hydrophilic polymers to promote axonal fusion. Neural Regen Res. 2016;11(4):525.
111. Ghergherehchi CL, et al. Effects of extracellular calcium and surgical techniques on restoration of axonal continuity by polyethylene glycol fusion following complete cut or crush severance of rat sciatic nerves. J Neurosci Res. 2016;94(3):231–45.
112. Bamba R, et al. Evaluation of a nerve fusion technique with polyethylene glycol in a delayed setting after nerve injury. J Hand Surg. 2018;43(1):82.e1–7.

2 Evaluation of the Patient with Postoperative Peripheral Nerve Issues

Maksim A. Shlykov, Katherine M. Velicki, and Christopher J. Dy

2.1 Intraoperative Nerve Injury Mechanisms

While it is difficult to obtain an accurate estimate of their incidence, iatrogenic peripheral nerve injuries are responsible for up to 20% of traumatic nerve lesions [1, 2]. Many of these injuries occur after orthopedic surgery due to the breadth and nature of procedures performed on the upper and lower extremities. A surgeon's best protective measures against intraoperative nerve injury are a detailed understanding of relevant anatomy (including potential variants) and understanding when these structures are at risk during each surgery (Table 2.1).

Iatrogenic nerve injuries can be broadly categorized into direct or indirect types. Direct injuries include nerve lacerations during dissection and injuries caused by insertion or removal of implants, such as the use of medial pins in unstable pediatric supracondylar humerus fractures. In revision or trauma settings, the relevant anatomy is more likely to be disrupted and may substantially increase the risk for direct nerve injury. Perioperative injection of local anesthetic, regional anesthetic, and steroids can cause neural injury if administered incorrectly or by way of neurotoxicity [3]. Indirect injuries are caused by stretch, compression, or thermal injury [3, 4]. Patient positioning and retractor placement deserve the same attention to detail as the critical portions of the case [5]. Meticulous soft tissue handling with avoidance of nerve stretch and direct nerve trauma is of utmost importance [5]. Direct visualization of nerves at risk can also minimize risk of injury. Thermal injury from electrocautery or during cementation may be irreversible but can be prevented with irrigation, adjustment of cautery settings, and protection of surrounding structures [1].

The mechanism and type of nerve injury are the major factors that shape prognosis. While 90% of "indirect" nerve injuries from stretch and compression due to improper patient positioning or aberrant retraction heal spontaneously, many lesions involving "direct" injury to a nerve require early repair or reconstruction to recover [1, 3]. Intraoperative or timely postoperative diagnosis of nerve injury is paramount to ensuring appropriate management, as delays in diagnosis can impact functional outcomes.

M. A. Shlykov
Department of Orthopedic Surgery, Washington University School of Medicine, St. Louis, MO, USA
e-mail: shlykovm@wustl.edu

K. M. Velicki
Washington University School of Medicine, St. Louis, MO, USA
e-mail: kvelicki@wustl.edu

C. J. Dy (✉)
Department of Orthopedic Surgery, Washington University, St. Louis, MO, USA
e-mail: dyc@wustl.edu

C. J. Dy et al. (eds.), *Peripheral Nerve Issues after Orthopedic Surgery*, https://doi.org/10.1007/978-3-030-84428-8_2

nicated. For direct injuries from a sharp/tidy mechanism, early repair should be performed by a surgeon with microsurgical capability [1, 3, 13]. For direct injuries with known partial or complete nerve discontinuity from a non-tidy mechanism (such as drills and reamers), nerve repair or reconstruction is performed after waiting an additional 2–3 weeks for the zone of injury to declare itself within the nerve. For suspected nerve injuries (when direct injury has not been visualized during the index surgery), nerve repair or reconstruction should be performed within 6 months after injury (and ideally within 3–4 months of injury) to maximize return of motor function [1–3, 14]. While the exact threshold upon which muscle fibrosis and atrophy are irreversible in humans is not clearly defined, a systematic review of the literature demonstrated improved outcomes with earlier intervention after known peripheral nerve injury [15]. Animal studies have demonstrated poorer motor reinnervation after prolonged denervation due to degeneration of the terminal ends of the distal nerve stump [16] and failure of the denervated muscle to recover from denervation atrophy [17]. While it is commonly believed that sensory nerve ends maintain the ability to regenerate for an indeterminate period of time [3], the degeneration of the distal nerve stump after prolonged denervation may compromise outcomes if reinnervation eventually occurs. Regardless of the decision whether to operate and the timing of operation, early referral to a peripheral nerve specialist allows the patient and surgeon to establish a trusting relationship and facilitates serial examination.

Unfortunately, delayed referrals to a peripheral nerve specialist are common following iatrogenic nerve injuries. Fewer than 40% of patients in two large retrospective studies underwent surgery within 6 months of their iatrogenic nerve injuries [2, 4]. There are many potential reasons for these delays in specialized care. First, peripheral nerve injuries may be difficult to diagnose due to either a lack of knowledge or failure to recognize the lesion [2]. Second, a prolonged observation period to see whether the clinical symptoms and EMG findings improve with conservative measures may delay appropriate referral [1, 18]. Out of hubris or hope, patients may be subjected to "therapeutic nihilism" and left unacceptably undertreated due to underlying skepticism that additional interventions would be helpful [19]. Third, patients with function-limiting nerve injuries are particularly vulnerable as they may be unable to return to work and continue to fund their treatment [1]. Lastly, shame, guilt, anxiety, possible professional repercussions, and fear of litigation that are experienced by the surgeon may discourage them from acknowledging errors and making timely referrals [3, 20–22].

Prompt referral to physical (PT) and/or occupational therapy (OT) after identification of a nerve injury can also improve prognosis until reinnervation of affected muscles is achieved [1]. Initial focus is placed on maintaining passive joint motion and incorporating strategies to alleviate neuropathic pain and maximize adjustment to altered or absent function. Once functional improvement begins either spontaneously or after surgical reconstruction, motor and sensory reeducation strategies are emphasized. In addition to the peripheral nerve specialist and PT/OT, pain management specialists experienced in the pharmacologic, procedural, and psychological treatments of neuropathic pain are critically important members of the treatment team. Social workers and vocational rehabilitation specialists are also incorporated into the treatment team, as the most severely affected patients may have difficulty with resuming their pre-injury employment.

2.4 Electrodiagnostic Studies

Electrodiagnostic studies (EDX) are useful to localize a peripheral nerve injury and predict prognosis. EDX should be considered an extension of the clinical assessment. EDX are composed of nerve conduction studies (NCS) and electromyography (EMG). NCS reflect function of the components of the nerve, specifically the axons and surrounding myelin. EMG indicates the integrity of the arc between the peripheral nerve and its associated muscle. Following axonal injury, Wallerian degeneration occurs to prepare the proximal and distal stumps for regeneration. EDX obtained earlier than 10 days after injury may be falsely "normal," as the effects of Wallerian degeneration will have not manifested on a macroscopic level. One potential use of early EDX is to evaluate for baseline nerve pathology, such as underlying radiculopathy or small fiber neuropathy. In most circumstances, the initial EDX assessment is obtained between 3 and 6 weeks after nerve injury. At this time, fibrillations and positive sharp waves are detectable during the resting phase of the EMG. These changes reflect the instability of the muscle membranes following nerve injury. The presence of a motor unit action potential (MUAP) during the activation phase of the EMG is a helpful indicator as to whether spontaneous muscle recovery will occur. In incomplete (axonotmetic) nerve injuries, the intact axons may collaterally sprout in order to reinnervate portions of the muscle "vacated" by the injured axons. These collateral sprouting MUAPs will have a distinct pattern from those MUAPs associated with regeneration of axons across the injured nerve segment. An experienced electromyographer may be able to discern the differences between these two MUAP patterns, but the signals are technically difficult to detect and the ultimate clinical implications are unclear. If MUAP are not detectable by 3 months, we typically recommend consideration of surgical treatment given the high unlikelihood of spontaneous recovery [18, 23–25]. If any MUAP activity is detected at 3 months, we will usually recommend continued observation with an additional clinical assessment with or without a follow-up EMG in 6 weeks. Serial EDX are best performed by the same electrodiagnostician to minimize technical variability, to maximize patient comfort, and to coordinate treatment plans with the peripheral nerve surgeon (such as including interrogation of potential donor neuromuscular units for nerve transfer). The motor portion of NCS will typically corroborate those findings seen on EMG, with losses in compound motor action potential (CMAP) amplitudes reflecting the amount of axonal injury. For sensory and mixed nerves, the latency and nerve conduction velocity measures can provide an assessment of function and can aid in lesion localization. In purely demyelinating injuries (neurapraxia), nerve conduction velocities are typically normal if measured distal to the lesion but will be decreased if measured across the lesion. Concomitant slowing is usually seen until recovery. CMAP amplitudes will be normal given that neurapraxic injuries are not associated with axonal loss. Partial nerve (axonetmetic) injuries and complete nerve (neurotmetic) injuries will have partial and complete loss of CMAP amplitudes, respectively. Comparison of CMAPs to the contralateral uninjured side can estimate degree of axonal loss, although the potential exists for changes associated with underlying (and possibly subclinical) compressive neuropathy [26].

2.5 Imaging

Evaluation of preoperative imaging can provide indications of cases with a high likelihood of postoperative peripheral nerve issues. For example, correction of a valgus knee deformity with total knee arthroplasty and fixation of a distal third humeral shaft fracture both have a higher chance of postoperative nerve palsy. Inspection of intraoperative fluoroscopy or postoperative radiographs can also suggest the likelihood of nerve palsies, such as lateralization of the glenohumeral joint after shoulder arthroplasty or leg lengthening after total hip arthroplasty. The reduction quality and location of osteosynthesis constructs and the surgical exposures necessary to position the constructs are useful in determining the risk and nature of nerve injury. Advanced imaging can be helpful in certain situations, such as using a CT scan or MRI to evaluate for the presence of a hematoma or other fluid collection. Ultrasound has the added benefit of being able to visualize nerves longitudinally, allowing for easier identification of nerve discontinuity. Ultrasound may also demonstrate neuromas and can be used to measure nerve cross-sectional area to assess for swelling [27–29].

2.6 Approach to Treatment

If a postoperative peripheral nerve issue is suspected, reversible causes of nerve injury, such as a tight-fitting cast or dressing, should be addressed [1]. If other potentially reversible causes, such as a hematoma or entrapment by implants, are suspected, early intervention is recommended. In most cases, the postoperative nerve injury is noted within the first 4–6 weeks after surgery. Motor and sensory loss are typically noticed after the initial pain from surgery subsides and the patient begins rehabilitation. Once suspicion arises for peripheral nerve injury, prompt referral to a clinician with experience caring for peripheral nerve injuries for the reasons stated above. While the duration of time to observe and await spontaneous recovery will vary based on the presumed nature and location of the injury, the absence of detectable MUAP on EMG at 3 months portends a relatively poor prognosis (Fig. 2.1). If operative intervention is considered, patient expectations should be set early, with repeated discussions between the patient and surgeon (as well as the patient and hand therapist) about the lengthy time duration for nerve recovery and the likely inability to restore "normal" or "perfect" function.

2.7 Early Nerve Repair

While the scenarios in which it arises are relatively uncommon, optimal results are obtained from immediate or early repair of a sharply transected nerve (Fig. 2.2). The primary goal of early nerve repair is to provide a supportive structure that guides sensory, motor, and autonomic axons distally toward their target organs. The proximal and distal ends of the nerve may need to be mobilized in order to facilitate a tension-free coaptation. This is technically much easier to accomplish, while the nerve ends are still "stuck" or scarred down. Following mobilization of the nerve ends, direct end-to-end epineural repair technique is typically used. In some cases where the nerve topography has been reliably established (such as the ulnar nerve in the distal forearm), a grouped fascicular repair technique is used. The nerve coaptation is performed using microsurgical technique. This attachment must be tension free, as excess stretch at the repair site can damage fragile endoneurial capillaries, devascularize the nerve, and lead to fibrosis at the repair site (Fig. 2.3) [23]. If a tension-free coaptation cannot be performed, nerve grafting is used (see below).

2.8 Staged Exploration and Neurolysis

The vast majority of cases undergoing surgical treatment weeks to months after the initial procedure are likely to be neuromas-in-continuity (i.e., axonotmetic injuries attempting to recover). Because of the technological limitations in preoperative assessment of the injured nerve, currently there is no substitute to the peripheral nerve surgeon assessing the neuroma-in-continuity intraoperatively via surgical exploration. Relatively crude measures are still used, with the nerve surgeon relying on visual inspection and palpation of the neuroma-in-continuity. External neurolysis is used to dissect away the scarred mesoneurial and external epineural tissue. Depending on the look and feel of the nerve, handheld nerve stimulators and/or nerve-to-nerve action potentials may be useful to assess function of the nerve. Both of these modalities are subject to technical difficulty and reliance on them may preclude the prolonged use of a limb tourniquet. Preoperative EDX can provide information about conduction loss across the site of injury. If MUAPs on EMG and CMAP amplitudes are present, neurolysis with scar excision can be highly successful (Fig. 2.4) [30]. If a more severe intraneural injury is suspected, internal neurolysis of the neuroma is performed using microsur-

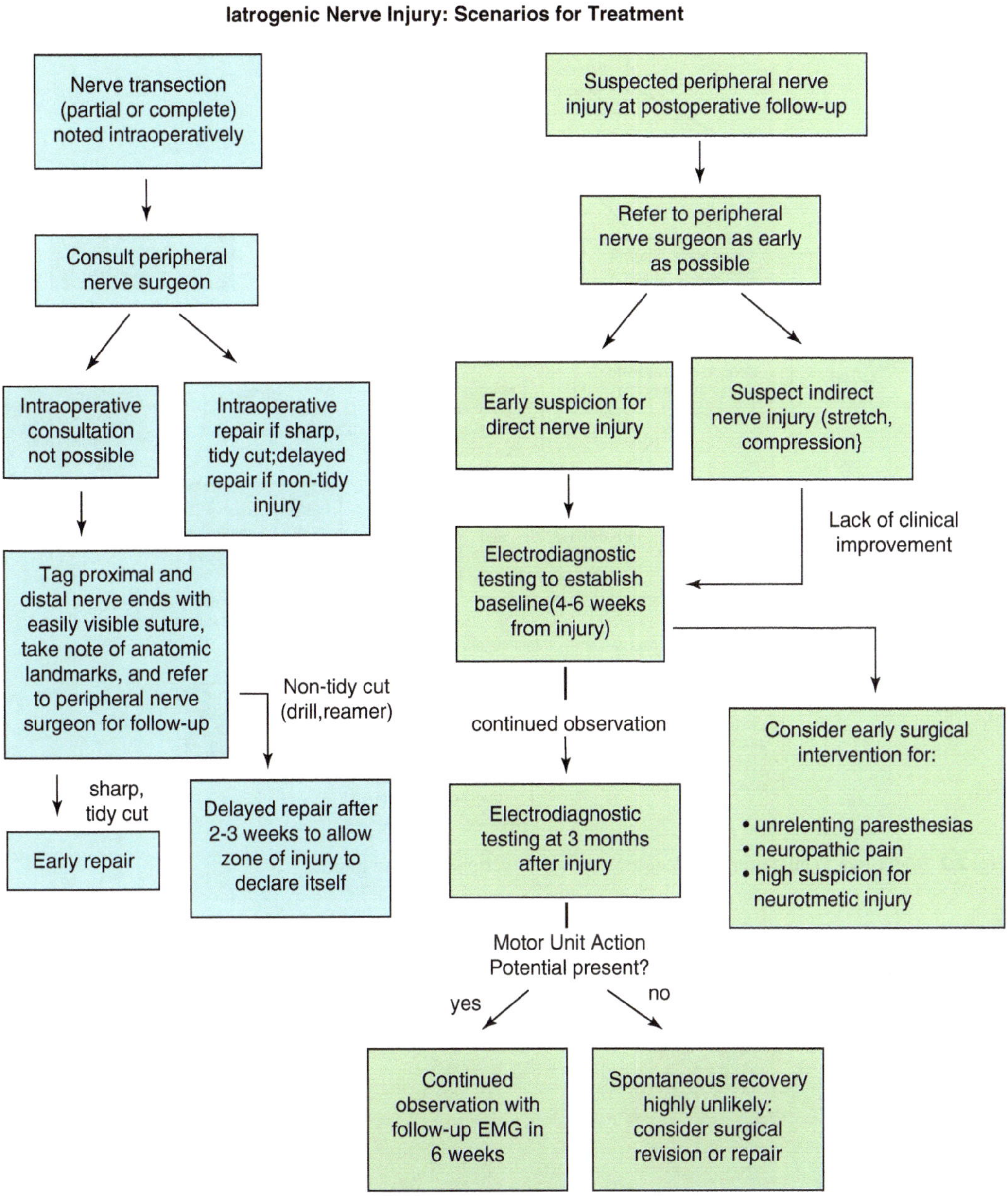

Fig. 2.1 Treatment algorithm to guide management of iatrogenic nerve injuries

gical technique to incise the perineurium and inspect individual fascicles. The individual fascicles are inspected, palpated, and can be interrogated with nerve-to-nerve action potentials. At this time, the surgeon makes a decision whether to excise scarred and unhealthy portions of nerve and how much to excise. If only portions of the nerve are thought to be diseased, then only these segments are removed and the healthy fascicles left intact. If the vast majority or entirety of the nerve is thought to be diseased, the neuroma is resected en bloc. In both situations, it is critically important to trim back to healthy, extruding fascicles. Performing neurorrhaphy within a diseased segment of the nerve is likely to lead to failure of nerve regeneration [31].

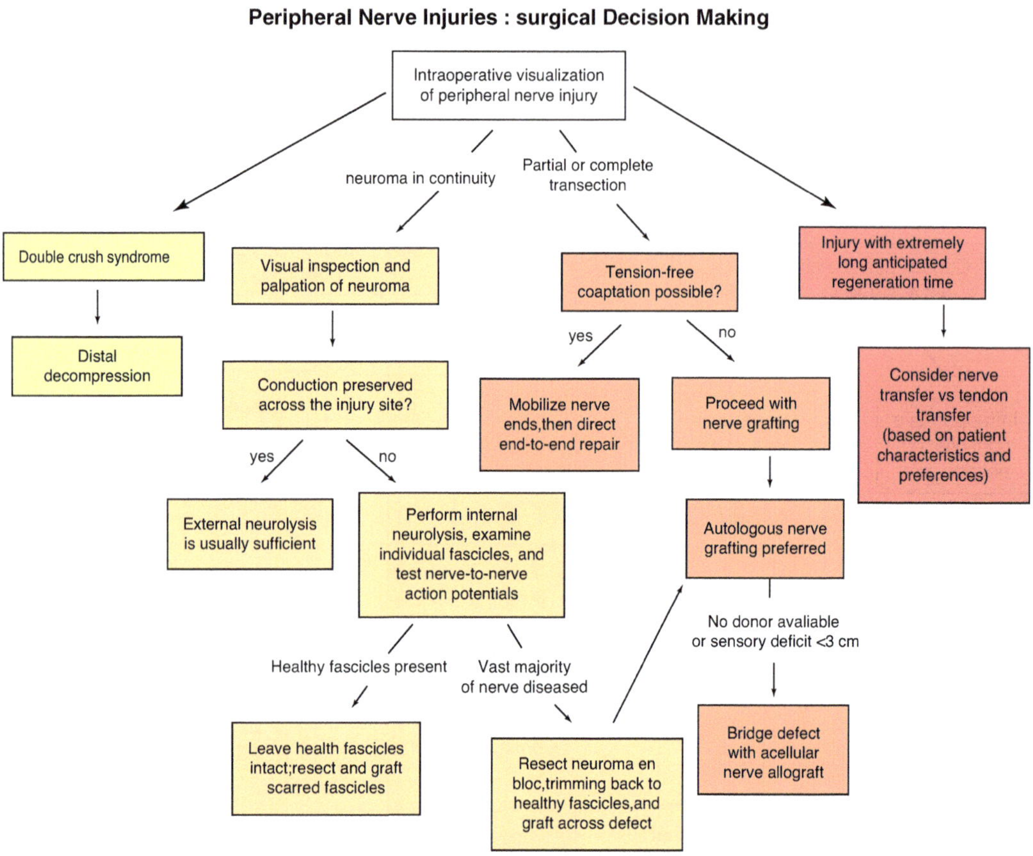

Fig. 2.2 Algorithm to guide surgical decision making for peripheral nerve injuries

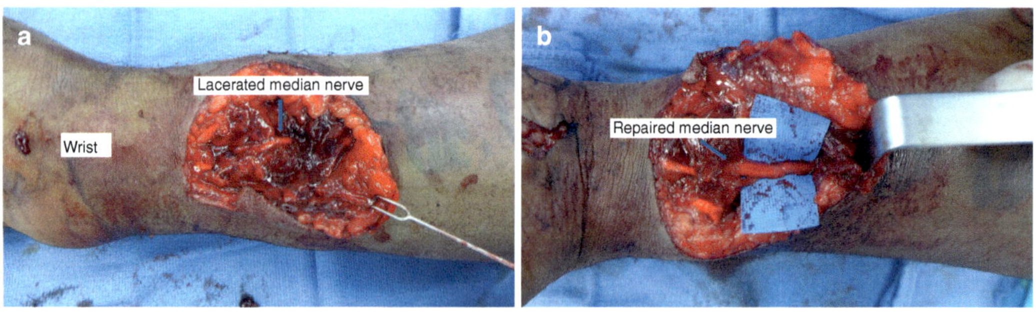

Fig. 2.3 Patient with a sharp median nerve laceration after being stabbed. (**a**) Distal aspect of median nerve is visualized. (**a**–**b**) Proximal aspect of median nerve is mobilized and tension-free end-to-end epineural coaptation is performed using microsurgical technique. (Photographs copyright Christopher J. Dy, MD MPH – used with permission)

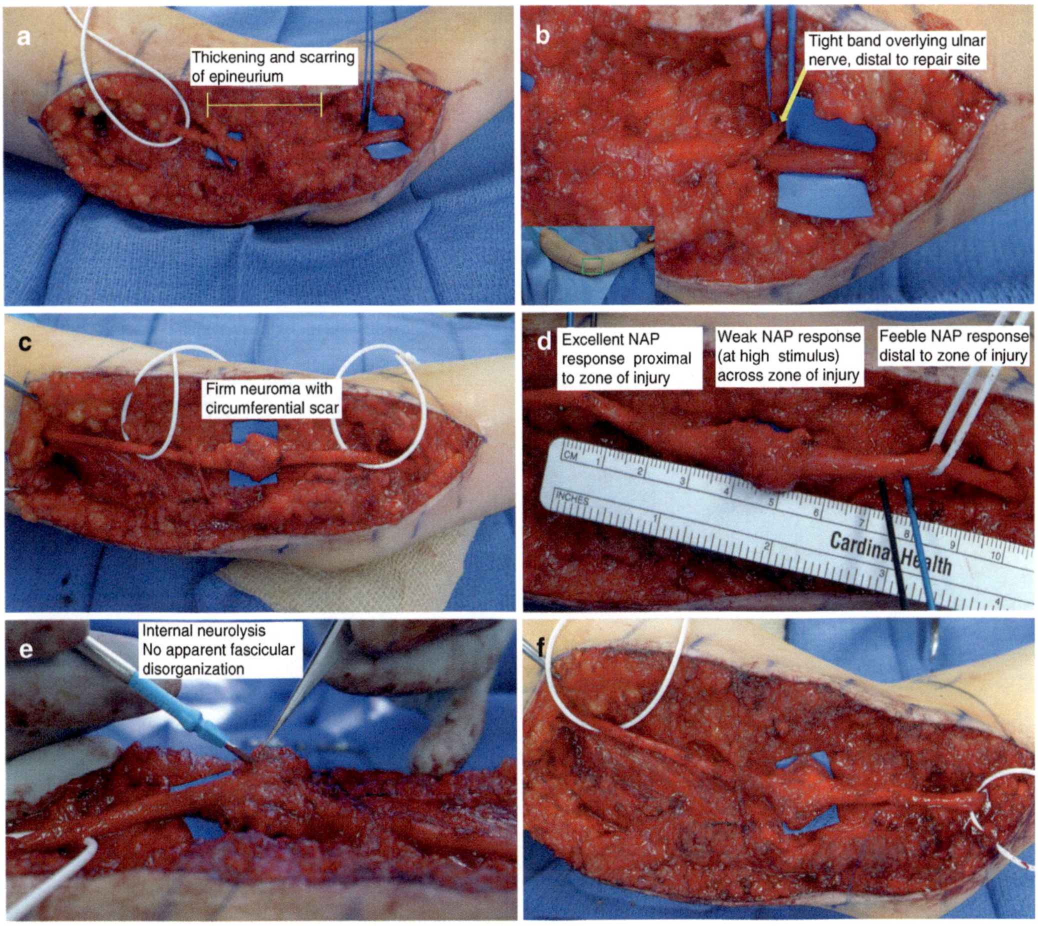

Fig. 2.4 Patient's 20 months status post primary repair of high ulnar nerve injury (sharp/tidy mechanism) at the elbow and primary supercharge end-to-side anterior interosseous to ulnar motor nerve transfer who presented with persistent pain and intrinsic weakness. (**a**) Thickening and scarring of ulnar nerve epineurium. (**b**) Tight band overlying ulnar nerve distal to repair site released. (**c**) Firm neuroma with circumferential scar encountered after performing external neurolysis. (**d**) Testing of nerve action potentials (NAP) demonstrated excellent NAP response proximal to zone of injury and weak responses across and distal to the zone of injury. (**e**) Internal neurolysis performed as no apparent fascicular disorganization was observed. (**f**) Ulnar nerve after external and internal neurolysis. (Photographs copyright Christopher J. Dy, MD MPH – used with permission)

2.9 Nerve Grafting

Autologous nerve grafting involves harvesting an expendable donor nerve segment from a patient to bridge a gap between proximal and distal ends of a nerve lesion [32]. The sural nerve is an easily accessible donor that can provide 30–35 cm of graft per leg with minimal donor site morbidity (Fig. 2.5) [3, 33]. Other potential donor sites include superficial peroneal, saphenous, and medial antebrachial cutaneous nerves [3]. The graft should extend approximately 15% longer than the lesion to minimize any potential tension from movement of the surrounding tissues and to account for contracture of the graft itself [33].

Prior to placing the graft, healthy fascicular architecture at the proximal and distal recipient nerve ends is confirmed. Single nerve grafts are used to span lesions when the donor and recipient nerves are similar in diameter. Cable grafts, or bundles of multiple small diameter nerves, are preferred for large-diameter nerves; this tech-

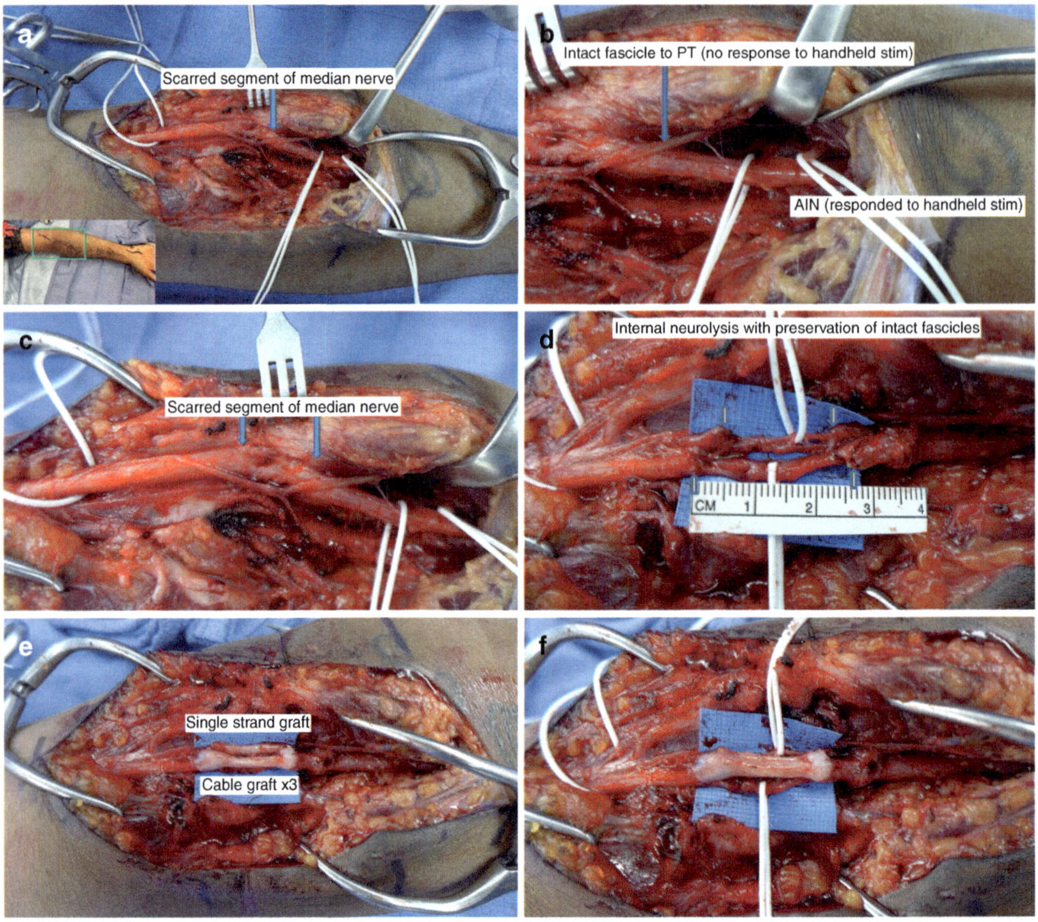

Fig. 2.5 Patient's status post gunshot wound to antecubital fossa with reported 85% median nerve transection on exploration and bascilic vein ligation by vascular surgery. (**a**) Zone of injury with significant scarring of the median nerve identified by working from known to unknown. (**b**) Intact fascicle to the pronator teres (PT) without response to handheld stimulation and anterior interosseous nerve (AIN) with response to handheld stimulation. (**c**) Close-up view of scarred portion of median nerve. (**d**) Internal neurolysis performed with preservation of intact fascicles with 3 cm gap in median nerve. (**e**) A 3 cm cabled sural nerve autograft using three fascicles and a 3 cm single fascicle graft were coapted. (**f**) Median nerve status post sural nerve autograft with vessel loops demonstrating preserved fascicles. (Photographs copyright Christopher J. Dy, MD MPH – used with permission)

nique maximizes the number of axons and enhances the viability of nonvascularized grafts [3, 23]. Although autologous nerve grafts undergo Wallerian degeneration after harvesting and interposition, the remaining Schwann cell basal laminae, neurotrophic factors, and adhesion molecules serve as a stimulating scaffold for distal axon migration [23].

One emerging alternative to autologous nerve grafting is the use of acellular nerve allografts. Acellular nerve allografts have been processed to minimize immunogenicity, but this process also removes the Schwann cells from the nerves. The endoneurial tubes, basal lamina, and laminin that remain in acellular nerve allografts provide an organized conduit for axon growth [23]. Allografts have the theoretical advantage of abundant supply, although they are not widely available outside of the United States. Advocates for nerve allograft contend that the additional cost of the tissue implant is minimal compared to the additional operative time and potential donor site morbidity associated with autograft harvest. While the current evidence has established it as a reliable option for treatment of small (<3 cm) sensory deficits, the role of acellular nerve allografts for mixed and motor nerves is in evolution.

2.10 Nerve Transfer

Nerve transfers have become a useful strategy in cases when the anticipated time to regeneration is extraordinarily long, either due to the distance between the nerve injury and the target muscle or due to a lengthy gap between nerve ends. In a nerve transfer, a healthy donor nerve is cut and sutured to the injured nerve's distal end (Fig. 2.6) [23]. Benefits of nerve transfers include only one neurorrhaphy site, short distance for nerve regen-

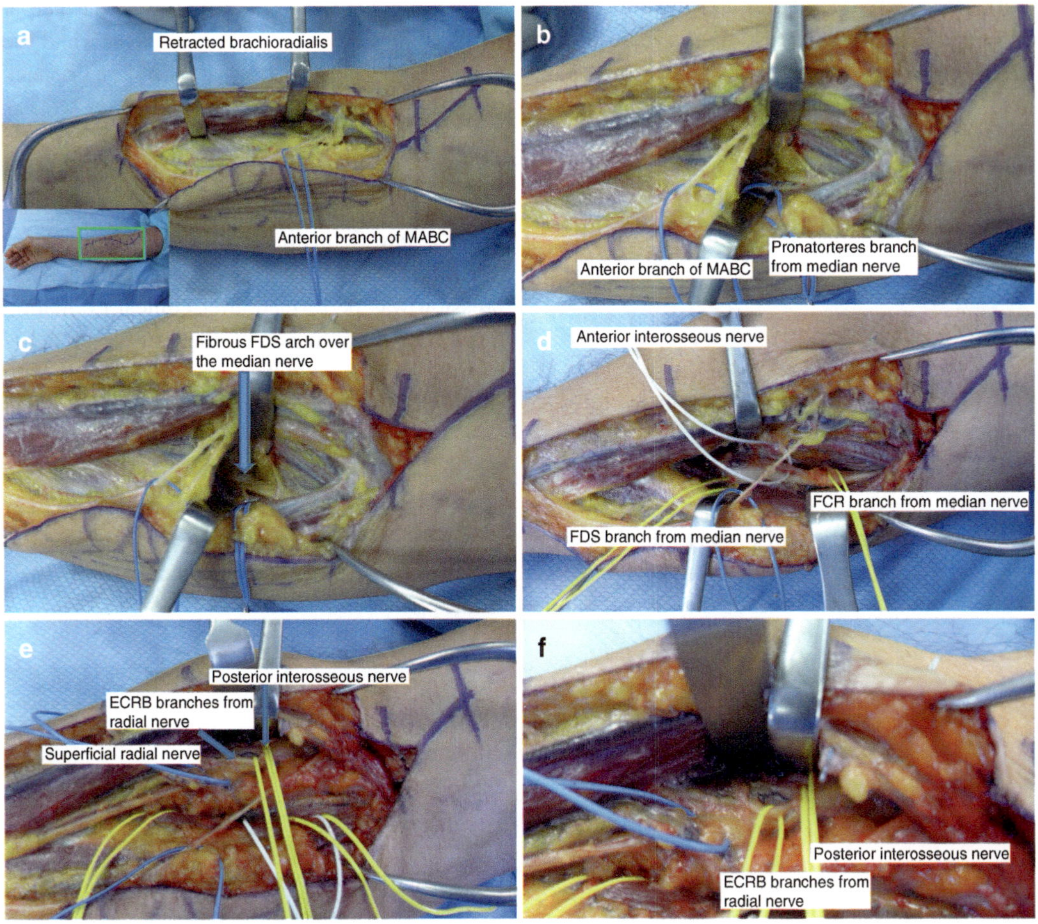

Fig. 2.6 Patient's 5 months status post radial shaft fracture open reduction internal fixation without resolution of preoperative radial nerve palsy. (**a**) The anterior branch of the medial antebrachial cutaneous nerve (MABC) is protected and brachioradialis is retracted. (**b**) Pronator teres branch from the median nerve is identified. (**c**) Flexor digitorum superficialis (FDS) aponeurotic arch is released. (**d**) Anterior interosseous nerve as well as the flexor carpi radialis (FCR) and FDS branches from the median nerve are identified. (**e**) Posterior interosseous nerve (PIN), superficial radial nerve, and extensor carpi radialis brevis (ECRB) branches from the radial nerve are identified. (**f**) Close-up view of PIN and ECRB branches. (**g**) Pronator teres (PT) and ECRB tendon transfer performed to help restore wrist extension. (**h**) Final coaptation of FDS to ECRB and FCR to PIN nerve transfers. (Photographs copyright Christopher J. Dy, MD MPH – used with permission)

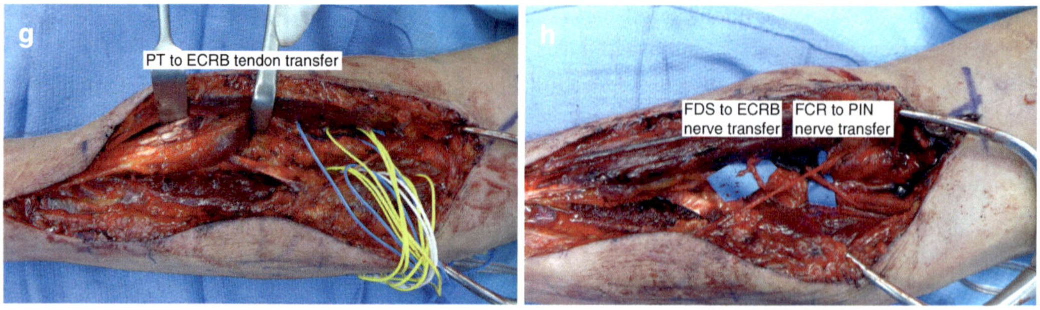

Fig. 2.6 (continued)

eration, rapid reinnervation and motor reeducation, and unaltered muscle biomechanics [23, 33]. Limitations of nerve transfers include their requirement for an expendable donor motor nerve in close proximity to the target and loss of the donor nerve's original function [23, 32, 33]. The latter may have implications in compromising options for subsequent tendon transfers.

2.11 Distal Decompression

Distal nerve decompression is based on the concept of double crush syndrome [11]. After surgery, swelling in the affected extremity increases due to the insult of surgery, but also immobility. Disruption of axoplasmic flow as a result of a proximal nerve injury may also create nerve swelling. Nerves particularly at risk in this setting include the median nerve at the carpal tunnel, ulnar nerve at the cubital tunnel, and the common peroneal nerve at the fibular neck (Fig. 2.7). Monitoring of Tinel's sign as well as ultrasound examination may be useful in this setting to evaluate nerve cross-sectional area. In a retrospective review of 142 patients undergoing nerve repair, Schoeller et al. demonstrated functional recovery in two cases where distal decompression was performed after clinical evaluation and EMG recordings were suggestive of nerve compression distal to the nerve repair [10]. A retrospective study evaluating common peroneal nerve decompression after proximal sciatic nerve injury sustained during total hip arthroplasty demonstrated recovery of dorsiflexion strength of ≥ 3 in 65% of patients compared to 50% of patients who were treated nonoperatively in other studies [34].

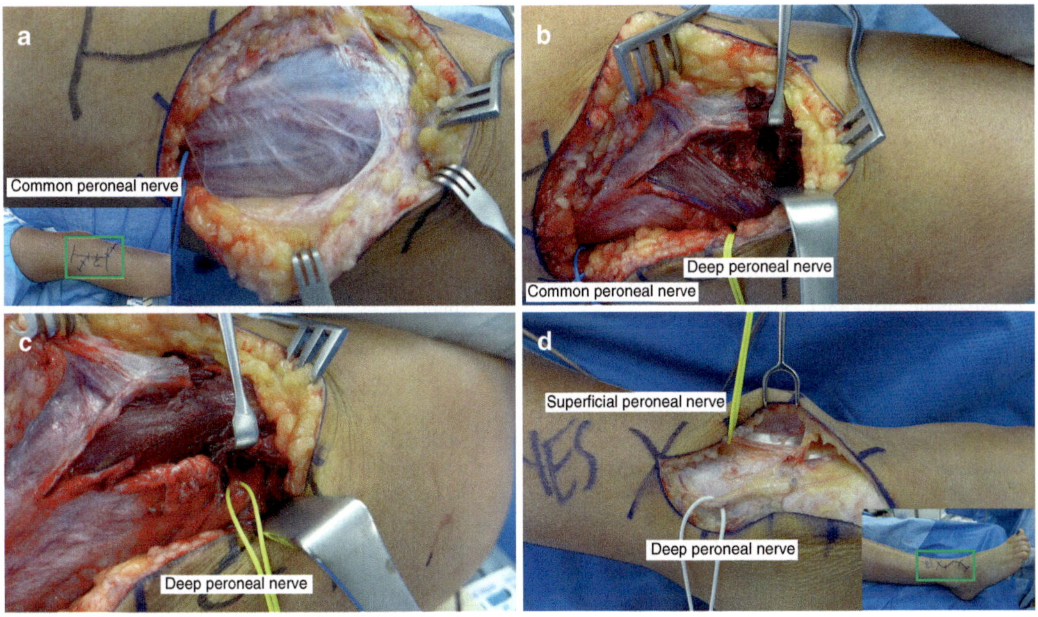

Fig. 2.7 Patient's 1 year and 3 months status post basketball injury and 8 months status post short head of biceps release, peroneal nerve release, and diagnostic knee arthroscopy with persistent foot drop. (**a**) An S-shaped incision (vs original longitudinal incision) was used demonstrating scarring overlying the common peroneal nerve. (**b**) The anterior crural, posterior crural, and deep intermuscular septa are released. (**c**) The deep peroneal nerve is sufficiently released. (**d**) Distal decompression of the deep peroneal nerve was performed due to concern for double crush syndrome. The patient had return of extensor hallucis longus function in the post-anesthesia care unit immediately after surgery. (Photographs copyright Christopher J. Dy, MD MPH – used with permission)

References

1. Antoniadis G, Kretschmer T, Pedro MT, Konig RW, Heinen CP, Richter HP. Iatrogenic nerve injuries: prevalence, diagnosis and treatment. Dtsch Arztebl Int. 2014;111(16):273–9.
2. Kretschmer T, Antoniadis G, Braun V, Rath SA, Richter HP. Evaluation of iatrogenic lesions in 722 surgically treated cases of peripheral nerve trauma. J Neurosurg. 2001;94(6):905–12.
3. Pulos N, Shin EH, Spinner RJ, Shin AY. Management of Iatrogenic nerve ijuries. J Am Acad Orthop Surg. 2019;27(18):e838–e48.
4. Rasulic L, Savic A, Vitosevic F, et al. Iatrogenic peripheral nerve injuries-surgical treatment and outcome: 10 years' experience. World Neurosurg. 2017;103:841–51 e6.
5. Winfree CJ, Kline DG. Intraoperative positioning nerve injuries. Surg Neurol. 2005;63(1):5–18; discussion.
6. James MA. Use of the Medical Research Council muscle strength grading system in the upper extremity. J Hand Surg Am. 2007;32(2):154–6.
7. Cuthbert SC, Goodheart GJ Jr. On the reliability and validity of manual muscle testing: a literature review. Chiropr Osteopat. 2007;15:4.
8. Shahgholi L, Bengtson KA, Bishop AT, et al. A comparison of manual and quantitative elbow strength testing. Am J Phys Med Rehabil. 2012;91(10):856–62.
9. Bertelli JA, Ghizoni MF. Abduction in internal rotation: a test for the diagnosis of axillary nerve palsy. J Hand Surg Am. 2011;36(12):2017–23.
10. Schoeller T, Otto A, Wechselberger G, Pommer B, Papp C. Distal nerve entrapment following nerve repair. Br J Plast Surg. 1998;51(3):227–9; discussion 30.
11. Kane PM, Daniels AH, Akelman E. Double crush syndrome. J Am Acad Orthop Surg. 2015;23(9):558–62.
12. Shin AY, Spinner RJ, Steinmann SP, Bishop AT. Adult traumatic brachial plexus injuries. J Am Acad Orthop Surg. 2005;13(6):382–96.
13. Ma J, Novikov LN, Kellerth JO, Wiberg M. Early nerve repair after injury to the postganglionic plexus: an experimental study of sensory and motor neuronal survival in adult rats. Scand J Plast Reconstr Surg Hand Surg. 2003;37(1):1–9.
14. Kim DH, Murovic JA, Tiel R, Kline DG. Management and outcomes in 353 surgically treated sciatic nerve lesions. J Neurosurg. 2004;101(1):8–17.
15. Martin E, Senders JT, DiRisio AC, Smith TR, Broekman MLD. Timing of surgery in traumatic brachial plexus injury: a systematic review. J Neurosurg. 2018;1:1–13.

16. Fu SY, Gordon T. Contributing factors to poor functional recovery after delayed nerve repair: prolonged denervation. J Neurosci. 1995;15(5 Pt 2):3886–95.
17. Gordon T, Tyreman N, Raji MA. The basis for diminished functional recovery after delayed peripheral nerve repair. J Neurosci. 2011;31(14):5325–34.
18. Campbell WW. Evaluation and management of peripheral nerve injury. Clin Neurophysiol. 2008;119(9):1951–65.
19. Mamede S, Schmidt HG. The twin traps of overtreatment and therapeutic nihilism in clinical practice. Med Educ. 2014;48(1):34–43.
20. Helo S, Moulton CE. Complications: acknowledging, managing, and coping with human error. Transl Androl Urol. 2017;6(4):773–82.
21. Chamberlain CJ, Koniaris LG, Wu AW, Pawlik TM. Disclosure of "nonharmful" medical errors and other events: duty to disclose. Arch Surg. 2012;147(3):282–6.
22. Schwappach DL, Koeck CM. What makes an error unacceptable? A factorial survey on the disclosure of medical errors. Int J Qual Health Care. 2004;16(4):317–26.
23. Grinsell D, Keating CP. Peripheral nerve reconstruction after injury: a review of clinical and experimental therapies. Biomed Res Int. 2014;2014:698256.
24. Finucane BT. Complications of regional anesthesia. Springer; 2007.
25. Katirji B. Electromyography in clinical practice E-book: a case study approach. Elsevier Health Sciences; 2007.
26. Robinson LR. Traumatic injury to peripheral nerves. Muscle Nerve. 2000;23(6):863–73.
27. Ashwell ZR, Froelich JM, Strickland CD. Unique utility of sonography for detection of an iatrogenic radial nerve injury. J Ultrasound Med. 2016;35(5):1101–3.
28. Bodner G, Harpf C, Gardetto A, et al. Ultrasonography of the accessory nerve: normal and pathologic findings in cadavers and patients with iatrogenic accessory nerve palsy. J Ultrasound Med. 2002;21(10):1159–63.
29. Cesmebasi A, Smith J, Spinner RJ. Role of sonography in surgical decision making for iatrogenic spinal accessory nerve injuries: a paradigm shift. J Ultrasound Med. 2015;34(12):2305–12.
30. Kim DH, Han K, Tiel RL, Murovic JA, Kline DG. Surgical outcomes of 654 ulnar nerve lesions. J Neurosurg. 2003;98(5):993–1004.
31. Millesi H, Meissl G, Berger A. The interfascicular nerve-grafting of the median and ulnar nerves. J Bone Joint Surg Am. 1972;54(4):727–50.
32. Bassilios Habre S, Bond G, Jing XL, Kostopoulos E, Wallace RD, Konofaos P. The surgical management of nerve gaps: present and future. Ann Plast Surg. 2018;80(3):252–61.
33. Panagopoulos GN, Megaloikonomos PD, Mavrogenis AF. The present and future for peripheral nerve regeneration. Orthopedics. 2017;40(1):e141–e56.
34. Wilson TJ, Kleiber GM, Nunley RM, Mackinnon SE, Spinner RJ. Distal peroneal nerve decompression after sciatic nerve injury secondary to total hip arthroplasty. J Neurosurg. 2018;130(1):179–83.

Part II

Nerve Injuries after Orthopedic Surgery of the Upper Extremity

Nerve Injury After Shoulder Arthroscopy, Stabilization, and Rotator Cuff Repair (Axillary, Musculocutaneous, Suprascapular Nerves)

3

Bridget P. Pulos and Nicholas Pulos

3.1 Introduction

Nerve injuries after orthopedic surgery can be related to surgical, patient, and anesthetic-related factors, or a combination of the three, and in many cases, it may be challenging to determine the causative factor. The inherent difficulty in assigning one cause for perioperative neuropathy has medico-legal implications for both surgeons and anesthesiologists. Common mechanisms of injury include positioning, stretch, retraction, direct trauma, laceration, or a postsurgical inflammatory etiology. Although the majority of nerve injuries after shoulder surgery are neuropraxias that will likely improve or resolve on their own, more severe nerve injuries that do not improve after serial examinations may warrant surgical treatment. Prompt referral within 3–6 months after the injury to a peripheral nerve surgeon is imperative for the best chance at a favorable outcome.

B. P. Pulos
Department of Anesthesiology, Mayo Clinic, Rochester, MN, USA
e-mail: Pulos.Bridget@mayo.edu

N. Pulos (✉)
Department of Orthopedic Surgery, Mayo Clinic, Rochester, MN, USA
e-mail: Pulos.Nicholas@mayo.edu

3.2 Incidence

The incidence of peripheral nerve issues after elective arthroscopic shoulder surgery is often thought to be quite low, but it has been reported to be between 0.1% and 10% [1–7]. Much of the incidence data come from small retrospective studies from the 1980s and 1990s, making it difficult to extrapolate to current practice. Data from large, multicenter, prospective studies are needed to better determine the true incidence of peripheral nerve issues after shoulder arthroscopy, stabilization, and rotator cuff repair. For example, in a nerve monitoring study during open Latarjet procedures, 76.5% of patients had a severe nerve alert during their procedure, with the majority involving the axillary or musculocutaneous nerve [8]. Fortunately, only 20% of these were clinically detectable, and all eventually spontaneously resolved, but this study highlights the high occurrence and risk of nerve injuries in these common shoulder procedures. In arthroscopic surgery, the incidence of nerve injury is potentially lower, but not clinically irrelevant. In one study using somatosensory evoked potentials, Pitman and colleagues found up to 10% of patients undergoing arthroscopic shoulder surgery in the lateral decubitus position experienced transient neuropraxia [5]. Fortunately, all resolved within 48 hours of the procedures.

Complications from regional anesthesia techniques used for shoulder surgery, such as interscalene nerve blocks, can also occur and

C. J. Dy et al. (eds.), *Peripheral Nerve Issues after Orthopedic Surgery*,
https://doi.org/10.1007/978-3-030-84428-8_3

may confound the postoperative clinical picture. However, it is very rare that these blocks cause permanent neurologic injury, with current estimates of 2–4 in 10,000 patients who receive nerve blocks [9]. Furthermore, studies show no increased risk for perioperative nerve injury in patients receiving peripheral nerve blocks compared to patients who do not; and in one study of shoulder arthroplasty patients, those who received a nerve block had a lower incidence of perioperative nerve injury [10, 11].

3.3 Clinical Evaluation

A thorough history and physical exam is the first step to define the affected nerves, which will help to determine next steps (Fig. 3.1). Further evaluation and treatment may also depend on the mechanism of injury. A history of severe neuropathic pain apparent immediately after surgery may indicate direct nerve trauma. On the other hand, a history of pain that starts several days after surgery followed by paralysis may be indicative of a brachial plexus neuritis (Fig. 3.2).

Proper evaluation of a shoulder patient begins well above the shoulder at the neck and extends on down through the hand. Patients who are considered for arthroscopic shoulder procedures, including stabilization procedures, may have a history of shoulder dislocations that could have been associated with transient or subclinical nerve injuries. Anterior shoulder dislocation, in particular, is associated with a 48% risk of nerve injury, with axillary nerve being the most common [12]. Naturally, it can be difficult to perform a thorough neurologic exam in some of these patients due to pain and distracting injuries. However, accurate documentation is essential and any nerve that cannot be evaluated should be documented as such (Fig. 3.3). Further, it may be difficult to assess whether a lack of active movement is caused by a neurologic lesion or a traumatic injury, such as a rotator cuff tear. Among patients with traumatic brachial plexus lesions, Brogan et al. found an 8.2% incidence of concomitant full-thickness rotator cuff tear [13]. Therefore, a complete work-up includes both a thorough physical examination and appropriate advanced imaging, which together, permit formulation of the correct diagnosis or diagnoses.

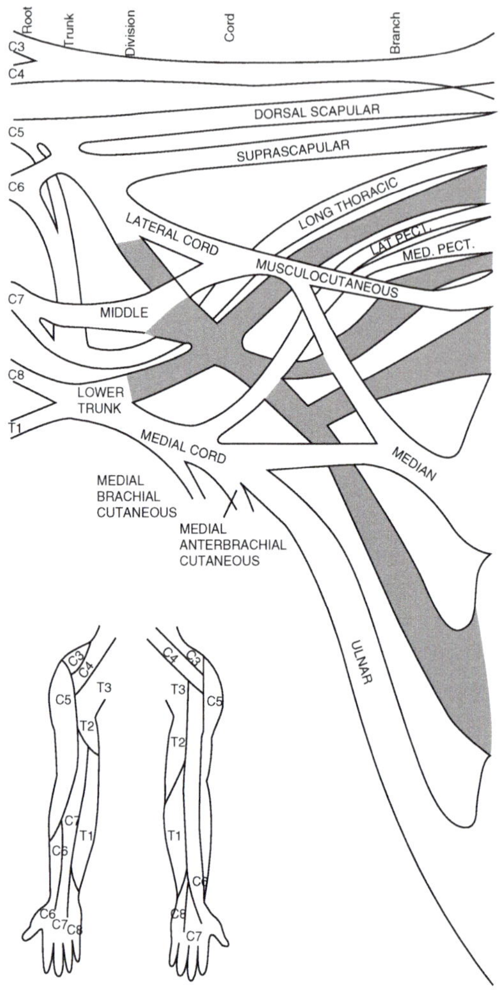

Fig. 3.1 Schematic of the brachial plexus. Motor and sensory components the upper extremity are assessed and recorded serially. (With permission of the Mayo Foundation for Medical Education and Research. All rights reserved)

Special consideration for performing a nerve block is warranted for patients who present for shoulder surgery with pre-existing nerve injury. There is the potential for the "double-crush" phenomenon where nerves that already have an abnormality are at increased risk to suffer a

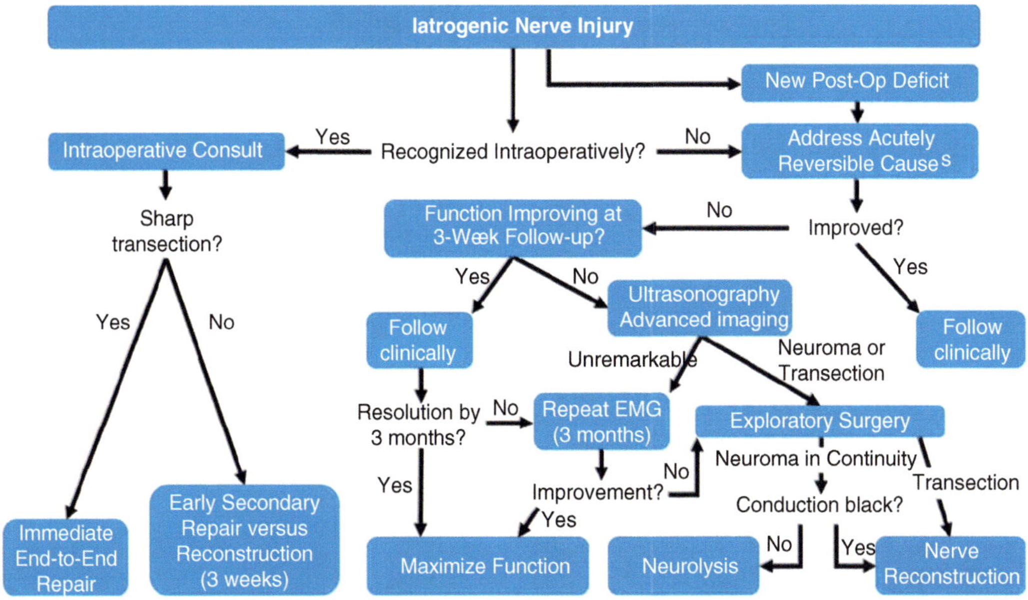

Fig. 3.2 Flow chart to guide evaluation and management of suspected iatrogenic nerve injury. (Pulos et al. [32])

"second-hit" from the nerve block that progresses to neuropraxia and potentially permanent neurologic injury [14]. A careful history (time course of prior neuropathy, whether symptoms are stable or progressing, mechanism of injury if known), physical exam (distribution of neuropathy), and discussion of risks and benefits are imperative before deciding whether to perform a nerve block on these patients. In cases of trauma and acute nerve injury, the affected distribution and extent of the injury should be well documented preoperatively. Regional anesthesia techniques can be performed safely in this patient population and may be beneficial to decrease perioperative opioid use; however, the potential for a nerve block to mask further nerve injury from surgery or postoperative compartment syndrome must be discussed among the surgeon, anesthesiologist, and patient.

If the patient did receive a peripheral nerve block, close communication with the anesthesia team is important to clarify which block and which local anesthetic was used in order to estimate expected duration of action. Advanced imaging will usually determine if the cause of limited motion is due to musculoskeletal injury or neurologic injury, but if there is any suspicion for a nerve lesion, electrodiagnostic studies should be performed at least 3 weeks following injury to allow for Wallerian degeneration and accurate assessment of the degree of muscle denervation. At this point, consultation with a neurologist may be warranted (Fig. 3.4).

3.4 Treatment

Many arthroscopic procedures are done on an outpatient basis, and so patients may not be evaluated for neurologic issues in the immediate postoperative period. Patients should be counseled before surgery to contact the surgical team if any neurologic issues arise, rather than wait for their next postoperative follow-up visit to avoid any potential delays in treatment. Further, in a patient with a suspected nerve injury, the surgeon should also ensure that the patient is not lost to follow-up in the early postoperative period. In a retrospective review from the Mayo Clinic Brachial Plexus Clinic over a 10-year period, the ultimate functional outcome was found to be

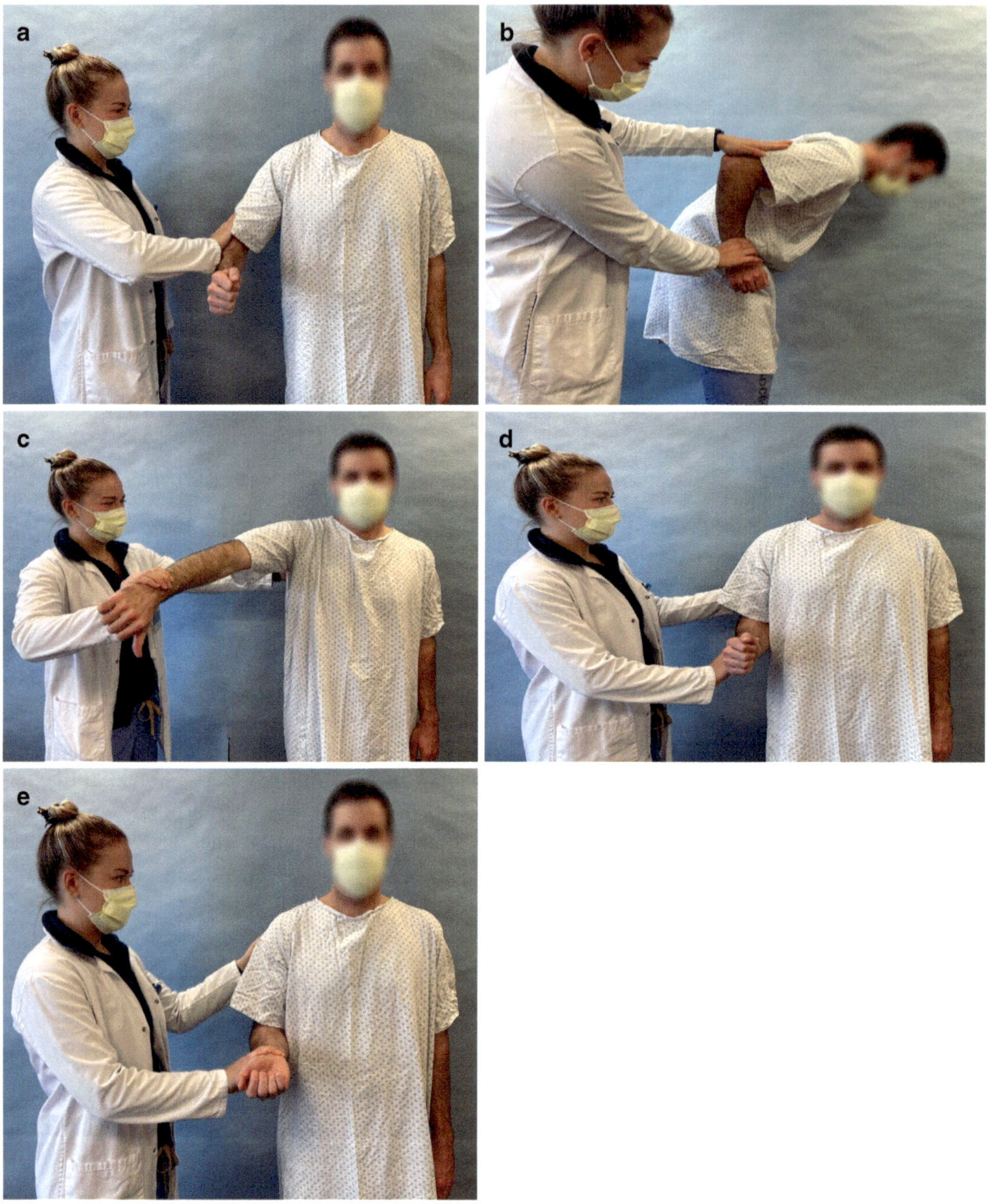

Fig. 3.3 Exam. Manual strength testing of (**a**) middle deltoid, (**b**) posterior deltoid, (**c**) supraspinatus, (**d**) infraspinatus, and (**e**) biceps muscles. (With permission of the Mayo Foundation for Medical Education and Research.)

worse in patients who presented 8 months or more from their shoulder procedure. After 12 months, the ability to perform nerve repairs and nerve transfers is limited and surgical treatment is largely relegated to tendon transfers and selective joint fusions [15].

Postsurgical inflammatory neuropathy, such as Pasonage-Turner syndrome, may be an under-

NERVE CONDUCTIONS

Nerve	Type	Record site	Rep stim	Side	Amp	Normal Amp	CV	Normal CV	Distal Lat	Normal Lat	F-Wave Lat	F-Wave Est	Temp (°C)
Median	Motor	APB		L	5.1	(> 4.0)	53	(> 48)	3.0	(> 4.5)	24.2	23.4	33.0
Radial	Motor	EDC		L	NR			(> 67)	NR	(> 3.1)			32.4
Radial	Motor	EDC		R	7.8			(> 67)	1.6	(> 3.1)			31.9
Ulnar	Motor	ADM		L	8.8	(> 6.0)	62	(> 51)	2.1	(> 3.6)	23.3	19.5	32.4
Median	Sensory	Dig II		L	36	(> 15.0)	58	(> 56)	3.1	(> 3.6)			32.7
Radial	Sensory	Wrist		L	NR	(> 20.0)		(> 49)	NR	(> 2.9)			32.7
Radial	Sensory	Wrist		L	20	(> 20.0)		(> 49)	2.3	(> 2.9)			31.7
Ulnar	Sensory	Dig V		R	38	(> 10.0)	59	(> 54)	2.3	(> 3.1)			32.6

Muscle	Side	Ins Act	Spont		Mup Normal	Activ	Recruitment		Duration		Amplitude		Phases	
			Fib	Fasc			Reduced	Rapid	Long	Short	High	Low		Turns
Ext digitorum communis	L	INC	+++	0		None								
First dorsal interosseous	L	INC	++	0		None								
Barchioradialis	L	INC	+++	0		None								
Biceps brachii	L	NL	0	0	NL									
Deltoid	L	NL	0	0					+		+		25%	++
Triceps brachii	L	NL	0	0	NL									

Fig. 3.4 EMG. Electrodiagnostic studies performed 3 months following proximal humerus open reduction and internal fixation demonstrating a severe left radial neuropathy with absent compound muscle action potentials (CMAPs) and no motor unit activation of radial nerve innervated muscles distal to the triceps. There is also a mild left axillary neuropathy with reinnervation

appreciated cause of postoperative neuropathy. These neuropathies often have a delayed presentation, and symptoms may occur outside of the expected distribution of the surgery or nerve block if one was performed [16]. If an inflammatory etiology is considered, patients should be referred for prompt evaluation by a neurologist for possible nerve biopsy and potential treatment with immune-modulating therapies (high-dose steroids, immunoglobulin). In the case of postsurgical inflammatory neuropathy, surgical treatment may in fact worsen the disease process.

3.5 Axillary Nerve Injury

3.5.1 Anatomy

The axillary nerve originates from the posterior cord of the brachial plexus and innervates the deltoid and teres minor muscles. Its terminal branch provides sensation to the lateral aspect of the upper brachium. The nerve lies in between 10 and 25 mm from the inferior glenoid rim en route to the quadrilateral space before dividing into anterior and posterior branches [17]. The anterior branch of the axillary nerve is reported to be found 4–7 cm inferior to the anterolateral corner of the acromion, but it may be as close as 3.1 cm. Shoulder abduction decreases the distance between the acromion and the nerve [18] (Fig. 3.5).

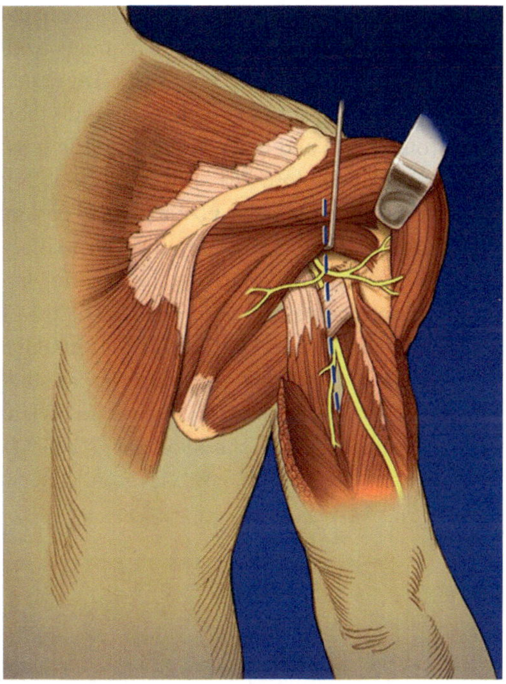

Fig. 3.5 Branching of the axillary and radial nerves through the quadrilateral and triangular spaces, respectively. (With permission of the Mayo Foundation for Medical Education and Research. All rights reserved)

3.5.2 Prevention

Axillary neuropathy is the most common neurologic complication following anterior shoulder dislocations [12]. The axillary nerve is, similarly, the most commonly injured nerve following shoulder surgery and has been reported with both open and arthroscopic procedures [15]. During arthroscopic surgery, there is a risk to the axillary nerve from insertion of portals in the anterior-inferior positions and the lateral position [19]. Its close proximity to the inferior shoulder capsule puts the axillary nerve at risk during arthroscopic Bankart repairs with inadvertent suture placement [15] and thermal shrinkage [20].

3.5.3 Evaluation

Some patients may be able to compensate remarkably well with deltoid paralysis and atrophy may not always be immediately appreciated on examination. For example, in patients with chronic deltoid paralysis, one study suggested some patients are able to compensate with their intact rotator cuff and other shoulder girdle muscles to regain close to full motion [21]. Furthermore, early in the postoperative period, protocols limiting motion may hide an axillary nerve palsy. However, injury to the superior lateral cutaneous nerve of the arm can lead to loss of sensation over the lateral aspect of the shoulder. Still, overlapping sensory innervation from other cutaneous nerves may mask the nerve deficit. Radiographically, often the shoulder is seen to sublux inferiorly on Grashey views in patients with axillary nerve injury. If an injury is suspected in the postoperative setting, an electrodiagnostic study should be performed ideally at 3–4 weeks following injury.

3.5.4 Treatment

In the rare event that an axillary nerve injury is observed in the operation, a consultation with a peripheral nerve surgeon intraoperatively is appropriate. In a sharp transection, the neve may be primarily repaired. However, if the nerve ends are damaged to the extent that they cannot be coapted and repaired without tension, then the nerve ends are tagged for later reconstruction with grafts.

More commonly, the nerve injury is identified postoperatively and requires serial clinical examinations to determine whether or not surgical exploration is warranted. Without evidence of clinical or electrodiagnostic recovery in the first 3–6 months, the nerve should be evaluated in the operating room. The timing depends on the index of suspicion for a penetrating injury or laceration to the nerve rather than a neurapraxia. Ultrasound can be a useful adjunct in this regard to assess the morphology of the axillary nerve at the potential site of injury. Once the decision to operate has been made, intraoperative neuromonitoring can assist in determining whether to perform neuroloysis or neuroma resection and nerve grafting (Fig. 3.6).

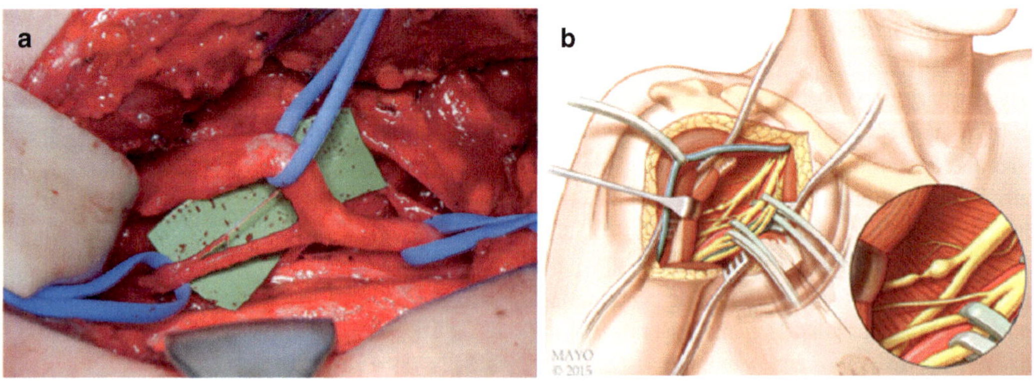

Fig. 3.6 Axillary nerve grafting. (**a**, **b**) Dissected infraclavicular plexus with medial retraction of the lateral and medial cords and the brachial artery and lateral reflection of the cephalic vein. A neuroma is identified within the axillary nerve, after it branches off the posterior cord (Used with permission of Mayo Foundation for Medical Education and Research. All rights reserved. (In: Baltzer et al. [47], Fig. 3.5))

Neuroma excision involves resecting the scarred portion of the nerve which leaves a defect in the nerve that does not permit neurorrhaphy. The gold stand for nerve graft remains autologous nerve. Typically this is harvested from the patient's sural nerve, which is purely sensory and leaves a permanent sensory deficit of the lateral border of the foot. When the diameter of the sural nerve does not match the diameter of the axillary nerve or its branches, the grafts can be laid in parallel to create a cable graft. Allograft nerve is available in larger diameters, but laboratory studies have demonstrated that the results for motor and mixed motor/sensory nerves are inferior to autograft, thus our choice to continue to use sural nerve autograft for reconstruction [22]. Options for neurorrhaphy include sutures, nerve wraps and cables, and or fibrin glue. Irrespective of the method used to coapt the nerve ends together, it is important to ensure that the nerve ends are brought into proximity to each other, but not overly approximated such that the nerve ends splay and are unable to permit axonal growth from the proximal donor nerve to the distal recipient. By 3 weeks, the tensile strength of the repair is such that the patient may begin gentle range of motion.

In cases where direct repair, neurolysis, or nerve grafting are not possible, Leechavengvongs described transfer of a triceps branch of the radial nerve to the anterior branch of the axillary nerve [23] (Fig. 3.7). There are several indications for this procedure including more proximal lesions or larger lesions, which after neuroma excision and grafting, will not permit axonal growth to reinnervate the deltoid within 1 year from injury and motor end plate death. Similarly in patients who present later, nerve transfer requires a shorter distance for axons to grow before reinnervating the target muscle. A contraindication to this procedure would be a patient with insufficient triceps strength to permit nerve transfer.

For patients evaluated more than 12 months from injury, nerve surgery is not likely to be

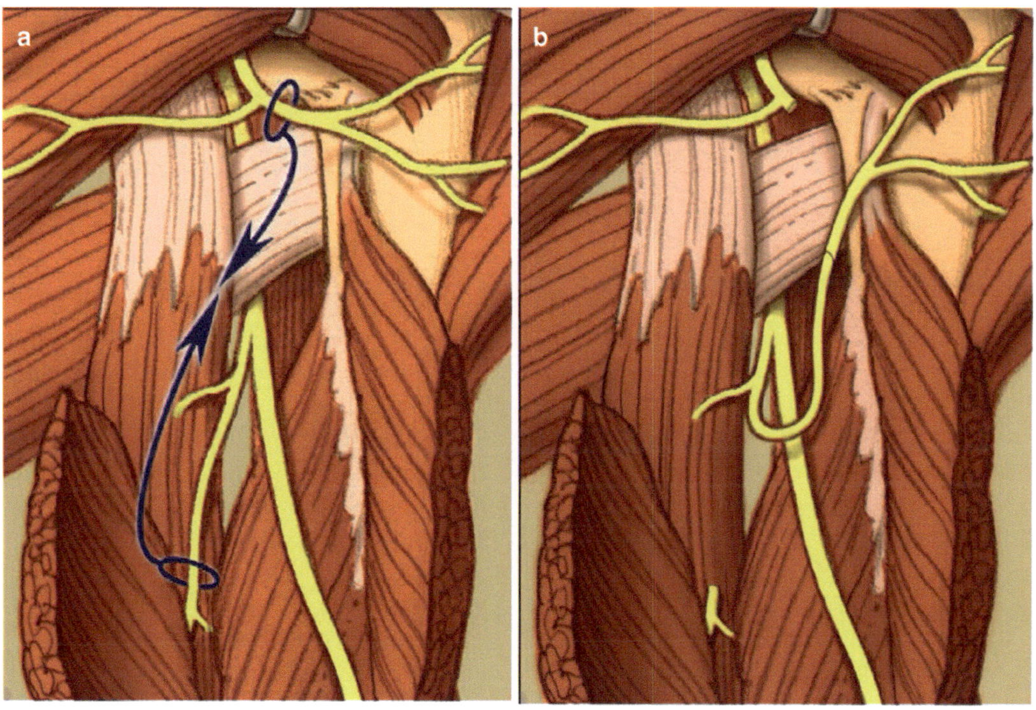

Fig. 3.7 Schematic illustration of the Leechavengvongs procedure (a) before and (b) after transfer to the anterior branch of the axillary motor nerve is performed. (Used with permission of Mayo Foundation for Medical Education and Research. All rights reserved. (In: Maldonado et al. [48], Figs. 3.5 and 3.6))

effective due to loss of the deltoid muscle motor end plates. In these cases, tendon transfers can be performed in patients with poor shoulder function. Pedicled pectoralis and latissimus dorsi muscle transfers have also been described [24, 25].

3.6 Musculocutaneous Nerve Injury

3.6.1 Anatomy

The musculocutaneous nerve originates from the lateral cord of the brachial plexus and innervates the coracobrachialis, biceps brachii, and brachialis muscles. Its terminal branch, the lateral antebrachial cutaneous nerve, provides sensation to the lateral aspect of the forearm all the way down to the wrist. The nerve travels obliquely inferior to the coracoid process before piercing the coracobrachialis muscle 5 cm distal to the coracoid and exiting the muscle belly approximately 7.5 cm distal. However, in over one-quarter of patients, the nerve enters the muscle proximal to this and small branches have been found inserting into the muscle as close as 1.7 cm from the coracoid [26, 27]. The nerve travels between the brachialis and biceps muscle before piercing the biceps approximately 11.5 cm distal to the coracoid (Fig. 3.8).

3.6.2 Prevention

Isolated musculocutaneous nerve injury is rare following trauma, but instead injury is more commonly injured during shoulder arthroscopy and open shoulder stabilization procedures [28]. Musculocutaneous nerve injury has been reported following Bristow-Latarjet procedure with transfer of the coracoid process to prevent recurrent glenohumeral instability [29] and subpectoral tenodesis [15]. For example, in a nerve monitoring study during open Latarjet procedures, 76.5% of patients had a severe nerve alert during their

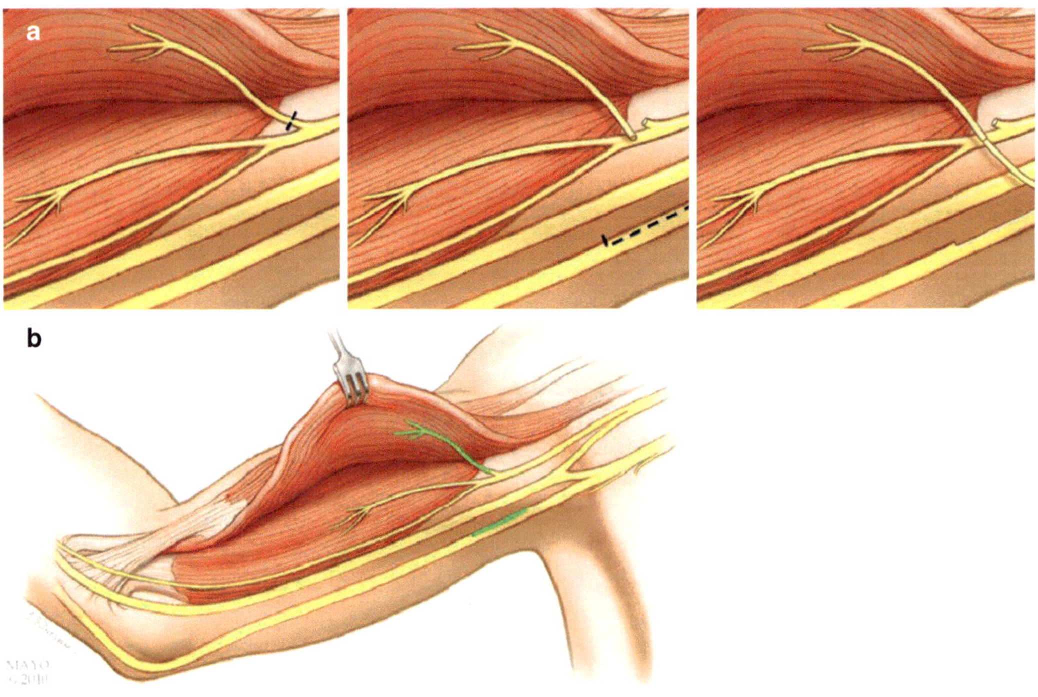

Fig. 3.8 Schematic illustration of the Oberlin procedure with a fascicle of the ulnar nerve transferred to the biceps branch of the musculocutaneous nerve. (Used with permission of Mayo Foundation for Medical Education and Research. All rights reserved. (In: Maldonado et al. [48], Fig. 3.1))

procedure, with the majority involving the axillary or musculocutaneous nerve [8]. Fortunately, all eventually spontaneously resolved postoperatively. A study of 1526 shoulders treated with biceps tenodesis noted musculocutaneous nerve complications in 9 patients all of which similarly resolved spontaneously [30]. In contrast, Rhee et al. reported a case where the distal aspect of the musculocutaneous nerve was transected and "tenodesed" to the humerus [49]. To prevent iatrogenic injury, the surgeon should maintain the origin of the coracobrachialis and short head of the biceps when dissecting around the shoulder and avoid excessive retraction into it. These muscles act as a tether to resist overzealous retraction. When detachment of the conjoined tendon is performed, either for surgical exposure or for transfer in the Latarjet procedure, re-attachment to the anterior glenoid takes tension off of the musculocutaneous nerve. However, excessive medial retraction should be avoided when the coracoid process and conjoint tendon are no longer there to act as a buffer to the musculocutaneous nerve.

Iatrogenic injury during arthroscopy is far less common and may be due to patient positioning or traction while in the lateral decubitus position. Medialization of anterior shoulder portals put the musculocutaneous nerve and other branches of the brachial plexus at risk. Furthermore, instruments placed through a low-anterior five o'clock portal travel within 10 mm of the musculocutaneous nerve [31]. Among seven reported injuries to the musculocutaneous nerve, Carofino et al. attributed two from open procedures, three from arthroscopic procedures, and two from combined open and arthroscopic procedures [15].

3.6.3 Evaluation

Patients with musculocutaneous neuropathy commonly complain of pain and sensory deficits over the lateral forearm down toward the base of the thumb. While many do not demonstrate weakness clinically, the majority will have some findings of motor involvement on electrodiagnostic studies. If an injury is suspected in the postoperative setting, an electrodiagnostic study should be performed 3–4 weeks following surgery. Furthermore, serial examinations are critical in the evaluation and monitoring of these injuries.

3.6.4 Treatment

When the musculocutaneous nerve is noted to be sharply transected during a surgical procedure, it may be amenable to immediate primary repair or nerve grafting. Otherwise, the majority of patients who present with a suspected injury to the musculocutaneous nerve should be observed initially with serial examinations concurrent with their postoperative visits at 2, 6, and 12 weeks. If no improvement is noted, nerve conduction and electromyography studies should be performed. Most postoperative musculocutaneous neuropathies are traction injuries that resolve over a period of weeks to months, depending on the extent of the injury.

Surgical options following injury to the musculocutaneous nerve includes neurolysis, neuroma resection and nerve grafting, nerve transfers, and tendon transfers. Surgical exploration should be conducted if no improvement in biceps and brachialis function is noted clinically or on serial electrodiagnostic studies. Ideally, this is performed within 6 months from injury.

If the nerve appears intact at the time of exploration, but is compressed by scar tissue and demonstrates electrical conduction across the lesion, neurolysis may be performed. This is performed with intraoperative electrodiagnostic studies evaluating nerve-to-nerve conduction. If surgical exploration reveals a neuroma in continuity that does not conduct a nerve action potential (NAP) or a rupture or transection of the nerve, neuroma excision with nerve grafting is preferred [32] (Fig. 3.9). The initial segment to be excised can be based on the electrodiagnostic data (between a conducting and non-conducting branch point), visual assessment of the extent of the lesion, and palpation. If there is any question as to the quality of the proximal nerve fascicles, a segment can be sent for frozen pathology to evaluate their viability.

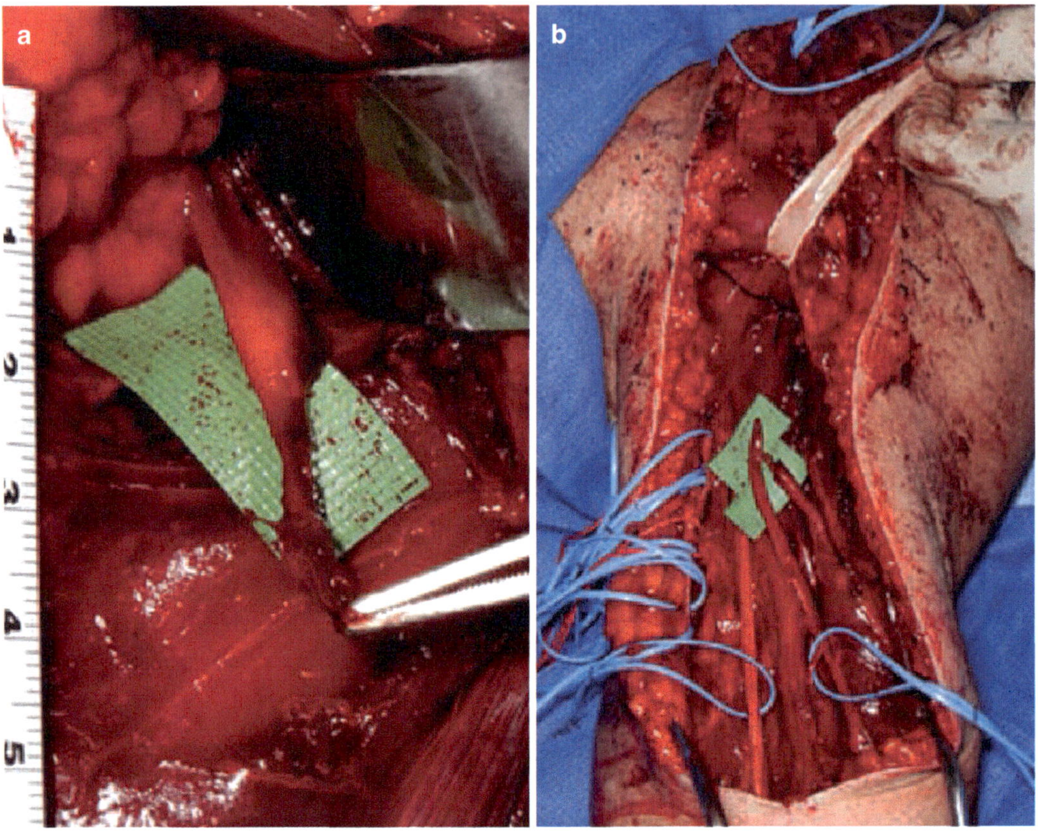

Fig. 3.9 Musculocutaneous nerve transection. Intraoperative photos of inadvertent tenodesis of the musculocutaneous nerve (**a**) and resultant transection of the musculocutaneous nerve (**b**). (Used with permission of Mayo Foundation for Medical Education and Research. All rights reserved. (In: Rhee et al. [49], Fig. 3.4))

Nerve transfers have increased in popularity for the treatment of brachial plexus and peripheral nerve injuries. These transfers may shorten the time to innervation and bypass the need to dissect in scarred or previously traumatized soft tissue. Oberlin's technique of transferring a fascicle of the ulnar nerve directly to the motor branch of the biceps muscle is one of the most common and most studied of these transfers [33] (Fig. 3.8). In a similar manner, a fascicle from the median and ulnar nerve can be used to innervate the brachialis and biceps muscles, respectively [34, 35]. With these nerve transfers, reinnervation of the biceps muscle may be seen as soon as 3 months following the procedure. In contrast, reinnervation following nerve grafting takes approximately 1 month for each inch, the nerve injury is proximal to the site of muscle innervation. Antigravity elbow flexion is reliably restored in over 80% of patients with either technique [36]. However, a recent systematic review found that more patients achieved M4 or greater elbow flexion strength following double nerve transfers compared to single fascicular nerve transfer for restoration of elbow flexion [37].

When patients present a year or more following musculocutaneous nerve injury, nerve repair and reconstruction is less likely to be successful. Some patients may still be able to actively flex their elbow through use of the brachioradialis alone. For those with insufficient elbow flexion strength, a variety of tendon transfers and other procedures have been described including Stiendler flexor plasty, triceps to biceps transfer, and pedicled latissimus transfer.

3.7 Suprascapular Nerve Injury

3.7.1 Anatomy

The suprascapular nerve originates from the C5 and C6 nerve roots at the junction of the upper trunk and its divisions and innervates the supraspinatus and infraspinatus muscles. In addition, it provides sensory innervation to the coracoacromial ligament and acromioclavicular and glenohumeral joint. The nerve follows the omohyoid muscle posteriorly and then runs inferiorly through the suprascapular notch. The roof of the suprascapular notch is the superior transverse suprascapular ligament. The suprascapular artery and vein pass superior to this ligament. After exiting the suprascapular notch, the nerve gives off branches to the supraspinatus muscle and travels medial to the superior edge of the glenoid across the floor of the supraspinatus fossa. At this point, as the nerve travels posteriorly, it may be less than 20 mm from the glenoid rim [38] (Fig. 3.10).

The suprascapular nerve enters the spinoglenoid notch at the posterolateral margin of the scapular spine. In the spinoglenoid notch, the spinoglenoid ligament can impinge on the nerve. However, the universal presence of a distinct spinoglenoid ligament is controversial [39]. After exiting the spinoglenoid notch, the nerve divides into two to four branches that enter the infraspinatus.

3.7.2 Prevention

The suprascapular nerve (SSN) is prone to injury during rotator cuff repair, particularly with massive tears. Some surgeons advocate for arthroscopic release of the SSN during rotator cuff repair to prevent secondary SSN compression [40, 41]. It can also be injured during other shoulder procedures, like reverse shoulder arthroplasty [42].

3.7.3 Evaluation

Patients with an injury to the suprascapular nerve often complain of pain over the posterior and lateral aspect of the shoulder. With an injury at the level of the suprascapular notch, pain may be elicited with deep palpation, and the patient may have weakness with abduction, external rotation, or both. Atrophy of the supraspinatus and infraspinatus can be noted on physical exam with prolonged denervation. However, a well-developed trapezius covers the supraspinatus muscle and

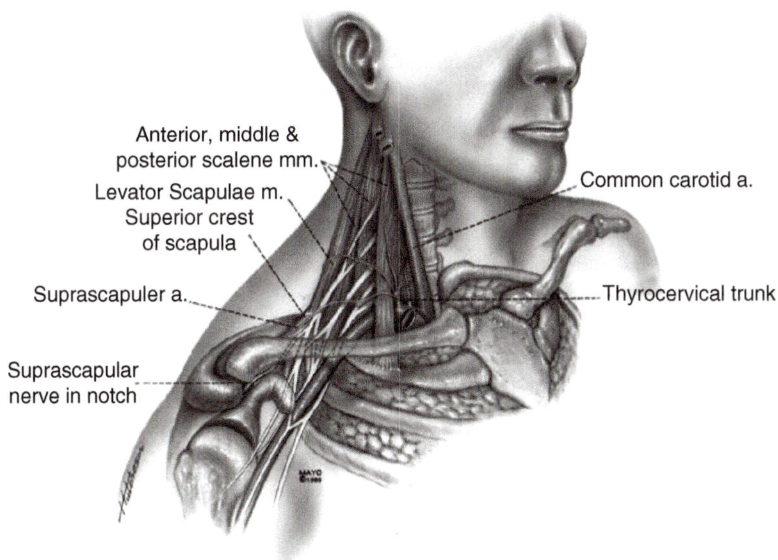

Fig. 3.10 Suprascapular nerve. Anatomy of the suprascapular nerve. (Used with permission of Mayo Foundation for Medical Education and Research. All rights reserved. (In: Shupeck et al. [50], Fig. 3.2))

posterior deltoid covers the infraspinatus, which may make it more difficult to appreciate any muscle wasting. Painless atrophy limited to the infraspinatus is more commonly associated with a lesion at the spinoglenoid notch, such as a cyst. Electrodiagnostic studies often detect suprascapular neuropathy.

3.7.4 Treatment

Rarely is an iatrogenic injury to the nerve recognized at the time of the initial surgery. Further, periods of immobilization and passive range of motion may mask any weakness resulting from injury to the suprascapular nerve.

When surgical exploration is warranted, the suprascapular nerve can be approached from an anterior, superior, or posterior direction. If compression alone is suspected, arthroscopic suprascapular nerve decompression within the suprascapular notch is another option [40]. A direct superior approach is performed by splitting the trapezius in line with its fibers allowing good visualization of the superior transverse scapular ligament, but only a small length of the nerve itself. The posterior approach detaches the trapezius from the spine of the scapula to the lateral edge of the acromion. The supraspinatus can be retracted to visualize the suprascapular nerve and the notch. If the suprascapular nerve needs to be explored into the spinoglenoid notch, the posterior deltoid can be detached from the spine of the scapula, allowing visualization of the nerve from the infraspinatus to the suprascapular notch.

A common extraplexal donor for suprascapular nerve injuries involves transfer of the spinal accessory nerve, which is a cranial nerve that innervates the trapezius muscle (Fig. 3.11). Much of the literature on the outcome of this nerve transfer is based on traumatic brachial plexus patients. Baltzer reported that while 85% of patients treated with spinal accessory to suprascapular nerve transfer demonstrated EMG evidence of re-innervation, less than a third had clinically meaningful external rotation. Results were better, however, in patients with isolated upper trunk injuries [43]. One potential limitation to utilizing the spinal accessory nerve is that the trapezius muscle may be better utilized for ipsilateral lower trapezius tendon transfers to improve external rotation [44, 45]. Therefore, it is advised to maintain some branching to the trapezius prior to transfer so as not to denervate the entire muscle. Other salvage options include reverse total shoulder arthroplasty for patients with good deltoid function, pedicled pectoralis transfer combined with reverse shoulder arthroplasty [25], or glenohumeral fusion [46] for patients with poor rotator cuff and deltoid function, but preserve periscapular motion.

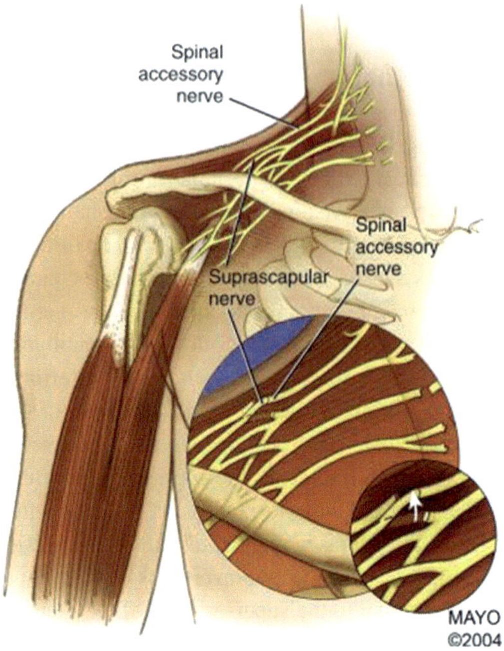

Fig. 3.11 Spinal accessory to suprascapular nerve transfer. Transfer of the distal spinal accessory nerve to the suprascapular nerve. (Used with permission of Mayo Foundation for Medical Education and Research. All rights reserved)

3.8 Conclusion

Perioperative nerve injury after shoulder arthroscopy is more common than often assumed and although more mild injury or neuropraxias may resolve spontaneously, severe injuries may cause significant patient pain and distress and even require surgical correction. Thorough knowledge of the anatomy is critical to help prevent nerve injury during arthroscopic surgery as the axillary, suprascapular, and musculocutaneous nerves have varying risks for injury during different surgical procedures. After a nerve issue is identified, the most important first steps are a thorough clinical history and physical examination to determine probable cause and to maintain a high index of suspicion for an iatrogenic cause. Timely referral to a peripheral nerve surgeon is paramount for achieving the best possible result should corrective surgery be required. Ultimately, surgical treatment involves either grafts or nerve transfers, requiring the surgeons to have an intimate knowledge of surrounding anatomy and technical variations.

References

1. Andrews JR, Carson WG. Shoulder joint arthroscopy. Orthopedics. 1983;6(9):1157–62. Epub 1983/09/01
2. Complications in arthroscopy: the knee and other joints. Committee on Complications of the Arthroscopy Association of North America. Arthroscopy. 1986;2(4):253–8. Epub 1986/01/01.
3. Ogilvie-Harris DJ, D'Angelo G. Arthroscopic surgery of the shoulder. Sports Med (Auckland, NZ). 1990;9(2):120–8. Epub 1990/02/01
4. Ellman H. Arthroscopic subacromial decompression: analysis of one- to three-year results. Arthroscopy. 1987;3(3):173–81. Epub 1987/01/01
5. Pitman MI, Nainzadeh N, Ergas E, Springer S. The use of somatosensory evoked potentials for detection of neuropraxia during shoulder arthroscopy. Arthroscopy. 1988;4(4):250–5. Epub 1988/01/01
6. Segmüller HE, Alfred SP, Zilio G, Saies AD, Hayes MG. Cutaneous nerve lesions of the shoulder and arm after arthroscopic shoulder surgery. J Shoulder Elb Surg. 1995;4(4):254–8. Epub 1995/07/01
7. Berjano P, González BG, Olmedo JF, Perez-España LA, Munilla MG. Complications in arthroscopic shoulder surgery. Arthroscopy. 1998;14(8):785–8. Epub 1998/12/16
8. Delaney RA, Freehill MT, Janfaza DR, Vlassakov KV, Higgins LD, Warner JJ. 2014 Neer Award Paper: neuromonitoring the Latarjet procedure. J Shoulder Elb Surg. 2014;23(10):1473–80.
9. Neal JM, Barrington MJ, Brull R, Hadzic A, Hebl JR, Horlocker TT, et al. The second ASRA practice advisory on neurologic complications associated with regional anesthesia and pain medicine: executive summary 2015. Reg Anesth Pain Med. 2015;40(5):401–30. Epub 2015/08/20
10. Welch MB, Brummett CM, Welch TD, Tremper KK, Shanks AM, Guglani P, et al. Perioperative peripheral nerve injuries: a retrospective study of 380,680 cases during a 10-year period at a single institution. Anesthesiology. 2009;111(3):490–7. Epub 2009/08/13
11. Sviggum HP, Jacob AK, Mantilla CB, Schroeder DR, Sperling JW, Hebl JR. Perioperative nerve injury after total shoulder arthroplasty: assessment of risk after regional anesthesia. Reg Anesth Pain Med. 2012;37(5):490–4. Epub 2012/06/19
12. Visser CP, Coene LN, Brand R, Tavy DL. The incidence of nerve injury in anterior dislocation of the shoulder and its influence on functional recovery. A prospective clinical and EMG study. J Bone Joint Surg Br. 1999;81(4):679–85. Epub 1999/08/27
13. Brogan DM, Carofino BC, Kircher MF, Spinner RJ, Elhassan BT, Bishop AT, Shin AY. Prevalence of rotator cuff tears in adults with traumatic brachial plexus injuries. J Bone Joint Surg Am. 2014;96(16):e139. https://doi.org/10.2106/JBJS.L.00420. PMID: 25143507.
14. The Second ASRA Practice Advisory on Neurologic Complications Associated With Regional Anesthesia and Pain Medicine Executive Summary 2015, https://rapm.bmj.com/content/rapm/40/5/401.full.pdf
15. Carofino BC, Brogan DM, Kircher MF, Elhassan BT, Spinner RJ, Bishop AT, et al. Iatrogenic nerve injuries during shoulder surgery. J Bone Joint Surg Am. 2013;95(18):1667–74. Epub 2013/09/21
16. https://www.mayoclinicproceedings.org/article/S0025-6196(19)30869-9/fulltext
17. Yoo JC, Kim JH, Ahn JH, Lee SH. Arthroscopic perspective of the axillary nerve in relation to the glenoid and arm position: a cadaveric study. Arthroscopy. 2007;23(12):1271–7. Epub 2007/12/08
18. Burkhead WZ Jr, Scheinberg RR, Box G. Surgical anatomy of the axillary nerve. J Shoulder Elb Surg. 1992;1(1):31–6. Epub 1992/01/01
19. Meyer M, Graveleau N, Hardy P, Landreau P. Anatomic risks of shoulder arthroscopy portals: anatomic cadaveric study of 12 portals. Arthroscopy. 2007;23(5):529–36. Epub 2007/05/05
20. Greis PE, Burks RT, Schickendantz MS, Sandmeier R. Axillary nerve injury after thermal capsular shrinkage of the shoulder. J Shoulder Elb Surg. 2001;10(3):231–5. Epub 2001/06/16
21. Werthel JD, Bertelli J, Elhassan BT. Shoulder function in patients with deltoid paralysis and intact rotator cuff. Orthop Traumatol Surg Res. 2017;103(6):869–73. Epub 2017/07/15
22. Rbia N, Shin AY. The role of nerve graft substitutes in motor and mixed motor/sensory peripheral nerve injuries. J Hand Surg Am. 2017;42(5):367–77. https://doi.org/10.1016/j.jhsa.2017.02.017. PMID: 28473159.
23. Leechavengvongs S, Witoonchart K, Uerpairojkit C, Thuvasethakul P. Nerve transfer to deltoid muscle using the nerve to the long head of the triceps, part II: a report of 7 cases. J Hand Surg Am. 2003;28(4):633–8. Epub 2003/07/25

24. Le Hanneur M, Lee J, Wagner ER, Elhassan BT. Options of bipolar muscle transfers to restore deltoid function: an anatomical study. Surg Radiol Anat. 2019;41(8):911–9. Epub 2018/12/14
25. Elhassan BT, Wagner ER, Werthel JD, Lehanneur M, Lee J. Outcome of reverse shoulder arthroplasty with pedicled pectoralis transfer in patients with deltoid paralysis. J Shoulder Elb Surg. 2018;27(1):96–103. Epub 2017/09/25
26. Flatow EL, Bigliani LU, April EW. An anatomic study of the musculocutaneous nerve and its relationship to the coracoid process. Clin Orthop Relat Res. 1989;244:166–71. Epub 1989/07/01
27. Eglseder WA Jr, Goldman M. Anatomic variations of the musculocutaneous nerve in the arm. Am J Orthop (Belle Mead, NJ). 1997;26(11):777–80. Epub 1997/12/24
28. Dwyer T, Henry PD, Cholvisudhi P, Chan VW, Theodoropoulos JS, Brull R. Neurological complications related to elective orthopedic surgery: part 1: common shoulder and elbow procedures. Reg Anesth Pain Med. 2015;40(5):431–42. Epub 2015/07/21
29. Bach BR Jr, O'Brien SJ, Warren RF, Leighton M. An unusual neurological complication of the Bristow procedure. A case report. J Bone Joint Surg Am. 1988;70(3):458–60. Epub 1988/03/01
30. McCrum CL, Alluri RK, Batech M, Mirzayan R. Complications of biceps tenodesis based on location, fixation, and indication: a review of 1526 shoulders. J Shoulder Elbow Surg. 2019;28(3):461–69. https://doi.org/10.1016/j.jse.2018.09.005. Epub 2018 Dec 18. PMID: 30573431.
31. Pearsall AW, Holovacs TF, Speer KP. The low anterior five-o'clock portal during arthroscopic shoulder surgery performed in the beach-chair position. Am J Sports Med. 1999;27(5):571–4. Epub 1999/09/25
32. Pulos N, Shin EH, Spinner RJ, Shin AY. Management of Iatrogenic Nerve Injuries. J Am Acad Orthop Surg. 2019;27(18):e838–e48. Epub 2019/02/06
33. Oberlin C, Béal D, Leechavengvongs S, Salon A, Dauge MC, Sarcy JJ. Nerve transfer to biceps muscle using a part of ulnar nerve for C5-C6 avulsion of the brachial plexus: anatomical study and report of four cases. J Hand Surg Am. 1994;19(2):232–7. Epub 1994/03/01
34. Liverneaux PA, Diaz LC, Beaulieu JY, Durand S, Oberlin C. Preliminary results of double nerve transfer to restore elbow flexion in upper type brachial plexus palsies. Plast Reconstr Surg. 2006;117(3):915–9. Epub 2006/03/10
35. Mackinnon SE, Novak CB, Myckatyn TM, Tung TH. Results of reinnervation of the biceps and brachialis muscles with a double fascicular transfer for elbow flexion. J Hand Surg Am. 2005;30(5):978–85. Epub 2005/09/27
36. Carlsen BT, Kircher MF, Spinner RJ, Bishop AT, Shin AY. Comparison of single versus double nerve transfers for elbow flexion after brachial plexus injury. Plast Reconstr Surg. 2011;127(1):269–76. https://doi.org/10.1097/PRS.0b013e3181f95be7. PMID: 20871484.
37. Sneiders D, Bulstra LF, Hundepool CA, Treling WJ, Hovius SER, Shin AY. Outcomes of single versus double fascicular nerve transfers for restoration of elbow flexion in patients with brachial plexus injuries: a systematic review and meta-analysis. Plast Reconstr Surg. 2019;144(1):155–66. Epub 2019/06/28
38. Bigliani LU, Dalsey RM, McCann PD, April EW. An anatomical study of the suprascapular nerve. Arthroscopy. 1990;6(4):301–5. Epub 1990/01/01
39. Plancher KD, Peterson RK, Johnston JC, Luke TA. The spinoglenoid ligament. Anatomy, morphology, and histological findings. J Bone Joint Surg Am. 2005;87(2):361–5. Epub 2005/02/03
40. Lafosse L, Piper K, Lanz U. Arthroscopic suprascapular nerve release: indications and technique. J Shoulder Elb Surg. 2011;20(2 Suppl):S9–13. Epub 2011/02/10
41. Savoie FH 3rd, Zunkiewicz M, Field LD, Replogle WH, O'Brien MJ. A comparison of functional outcomes in patients undergoing revision arthroscopic repair of massive rotator cuff tears with and without arthroscopic suprascapular nerve release. Open Access J Sports Med. 2016;7:129–34. Epub 2016/11/02
42. Wang J, Singh A, Higgins L, Warner J. Suprascapular neuropathy secondary to reverse shoulder arthroplasty: a case report. J Shoulder Elb Surg. 2010;19(3):e5–8. Epub 2010/01/09
43. Baltzer HL, Wagner ER, Kircher MF, Spinner RJ, Bishop AT, Shin AY. Evaluation of infraspinatus reinnervation and function following spinal accessory nerve to suprascapular nerve transfer in adult traumatic brachial plexus injuries. Microsurgery. 2017;37(5):365–70. Epub 2016/05/22
44. Elhassan BT, Sanchez-Sotelo J, Wagner ER. Outcome of arthroscopically assisted lower trapezius transfer to reconstruct massive irreparable posterior-superior rotator cuff tears. J Shoulder Elb Surg. 2020;29(10):2135–42. Epub 2020/06/24
45. Elhassan BT, Wagner ER, Werthel JD. Outcome of lower trapezius transfer to reconstruct massive irreparable posterior-superior rotator cuff tear. J Shoulder Elb Surg. 2016;25(8):1346–53. Epub 2016/03/13
46. Wagner ER, McLaughlin R, Sarfani S, Cofield RH, Sperling JW, Sanchez-Sotelo J, et al. Long-term outcomes of glenohumeral arthrodesis. J Bone Joint Surg Am. 2018;100(7):598–604. Epub 2018/04/04
47. Baltzer HL, et al. Axillary nerve reconstruction: anterior-posterior exposure with sural nerve cable graft pull-through technique. Tech Hand Surg. 2015;19:168–75.
48. Maldonado AA, et al. Five operations that give the best results after brachial plexus injury. Plast Reconstr Surg. 2017;140:545–56.
49. Rhee PC, et al. Iatrogenic brachial plexus injuries associated with subpectoral biceps tenodesis. Am J Sports Med. 2013;41(9):2048–53.
50. Shupeck M, et al. An anterior approach for decompression of the suprascapular nerve. J Neurosurg. 1990;73(1):53–6.

4 Nerve Injury After Shoulder Arthroplasty

Matthew Florczynski, Ryan Paul, and Heather Baltzer

4.1 Introduction

Shoulder arthroplasty is a highly successful procedure but is carried out in close proximity to the brachial plexus. Injuries to the plexus itself, as well as to individual nerves including the axillary, suprascapular, musculocutaneous, radial, and subscapular nerves are reported complications of shoulder arthroplasty (Illustration 4.1) [1–6]. Severity of injury ranges on a spectrum from neuropraxia to neurotmesis and can have potentially permanent and devastating consequences.

Historically, nerve injuries during shoulder arthroplasty were thought to be rare [7, 8]. Recent estimates suggest that the prevalence of clinically significant nerve injury is 0.63% in anatomic total shoulder arthroplasty (TSA) and 1.2% in reverse total shoulder arthroplasty (RSA) [2]. However, subclinical injury and intraoperative nerve trauma appear to occur at a much higher rate. One study found that the rate of subclinical axillary nerve injury detectable on electromyography (EMG) after RSA was 10.9 times greater than the rate of nerve injury after TSA, although electrophysiologic abnormalities resolved in all but one patient by 6 months after surgery [5]. Another study used intraoperative neuromonitoring to detect changes in motor-evoked potentials (MEPs) and somatosensory-evoked potentials (SSEPs) corresponding to transient nerve trauma during shoulder arthroplasty [9]. The investigators found that such changes occurred in 35 of 36 patients, but only 2 patients had clinically detectable neurologic deficits that resolved by 6 months postoperatively. In these and other studies, it appears the nerves are at highest risk of traction injury when the arm is in extension and external rotation. While subclinical nerve trauma is unlikely to translate into lasting deficits, these findings show that nerve structures are routinely at risk during shoulder arthroplasty. A thorough knowledge of these structures and the surgical steps that place them at risk is necessary to prevent rare but significant complications.

Nerve injury can result through direct or indirect mechanisms. Direct mechanisms include laceration of nerves with a scalpel, thermal injuries with electrocautery, as well as compression resulting from retractor placement, postoperative

M. Florczynski
Department of Orthopaedic Surgery, University of Toronto, Toronto, ON, Canada
e-mail: matt.florczynski@mail.utoronto.ca

R. Paul
Department of Orthopaedic Surgery, University of Toronto, Toronto, ON, Canada

Department of Plastic and Reconstructive Surgery, University of Toronto, Toronto, ON, Canada
e-mail: ryan.paul2@uhn.ca

H. Baltzer (✉)
Department of Plastic and Reconstructive Surgery, University of Toronto, Toronto, ON, Canada
e-mail: heather.baltzer@uhn.ca

C. J. Dy et al. (eds.), *Peripheral Nerve Issues after Orthopedic Surgery*,
https://doi.org/10.1007/978-3-030-84428-8_4

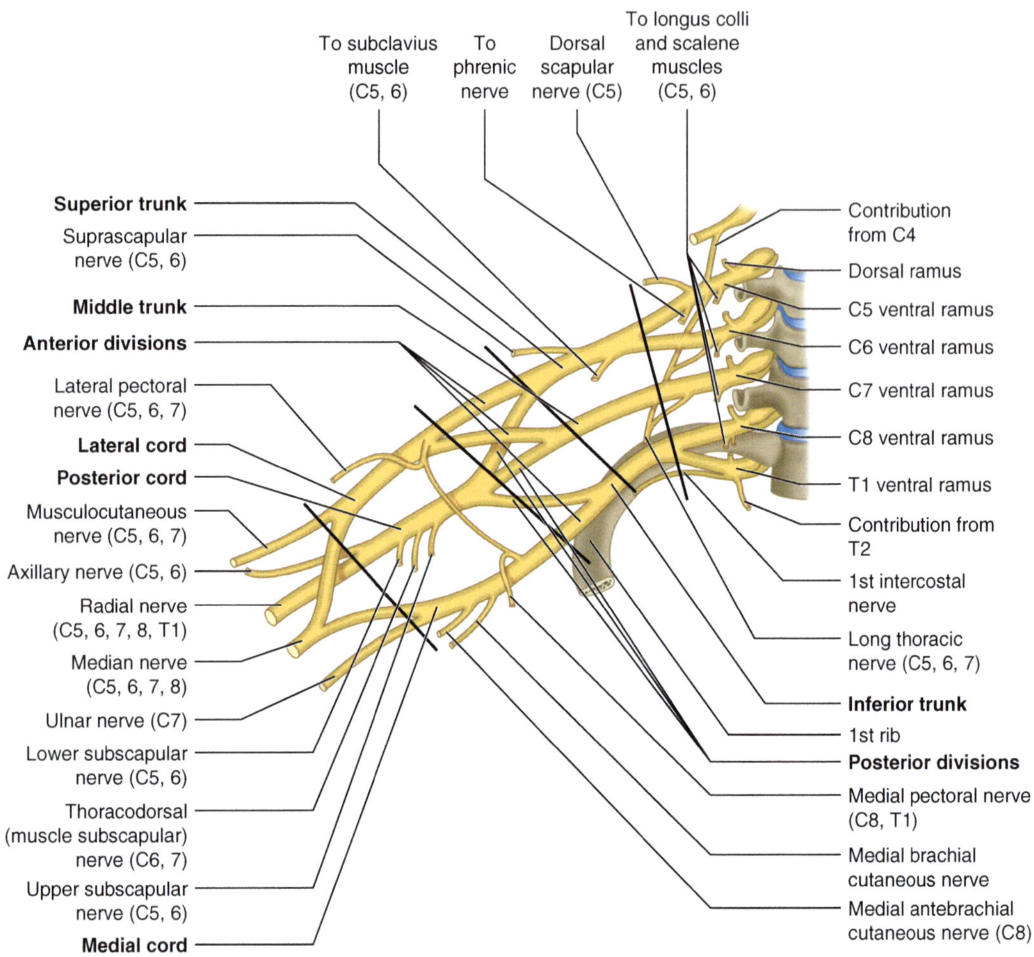

Illustration 4.1 Brachial plexus with branches vulnerable during shoulder arthroplasty bolded

hematomas, or cement extrusion from the humeral shaft [10]. During shoulder arthroplasty, dissection and instrumentation are performed lateral to the coracoid process. Therefore, direct injury at this level typically involves the cords and terminal branches of the brachial plexus. Indirect mechanisms (which typically involve the division or cord level of the brachial plexus) include aggressive intraoperative positioning and manipulation of the arm in extension and external rotation [9], alteration of the native shoulder joint or lengthening of the arm [4, 6, 11], vascular injury [12], intraoperative humeral shaft fracture [13], and interscalene regional anesthesia [14]. Specific mechanisms of injury, risk factors, and pertinent anatomic and surgical considerations for each nerve at risk are discussed in the sections that follow.

4.2 Pertinent Surgical Anatomy

Modern shoulder prostheses can be divided into three categories of implants: hemiarthroplasty, TSA, and RSA [15]. Hemiarthroplasties are unconstrained prostheses that replace the proximal humeral articulation with a stemmed or stemless metal implant. Anatomic TSA further adds replacement of the native glenoid surface, requiring more extensive retraction for exposure. The RSA is a semi-constrained implant useful for reconstruction in patients with severely comminuted proximal humerus fractures or with arthropathy in the setting of irreparable rotator cuff deficiency, chronic instability, extensive glenoid deformity, or prior failed arthroplasties [16–20]. The RSA reverses the traditional relationship between the humeral head and glenoid, requiring relative lengthening of the humerus and replacing the dynamic stability of the rotator cuff with a semi-constrained articulation to generate motion through the deltoid. This warrants special attention as it significantly alters the native proportions of the glenohumeral joint and has the potential to apply traction to local neurovascular structures and the brachial plexus both intraoperatively and postoperatively. As we proceed to discuss the key anatomic landmarks and surgical steps in shoulder arthroplasty, we will highlight unique features of the RSA that pose risks for nerve injury.

4.2.1 Surgical Approach

The workhorse approach in shoulder arthroplasty procedures is the deltopectoral approach (Fig. 4.1). Surgery is performed with the patient in beach chair position under general anesthesia, often supplemented by a preoperative regional block. Many variations of the skin incision exist, but all exploit the superficial intermuscular interval between the deltoid laterally and pectoralis major medially. As one develops skin flaps by releasing the retinacular tissue just under the skin, these muscles are easily visualized. The anatomic landmarks for identifying the deltopectoral interval are the cephalic vein and coracoid, which are identified within the clavipectoral triangle and often marked by a fatty stripe of tissue (Fig. 4.1b). Properly identifying the superficial interval and keeping dissection within this plane will ensure that neurovascular structures, including the cephalic vein, are avoided.

Separation of the deltoid and pectoralis major will reveal several important landmarks. The coracoacromial ligament and conjoint tendon make up the superior and medial borders of the deep surgical field, respectively (Fig. 4.1c). The conjoint tendon is an important landmark originating from the coracoid and consisting of the short head of the biceps brachii and coracobrachialis. Once the lateral border of the conjoint tendon has been identified, there is no need to venture further medially beyond gentle mobilization as this endangers the musculocutaneous and subscapular nerves. The conjoint tendon also serves to protect the medial structures of the brachial plexus from excessive retraction.

The deep surgical field includes the bicipital groove of the humerus, which is covered by the bicipital aponeurosis and contains the long head of the biceps brachii tendon. The tendinous insertion of the subscapularis muscle is just medial to this groove. The long head of biceps is reliably found passing under the upper border of the pectoralis major muscle just medial to its insertion on the humerus. The bicipital aponeurosis is opened and the long head of the biceps tendon is released (Fig. 4.1d); a soft tissue tenodesis is often performed, tethering the released tendon to the pectoralis major. The subscapularis is then further defined with its superior border found at the rotator interval and its inferior border identified by a branch of the posterior humeral circumflex artery and its two venae comitantes (known as the "three sisters"). These vessels may be ligated as necessary. Importantly, the axillary nerve passes along the inferior edge of subscapularis at the level of the glenoid neck in this region.

The next critical step involves exposing the glenohumeral joint by releasing the subscapularis tendon. The tendon is often indistinguishable from the joint capsule and they are released as a single layer. The tendon can be tenotomized, peeled together with periosteum off of its insertion or mobilized by a lesser tuberosity osteotomy (Fig. 4.1e, f). It is reattached at the end of surgery. The humeral head and glenoid can now be visualized with appropriate retraction.

4.2.2 Joint Preparation and Implants

Once the shoulder capsule has been opened, the joint surfaces must be adequately exposed. The humeral head is best accessed by placing the arm

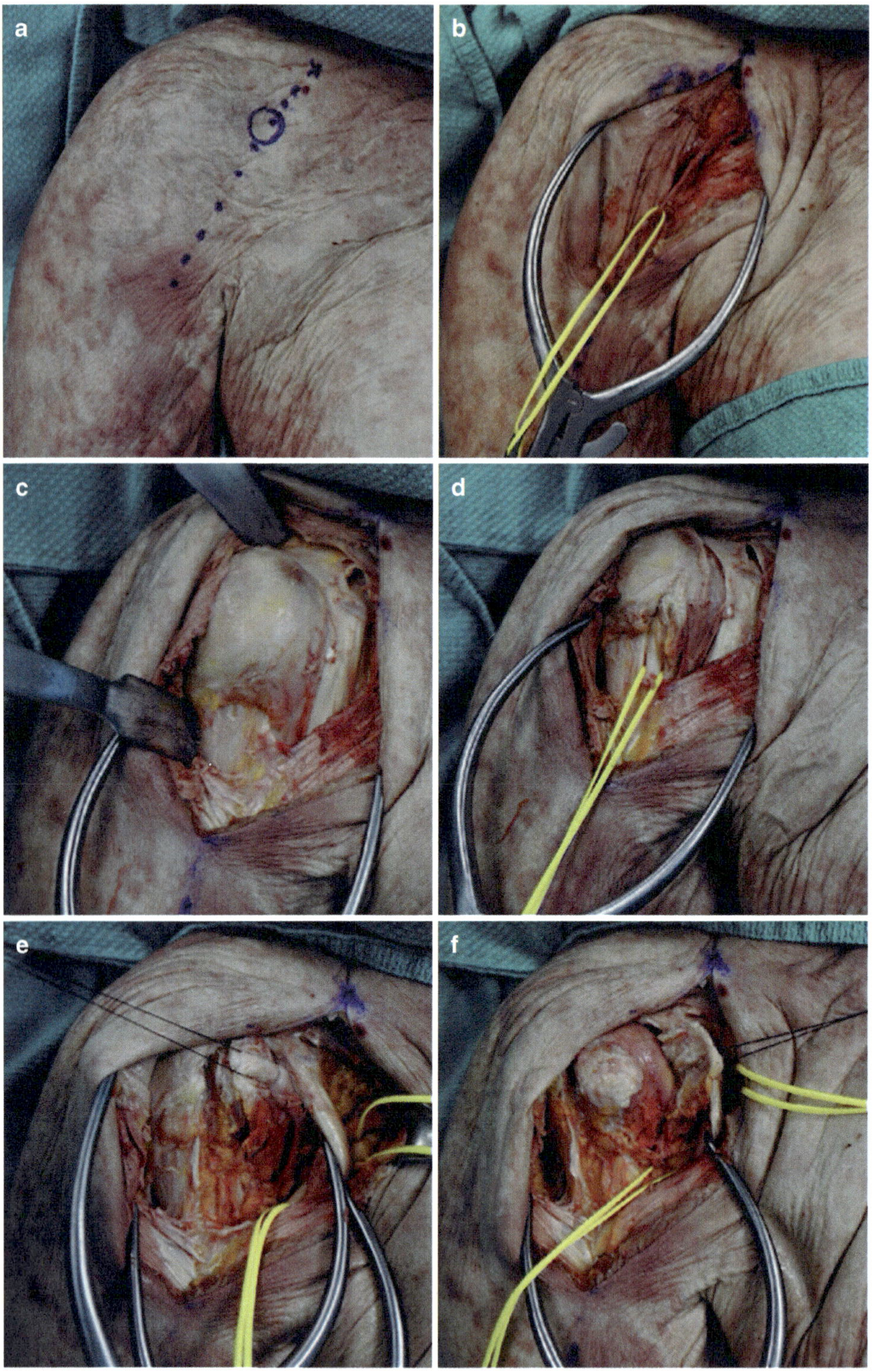

Fig. 4.1 Cadaveric images of the deltopectoral approach. Image (**a**) demonstrates the typical incision and image (**b**) shows the superficial interval between the deltoid and pectoralis major separated by the cephalic vein. Image (**c**) demonstrates the deep exposure of the proximal humerus covered by the rotator cuff, with the coracoacromial ligament superiorly and conjoint tendon medially. In image (**d**), the long head of the biceps has been exposed and tagged. Images (**e**, **f**) show the tagged subscapularis after initial release and retraction, respectively

in adduction and maximal external rotation. The glenoid is later visualized and prepared by dislocating the shoulder posteroinferiorly. With the aid of leverage style retractors on the glenoid, exposure can be accomplished by placing the arm in abduction and internal rotation or adduction and external rotation. The significant joint translation of these maneuvers may create traction on the brachial plexus, particularly the axillary nerve [9, 21].

In TSA, emphasis is placed on restoring the native shoulder anatomy and a cemented glenoid component is utilized. Obtaining satisfactory glenoid exposure is the most challenging and crucial step. A glenoid with advanced posterior wear and retroversion may require more extensive exposure for adequate reconstruction. In RSA, the center of rotation is medialized and distalized to give a mechanical advantage to the deltoid [19], which increases traction on the bony and soft tissue structures around the shoulder girdle including traction to the brachial plexus and its terminal branches. In addition, multiple screws are required to stabilize the glenoid component.

4.2.3 Nerves at Risk

4.2.3.1 Axillary Nerve

The axillary nerve is the most commonly injured nerve during shoulder surgery [22, 23]. It is susceptible to direct injury during the deltopectoral approach at the inferior border of the subscapularis, particularly when a subscapularis tenotomy is performed. It is also susceptible to direct injury below the inferior rim of the glenoid during inferior mobilization of the subscapularis, debridement of glenoid osteophytes, and implantation of the glenoid component during RSA. Humeral component preparation and implantation also endanger the nerve due to its close proximity to the posterior metaphysis of the proximal humerus. The nerve is further vulnerable to traction injury during dislocation and reduction of the proximal humerus, as well as stretch injury when the arm is extended and externally rotated during glenoid preparation (Fig. 4.2).

The axillary nerve originates from the posterior cord of the brachial plexus, formed by the confluence of the C5 and C6 ventral rami. It lies posterior to the axillary artery and vein and is typically the superior-most branch of the brachial plexus at its origin, superior to the radial nerve and lateral to the median and ulnar nerves [24]. The anatomy with respect to other nerves is consistent with the exception of the musculocutaneous nerve, which is the superior-most branch in 20% of cases [25]. Distally, the axillary nerve divides into anterior and posterior divisions [22, 26, 27]. The anterior division supplies motor function to the anterior third of the deltoid and

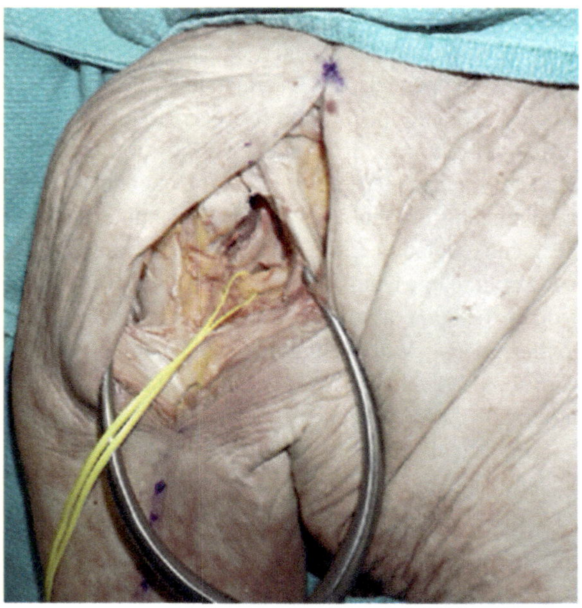

Fig. 4.2 Cadaveric image demonstrating the proximity of the axillary nerve (yellow vessel loop) relative to the subscapularis and inferior glenoid neck after exposure of the glenohumeral joint

middle third of the deltoid in approximately 54% of cases. The posterior branch supplies motor function to the teres minor and the posterior third of the deltoid in 92% and gives off sensory fibers to the skin overlying the shoulder. It further branches into the superior lateral cutaneous nerve of the arm, which supplies sensation to the proximal lateral arm. (Illustration 4.2) [28].

The axillary nerve is potentially susceptible to direct injury during subscapularis tenotomy. From its point of origin, it runs in the lateral direction obliquely over the anterior surface of subscapularis and posterior to the conjoint tendon. As it passes below the inferior border of subscapularis, it is located at a mean distance of 7.7 mm (range 0–12 mm) from the musculotendinous junction [29, 30]. Injuries to the axillary nerve in this region have been reported during open Latarjet procedures [31, 32]. Once it has passed below the subscapularis, the axillary nerve enters the quadrangular space with the posterior humeral circumflex artery and vein, where it divides into its anterior and posterior branches [26].

The anterior division of the axillary nerve is susceptible to injury due to its close proximity to the posterior humeral metaphysis. It winds posteriorly, circling along the medial surface of the surgical neck of the humerus and eventually emerging laterally 5–6 cm distal to the acromion [33, 34]. During preparation of the proximal humerus, an osteotomy of the humeral head is first performed, followed by serial broaching and reaming trial components and eventually the final humeral components are inserted. In cadaveric studies, the anterior division has been found to reside 5.2–8.1 mm from the final position of humeral implants but was found in direct contact with implants in some cases [5, 35]. Low humeral neck cuts, violation of the posterior metaphyseal cortex with large reamers, and excessive retroversion of the humeral implant can all endanger the axillary nerve. When using cemented implants, care should be taken to avoid extrusion of cement around the humeral neck.

The articular branch of the axillary nerve is vulnerable to injury during several surgical steps. This branch originates from the main nerve trunk in 30% of cases, posterior division in 33.3% of cases, and anterior division in 16.6% of cases [28]. It passes below the inferior rim of the glenoid between the 5:30 and 6:30 positions relative to the glenoid face [36]. On average, its distance from the glenoid rim is 13.6 mm [35]. This distance decreases with arm abduction angles greater than 45° but does not change significantly with external rotation [37]. In an effort to improve visualization of the glenoid during arthroplasty surgery, soft tissue releases of the capsule and subscapularis are performed around the inferior rim, potentially endangering the axillary nerve. Similarly, debridement of osteophytes around the inferior glenoid rim must be performed with care. During RSA, the glenosphere is often situated at an inferior position on the glenoid in order to prevent the humeral component from abutting and "notching" the medial scapula. Despite the hypothetical danger to the axillary nerve, inferior positioning of the glenosphere does not appear to bring the nerve into direct contact with the implant [5].

Finally, positioning of the arm during surgery is an important consideration with respect to the anatomy of the axillary nerve. In a cadaveric study, applying traction to the shoulder resulted in macroscopic changes to the axillary nerve below the glenoid rim, causing it to lose its natural rounded contour [21]. These changes first became evident when the head of the humerus was distracted inferiorly below the mid glenoid level. The nerve was stretched by 34% when the humerus was distracted all the way to the level of the inferior glenoid rim. Traction to distract the humerus may be necessary during exposure and preparation of both the humerus and glenoid components and must be performed with caution. Reduction of the humerus after implantation can be another source of nerve trauma, as revealed by intraoperative neuromonitoring [9]. This may be especially important in RSA, which involves increasing soft tissue tensioning. During reduction of RSA, the number of electrophysiologically detectable nerve traumas was increased fivefold compared to TSA. Interestingly, lateralization of the humeral head relative to the gle-

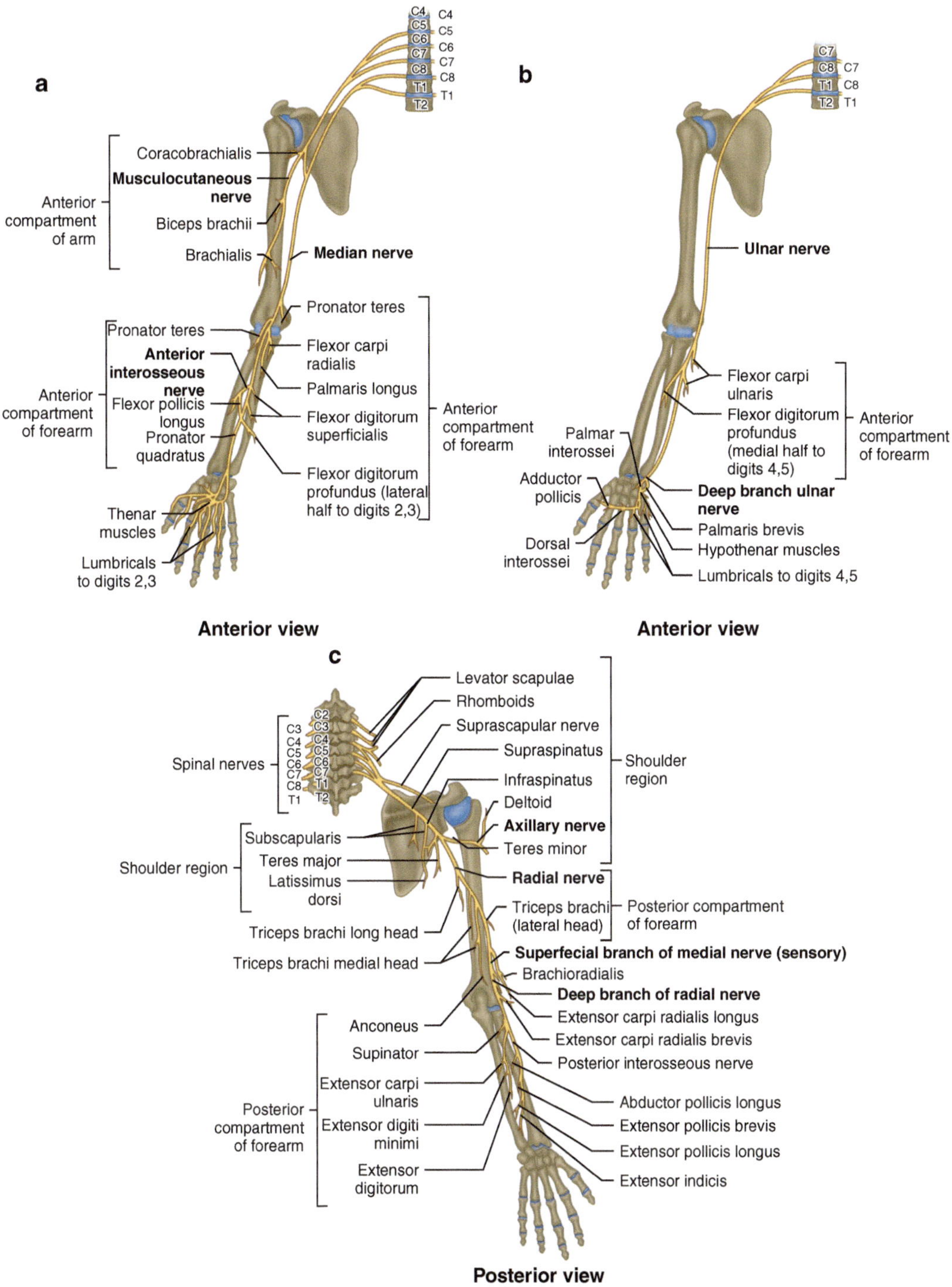

Illustration 4.2 Topographic anatomy of nerves vulnerable to injury during shoulder arthroplasty. The anterior view illustrates the paths of the suprascapular, musculocutaneous, and subscapular nerves. The posterior view illustrates the paths of the axillary and radial nerves

noid by as much as 2 cm was not shown to cause macroscopic changes to the axillary nerve and caused minimal stretch in cadaveric shoulders [21]. Some degree of relative lateralization is commonly used to maximize stability and improve impingement-free motion in RSA and contributes to soft tissue tensioning. Lengthening of the arm has been proposed as an important mechanism of axillary nerve and brachial plexus trauma in RSA [11], but the hypothesis requires further investigation to clearly define this relationship.

4.2.3.2 Suprascapular Nerve

Suprascapular nerve injury has recently been described as an uncommon complication of RSA [38, 39]. Unlike TSA, in which a polyethylene glenoid component is secured to the scapula by a relatively shallow keel or multiple small pegs, RSA requires screws to secure the glenoid component. Direct injury from screw insertion can occur at two important anatomic points: as the nerve traverses the suprascapular notch or the spinoglenoid notch (Illustration 4.2) [39, 40].

The suprascapular nerve originates from the superior trunk of the brachial plexus, formed by the confluence of C5, C6, and infrequently C4 [27, 40]. It descends through the posterior triangle of the neck between the trapezius posteriorly and omohyoid anteriorly. It travels in a posterior and lateral direction toward the scapula, entering the supraspinatus fossa via the suprascapular notch. This notch between the posterior aspect of the coracoid process and medial scapula is contained by the superior transverse scapular ligament. The nerve then courses laterally under the supraspinatus to the lateral border of the scapular spine, giving off motor branches to the supraspinatus. It dives posteriorly through the spinoglenoid notch, contained by the inferior transverse scapular ligament, and into the infraspinatus fossa. Here it gives off sensory branches to the posterior and superior aspect of the glenohumeral joint before terminating in motor branches to the infraspinatus.

Awareness of the anatomic properties of the scapular bony anatomy in relation to the suprascapular nerve is needed to avoid nerve injury. Safe zones for screw placement have been described, with posteriorly directed screws greater than 14 mm in length endangering the nerve in the spinoglenoid notch and superiorly directed screws greater than 23 mm in length endangering the nerve in the suprascapular notch (Illustration 4.3) [41]. A more recent cadaveric study investigated this issue further [40]. Posteriorly directed screws were found to be the biggest liability, coming into contact with the nerve in the spinoglenoid notch in 90% of cases, but the shortest screw length used was 18 mm. Superiorly directed screws came into contact with the nerve in 40% of cases but screw lengths of 32 mm or longer did not necessarily endanger the nerve, making this anatomic relationship less clear. Screws directed anteriorly toward the subscapularis fossa or inferiorly were found to be safe. Some additional considerations are that supraspinatus and infraspinatus tears have been associated with suprascapular

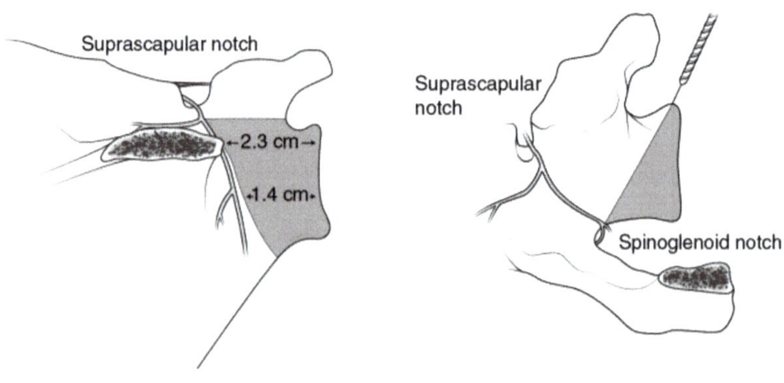

Illustration 4.3 Safe zones for glenoid screw placement during RSA. (Adapted from Shishido and Kikuchi [41])

nerve injury, possibly due to tension on the nerve from retraction of the torn tendons [42, 43]. Preexisting injuries to the suprascapular nerve also appear to be a risk factor for new acute injuries during shoulder arthroplasty [35]. Whether this can be explained by abnormal anatomy in patients with preexisting injuries remains to be determined.

4.2.3.3 Musculocutaneous Nerve

Injuries to the musculocutaneous nerve have been described due to traction during the deltopectoral approach and due to entrapment during subpectoral biceps tenodesis [32, 44]. Although their prevalence in shoulder arthroplasty is unknown, a study using intraoperative neuromonitoring suggested that subclinical trauma is common [45]. The musculocutaneous nerve receives contributions from C5, C6, and C7 and originates from the lateral cord of the brachial plexus (Illustration 4.2) [46]. It travels anteriorly from its origin and gives off a motor branch to the coracobrachialis before piercing between the two vestigial heads of the muscle, which form a single mass in early development. The musculocutaneous nerve emerges anteriorly through the coracobrachialis an average of 56 mm below the inferior border of the coracoid, but this distance can be as close as 20 mm [47]. The nerve then descends laterally between the short head of the biceps and brachialis, giving off motor branches before traversing the deep fascia at the elbow to become the lateral antebrachial cutaneous nerve of the forearm. During arthroplasty, direct injury to the nerve can be avoided by keeping dissection lateral to the conjoint tendon. Overzealous retraction of the tendon or errant placement of instruments within the tendon itself must also be avoided. Finally, it is worth noting that the nerve can potentially become entrapped by the long head of the biceps so the muscle should not be extensively manipulated or twisted prior to tenodesis [44].

4.2.3.4 Radial Nerve

Radial nerve injury is a rare complication of shoulder arthroplasty limited to the setting of peri-prosthetic humeral shaft fractures [13]. Reported combined rates of intraoperative and postoperative humeral shaft fractures during shoulder arthroplasty range from 1.2% to 19.4% [48]. Intraoperatively, they occur most often during implant removal for revision arthroplasty, during humeral component preparation, and during reduction of the implants due to excessive torque on the humerus. The radial nerve is vulnerable to injury as it comes into contact with the humeral diaphysis in the spiral groove (Illustration 4.2, Fig. 4.5b) [49]. On average, this location is 101.9 mm distal to the inferior subscapularis insertion and 39.6 mm distal to the inferior latissimus dorsi insertion and, therefore, not susceptible to injury during routine exposures in shoulder arthroplasty, and only occasionally in revision arthroplasty. Care must be taken to avoid entrapping the nerve during fixation of periprosthetic humeral shaft fractures with cerclage cables distal to the insertion of the latissimus dorsi or when using cemented implants in the setting of humeral shaft fractures as distal extrusion of cement can cause thermal injury to the radial nerve [10].

4.2.3.5 Subscapular Nerves

The integrity of the subscapularis muscle is important for stability and function of the shoulder. Subscapularis muscle deficiency manifesting as a deficit of internal rotation power is common after shoulder arthroplasty despite satisfactory repair at the time of surgery, as is progression of fatty degeneration [50, 51]. These observations raise the concern that dysfunction of the nerves supplying the muscle, rather than the integrity of the intraoperative repair, could be responsible [27]. Excessive mobilization of the subscapularis muscle and retraction of the conjoint tendon are potential mechanisms of nerve injury [52, 53]. The subscapularis is innervated by the upper and lower subscapular nerves. These nerves originate from the posterior cord of the brachial plexus, bisected by the thoracodorsal nerve, and receive variable contributions from C5, C6, and C7. They descend laterally superficial to the subscapularis muscle before terminating in motor branches medial to the conjoint tendon [54]. With the arm in neutral rotation, the ends of the upper subscapular and lower subscapular nerves are located 52 mm and 47 mm medial to the lateral border of the conjoint tendon, respectively. Avoidance of direct injury can thus be ensured by keeping dissection lateral to the conjoint tendon. Traction injury can be avoided by limiting retraction of the conjoint tendon and the tenotomized subscapularis.

4.2.3.6 Other Nerve Injuries

Traction injuries to the brachial plexus can result from many of the steps previously described, including errant retraction, excessive manipulation of the arm, reduction of components, and overlengthening of the arm during RSA. Electrophysiologic studies suggest that intra-operative trauma to the brachial plexus is common [9, 45]. Injuries may occur in nerve distributions not normally linked to shoulder arthroplasty, such as the median or ulnar nerves. Worsening of preexisting compression neuropathies such as carpal tunnel syndrome or cubital tunnel syndrome may also occur [11]. Since these injuries are indirect, they are typically neuropraxias that improve spontaneously [3, 4]. The same precautionary measures should be taken to avoid these injuries as described above.

Overlengthening of the arm during RSA has been proposed as a mechanism of brachial plexus traction injury, although no clear correlation between the extent of lengthening and nerve injury has been established [11]. This topic has garnered attention recently. In their retrospective analysis, Kim et al. [4] showed a significant increase in arm length based on acromiohumeral distance in patients demonstrating EMG evidence of neurologic injury after RSA compared to patients who did not. Overall, 19% of patients showed evidence of nerve injury, but all recovered nonoperatively. Meanwhile, Lowe et al. [6] showed no difference in neurologic complications in RSA compared to TSA, despite significantly greater arm lengths in patients who underwent RSA. The rate of postoperative nerve injury in this study was only 4%, and all recovered nonoperatively. The authors concluded that the risk of neurologic injury in RSA is no greater than TSA when new implant designs with a 135° neck-shaft angle and lateralized glenosphere are used.

Distalizing the center of rotation of the glenohumeral joint in RSA is an important step in tensioning the deltoid muscle and optimizing its mechanical advantage in the absence of a functional rotator cuff [19]. This is accomplished through inferior positioning and slight downward tilt of the glenoid baseplate, which is thought to improve stability of the prosthesis [55], maximize impingement-free range of motion [56], and minimize the risk of scapular notching [57]. Despite this, increasing inferior offset of the glenoid baseplate by more than 2.5 mm was shown to be detrimental to deltoid function, resulting in a nearly 50% reduction in the ability of the muscle to elongate under tension [58]. In addition, overall deltoid lengthening greater than 26 mm may be associated with increased risk of acromial fractures, deltoid dehiscence, or deltoid-related pain [59]. As such, when implanting the baseplate in RSA, we suggest using a modest inferior tilt of 10–15°, distalizing the center of the baseplate no more than 2.5 mm, and limiting overall arm lengthening to less than 25 mm in order to reduce the likelihood of deltoid dysfunction and traction-related complications [55, 58].

4.3 Prevention Strategies

The following tips can be used to prevent nerve injuries in shoulder arthroplasty:

- *Use caution when releasing the inferior border of the subscapularis.*
  Whether using a subscapularis tenotomy, subscapularis peel or lesser tuberosity osteotomy technique, care must be taken to avoid injuring the axillary nerve just below the lower border of the subscapularis. The lower border of the subscapularis is identified by a branch of the posterior humeral circumflex artery and its venae comitantes ("the three sisters") and dissection should be carried further distal with

extreme caution. A 270° release of the subscapularis, which avoids dissection along the inferior 90° arc, can achieve adequate visualization while avoiding iatrogenic nerve injury. If more extensive release is required due to scarring, chronic retraction, or revision surgery, an axillary neurolysis may be necessary.

- *Stay lateral to the conjoint tendon.*
  The musculocutaneous nerve and upper and lower subscapular nerves descend well medial to the lateral border of the conjoint tendon and can be easily avoided. When retraction of the tendon is necessary, it should be done gently, and instruments should never penetrate the tendon.
- *Release the inferior portion of the glenoid under direct visualization.*
  The axillary nerve is located approximately 10–15 mm inferior to the glenoid rim. Circumferential capsular release may be performed with caution. Tissue may be pulled onto the glenoid face to ensure no tethering of the axillary nerve prior to resection. In addition, radial relaxing incisions in the labrum may safely increase visualization. Particular care must be used along the inferior glenoid rim, with no plunging of sharp instruments and judicious use of periosteal elevators to ensure safety. Peripheral osteophytes should be debrided only once satisfactory exposure of the glenoid has been achieved. Humeral abduction greater than 45° reduces the distance between the axillary nerve and the inferior glenoid rim. Finally, identification of the axillary nerve can help to ensure any work around the inferior glenoid is safe from iatrogenic injury.
- *Take time to plan the humeral component.*
  Preoperative planning for shoulder arthroplasty often focuses on version of the glenoid component, but care should go into planning the humeral implant as well. The axillary nerve is vulnerable to injury as it comes into contact with the posterior humeral metaphysis. Respecting the native version of the humerus can limit the chance of injury, and anatomic references such as the humeral bare area should be used prior to osteotomizing the humeral head. Injury can be further prevented by avoiding low humeral cuts, excessive reaming, and oversized implants.
- *Limit glenoid screw length in RSA.*
  When securing the glenoid baseplate, posteriorly and superiorly directed screws risk injury to the suprascapular nerve in the spinoglenoid and suprascapular notches, respectively. Posterior screws greater than 14 mm may increase risk. Although longer superior screws do not necessarily endanger the nerve, screw lengths less than 23 mm are generally considered safe.
- *Finally, take care when handling the arm.*
  Nerve trauma resulting from traction and arm positioning is common. Limit the length and duration of positioning in extremes of motion when not critical. This is particularly important during glenoid exposure in extension and external rotation. Relax the soft tissues frequently.

4.4 Natural History of Nerve Injuries During Shoulder Arthroplasty

The vast majority of nerve injuries during shoulder surgery are transient neuropraxias that resolve spontaneously in clinical and electrophysiologic studies [1, 2, 60]. A prospective study investigating 30 patients who underwent TSA, hemiarthroplasty, or revision arthroplasty found that 4 patients demonstrated clinical and electromyographic evidence of neurologic deficits postoperatively, all of which resolved within 6 months [45]. In another study, 2 of 36 patients undergoing TSA or RSA were found to have clinical and electromyographic neurologic deficits postoperatively, which also resolved spontaneously within 6 months [9].

Few studies have attempted to characterize the long-term prognoses of these injuries. A retrospective case series of 417 shoulders that underwent TSA found a 4.3% prevalence of neurologic deficits, mostly involving the upper and middle trunks of the brachial plexus [61]. All but one of the injuries involved mixed sensory and motor deficits. All of the patients demonstrated recovery of function at 1 year of follow-up, even though recovery was only graded as "fair" in 5 of 16 shoulders. Another retrospective series followed 26 patients with neurologic injuries after shoulder surgery, presenting on average 5.4 months after their surgery [3]. Four patients had undergone arthroplasty procedures. In this study, 58% of patients did not recover nerve function and required surgical management. Patients with structural peripheral nerve injuries due to laceration or entrapment with a suture were more likely to require surgery. In a portion of these cases, optimal surgical management could not be offered due to delayed presentation, highlighting the importance of prompt recognition of neurologic injuries.

Little is known about the natural history of specific peripheral nerve injuries in shoulder arthroplasty. Axillary nerve injury is most commonly reported both clinically and in electrodiagnostic studies, but recent evidence suggests that suprascapular nerve injury is relatively common and slower to recover [38]. In a prospective study of 20 patients undergoing RSA, the prevalence of acute injury on postoperative EMG was 31.5%. Of the nine axillary nerve lesions, seven recovered fully by 6 months of follow-up, while all six suprascapular nerve lesions had persistent EMG changes even after 6 months. Importantly, many of the lesions caught on postoperative EMG occurred in patients with previous chronic EMG changes. There were no significant differences in range of motion or constant score in patients with nerve lesions, calling the clinical importance of these findings into question. Even less is known about the natural history of other peripheral nerve injuries because they are so rare. Case reports of musculocutaneous nerve entrapment during biceps tenodesis and radial nerve thermal injury due to cement extrusion both described full recovery after surgical decompression of the nerves [10, 44]. Brachial plexus injuries appear to carry the best prognosis for spontaneous recovery, as they are more likely to result from indirect injury due to traction or arm positioning [3]. The natural course of injuries to specific nerves is an interesting topic that warrants further research. In the following sections, we will discuss the evaluation and treatment of specific neurologic injuries.

4.5 Clinical Evaluation

Evaluation of neurologic function should be performed at every postoperative clinic visit. Most clinically significant deficits are evident on physical exam within 7 days of surgery, but the exam should be repeated at subsequent visits to ensure that injuries are not missed [61]. A complete history includes asking the patient about pain, weakness, paresthesias, and sensory deficits since surgery. General physical exam should include inspection for muscle atrophy. A comprehensive motor and sensory exam of the entire brachial plexus, and assessment of reflexes and vascular status should be performed. In cases of suspected brachial plexus injuries, a pre-ganglionic or post-ganglionic location for the lesion should be identified. Below we highlight useful steps for diagnosing specific peripheral nerve injuries.

4.5.1 Axillary Nerve

- History may be suggestive of weakness or numbness in the "sergeant's patch" distribution. In patients with pre-existing rotator cuff tears, a history of baseline shoulder function should be obtained since these patients will have pre-existing weakness.
- Motor exam may initially demonstrate absence or weakness of active shoulder abduction due to disruption of innervation to the deltoid. Palpation of the deltoid may reveal an absence of contraction and should be tested to isolate the anterior, middle, and posterior deltoid, respectively. Abduction power should be graded with the shoulder in internal rotation to diminish the ability of the supraspinatus to compensate [62]. The posterior deltoid can be isolated by extending the shoulder while keep-

ing the elbow flexed to prevent compensation from the triceps. The middle deltoid is isolated with abduction in line with the body, while the anterior deltoid is isolated with the arm in line with the scapula or in forward flexion.

- Motor testing of external rotation with the arm in 90° of abduction isolates the teres minor (axillary nerve) from the infraspinatus (suprascapular nerve). Axillary nerve injury can manifest as inability to maintain this position actively, known as the "Hornblower's sign."
- Sensory exam may reveal diminished sensation on the surface of the deltoid or over the proximal upper arm. Sensory loss may be incomplete and present in only a segment of the deltoid [63].
- Atrophy of the deltoid will be visible with chronic injuries.

4.5.2 Suprascapular Nerve

- History may reveal persistent weakness in abduction or external rotation. Patients with preexisting rotator cuff tears will have a history of weakness at baseline and significant deficits may be difficult to determine in the early postoperative period. Deep aching pain in the superior or posterior shoulder is a rare presentation [39].
- Motor exam of the supraspinatus may reveal an inability to initiate active abduction of the shoulder with the arm in neutral position.
- Motor testing of external rotation with the arm in 0° of abduction isolates the infraspinatus muscle. The patient may also demonstrate an external rotation "lag sign" by being unable to maintain arm position after it is passively positioned in external rotation.
- No sensory deficits are anticipated in isolated suprascapular nerve injury. A sensory deficit may indicate injury to a different nerve or concomitant injury.
- Atrophy in the supraspinatus or infraspinatus fossa will be visible with chronic injury.

4.5.3 Musculocutaneous Nerve

- History may reveal purely sensory or mixed sensorimotor deficits.
- Motor exam may reveal weakness of elbow flexion and forearm supination, due to disrupted innervation of the biceps and brachialis.
- A sensory deficit is expected in the lateral forearm.
- Atrophy in the biceps will be visible with chronic injury.

4.5.4 Radial Nerve

- A history of peri-prosthetic fracture should be apparent since the radial nerve is not endangered during routine shoulder arthroplasty. If there is no history of trauma postoperatively, there should be a high index of suspicion for intraoperative fracture of the humeral shaft, and X-rays should be reviewed.
- Since the injury occurs at the level of the spiral groove, distal to proximal branches of the nerve, motor exam is likely to reveal sparing of active elbow extension. Weakness of elbow flexion with the forearm in neutral rotation ("hammer curl position") indicates disrupted innervation to the brachioradialis and is consistent with an injury at the midshaft level of the humerus.
- Motor exam will further reveal weakness of wrist and finger extension.
- Diminished sensation in the distribution of the lateral antebrachial cutaneous nerve of the forearm and possibly the posterior cutaneous nerve will be present in radial nerve palsy and distinguishes this from posterior interosseous nerve (PIN) palsy.
- A Tinel sign can be elicited by tapping the skin overlying the injured nerve. Migrating Tinel sign, which can be elicited increasingly distal in the arm on serial exams, is a good prognostic sign for spontaneous recovery [64].
- Atrophy in the mobile wad or posterior forearm may be visible with chronic injury.

4.5.5 Subscapular Nerves

- Challenging to diagnose early, most likely to become apparent months after surgery.
- History and review of operative records may be most useful in diagnosis. Key historical feature is a lack of resolution of internal rotation weakness over time despite documentation of adequate intraoperative repair of the subscapularis.
- Internal rotation range of motion and strength should be graded.
- The "lift-off," "belly-press," and "bear-hug" tests can all be used to elicit subscapularis weakness.
- No sensory deficit should be noted; a sensory deficit indicates injury to a different nerve or concomitant injury.
- Atrophy is not visible as the subscapularis is deep to the larger pectoralis major muscle.
- Excessive external rotation may indicate failure of subscapularis repair as a cause of persistent weakness. In TSA, this can result in joint dislocation.

4.6 Diagnostic Testing

Nerve injuries in the context of shoulder arthroplasty warrant an initial observation period of 4–6 weeks, followed by electrodiagnostic studies (EMG and nerve conduction), followed by early referral (within 3 months) to a peripheral nerve surgeon [2, 3, 60]. EMG can be used to confirm the diagnosis of peripheral nerve injury, rule out other diagnoses, and determine the severity of axonal loss, completeness of the lesion, and prognosis for recovery [65, 66]. These studies can also differentiate acute injuries from chronic injuries or disuse and identify preexisting or unrelated peripheral nerve lesions [38]. Optimal timing for EMG studies must be determined based on knowledge of neurologic reinnervation patterns after injury and the urgency of surgical intervention. Early EMG testing within 3-4 weeks of surgery can yield false-negative results as Wallerian degeneration has not yet occurred [65]. Denervation changes may become apparent as early as 10–14 days after injury in proximal muscles and 3–6 weeks after injury in distal muscles [66]. Optimal surgical timing for exploration and reinnervation is between 3 and 6 months, so the time interval between 6 weeks and 3 months after arthroplasty surgery is most appropriate for performing electrodiagnostic studies in patients with unresolving neurologic lesions.

Plain radiography is generally unhelpful but should be used in specific cases. Radial nerve injury after arthroplasty should be investigated with radiographs to rule out peri-prosthetic fracture, as this is the most likely cause of injury [48]. Radiographs can also be used to rule out an acromial stress fracture, which is a relatively common complication of shoulder arthroplasty that can present with a pain pattern similar to suprascapular nerve injury or limitation in motion similar to axillary nerve injury [38]. Radiographs in a patient with axillary nerve injury often demonstrate inferior pseudosubluxation of the humeral head as a result of deltoid atony [63].

Advanced imaging studies are not essential but may provide useful information for preoperative planning [67]. Magnetic resonance neurography (MRN) utilizes high-resolution MR sequences optimized to image nerves. It is superior to CT myelography in visualizing postganglionic and peripheral nerve lesions. The location and severity of the lesion as well as the length of nerve affected can be directly visualized using this technique. MRN can also be used to evaluate potential donor nerves for nerve transfer. The main disadvantage of MR imaging in the context of shoulder arthroplasty is the artifact introduced by metal implants, which may limit visualization. On the other hand, advanced ultrasonography techniques can visualize nerve lesions in even higher resolution than MRN in real time, are generally more accessible, and are not limited by metal artifact. Ultrasound can thus be used preoperatively to identify the specific location of injury and differentiate between neurotmetic and axonotmetic injuries. Other investigations such as CT myelography and vascular studies are usually unnecessary except in select cases [65, 66].

4.7 Nerve Reconstruction

Reports on operative repair or reconstruction of nerve injuries associated with shoulder arthroplasty are rare, with outcomes limited to case reports. Surgical strategies can be extrapolated from the literature on traumatic peripheral nerve and brachial plexus injuries with recognition that these injuries may differ in severity, location, and prognosis from those associated with arthroplasty. Once a peripheral nerve injury has been diagnosed, optimal timing for surgical intervention is 3–6 months after the injury if there are no signs of recovery. If there has been a known transection of a nerve, reconstruction should be performed as early as possible after the arthroplasty.

Nerve injuries that fail to show clinical or electrodiagnostic evidence of recovery after an initial period of observation and serial examinations should be treated surgically [65, 66]. If a damaged nerve is not reinnervated within 6 months of injury, irreversible changes begin to occur at the motor endplates and the prognosis for recovery deteriorates [1, 63, 68]. We recommend prompt clinical and electrodiagnostic evaluation of these injuries, aiming to perform surgery 3–6 months after injury when necessary. Intraoperative EMG can be used to confirm the injury and type of reconstruction.

We will now discuss primary surgical treatment in the form of nerve reconstruction. Nerves transected intraoperatively should undergo acute direct repair. However, almost all nerve injuries related to shoulder arthroplasty are only recognized in the postoperative period. Neuroma formation occurs in the weeks following injury, and subsequent treatment must include excision of the segment of devitalized nerve. In this setting, a direct tension-free repair is rarely an option. We will focus on three modalities of treatment: neurolysis, nerve grafting, and nerve transfers. Neurolysis is the debridement of scar tissue around a nerve and is indicated when the nerve is in continuity [63]. Nerve grafting is the use of a conduit to bridge a devitalized segment of the damaged nerve. Ideally, autograft nerve harvested from the patient is used, but this carries potential donor site morbidity. Nerve transfers have become increasingly popular over recent decades [69]. Their goal is to restore function to an injured nerve by transferring an expendable nerve branch from another functional nerve. Key elements for a successful nerve transfer include close proximity of the donor nerve to the motor endplates of the target muscle, expendability of the donor branch, good size match and a comparable number of axons to the target nerve, and synergistic muscle action between the donor and recipient.

4.7.1 Axillary Nerve

Surgery for axillary nerve injuries should be performed within 3–6 months to optimize outcomes [1, 63, 70]. Most traumatic injuries to the axillary nerve occur just distal to its origin in the brachial plexus or just proximal to the quadrilateral space [71–74]. Preoperative MRI or MR neurography can be helpful to identify the location of the lesion but will be limited by metal artifact due to the preexisting shoulder arthroplasty. Intraoperative nerve stimulation is critical and should be made available.

For all of the following procedures, a combined anterior and posterior approach may be necessary (Figs. 4.3 and 4.4). We recommend beginning with the anterior approach, which is used to explore the origin and proximal part of the axillary nerve. The previous deltopectoral approach may need to be extended along the inferior border of the clavicle medially. The pectoralis minor, which is attached medially on the coracoid, should be identified and gently separated from the adjacent conjoint tendon. Pectoralis minor is then tenotomized within 1 cm of its origin. Alternatively, the tip of the coracoid can be osteotomized and later reattached [70]. Gentle retraction will reveal the axillary sheath encasing the infraclavicular brachial plexus in adipose tissue.

If the zone of injury of the axillary nerve cannot be demarcated through the anterior approach, a second posterior approach is used. An incision is made along the posterior border of the deltoid

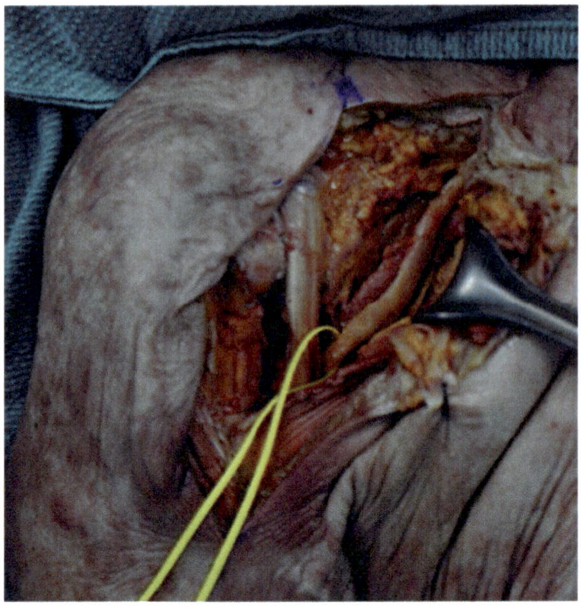

Fig. 4.3 Cadaveric image of the infraclavicular brachial plexus. The pectoralis minor tendon has been released but the conjoint tendon is intact lateral to the plexus. The musculocutaneous loop (yellow vessel loop) is shown entering the coracobrachialis muscle

and skin and subcutaneous flaps are elevated in the subfascial plane. Sensory fibers from the posterior division of the axillary nerve can be identified superficially and used to trace its path to the main nerve trunk. The posterior head of the deltoid is elevated and the axillary nerve is followed to the quadrangular space between the teres minor and teres major. It is important to identify and protect the posterior humeral circumflex artery branches running alongside the axillary nerve at this point.

4.7.1.1 Neurolysis

Neurolysis is the treatment of choice when intraoperative stimulation of the injured axillary nerve demonstrates nerve action potentials (NAPs) or motor unit action potentials (MUAPs). Favorable outcomes have been demonstrated using neurolysis alone during surgical exploration of nerve traction injuries and contusions that have not shown signs of clinical or electrodiagnostic recovery after several months of observation [72].

4.7.1.2 Interpositional Nerve Grafting

Interpositional nerve grafting using sural nerve autograft can restore function in the setting of an isolated axillary nerve injury. This technique is indicated when intraoperative EMG confirms discontinuity of the axillary nerve, and there is easily visible and demarcated neuroma precluding a tension-free repair. The main advantage of this technique compared to nerve transfer is the ability to restore native anatomic proportions of the anastomosed nerve ends [75]. If the interval between nerve injury and surgery is approaching 1 year, a nerve transfer may be preferable due to the relative proximity to the motor endplates, easily bypassing the zone of injury, and the axonal regeneration only having to bypass one nerve coaptation site. The relationship between length of the nerve graft and outcomes remains controversial, but good outcomes can be achieved even when long nerve grafts are necessary [68, 76, 77]. We prefer a two-incision pull-through technique as described by Baltzer et al. [78] (Illustration 4.4). Key steps are described below.

- *Anterior exposure:* Using the anterior approach, the released pectoralis minor tendon is retracted medially to expose the infraclavicular brachial plexus. The axillary and musculocutaneous nerves make up the two superior-most branches at the level of the cor-

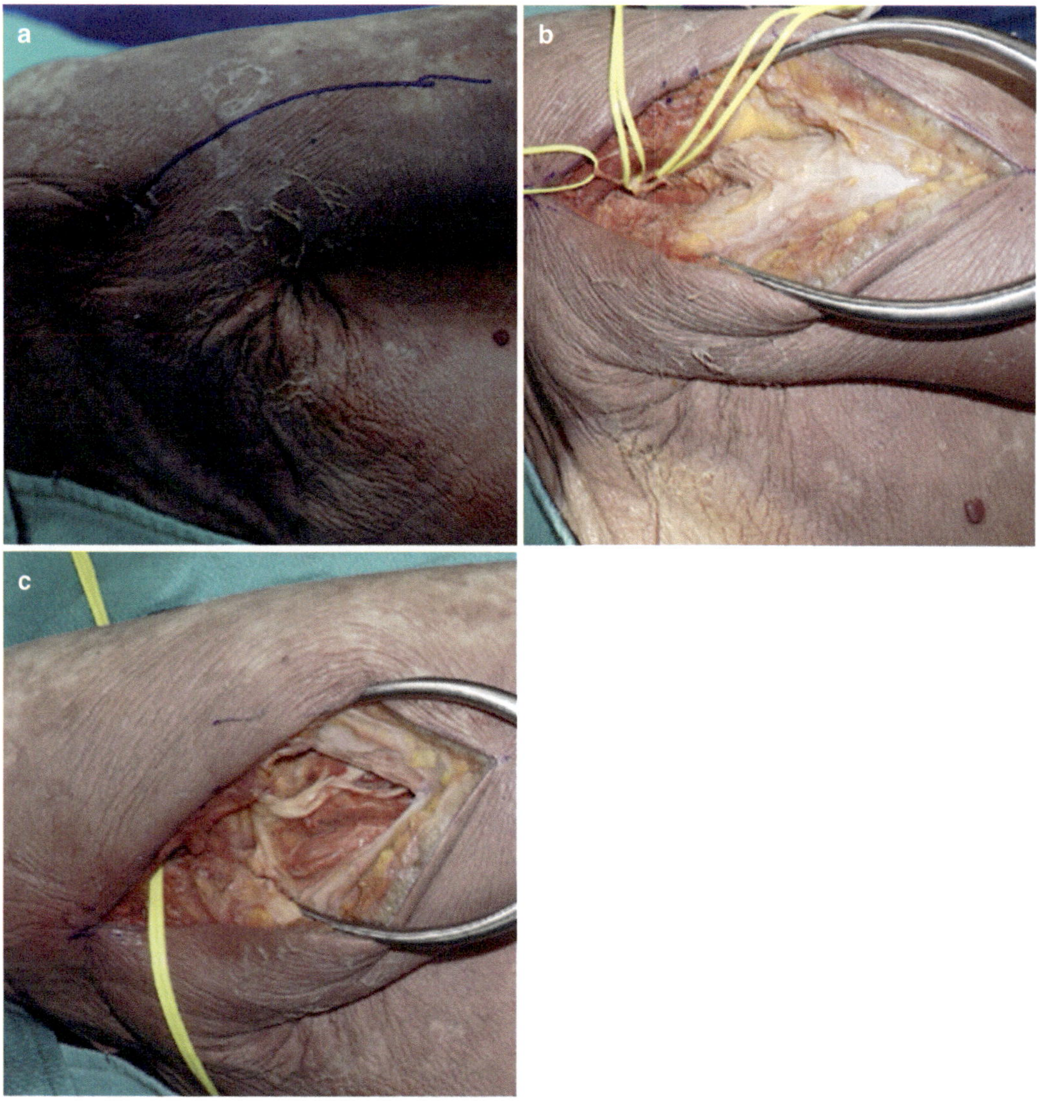

Fig. 4.4 Cadaveric images illustrating the posterior exposure of the axillary nerve used in reconstruction procedures. Image (**a**) shows the typical posterior incision. Image (**b**) shows the trifurcation of the axillary nerve into its anterior, posterior, and sensory branches prior to entering the quadrangular space. Image (**c**) demonstrates a vessel loop pulled through the quadrangular space to join the anterior and posterior exposures

acoid and can be traced back to their origins in the brachial plexus. The larger radial nerve can be found inferiorly. These three nerves are dissected circumferentially, and the axillary nerve exposed distally to the quadrangular space.

– Key decision point: Nerve stimulation is performed and the neuroma is inspected proximally. If muscle activity is present, simple neurolysis can be performed [70]. If muscle activity is absent, but the neuroma extends into the posterior cord of the brachial plexus, a nerve transfer should be performed to avoid injury to the brachial plexus during proximal dissection [78]. Neuroma excision and nerve grafting should be performed if muscle activity is

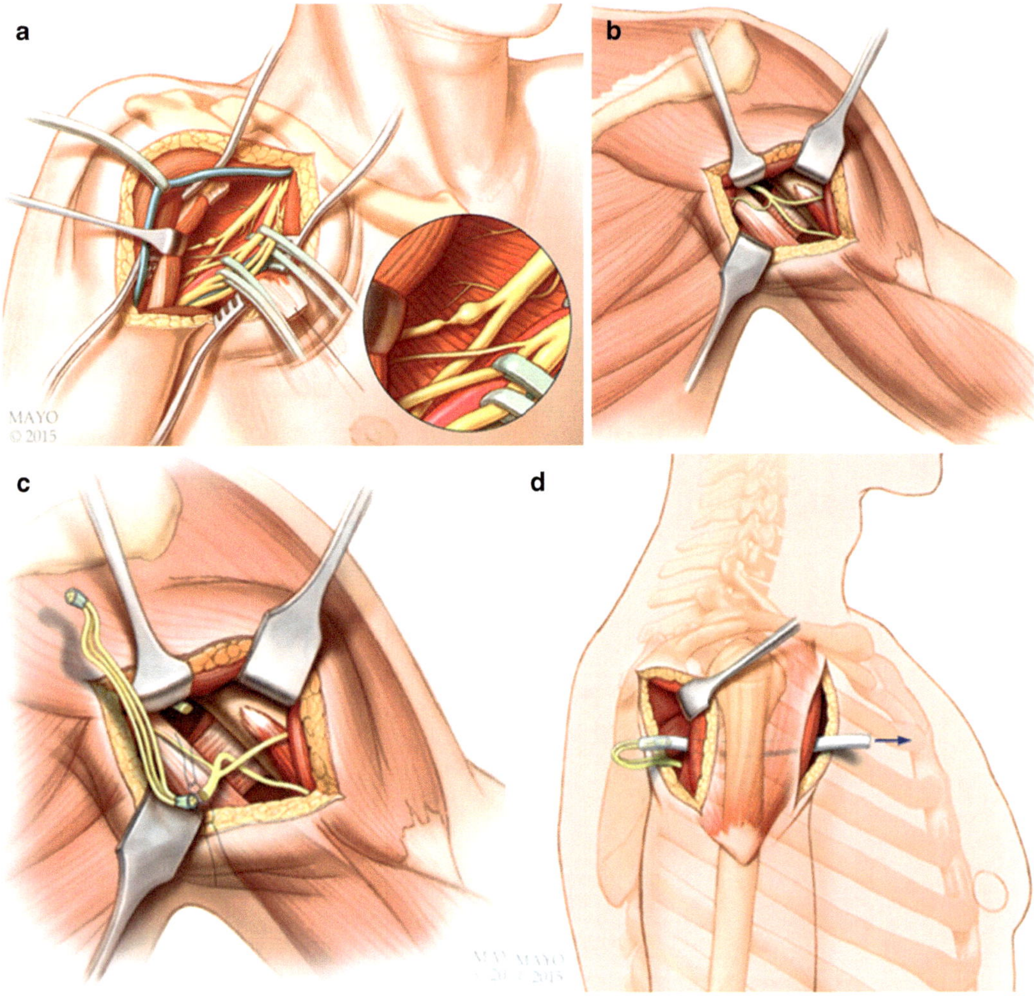

Illustration 4.4 Schematic of interpositional sural nerve grafting using the pull-through technique described in Baltzer et al. [71, 78]. Image (**a**) demonstrates the anterior exposure of the infraclavicular brachial plexus with axillary nerve neuroma illustrated. Image (**b**) shows the posterior exposure with the axillary nerve emerging through the quadrangular space. Images (**c**, **d**) show the distally transected axillary nerve anastomosed to a nerve graft and being pulled from the posterior to anterior exposure using a penrose drain. (With permission of the Mayo Foundation for Medical Education and Research. All rights reserved.)

absent and the neuroma originates distal to the brachial plexus.

- *Posterior exposure:* Through the posterior approach, motor fascicles of the deltoid as well as the branch to teres minor and posterior lateral cutaneous nerve fibers are identified. The entire nerve is used in the graft anastomosis.
- *Delineating the zone of injury:* The proximal end of the neuroma is removed through the anterior incision, and the axillary nerve cut back until healthy fascicles are seen. The distal end of the neuroma is then removed through the posterior incision.
- *Graft harvest :* Both legs should be prepped and draped free in case two grafts are required. The sural nerve is found using a transverse incision just distal to the popliteal fossa. The nerve is harvested to the level of the lateral malleolus distally, as it splits off into branches

thereafter. Harvest is accomplished using a nerve stripper and step-cuts as necessary between the proximal and distal incisions. Alternatively, the distal end of the nerve can be found. Typically, a 25–30 cm graft can be collected from each leg.

- *Sizing the graft:* A penrose drain is placed in the gap between the two ends of the truncated axillary nerve and the length measured. The sural nerve graft is divided and cut into multiple segments of this length, called "cables." Three or four cables are needed to match the cross-sectional size of the graft to the axillary nerve. The directionality of the nerve graft is reversed for inset to prevent loss of axons through side branches.
- *Axillary nerve reconstruction:* Anastomosis of the graft to the distal stump of the axillary nerve is performed through the posterior exposure. The proximal end of the graft is then fastened to the penrose drain and pulled through the quadrangular space and into the anterior field of view. Anastomosis to the proximal stump is then completed.

4.7.1.3 Radial to Axillary Nerve Transfer

The main advantage of nerve transfer is the close proximity of the donor nerve to the injured nerve, resulting in faster reinnervation than nerve grafting [79, 80]. In proximal lesions involving the posterior cord of the brachial plexus, nerve transfers do not require intraneural neurolysis, which endangers the adjacent radial nerve [71]. Therefore, triceps branch transfer to the axillary nerve is our preferred treatment when surgery has been delayed (beyond 9–12 months) and for proximal lesions. We use the technique described by Leechavengvongs et al. [81] (Illustration 4.5).

- *Posterior exposure:* The posterior approach to the deltoid may need to be extended distally in the upper third of the arm in line with the humerus. The deltoid is elevated and the interval between the long and lateral heads of triceps is developed to expose the quadrangular space superiorly and triangular interval inferiorly, separated by teres major.

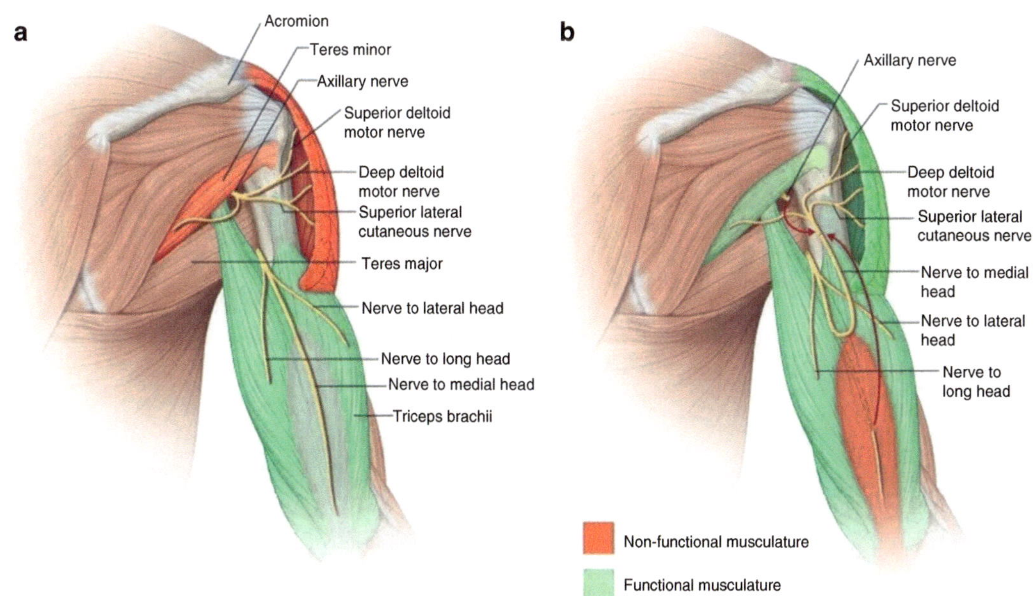

Illustration 4.5 Transfer of the radial nerve motor branch innervating the medial head of the triceps to the distal axillary nerve. Image (**a**) depicts the axillary (above) and radial nerves (below) prior to transfer. Image (**b**) depicts the completed transfer

- *Axillary nerve dissection:* Motor fascicles of the deltoid are separated from the branch to teres minor and posterior lateral cutaneous nerve fibers. They are followed to the posterior branch of the axillary nerve and then eventually to the main nerve trunk through the quadrangular space. Nerve stimulation is performed.
- *Radial nerve dissection:* The radial nerve gives off its first motor branch to the long head of the triceps just proximal to the inferior edge of teres major, which can be partially released and elevated to improve visualization. The nerve is followed distally and cut as close as possible to its insertion into the triceps muscle (Fig. 4.5a).
  - Key decision point: Alternatively, the branch to the medial or lateral head can be used [68]. Classically, the branch to the long head is chosen because it is the first motor branch and contributes minimally to triceps strength. We recommend selecting the branch with the best size match and length.
- *Nerve transfer:* The donor triceps branch is cut as distally as possible and the axillary nerve is cut as proximally as possible. Anastomosis is performed under microscopic visualization.

4.7.2 Suprascapular Nerve

The suprascapular nerve powers the supraspinatus and infraspinatus muscles, which are important for glenohumeral joint dynamic stability in the native shoulder, as well as in hemiarthroplasty and TSA [82]. The importance of these muscles in RSA is less clear, as RSA is often performed in patients with severely deficient or nonfunctional supraspinatus and infraspinatus muscles. Therefore, injury to the suprascapular nerve in RSA may not have significant functional manifestations but may contribute to persistent pain due to the sensory components of the nerve [39]. It is vulnerable during glenoid drilling and superior or posterior screw insertion in RSA as it passes through the suprascapular and spinoglenoid notches [40]. When entrapment of the nerve is suspected, radiographs and CT imaging should be obtained to confirm the location of the errant screw. The culprit screw will protrude outside the glenoid vault either posteri-

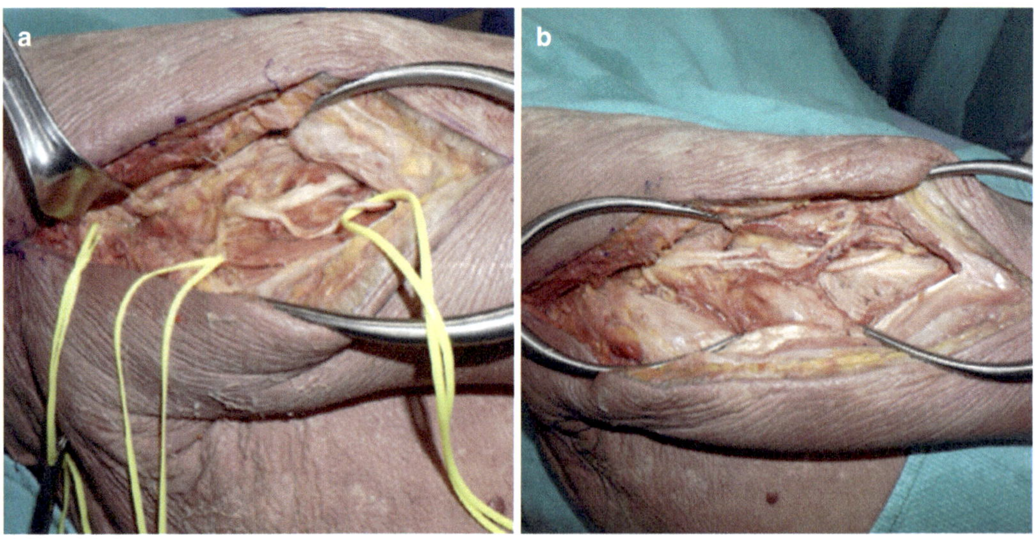

Fig. 4.5 Cadaveric images of the radial nerve visualized through an extended posterior exposure. Image (**a**) illustrates the proximity of the axillary nerve in the quadrangular space (left) to the branches of the radial nerve emerging from the triangular interval (right). Image (**b**) shows the path of the radial nerve passing across the spiral groove of the humerus

orly or superiorly, as extraosseous inferior and anterior screws do not endanger the suprascapular nerve. Screw removal from the suprascapular notch and neurolysis fully restored suprascapular nerve function in one case report [39]. The authors used a superior trapezius-splitting approach to access the supraspinatus fossa and directly visualize the entrapped nerve. They amputated the protruding screw tip using a high-speed burr and debrided the scar tissue formed around the nerve. Screw removal with neurolysis should be the treatment of choice for most suprascapular nerve injuries in RSA. In patients with persistent severe external rotation weakness after hemiarthroplasty or TSA with an intact rotator cuff, or in those with humeral head elevation, suprascapular nerve palsy should be evaluated. In these cases, nerve or tendon reconstructive procedures may be considered in addition to conversion to RSA.

4.7.2.1 Spinal Accessory to Suprascapular Nerve Transfer

Transection of the suprascapular nerve has been reported in the context of arthroscopic subacromial decompression and ganglion cyst removal from the supraspinatus muscle [3]. Concomitant suprascapular and axillary nerve injuries were treated with nerve transfers, demonstrating full recovery in follow-up. Transfer of the spinal accessory nerve to the suprascapular nerve from the posterior approach is a viable option for injuries at or proximal to the suprascapular notch due to the proximity of the spinal accessory nerve. Injury distal to the notch is a contraindication to this nerve transfer. This transfer can be performed through either an anterior [82, 83] or a posterior approach [84]. We prefer a posterior approach as this allows for identification of the suprascapular nerve at the suprascapular notch (Illustration 4.6),

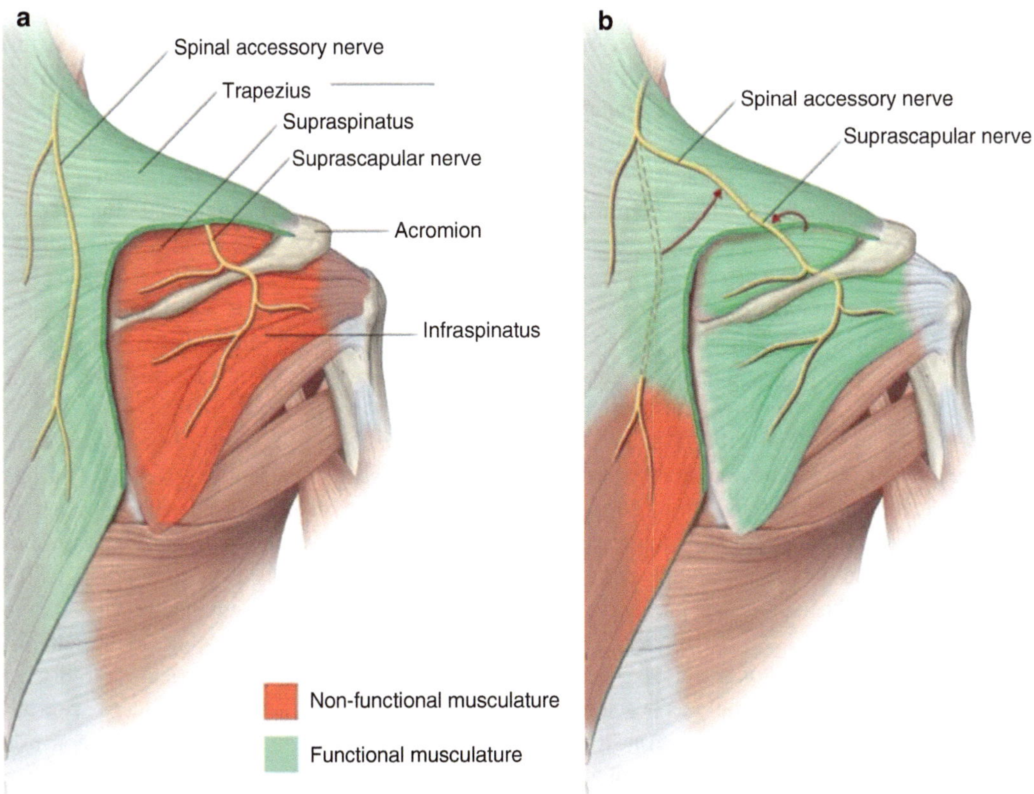

Illustration 4.6 Transfer of the spinal accessory nerve to the suprascapular nerve from the posterior approach. Image (**a**) depicts the spinal accessory (medial) and suprascapular nerves (lateral) prior to transfer. Image (**b**) depicts the completed transfer

whereas an anterior approach may not allow visualization of the nerve at the location of injury.

- *Exposure:* A transverse incision is planned along the superior border of the scapula. The spinal accessory nerve is identified along this line, approximately 44% of the way between the superomedial corner of the scapula and the posterior corner of the acromion [84]. After skin incision, the fascia of the trapezius is released and careful dissection is carried out through the trapezius until in the fatty areolar plane deep to this for nerve identification.
- *Suprascapular nerve dissection:* The suprascapular nerve is identified along the superior border of the scapula as it traverses through the notch. The ligament is palpated along the superior border of the scapula. The ligament is visualized and released, taking care not to injure the suprascapular artery. The suprascapular nerve can then be dissected from distal to proximal. It is important to ensure that adequate length is available for the nerve transfer to be carried out in a tension-free manner. Nerve grafts should not be necessary and will limit the potential for recovery.

  – Key decision point: A nerve stimulator or intraoperative EMG should be used to confirm that the supraspinatus is denervated and that there is no evidence of suprascapular nerve recovery.
- *Spinal accessory nerve dissection:* During the dissection of the trapezius muscle, nerve stimulation is critical to identify the precise location of the nerve. Once in the areolar fatty plane beneath the trapezius, the spinal accessory nerve can be identified and should be dissected distally. On some occasions, more than one branch is identified and allows for preservation of partial innervation of the trapezius. The spinal accessory nerve should not be transected until the suprascapular nerve has been identified.
- *Nerve transfer:* The donor spinal accessory nerve branch is cut as distally as possible and moved to the suprascapular fossa. Anastomosis is performed under microscopic visualization.

4.7.3 Musculocutaneous Nerve

Among the few musculocutaneous nerve injuries that have been described in the shoulder surgery literature, most appear to resolve spontaneously [27, 32]. Persistent injuries are usually caused by entrapment and can be effectively treated with neurolysis [44].

4.7.3.1 Oberlin Transfer

One study describing a laceration of the musculocutaneous nerve during arthroscopic shoulder surgery showed a partial recovery of function after delayed treatment with Oberlin nerve transfer [3]. In the context of a distal peripheral nerve injury, a distal nerve transfer, specifically an Oberlin transfer or double fascicular transfer, is an appropriate choice for isolated iatrogenic musculocutaneous nerve injuries [85–87]. Oberlin transfer has shown superior outcomes to conventional nerve grafting of the musculocutaneous nerve [88]. A prospective study showed no difference in outcomes between single and double fascicular Oberlin transfer and no added morbidity of the double transfer [89]. We suggest using the double transfer when possible to maximize the potential for reinnervation.

- *Approach:* An incision is made along the bicipital groove to allow for dissection of the musculocutaneous, median, and ulnar nerves. The median nerve is the first structure identified, followed by the brachial artery. The musculocutaneous nerve is identified under the biceps muscle. The ulnar nerve is identified more posteriorly as it traverses toward the cubital tunnel.
- *Distal musculocutaneous nerve dissection:* The musculocutaneous nerve is identified deep to the biceps muscle. The branch to biceps is located approximately at the midpoint of the humerus. Continuing distally, the lateral antebrachial cutaneous nerve and branch to brachialis must be identified. An intraneural neurolysis is carried out to dissect the branches to brachialis and biceps as proximal as possible to allow for a tension-free transfer to the donor nerves. Intraoperative

nerve stimulation and, if available, EMG are performed to ensure that there is no conductivity of the nerve or evidence of muscle contraction or MUAPs.

- *Ulnar nerve transfer:* The epineurium of the ulnar and median nerves is carefully opened in the distal half of the arm to allow for adequate length of the donor nerve. Nerve stimulation is used to identify the appropriate fascicle for transfer. Classically, the ulnar nerve fascicle with maximal stimulation to the FCU and least intrinsic muscle involvement is selected and anastomosed to the branch of the musculocutaneous nerve to the biceps [87]. This fascicle is often located on the medial border of the ulnar nerve. Once the fascicle is identified, an intrafascicular dissection is carried out from distal to proximal to allow for a tension-free nerve coaptation.

  – Key decision points: Selecting donor fascicles at random with attention to appropriate size match rather than function has been shown to be an acceptable strategy [90]. The ulnar nerve branch can be transferred to the nerve innervating the brachialis instead [86]. In proximal injuries, supplementary nerve grafting of the musculocutaneous nerve may be preferred to double Oberlin transfer [68].
- *Median nerve transfer:* In the double Oberlin transfer, fascicles of the median nerve are anastomosed to the branch of the musculocutaneous nerve innervating brachialis [86]. Fascicles to the flexor carpi radialis (FCR), flexor digitorum superficialis (FDS), or palmaris longus can be selected based on size match using a similar intrafascicular dissection as described for the ulnar nerve. All nerve coapations should be performed under microscope assistance. The authors suture the nerves and secure the coaptations with fibrin glue.

4.7.4 Radial Nerve

In shoulder arthroplasty, radial nerve injuries have been reported in the context of periprosthetic humeral shaft fractures and cement extrusion from the humerus [10, 13]. Treatment of radial nerve palsy resulting from humeral shaft fractures continues to be controversial, but important insights can be extrapolated from the extensive literature on this topic [91–93]. In the general context of humeral shaft fractures, the rate of spontaneous recovery is approximately 70%, but this may be higher for low-energy periprosthetic fractures [94]. The majority of these injuries are contusions rather than frank lacerations [95]. Early surgical exploration does not appear to improve outcomes compared to expectant management [93, 96]. Therefore, a period of observation followed by electrodiagnostic studies 6 weeks to 3 months after injury is a reasonable treatment strategy for these injuries. Many consider 4–6 months to be an appropriate duration of observation [92].

Peri-prosthetic humeral shaft fractures in shoulder arthroplasty require surgical management, either with stabilization of the fracture alone or stabilization and revision of the stemmed humeral component [48]. This provides an opportunity to explore the radial nerve, which is prudent if plates and screws or cerclage cables are to be applied around the humeral shaft. The lower border of the latissimus dorsi can be used as a landmark for where the radial nerve enters the spiral groove. If the fracture and radial nerve palsy are identified postoperatively, additional ultrasound examination may be helpful to identify a location of nerve entrapment and whether the nerve is in continuity [97]. Findings during surgical exploration can then guide further treatment.

Acute management of the radial nerve injury will depend on intraoperative findings. Observation alone is a reasonable option if the nerve is found to be mildly contused and in continuity [98]. The nerve should be liberated from entrapment, and neurolysis should be performed if there is scarring around the nerve. Neuromonitoring should be available to confirm the presence of nerve action potentials. If the nerve is transected, direct nerve repair or reconstruction with a nerve graft should be performed [99].

Management is more controversial for injuries that fail to resolve after a period of 6 months despite these interventions. Historically, radial nerve injuries failing to improve after 6–12 months of conservative treatment have been treated with tendon transfers with good outcomes [69, 100]. Although nerve transfers have been described, they compromise donor muscles that would be used for tendon transfers should the procedure fail. Theoretical advantages of nerve transfers are improved ergonomics, grip strength, muscle endurance, and dexterity [69]. Nerve transfers should be considered more strongly in young, active patients or in those whose lifestyles require a high level of finger dexterity, particularly in scenarios where there is a shorter interval since nerve injury. There is no agreed upon interval since injury, but the authors would consider nerve transfers if less than 9 months have passed; otherwise tendon transfers should be favored. Several variations of nerve transfers using donor branches from the median nerve have been described [101–104]. The procedure is performed through a curvilinear incision beginning at the antecubital fossa and extending distally in the interval between pronator teres (PT) and brachioradialis (BR). Proximally, proposed target nerves include radial nerve branches to extensor carpi radialis longus (ECRL) or brevis (ECRB) and potential donors include median nerve branches to PT or FDS. Distally, a second transfer is performed to the PIN with potential donors including nerve branches to FCR, FDS, or palmaris longus (PL). More research is needed to determine the optimal donor–target combinations and compare functional results with the tendon transfer procedures discussed in the following section.

4.7.5 Subscapular Nerves

It is unclear to what extent, if any, injury to the subscapular nerves contributes to internal rotation weakness and progression of fatty atrophy of the subscapularis after shoulder arthroplasty. Direct injuries of the nerves have not been reported, and they are well medial to the surgical field in shoulder arthroplasty. Furthermore, their impact, particularly on RSA, is not known to cause a functional deficit that requires surgical intervention. While further attention to this topic is warranted, there is currently insufficient evidence to recommend nerve reconstruction.

4.8 Salvage Surgical Techniques

Salvage procedures are indicated when nerve reconstruction has failed and functional deficits persist, or when more than 12 months have elapsed since the injury, reducing the likelihood of successful nerve reconstruction [63, 68, 105].

4.8.1 Tendon Transfers

Tendon transfers restore functional deficits, such as those incurred by nerve injury, by rerouting other functional muscles. Unlike nerve transfers, the recovery of function does not depend on muscle reinnervation but rather motor retraining during rehabilitation [69]. Key principles underlying the success of tendon transfers include soft tissue equilibrium around the affected joint, expendability of the donor muscle, direct line of pull, singular function, sufficient power, similar excursion, and synergistic function between the donor and recipient muscles [69, 106, 107]. Tendon transfers have only rarely been described in the context of nerve injuries resulting from shoulder arthroplasty.

Transfers of the trapezius and latissimus dorsi have been used to address specific deficits in shoulder function or stability [108]. Below we discuss the important technical points and potential applications for each procedure after nerve injury.

4.8.1.1 Trapezius Transfer

Trapezius transfers are a well-described technique for restoring shoulder abduction, external rotation, and stability [106, 109, 110]. The upper and middle thirds of the trapezius can be used to restore the initiation of shoulder abduction and help with glenohumeral joint coronal plane stability, while the lower third of the trapezius is particularly well suited to restore shoulder external rotation due to its direct line of pull and synergistic in-phase activation with the infraspinatus (Illustration 4.7) [111, 112]. In the context of shoulder arthroplasty, potential indications include injury to the axillary nerve or suprascapular nerve.

Like all other tendon transfers, a functional donor muscle group with British Medical Research Council (MRC) grade 4 power or higher is recommended. Biomechanical studies have shown that the supraspinatus contributes only 14% of the shoulder abduction moment arm, whereas the infraspinatus and teres minor contribute 32% in addition to providing 45% of external rotation [113, 114]. Furthermore, the infraspinatus and teres minor contribute to the posterior aspect of the shoulder axial plane anterior–posterior force couple, providing dynamic stability to the glenohumeral joint. This has increasingly led to recognition of the importance of adequately restoring both shoulder abduction and external rotation with tendon transfers [106, 108, 115]. We present our preferred techniques for upper and lower trapezius transfers below.

Upper Trapezius Transfer for Restoration of Shoulder Abduction:

- *Approach and exposure:* The patient is positioned in the lateral decubitus position or beach chair position. A sabrecut incision is made along the lateral edge of the acromion extending anteriorly to the level of the coracoid and posteriorly over the scapula. Full thickness flaps are created to expose the trapezius medially and deltoid laterally including their attachments to the clavicle and scapular spine.
- *Preparation of tendons for transfer:* The deltoid is released and mobilized from the lateral third of the clavicle, acromion, and lateral third of the scapular spine. An oblique osteot-

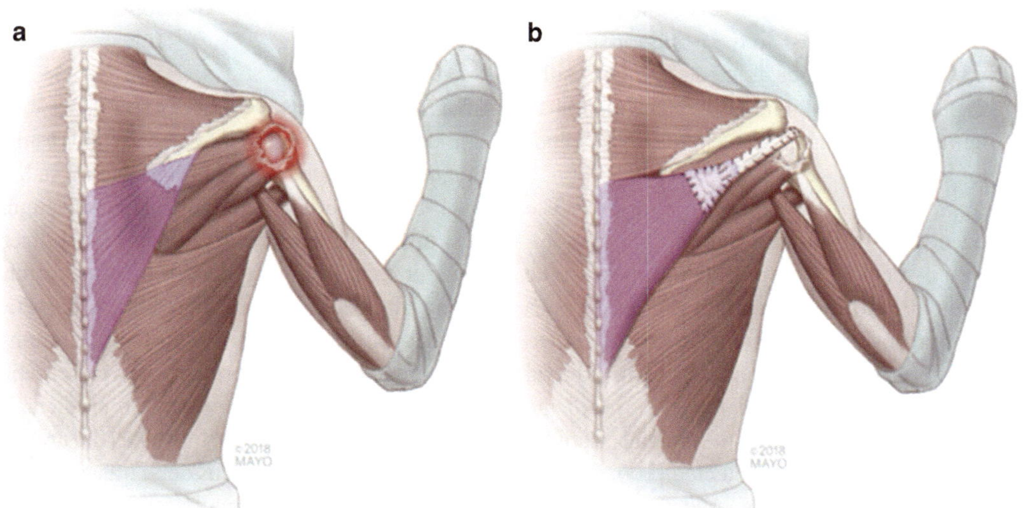

Illustration 4.7 Lower trapezius tendon transfer to restore external rotation in suprascapular nerve injury. Image (**a**) depicts the desired insertion for the transferred tendon on the proximal humerus. Image (**b**) depicts the completed transfer with a supplementary tendon graft (Adapted from Burnier et al. [108]). (With permission of the Mayo Foundation for Medical Education and Research. All rights reserved)

omy of the acromion is then performed and the upper trapezius is mobilized from the scapular spine and clavicle, leaving the coracoclavicular ligaments intact [116].

  - Key decision point: The insertion of the transferred trapezius muscle relative to the greater tuberosity of the proximal humerus is crucial in determining postoperative shoulder motion and stability. We recommend a position just below the greater tuberosity [110, 116].

- *Completion of tendon transfer:* The acromion osteotomy is secured in position using two 6.5-mm cancellous screws. It is secured with the shoulder in 70–80° of abduction to ensure appropriate tensioning. As advocated by Rühmann et al. [110], the deltoid muscle should then be sutured to the trapezius as far medially as possible. This medial repair potentially results in some transfer of contraction through the deltoid muscle fibers when the trapezius contracts.

Lower Trapezius Transfer for Restoration of Shoulder External Rotation:

- *Approach and exposure:* Surgery is performed in the lateral decubitus or beach chair position with adequate access to the posterior scapula. A horizontal incision is made just below the scapular spine, beginning 1–2 cm medial to the medial border of the scapula and extending laterally.
- *Preparation of tendons for transfer:* The lower third of the trapezius muscle is mobilized by detaching it from its insertion on the scapular spine and separating it from the middle third of the trapezius. The spinal accessory nerve may be encountered in the interval between the middle and lower thirds of the trapezius just medial to the medial scapular border and should be protected [106, 115]. A nerve stimulator can be used to identify its location if necessary. Alternatively, keeping the dissection lateral to the medial border of the scapula or carefully dissecting medial to the medial border can avoid injury to this nerve.
- *Completion of tendon transfer:* Laterally, the infraspinatus is exposed by detaching a portion of the posterior deltoid from the scapular spine. Some of the paralyzed infraspinatus muscle may need to be peeled off to expose the full extent of the infraspinatus tendon [117]. The lower trapezius tendon can then be attached directly onto the tendinous portion of the infraspinatus. The shoulder is held in maximal external rotation and abduction during tensioning.
  - Key decision point: Attaching the transferred trapezius muscle to the infraspinatus maintains the attachment to the greater tuberosity and can have the inadvertent effect of depressing the humeral head and limiting ultimate external rotation range of motion. This can be avoided by bypassing the infraspinatus with a tendon graft (usually Achilles tendon) and attaching the transferred trapezius to the anterior humerus (just posterior to the bicipital groove and wrapping laterally/inferiorly around the greater tuberosity. This technique is especially useful when infraspinatus tendon quality is poor or severely contracted.

4.8.1.2 Latissimus Dorsi Transfer

Latissimus dorsi transfers are also used to restore shoulder abduction, external rotation, and stability [118]. The broad insertion of the latissimus dorsi makes it a particularly effective stabilizer. However, lack of synergy, out of phase function, and an altered line of pull creating a humeral head depression moment make motor retraining challenging. For these reasons, achieving acceptable functional results may be less predictable than with lower trapezius transfers (Illustration 4.8). Nevertheless, latissimus dorsi transfers have been performed concurrently with RSA with good results in the setting of severe active abduction and external rotation deficit [119]. Similar to

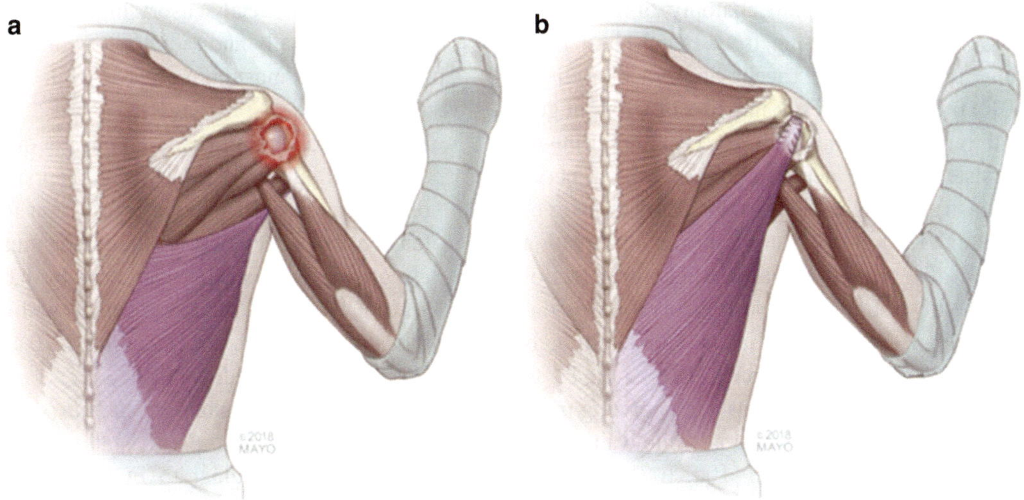

Illustration 4.8 Latissumus dorsi tendon transfer to restore external rotation in suprascapular nerve injury. Image (**a**) depicts the desired insertion for the transferred tendon on the proximal humerus. Image (**b**) depicts the completed tendon transfer (Adapted from Burnier et al. [108]). (With permission of the Mayo Foundation for Medical Education and Research. All rights reserved)

trapezius transfers, this technique could be used in the setting of persistent axillary or suprascapular nerve injury. Numerous open and arthroscopic techniques have been described [120–123]. Our preferred technique is that of Ghosh et al. [122] and is discussed below.

- *Approach and exposure:* With the patient in lateral decubitus position, an oblique incision is made along the lateral border of the scapula, starting at the posterolateral corner of the acromion. Subcutaneous flaps are developed medially to identify the distinct muscle bellies of the teres major superiorly and latissimus dorsi inferiorly. Their respective neurovascular bundles, including the lower subscapular nerve and thoracodorsal nerve, are identified and protected.
- *Preparation of tendons for transfer:* Flaps are then developed laterally and proximally into the posterior axillary fold, following the muscle bellies to identify their tendinous attachments onto the humerus. In the posterior axillary fold, the tendon belongs to the latissimus while the muscle belongs to the teres major. The tendinous insertion of the latissimus dorsi is detached and mobilized together with its neurovascular bundle.
- *Completion of tendon transfer:* Superiorly, the posterior third of the deltoid muscle is split from the middle third in line with the muscle fibers. The infraspinatus is then exposed through this interval. The mobilized latissimus dorsi is then routed below the deltoid and attached to the tendon of the infraspinatus with the arm in maximal external rotation and abduction. Alternatively, the tendon may be attached through an arthroscopic assisted approach on the lateral aspect of the greater tuberosity, which limits the posterior incision and does not require a deltoid-splitting exposure.

4.8.1.3 Tendon Transfers for Radial Nerve Injury

Transfer of musculotendinous units from the median nerve is a well-established treatment for persistent radial nerve injuries [65, 69, 100, 107].

Due to the topographic anatomy of the radial nerve, injuries resulting from radial shaft fractures typically spare triceps and brachioradialis (BR) function and result in a loss of wrist, finger, and thumb extension [100, 107]. In the setting of persistent radial nerve injury in which nerve reconstruction is not being considered in favor of eventual tendon reconstruction, an observation period of 6 months is reasonable before electrodiagnostic testing of nerve reinnervation potential [91]. If evidence of latent reinnervation is detected, end-to-side tendon transfer of the PT to ECRB has been advocated as a temporizing measure to provide wrist extension while waiting for the muscles to reinnervate [100, 107]; however, this is controversial.

Several variations of tendon transfers have been described for radial nerve injuries that fail to show reinnervation after 6 months or longer of observation [65, 69, 100, 107]. Most of these involve transfer of PT to ECRB to restore wrist function. Restoration of thumb extension is most commonly accomplished with transfer of PL or FDS II to extensor pollicis longus (EPL). Restoration of finger extension is most controversial, with potential donors to extensor digitorum communis (EDC) being FCR (*Brand transfer*), FCU (*Jones transfer*), or FDS (*modified Boyes transfer*). The Brand transfer is our preferred method as this muscle has similar donor strength to its recipient EDC. The relative strength of FCU to EDC is 2:1, and thus, FCU transfer may generate greater donor site morbidity than necessary in terms of power grip. The modified Boyes transfer is a nonsynergistic transfer (donor FDS and recipient EDC), which may require more cognitive retraining. Key steps in the Brand transfer technique are outlined below:

- *Approach and exposure:* Typically, separate volar radial and dorsal radial approaches are needed to access the donor and recipient muscle groups, respectively.
- *Preparation of donor tendons – pronator teres:* Proximally, PT is exposed by mobilizing BR together with the mobile wad and lateral antebrachial cutaneous nerve radially. Just deep to this, PT is reliably located between the superficial sensory branch of the radial nerve radially and radial artery ulnarly. These structures must be protected while harvesting PT.
  – Key technical point: Since PT inserts onto the radius quite proximally, the excursion of the tendon itself may be insufficient for tension-free attachment to the donor muscle group. This can be overcome by harvesting the distal tendon together with a thin strip of periosteum extending 5–10 cm further down the radius [100].
- *Preparation of donor tendons – palmaris longus and flexor carpi radialis:* Distally, PL is a superficial structure ulnar to FCR. It is the thinner tendon, and care must be taken to protect the median nerve, which is deep to it. PL and FCR should both be released as distally as possible. It is also important to mobilize them from surrounding adhesions proximally to their musculotendinous junctions.
- *Preparation of recipient tendons – extensor carpi radialis brevis:* ECRB can be accessed through the volar incision by elevating the radial skin flap and retracting FCR ulnarly. ECRB is preferred over ECRL because of its more central insertion (onto the third metacarpal base), resulting in a central vector of wrist flexion [107]. The tendon is released as proximally as possible (at the level of the musculotendinous junction).
- *Preparation of recipient tendons – extensor pollicis longus and extensor digitorum communis:* A dorsal incision is used to access EPL and EDC. Distally, EPL and EDC are superficial tendons located in the third and fourth extensor compartments, respectively. The third compartment lies deep to the second and fourth compartments. The tendons should be mobilized and released as proximally as possible. Caution should be taken not to cut the extensor retinaculum distally, which would destabilize the tendon transfers and potentially lead to bowstringing and instability.
  – Key decision point: Various sequences can be used when performing the tendon transfers. We recommend performing transfers to the thumb and fingers first in order to

ensure appropriate tensioning by allowing the surgeon to move the wrist freely [100].

- *Tendon transfers – fingers:* EPL is transposed out of the third extensor compartment to the volar exposure by tunneling it under the radial skin flap. FCR is transposed from the volar exposure to the dorsal exposure. Pulvertaft weaves are used to weave EPL into PL and FCR into EDC.
  - Key technical point: Appropriate tensioning is crucial for the functional outcome. The transfers should be tensioned such that full finger extension can be achieved with the wrist in 30° of flexion, and the fingers can be passively curled into the palm with the wrist extended [100].
- *Tendon transfer – wrist:* PT is finally woven into ECRB. Tension is assessed by examining the wrist cascade, which should be compared to the passive cascade of the other wrist. Range of motion should be tested prior to immobilization once skin closure is complete.

4.8.2 Free Functioning Muscle Transfer

Free functioning muscle transfer (FFMT) using a pedicled gracilis graft has shown promising results in restoring elbow function in delayed brachial plexus reconstruction (Illustration 4.9) [65]. In fact, when treatment has been delayed by more than 12 months, FFMT consistently outperforms nerve transfers in improving elbow flexion strength [124–126]. Staged double free gracilis muscle transfer (DFMT) procedures have also been described, with potential to help restore flexion at the elbow, wrist, and fingers in patients with complete brachial plexus injuries [127,

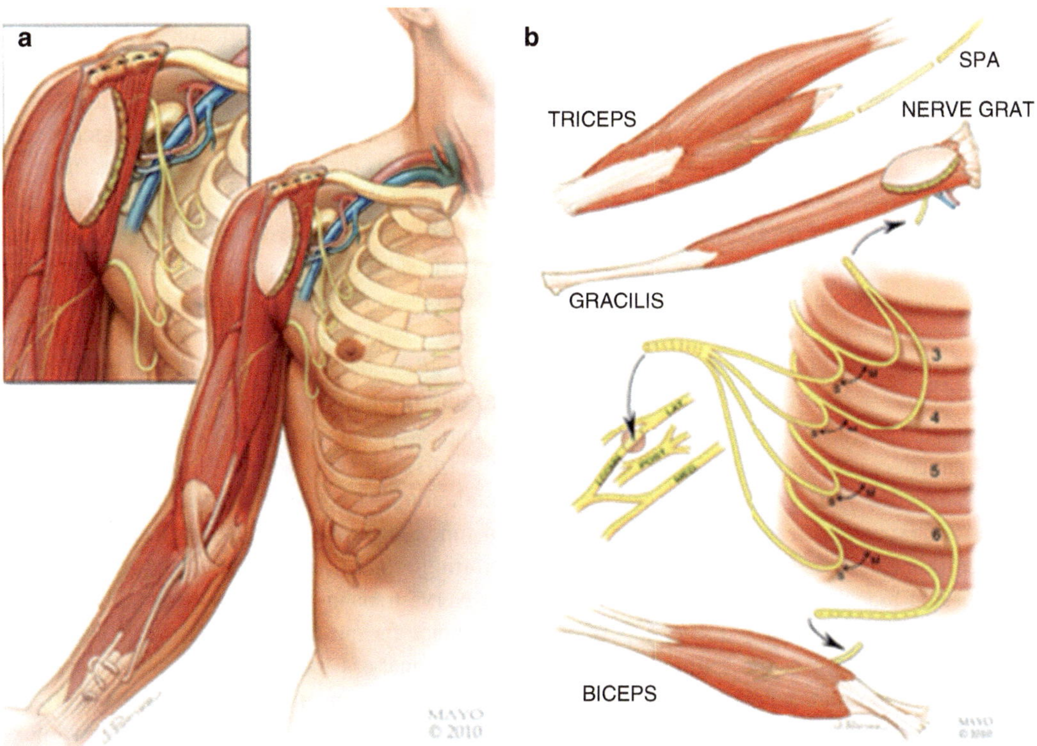

Illustration 4.9 Free-functioning muscle transfer of the gracilis muscle, supercharged with intercostal nerve transfers. Image (**a**) depicts the gracilis muscle and skin flap after inset onto the clavicle proximally and woven into the flexor tendons at the wrist distally. Image (**b**) depicts individual components of the transfer (Adapted from Noland et al. [65]). (With permission of the Mayo Foundation for Medical Education and Research. All rights reserved)

128]. In the context of shoulder arthroplasty, FFMT could lend itself to delayed presentations of musculocutaneous nerve injuries.

4.8.3 Shoulder Arthrodesis

Glenohumeral arthrodesis is an end-of-line salvage procedure used in the treatment of severe brachial plexus injuries [129, 130]. Its potential use after shoulder arthroplasty would be limited to situations in which severe nerve injury has resulted in persistent shoulder instability that cannot be restored with nerve or tendon transfers. Nerve injury in the setting of a chronically infected arthroplasty could also warrant such management. Some residual motion can be retained through the scapulothoracic joint, and limited scapulothoracic motion is a relative contraindication to shoulder arthrodesis [106]. While patients can expect to experience pain relief, function after shoulder arthrodesis remains poor, and a recently published retrospective series with 29 patients found rates of major complications and reoperation to be 41% and 38%, respectively [130].

4.9 Outcomes of Treatment

The prognosis of nerve injuries resulting from shoulder arthroplasty is excellent and few go on to require surgery [1, 2, 60]. Those that have required nerve reconstructive or salvage operations have generally had favorable outcomes, with patients achieving complete or near-complete recovery [3]. Our knowledge of the outcomes of specific nerve reconstructive and salvage procedures is largely derived from the literature on brachial plexus injuries, where they are most commonly employed. It is important to recognize that injury in the setting of shoulder arthroplasty represents an entirely different paradigm than brachial plexus injury. Whereas the latter results from significant high-energy trauma, shoulder arthroplasty is an elective procedure and a permanent nerve injury is a devastating complication.

Favorable results can be expected from nerve reconstruction provided it is performed within an appropriate timeframe. The prognosis of axillary nerve injuries has been well studied. In 99 patients with isolated stretch injuries to the axillary nerve, patients treated with neurolysis achieved a mean deltoid MRC grade of 4.0, those requiring nerve repair had a mean grade of 3.8 and those requiring nerve grafting had a mean grade of 3.7 [72]. In a series of 176 patients with posttraumatic brachial plexopathies, in which the majority were treated with a combination of nerve transfers and grafting of the axillary nerve, good or excellent results were only obtained in 46% of patients [76]. However, patients with infraclavicular brachial plexus lesions had significantly better outcomes (mean deltoid MRC grade of 3.85) than patients with more proximal lesions (mean deltoid MRC grade of 2.74). A retrospective series of 27 patients who underwent radial to axillary nerve transfers found that 63% of patients achieved a deltoid MRC grade of 4 or higher, and shoulder abduction increased from 12° preoperatively to 112° after surgery [131]. Baltzer et al. [71] compared 21 patients who underwent radial to axillary nerve transfers and 8 patients who underwent sural nerve grafting for isolated axillary nerve lesions. Clinical recovery first became apparent 10–11 months after surgery. Disability of the arm, shoulder, and hand (DASH) scores, deltoid strength, and range of motion improved after surgery in both groups. Average deltoid strength was grade 4 in the nerve grafting group and grade 3 in the nerve transfer group, differing significantly. However, the sample size in this study was small, and taken together the literature suggests that a substantial recovery of function can be expected whether using nerve grafting or nerve transfers.

Nerve transfer is the reconstructive treatment of choice for musculocutaneous nerve lesions. In a meta-analysis including 356 patients, 83% of patients who underwent nerve transfers to the musculocutaneous nerve achieved an elbow flexion MRC grade of 4 or higher compared to only 56% of patients who underwent nerve grafting [79]. This study also compared patients with combined axillary and suprascapular nerve deficits undergoing nerve transfers to address one or both nerves. Of the 54 patients who underwent dual transfers, 74% achieved a deltoid MRC grade of 4 or higher with mean postoperative shoulder abduction of 122°. Interestingly, patients who underwent nerve transfers to both the axillary and suprascapular nerves had significantly better strength and range of motion in shoulder abduction and external rotation than patients who underwent spinal accessory nerve to suprascapular nerve transfer alone. Albeit somewhat indirectly, these results suggest a poorer outlook for nerve reconstruction of the suprascapular nerve than other peripheral nerves. Concerningly, isolated suprascapular nerve lesions also appear to be less likely to recover spontaneously than axillary nerve lesions [38, 72]. Early surgical treatment of suprascapular nerve injuries within 6 months has also been shown to improve outcomes, and better results have been achieved with nerve transfers than with nerve grafting [82].

While MRC strength of 3–4 and a functional range of motion can be expected after nerve reconstructive procedures, the prognosis of salvage operations is more guarded. In a study of 52 patients who underwent lower trapezius transfer for paralytic shoulder injuries, mean shoulder abduction increased from 10° to 60° and external rotation increased from 0° to 20° [112]. Notably, this was a heterogeneous population where most patients underwent multiple simultaneous tendon transfers in addition to lower trapezius transfer. The relatively poor results are likely attributable to the severity of the preexisting injuries, making it difficult to generalize these findings to the context of shoulder arthroplasty. In fact, these results are not dissimilar from a series of 54 patients with severe brachial plexus injuries who underwent shoulder arthrodesis, as 75% of patients achieved shoulder abduction greater than 45° and 65% achieved external rotation greater than 45° with a 73% rate of successful fusion [129]. On the other hand, a series of 35 patients with incomplete injuries to C5 and C6 who underwent combined latissimus dorsi and teres major transfers showed an improvement in abduction from 74° preoperatively to 120° postoperatively, while external rotation improved from 5° to 31° [123]. External rotation strength increased in 83% of patients but abduction strength increased in only 37%. Nevertheless, the functional results were much better than in patients with pan-plexus injuries as in the studies above.

A recent systematic review showed a promising impact of lower trapezius transfers in patients with paralyzing shoulder conditions [115]. Across three studies including 69 patients with brachial plexus injuries, patients gained an average of 79.2° of external rotation, 43.4° of abduction, and 35.3° of forward elevation after tendon transfer surgery. Across two studies including 48 patients with massive irreparable rotator cuff tears and shoulder pseudoparalysis, patients gained 34.3° of external rotation, 50.0° of abduction, and 37.5° of forward elevation postoperatively. DASH scores also improved substantially in both patient populations.

Although tendon transfers remain the mainstay of treatment for late reconstruction of radial nerve injuries, recent findings suggest that early nerve transfer may afford better outcomes [132]. In this retrospective study by Bertelli, 14 patients underwent nerve transfer of the anterior interosseous nerve (AIN) to the motor branch of ECRB and FCR to the PIN and 13 patients underwent tendon transfers of PT to ECRB, FCU to EDC, and PL to EPL. Patients in the nerve transfer group achieved an average 67° of wrist extension, 66° of wrist flexion, and 58% recovery of grip strength, while patients in the tendon transfer group only achieved 35° of wrist extension, 37° of wrist flexion, and 43% recovery of grip strength. The nerve transfer group also performed better in terms of finger extension power and thumb range of motion. The outcomes of nerve transfer were consistent with previous studies grading mostly good to excellent outcomes for wrist power, with somewhat more variable results for finger and thumb power [103, 104]. Importantly, in the study by Bertelli [132], nerve transfers were performed at an average of 6 months after injury, while tendon transfers were performed on patients who presented more than 15 months after injury to the radial nerve. It is unclear whether earlier intervention with tendon transfers would have affected outcomes.

When it comes to tendon transfers, a study comparing the Brand, Jones, and modified Boyes tendon transfers found no significant differences in outcomes between groups, with 95% patient satisfaction overall [133]. Results for wrist motion were largely graded good to excellent, while outcomes were variable for finger and thumb motion. Currently, reconstruction of radial nerve injuries with nerve transfers or tendon transfers both appear to be viable options [134], and more studies directly comparing the treatments are needed.

Overall, the functional results of delayed salvage procedures are less consistent than the favorable outcomes seen with early reconstruction. While it is difficult to generalize the results of each procedure in the context of shoulder arthroplasty, it can be concluded that patients will be best served by prompt recognition and monitoring of injuries. Consideration of nerve reconstruction versus tendon transfer or alternative procedures should be made on an individual patient basis in consultation with an interdisciplinary team with expertise in each of the various techniques.

4.10 Technical Pearls and Pitfalls

Overview

- Nerve injuries during shoulder arthroplasty are rare but potentially devastating injuries, ranging on a spectrum from neuropraxia to neurotmesis.
- The prevalence of subclinical nerve trauma is common, indicating that neurologic structures are routinely endangered during surgery.

Prevention Strategies

- The axillary nerve is endangered during subscapularis tenotomies, dissection around the inferior margin of the glenoid, and forceful positioning of the arm. Injury can be avoided by careful releases of the subscapularis tendon and around the glenoid, with shoulder abduction less than 45°, dissecting under direct visualization and limiting traction and manipulation of the arm.
- The suprascapular nerve is endangered during placement of posterior and superior glenoid screws in RSA. Posterior and superior screws should be limited to less than 14 mm and 23 mm in length, respectively.
- The musculocutaneous nerve is vulnerable to injury during excessive retraction and far medial dissection of the conjoint tendon, which should be avoided.
- The *radial and subscapular nerves* are not routinely endangered during shoulder arthroplasty. Radial nerve injury should raise concern for peri-prosthetic fracture or cement extrusion in the setting of revision arthroplasty.

History and Clinical Evaluation

- The vast majority of nerve injuries resolve spontaneously after a period of observation.
- Nerve injuries can be detected on clinical exam within 7 days of surgery. A thorough neurologic history and physical assessment should be completed at every clinic visit.
- Electrodiagnostic testing should be performed between 6 weeks and 3 months after surgery for injuries that do not improve clinically.

Surgical Management

- Surgery is indicated when there is no evidence of clinical or electrophysiologic recovery after 3 months of observation.
- Nerve repair or neurolysis is favored over more complex procedures when feasible.
- Nerve reconstructive procedures are ideally performed within 3–6 months of injury, whereas salvage procedures are required if treatment is delayed by more than 12 months.
- Interpositional nerve grafting or radial to axillary nerve transfer are well-established primary reconstructive options for *axillary nerve* injuries with successful outcomes. Salvage options include upper trapezius tendon transfer or joint arthrodesis for a persistently unstable shoulder joint.
- Screw removal with neurolysis is the initial treatment for persistent *suprascapular nerve* injuries in the setting of RSA. Although rarely

necessary, the best reconstructive option is spinal accessory to suprascapular nerve transfer. Salvage options include lower trapezius and latissimus dorsi transfers.

- Oberlin transfer is a reliable primary reconstructive option for *musculocutaneous nerve* injuries and has better outcomes than nerve grafting. FFMT is a promising salvage option when treatment has been delayed for more than 12 months.
- Although nerve transfers for *radial nerve* injuries have shown promise, tendon transfers remain the preferred treatment for injuries that do not resolve after nerve exploration and neurolysis.

Outcomes

- Results of nerve reconstruction are generally favorable, and recovery of MRC grade 3–4 strength and a functional range of motion can be expected for most injuries.
- Suprascapular nerve injuries have a poorer prognosis for nonoperative recovery and nerve reconstruction than axillary nerve injuries.
- Salvage operations are generally inferior to nerve reconstruction, highlighting the importance of early diagnosis and treatment.

References

1. Boardman ND 3rd, Cofield RH. Neurologic complications of shoulder surgery. Clin Orthop Relat Res. 1999;368(368):44–53.
2. Bohsali KI, Bois AJ, Wirth MA. Complications of shoulder arthroplasty. J. Bone Joint Surg Am Vol. 2017;99(3):256–69.
3. Carofino BC, et al. Iatrogenic nerve injuries during shoulder surgery. J. Bone Joint Surg Am Vol. 2013;95(18):1667–74.
4. Kim HJ, et al. Neurologic deficit after reverse total shoulder arthroplasty: correlation with distalization. J Shoulder Elb Surg. 2020;29:1096–103.
5. Ladermann A, et al. Injury to the axillary nerve after reverse shoulder arthroplasty: an anatomical study. Orthop Traumatol Surg Res: OTSR. 2014;100(1):105–8.
6. Lowe JT, et al. Lateralization of the glenosphere in reverse shoulder arthroplasty decreases arm lengthening and demonstrates comparable risk of nerve injury compared with anatomic arthroplasty: a prospective cohort study. J Shoulder Elb Surg. 2018;27(10):1845–51.
7. Boileau P, et al. Neer Award 2005: the Grammont reverse shoulder prosthesis: results in cuff tear arthritis, fracture sequelae, and revision arthroplasty. J Shoulder Elb Surg. 2006;15(5):527–40.
8. Wirth MA, Rockwood CA Jr. Complications of total shoulder-replacement arthroplasty. J Bone Joint Surg Am Vol. 1996;78(4):603–16.
9. Parisien RL, et al. The risk of nerve injury during anatomical and reverse total shoulder arthroplasty: an intraoperative neuromonitoring study. J Shoulder Elb Surg. 2016;25(7):1122–7.
10. Sherfey MC, Edwards TB. Cement extrusion causing radial nerve palsy after shoulder arthroplasty: a case report. J Shoulder Elb Surg. 2009;18(3):e21–4.
11. Ladermann A, et al. Prevalence of neurologic lesions after total shoulder arthroplasty. J Bone Joint Surg Am Vol. 2011;93(14):1288–93.
12. Wingert NC, Beck JD, Harter GD. Avulsive axillary artery injury in reverse total shoulder arthroplasty. Orthopedics. 2014;37(1):e92–7.
13. Athwal GS, et al. Periprosthetic humeral fractures during shoulder arthroplasty. J Bone Joint Surg Am Vol. 2009;91(3):594–603.
14. Conn RA, et al. Interscalene block anesthesia for shoulder surgery. Clin Orthop Relat Res. 1987;(216):94–8.
15. Wiater JM, Fabing MH. Shoulder arthroplasty: prosthetic options and indications. J Am Acad Orthop Surg. 2009;17(7):415–25.
16. Cerciello S, et al. Shoulder arthroplasty to address the sequelae of anterior instability arthropathy and stabilization procedures: systematic review and meta-analysis. Arch Orthop Trauma Surg. 2020;140:1891–900.
17. Cho CH, Kim DH, Song KS. Reverse shoulder arthroplasty in patients with rheumatoid arthritis: a systematic review. Clin Orthop Surg. 2017;9(3):325–31.
18. Ferrel JR, Trinh TQ, Fischer RA. Reverse total shoulder arthroplasty versus hemiarthroplasty for proximal humeral fractures: a systematic review. J Orthop Trauma. 2015;29(1):60–8.
19. Gerber C, Pennington SD, Nyffeler RW. Reverse total shoulder arthroplasty. J Am Acad Orthop Surg. 2009;17(5):284–95.
20. Sears BW, et al. Glenoid bone loss in primary total shoulder arthroplasty: evaluation and management. J Am Acad Orthop Surg. 2012;20(9):604–13.
21. Marion B, et al. Potential axillary nerve stretching during RSA implantation: an anatomical study. Anat Sci Int. 2014;89(4):232–7.
22. Apaydin N, et al. Review of the surgical anatomy of the axillary nerve and the anatomic basis of its iatrogenic and traumatic injury. Surg Radiol Anat: SRA. 2010;32(3):193–201.
23. Perlmutter GS. Axillary nerve injury. Clin Orthop Relat Res. 1999;(368):28–36.

24. Tubbs RS, et al. Surgical landmarks for the proximal portion of the axillary nerve. J Neurosurg. 2001;95(6):998–1000.
25. Apaydin N, et al. The anatomic relationships of the axillary nerve and surgical landmarks for its localization from the anterior aspect of the shoulder. Clin Anat (New York, N.Y.). 2007;20(3):273–7.
26. Gurushantappa PK, Kuppasad S. Anatomy of axillary nerve and its clinical importance: a cadaveric study. J Clin Diagn Res. 2015;9(3):AC13–7.
27. Scully WF, et al. Iatrogenic nerve injuries in shoulder surgery. J Am Acad Orthop Surg. 2013;21(12):717–26.
28. Uz A, et al. The anatomic branch pattern of the axillary nerve. J Shoulder Elb Surg. 2007;16(2):240–4.
29. Duparc F, et al. Anatomical basis of the variable aspects of injuries of the axillary nerve (excluding the terminal branches in the deltoid muscle). Surg Radiol Anat: SRA. 1997;19(3):127–32.
30. Loomer R, Graham B. Anatomy of the axillary nerve and its relation to inferior capsular shift. Clin Orthop Relat Res. 1989;(243):100–5.
31. Delaney RA, et al. 2014 Neer Award Paper: neuromonitoring the Latarjet procedure. (1532–6500 (Electronic)).
32. Shah AA, et al. Short-term complications of the Latarjet procedure. J Bone Joint Surg Am Vol. 2012;94(6):495–501.
33. Cetik O, et al. Is there a safe area for the axillary nerve in the deltoid muscle? A cadaveric study. J Bone Joint Surg Am Vol. 2006;88(11):2395–9.
34. Cheung S, Fitzpatrick M, Lee TQ. Effects of shoulder position on axillary nerve positions during the split lateral deltoid approach. J Shoulder Elb Surg. 2009;18(5):748–55.
35. Leschinger T, et al. The risk of suprascapular and axillary nerve injury in reverse total shoulder arthroplasty: an anatomic study. Injury. 2017;48(10):2042–9.
36. Yoo JC, et al. Arthroscopic perspective of the axillary nerve in relation to the glenoid and arm position: a cadaveric study. Arthrosc: J Arthrosc Relat Surg. 2007;23(12):1271–7.
37. Simone JP, et al. Change in the distance from the axillary nerve to the glenohumeral joint with shoulder external rotation or abduction position. Hand (New York, N.Y.). 2017;12(4):395–400.
38. Lopiz Y, et al. Injury to the axillary and suprascapular nerves in rotator cuff arthropathy and after reverse shoulder arthroplasty: a prospective electromyographic analysis. J Shoulder Elb Surg. 2018;27(7):1275–82.
39. Wang J, et al. Suprascapular neuropathy secondary to reverse shoulder arthroplasty: a case report. J Shoulder Elb Surg. 2010;19(3):e5–8.
40. Molony DC, et al. A cadaveric model for suprascapular nerve injury during glenoid component screw insertion in reverse-geometry shoulder arthroplasty. J Shoulder Elb Surg. 2011;20(8):1323–7.
41. Shishido H, Kikuchi S. Injury of the suprascapular nerve in shoulder surgery: an anatomic study. J Shoulder Elb Surg. 2001;10(4):372–6.
42. Albritton MJ, et al. An anatomic study of the effects on the suprascapular nerve due to retraction of the supraspinatus muscle after a rotator cuff tear. J Shoulder Elb Surg. 2003;12(5):497–500.
43. Shi LL, et al. Association of suprascapular neuropathy with rotator cuff tendon tears and fatty degeneration. J Shoulder Elb Surg. 2014;23(3):339–46.
44. Ma H, et al. Musculocutaneous nerve entrapment: an unusual complication after biceps tenodesis. Am J Sports Med. 2009;37(12):2467–9.
45. Nagda SH, et al. Neer Award 2005: peripheral nerve function during shoulder arthroplasty using intraoperative nerve monitoring. J Shoulder Elb Surg. 2007;16(3 Suppl):S2–8.
46. Guerri-Guttenberg RA, Ingolotti M. Classifying musculocutaneous nerve variations. Clin Anat (New York, N.Y.). 2009;22(6):671–83.
47. Clavert P, et al. Relationships of the musculocutaneous nerve and the coracobrachialis during coracoid abutment procedure (Latarjet procedure). Surg Radiol Anat: SRA. 2009;31(1):49–53.
48. Fram B, Elder A, Namdari S. Periprosthetic humeral fractures in shoulder arthroplasty. JBJS Rev. 2019;7(11):e6.
49. Fu MC, et al. Surgical anatomy of the radial nerve in the deltopectoral approach for revision shoulder arthroplasty and periprosthetic fracture fixation: a cadaveric study. J Shoulder Elb Surg. 2017;26(12):2173–6.
50. Gerber C, et al. Subscapularis muscle function and structure after total shoulder replacement with lesser tuberosity osteotomy and repair. J Bone Joint Surg Am Vol. 2005;87(8):1739–45.
51. Miller SL, et al. Loss of subscapularis function after total shoulder replacement: a seldom recognized problem. J Shoulder Elb Surg. 2003;12(1):29–34.
52. Sager B, et al. Innervation of the subscapularis: an anatomic study. JSES Open Access. 2019;3(2):65–9.
53. Walley KC, et al. Characterization of an anatomic safe zone surrounding the lower subscapular nerve during an open deltopectoral approach. J Shoulder Elb Surg. 2019;28(4):671–7.
54. Kasper JC, et al. Human cadaveric study of subscapularis muscle innervation and guidelines to prevent denervation. J Shoulder Elb Surg. 2008;17(4):659–62.
55. Gutierrez S, et al. Biomechanical comparison of component position and hardware failure in the reverse shoulder prosthesis. J Shoulder Elb Surg. 2007;16(3 Suppl):S9–S12.
56. Gutierrez S, et al. Range of impingement-free abduction and adduction deficit after reverse shoulder arthroplasty. Hierarchy of surgical and implant-design-related factors. J Bone Joint Surg Am Vol. 2008;90(12):2606–15.
57. Simovitch RW, et al. Predictors of scapular notching in patients managed with the Delta III reverse total

shoulder replacement. J Bone Joint Surg Am Vol. 2007;89(3):588–600.
58. Wright J, et al. A quantitative analysis of the effect of baseplate and glenosphere position on deltoid lengthening in reverse total shoulder arthroplasty. Int J Shoulder Surg. 2015;9(2):33–7.
59. Acott TR, et al. A quantitative analysis of deltoid lengthening and deltoid-related complications after reverse total shoulder arthroplasty: a retrospective case-control study. Curr Orthop Pract. 2020;31(2):126–32.
60. Rahmi H, Jawa A. Management of complications after revision shoulder arthroplasty. Curr Rev Musculoskelet Med. 2015;8(1):98–106.
61. Lynch NM, et al. Neurologic complications after total shoulder arthroplasty. J Shoulder Elb Surg. 1996;5(1):53–61.
62. Bertelli JA, Ghizoni MF. Abduction in internal rotation: a test for the diagnosis of axillary nerve palsy. J Hand Surg Am. 2011;36(12):2017–23.
63. Mitchell JJ, et al. Axillary nerve palsy and deltoid muscle atony. JBJS Rev. 2017;5(7):e1.
64. Elton SG, Rizzo M. Management of radial nerve injury associated with humeral shaft fractures: an evidence-based approach. J Reconstr Microsurg. 2008;24(8):569–73.
65. Noland SS, et al. Adult traumatic brachial plexus injuries. J Am Acad Orthop Surg. 2019;27(19):705–16.
66. Shin AY, et al. Adult traumatic brachial plexus injuries. J Am Acad Orthop Surg. 2005;13(6):382–96.
67. Holzgrefe RE, et al. Imaging of the peripheral nerve: concepts and future direction of magnetic resonance neurography and ultrasound. J Hand Surg Am. 2019;44(12):1066–79.
68. Isaacs J, Cochran AR. Nerve transfers for peripheral nerve injury in the upper limb: a case-based review. Bone Joint J. 2019;101-B(2):124–31.
69. Giuffre JL, et al. The best of tendon and nerve transfers in the upper extremity. Plast Reconstr Surg. 2015;135(3):617e–30e.
70. Steinmann SP, Moran EA. Axillary nerve injury: diagnosis and treatment. J Am Acad Orthop Surg. 2001;9(5):328–35.
71. Baltzer HL, et al. A comparison of outcomes of triceps motor branch-to-axillary nerve transfer or sural nerve interpositional grafting for isolated axillary nerve injury. Plast Reconstr Surg. 2016;138(2):256e–64e.
72. Kline DG, Kim DH. Axillary nerve repair in 99 patients with 101 stretch injuries. J Neurosurg. 2003;99(4):630–6.
73. McAdams TR, Dillingham MF. Surgical decompression of the quadrilateral space in overhead athletes. Am J Sports Med. 2008;36(3):528–32.
74. Petrucci FS, Morelli A, Raimondi PL. Axillary nerve injuries--21 cases treated by nerve graft and neurolysis. J Hand Surg Am. 1982;7(3):271–8.
75. Mackinnon SE, et al. Selection of optimal axon ratio for nerve regeneration. Ann Plast Surg. 1989;23(2):129–34.
76. Terzis JK, Barmpitsioti A. Axillary nerve reconstruction in 176 posttraumatic plexopathy patients. Plast Reconstr Surg. 2010;125(1):233–47.
77. Wolfe SW, et al. Long-nerve grafts and nerve transfers demonstrate comparable outcomes for axillary nerve injuries. J Hand Surg Am. 2014;39(7):1351–7.
78. Baltzer HL, et al. Axillary nerve reconstruction: anterior-posterior exposure with sural nerve cable graft pull-through technique. Tech Hand Up Extrem Surg. 2015;19(4):168–75.
79. Garg R, et al. Comparison of nerve transfers and nerve grafting for traumatic upper plexus palsy: a systematic review and analysis. J Bone Joint Surg Am Vol. 2011;93(9):819–29.
80. Lee JY, et al. Factors affecting outcome of triceps motor branch transfer for isolated axillary nerve injury. J Hand Surg Am. 2012;37(11):2350–6.
81. Leechavengvongs S, et al. Nerve transfer to deltoid muscle using the nerve to the long head of the triceps, part II: a report of 7 cases. J Hand Surg Am. 2003;28(4):633–8.
82. Terzis JK, Kostas I. Suprascapular nerve reconstruction in 118 cases of adult posttraumatic brachial plexus. Plast Reconstr Surg. 2006;117(2):613–29.
83. Dailiana ZH, Mehdian H, Gilbert A. Surgical anatomy of spinal accessory nerve: is trapezius functional deficit inevitable after division of the nerve? J Hand Surg (Edinb, Scotl). 2001;26(2):137–41.
84. Colbert SH, Mackinnon S. Posterior approach for double nerve transfer for restoration of shoulder function in upper brachial plexus palsy. Hand (New York, N.Y.). 2006;1(2):71–7.
85. Leechavengvongs S, et al. Nerve transfer to biceps muscle using a part of the ulnar nerve in brachial plexus injury (upper arm type): a report of 32 cases. J Hand Surg Am. 1998;23(4):711–6.
86. Mackinnon SE, et al. Results of reinnervation of the biceps and brachialis muscles with a double fascicular transfer for elbow flexion. J Hand Surg Am. 2005;30(5):978–85.
87. Oberlin C, et al. Nerve transfer to biceps muscle using a part of ulnar nerve for C5-C6 avulsion of the brachial plexus: anatomical study and report of four cases. J Hand Surg Am. 1994;19(2):232–7.
88. Bhandari PS, Deb P. Management of isolated musculocutaneous injury: comparing double fascicular nerve transfer with conventional nerve grafting. J Hand Surg Am. 2015;40(10):2003–6.
89. Martins RS, et al. A prospective study comparing single and double fascicular transfer to restore elbow flexion after brachial plexus injury. Neurosurgery. 2013;72(5):709–14; discussion 714–5; quiz 715.
90. Bhandari PS, Deb P. Fascicular selection for nerve transfers: the role of the nerve stimulator when restoring elbow flexion in brachial plexus injuries. J Hand Surg Am. 2011;36(12):2002–9.
91. Carroll EA, et al. Management of humeral shaft fractures. J Am Acad Orthop Surg. 2012;20(7):423–33.
92. Ljungquist KL, Martineau P, Allan C. Radial nerve injuries. J Hand Surg Am. 2015;40(1):166–72.

93. Rocchi M, et al. Humerus shaft fracture complicated by radial nerve palsy: is surgical exploration necessary? Musculoskelet Surg. 2016;100(Suppl 1):53–60.
94. Shao YC, et al. Radial nerve palsy associated with fractures of the shaft of the humerus: a systematic review. J Bone Joint Surg Br Vol. 2005;87(12):1647–52.
95. Sonneveld GJ, et al. Treatment of fractures of the shaft of the humerus accompanied by paralysis of the radial nerve. Injury. 1987;18(6):404–6.
96. Bishop J, Ring D. Management of radial nerve palsy associated with humeral shaft fracture: a decision analysis model. J Hand Surg. 2009;34(6):991–6.e1.
97. Bodner G, et al. Sonographic detection of radial nerve entrapment within a humerus fracture. J Ultrasound Med. 1999;18(10):703–6.
98. Thes A, et al. Cortical onlay strut allograft with cerclage wiring of periprosthetic fractures of the humerus without stem loosening: technique and preliminary results. Eur J Orthop Surg Traumatol: Orthop Traumatol. 2017;27(4):553–7.
99. Lowe JB 3rd, Sen SK, Mackinnon SE. Current approach to radial nerve paralysis. Plast Reconstr Surg. 2002;110(4):1099–113.
100. Ratner JA, Peljovich A, Kozin SH. Update on tendon transfers for peripheral nerve injuries. J Hand Surg Am. 2010;35(8):1371–81.
101. Brown JM, Tung TH, Mackinnon SE. Median to radial nerve transfer to restore wrist and finger extension: technical nuances. Neurosurgery. 2010;66(3 Suppl Operative):75–83; discussion 83.
102. Davidge KM, et al. Median to radial nerve transfers for restoration of wrist, finger, and thumb extension. J Hand Surg Am. 2013;38(9):1812–27.
103. Garcia-Lopez A, et al. Nerve transfers from branches to the flexor carpi radialis and pronator teres to reconstruct the radial nerve. J Hand Surg Am. 2014;39(1):50–6.
104. Ray WZ, Mackinnon SE. Clinical outcomes following median to radial nerve transfers. J Hand Surg Am. 2011;36(2):201–8.
105. Coulet B. Principles of tendon transfers. Hand Surg Rehabil. 2016;35(2):68–80.
106. Elhassan B, et al. Shoulder tendon transfer options for adult patients with brachial plexus injury. J Hand Surg Am. 2010;35(7):1211–9.
107. Sammer DM, Chung KC. Tendon transfers: part I. Principles of transfer and transfers for radial nerve palsy. Plast Reconstr Surg. 2009;123(5):169e–77e.
108. Burnier M, Elhassan BT, Sanchez-Sotelo J. Surgical management of irreparable rotator cuff tears: what works, what does not, and what is coming. J Bone Joint Surg Br Vol. 2019;101(17):1603–12.
109. Aziz W, Singer RM, Wolff TW. Transfer of the trapezius for flail shoulder after brachial plexus injury. J Bone Joint Surg Br Vol. 1990;72(4):701–4.
110. Ruhmann O, et al. Trapezius transfer in brachial plexus palsy. Correlation of the outcome with muscle power and operative technique. J Bone Joint Surg Br Vol. 2005;87(2):184–90.
111. Crepaldi BE, et al. Lower trapezius transfer for patients with brachial plexus injury. Hand (New York, N.Y.). 2019;14(2):179–86.
112. Elhassan B, et al. Tendon transfer options about the shoulder in patients with brachial plexus injury. J Bone Joint Surg Br Vol. 2012;94(15):1391–8.
113. Bassett RW, et al. Glenohumeral muscle force and moment mechanics in a position of shoulder instability. J Biomech. 1990;23(5):405–15.
114. Keating JF, et al. The relative strengths of the rotator cuff muscles. A cadaver study. J Bone Joint Surg Br Vol. 1993;75(1):137–40.
115. Clouette J, et al. The lower trapezius transfer: a systematic review of biomechanical data, techniques, and clinical outcomes. J Shoulder Elbow Surg. 2020;29:1505–12.
116. Saha AK. Surgery of the paralysed and flail shoulder. Acta Orthop Scand. 1967;38(Suppl 97):5–90.
117. Elhassan B. Lower trapezius transfer for shoulder external rotation in patients with paralytic shoulder. J Hand Surg Am. 2014;39(3):556–62.
118. Checchia C, et al. Current options in tendon transfers for irreparable rotator cuff tears. JBJS Rev. 2019;7(2):e6.
119. Popescu IA, et al. Functional improvements in active elevation, external rotation, and internal rotation after reverse total shoulder arthroplasty with isolated latissimus dorsi transfer: surgical technique and midterm follow-up. J Shoulder Elb Surg. 2019;28(12):2356–63.
120. Cutbush K, Peter NA, Hirpara K. All-arthroscopic latissimus dorsi transfer. Arthrosc Tech. 2016;5(3):e607–13.
121. Gerber C, et al. Latissimus dorsi transfer for the treatment of massive tears of the rotator cuff. A preliminary report. Clin Orthop Relat Res. 1988;(232):51–61.
122. Ghosh S, et al. Isolated latissimus dorsi transfer to restore shoulder external rotation in adults with brachial plexus injury. Bone Joint J. 2013;95-B(5):660–3.
123. Phipps GJ, Hoffer MM. Latissimus dorsi and teres major transfer to rotator cuff for Erb's palsy. J Shoulder Elb Surg. 1995;4(2):124–9.
124. Hoang D, Chen VW, Seruya M. Recovery of elbow flexion after nerve reconstruction versus free functional muscle transfer for late, traumatic brachial plexus palsy: a systematic review. Plast Reconstr Surg. 2018;141(4):949–59.
125. Maldonado AA, et al. Free functioning gracilis muscle transfer versus intercostal nerve transfer to musculocutaneous nerve for restoration of elbow flexion after traumatic adult brachial pan-plexus injury. Plast Reconstr Surg. 2016;138(3):483e–8e.
126. Maldonado AA, et al. Free functioning gracilis muscle transfer with and without simultaneous intercostal nerve transfer to musculocutaneous

nerve for restoration of elbow flexion after traumatic adult brachial pan-plexus injury. J Hand Surg. 2017;42(4):293.e1–7.
127. Doi K, et al. Current procedure of double free muscle transfer for traumatic total brachial plexus palsy. JBJS Essent Surg Tech. 2013;3(3):e16.
128. Elzinga K, et al. Double free gracilis muscle transfer after complete brachial plexus injury: first Canadian experience. Plast Surg (Oakville, Ont.). 2014;22(1):26–9.
129. Atlan F, et al. Functional outcome of glenohumeral fusion in brachial plexus palsy: a report of 54 cases. J Hand Surg Am. 2012;37(4):683–8.
130. Wagner ER, et al. Long-term outcomes of glenohumeral arthrodesis. J Bone Joint Surg Am Vol. 2018;100(7):598–604.
131. Desai MJ, et al. Radial to axillary nerve transfers: a combined case series. J Hand Surg Am. 2016;41(12):1128–34.
132. Bertelli JA. Nerve versus tendon transfer for radial nerve paralysis reconstruction. J Hand Surg Am. 2020;45:418–26.
133. Moussavi AA, Saied A, Karbalaeikhani A. Outcome of tendon transfer for radial nerve paralysis: comparison of three methods. Indian J Orthop. 2011;45(6):558–62.
134. Compton J, et al. Systematic review of tendon transfer versus nerve transfer for the restoration of wrist extension in isolated traumatic radial nerve palsy. J Am Acad Orthop Surg Glob Res Rev. 2018;2(4):e001.

Nerve Injury After Humerus, Elbow, and Forearm Fractures (Radial, Posterior Interosseous, and Ulnar Nerves)

5

Charles A. Daly and Michael B. Gottschalk

5.1 Introduction

Peripheral nerve injuries are common due to the nature of the practice of orthopedic surgery. These lesions span a spectrum between neurapraxia sustained at the time of injury to iatrogenic nerve lacerations. Our understanding of peripheral nerve pathology and surgery has undergone dramatic growth within the last decade. Despite this, there is still considerable opportunity for continued improvement. Not only is timely treatment of many of these peripheral nerve injuries paramount, but this treatment varies dramatically based on patient characteristics and injury patterns. Injury characteristics play a significant role within the treatment paradigm for nerve repair/reconstruction, and surgeons should be aware of the concomitant pathology associated with fractures/dislocations, as well as the potential pitfalls during operative intervention of these injuries. When a nerve injury is encountered, an appropriate treatment plan can vary from conservative management with maintenance of passive range of motion to urgent nerve grafting and nerve transfers. When combined with the disability of the associated musculoskeletal injury, these peripheral nerve complications can be particularly onerous on the patient as well as the practitioner. The principles that follow will provide guidance to treat and mitigate the morbidity from these complex pathologies.

5.2 Humeral Shaft Fractures: Radial Nerve

Humeral shaft fractures are one of the most common orthopedic injuries, accounting for nearly 3% of all fractures [1]. Studies have demonstrated an incidence of about 3 per 100,000 per year with recent trends toward surgeons performing more surgical fixation than previous years [2–4]. Radial nerve palsy after humeral shaft fractures has been reported as the most common neurovascular complication of any long bone fracture. The incidence varies based on the location of the fracture with Mangan et al. reporting rates as low as 1.5% in proximal third, 41.5% in middle third, and 56.9% in distal third fractures. With preoperative rates of radial nerve palsy approaching 12% for humeral shaft fractures, operative intervention further poses an additional risk of radial nerve injury [5–7].

The proposed mechanism for radial nerve palsy following a distal humerus fracture was originally described by Holstein and Lewis [8]. The initial rationale was based on its proximity to the bone and entrapment of the nerve between

C. A. Daly (✉) · M. B. Gottschalk
Division of Upper Extremity Surgery, Department of Orthopedic Surgery, Emory University, Atlanta, GA, USA
e-mail: cadaly@emory.edu; Michael.gottschalk@emoryhealthcare.org

C. J. Dy et al. (eds.), *Peripheral Nerve Issues after Orthopedic Surgery*, https://doi.org/10.1007/978-3-030-84428-8_5

the two fracture fragments. However, several studies have investigated the course of the radial nerve about the humerus and its spiral groove, suggesting that it is more likely the amount of displacement of the fracture, instead of the nerve's relative proximity to the bone; given the nerve is 1–5 cm away from the bone at level of the distal 1/3 of the humerus (Fig. 5.1) [9–15]. To further substantiate this corollary, Carlan et al. have provided a more detailed description of when the nerve is most in contact with the humerus [10]. There is a 6.3 cm area of contact within the spiral groove located between 17.1 and 10.9 cm proximal to the lateral epicondyle, and between the exit of the spiral groove (10.9 cm from the lateral epicondyle) and the proximal aspect of the metaphyseal flare [16]. Given the nerve is directly adjacent to the bone at these locations, any surgical fixation must ensure that the nerve has been freed completely prior to passing any plate.

Injury to the radial nerve in the brachium can place several structures at risk. The nerve is responsible for providing innervation to all three heads of the triceps (from which the motor branches exit the nerve in the proximal third of the brachium), the lateral cutaneous sensation of the brachium, motor for the radial half of the brachialis, the wrist, finger, and thumb extensors, and the posterior cutaneous sensation of the forearm and hand. Functional loss of any of the motor fibers of the nerve can render the limb significantly impaired.

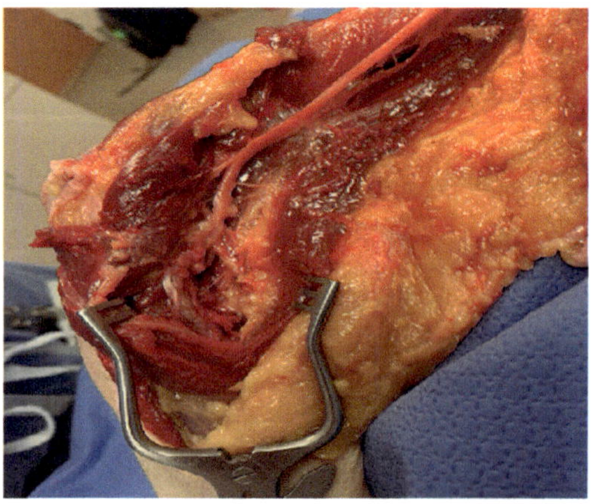

Fig. 5.1 Course of the radial nerve about the distal humerus

5.2.1 Humeral Shaft: Anatomic Considerations

The radial nerve proper receives contributions from C5 to T1, travels dorsal to the axillary artery and vein, passes deep to the lateral head of the triceps, and at this point provides motor branches to the triceps. The nerve travels in the spiral groove, typically directly posterior at the level of the deltoid tuberosity. The posterior cutaneous nerve to the arm and the posterior cutaneous nerve to the forearm branch off and the radial nerve proper continues deep crossing the humerus in the spiral groove and pierces the lateral intramuscular septum just over 10 cm proximal to the lateral epicondyle. Distal to this point, the radial nerve lies between the brachialis and brachioradialis providing a reproducible location for identification.

Several factors must be taken in to account when determining the appropriate surgical approach for the treatment of humerus fractures, including the location and extent of fracture, and any associated open wounds. In most cases, the extent of the exposure needed and the location of the fracture (proximal, middle, or distal) dictates the surgical approach and associated neurovascular risks [12, 15]. The most common surgical approaches include the anterolateral (e.g., deltopectoral) and direct lateral (e.g., deltoid split) for proximal fractures, either the anterolateral or posterior/posterolateral for midshaft fractures, and the posterior/posterolateral for distal fractures.

The anterolateral approach is a more distal extension of the deltopectoral exposure in the internervous *plane* between muscles innervated by the radial and axillary nerves. As the exposure moves distally, the biceps brachii may be retracted medially exposing the brachialis and more distally the brachioradialis. The lateral antebrachial cutaneous nerve should be identified between the brachialis and the brachioradialis and is the terminal extension of the musculocutaneous nerve. As the approach is deepened, the radial nerve can be identified piercing the lateral intermuscular septum at an average of 12.8 cm proximal to the lateral epicondyle as it innervates the lateral aspect of the brachialis and the brachioradialis [16]. Alternatively, the brachialis may be incised through the midline of the humerus and the radial half retracted thus protecting the radial nerve during midshaft plating of the humerus. Any injury to the nerve at this location will spare the triceps branches of the nerve but will include all wrist and finger extensors. The authors prefer this approach for simple midshaft fractures as it poses minimal risk to the radial or median nerves at this location as the nerve is often directly posterior to the humerus at the level of the deltoid tuberosity. An anatomic study showed from this anterior approach, the radial nerve was estimated to enter the spiral groove approximately 4 cm from the lower border of the latissimus dorsi insertion [17].

For more distal fractures or those that include the entirety of the humerus, with the exception of the proximal portion, a posterior or modified posterolateral approach can provide up to 94% exposure of the humerus [12]. The posterior or triceps splitting approach requires intramuscular dissection, and its distal extension is limited due to triceps attachment on the olecranon. The posterolateral approach to humerus allows dissection through an intramuscular, intranervous plane between the triceps and the anterior compartment of the brachium, just posterior to the lateral intramuscular septum. This approach is most safe for distal fractures that are less than 7.5–10 cm from the lateral epicondyle as these fall within the safe zone of injury of the radial nerve [15]. However, for midshaft fractures that are more proximal than this area, the radial nerve will require dissection and mobilization for adequate fracture repair. The lower lateral brachial cutaneous nerve is often easily identified in the subcutaneous tissues of the lateral aspect of the midbrachium and may be used to help trace the nerve proximally to the radial nerve proper (Fig. 5.2). The exposure may be taken up proximally all the way up to the axillary nerve by medially retracting the triceps muscles and elevating them off the humerus proximally. The radial nerve will have several triceps branches proximally which can make mobilization and fracture reduction challenging in cases of very proximal fractures. Care must be taken with both retractor placement and fracture reduction, as these are common causes of nerve injury. As the nerve courses laterally over the humerus, internal rotation of the distal fracture fragment will cause excess undue tension on the radial nerve and has a high possibility of causing radial nerve palsy (Fig. 5.3). External rotation of the distal fragment can be performed without similar risks of radial nerve palsy as it will decrease tension on radial nerve. The authors recommend this approach for

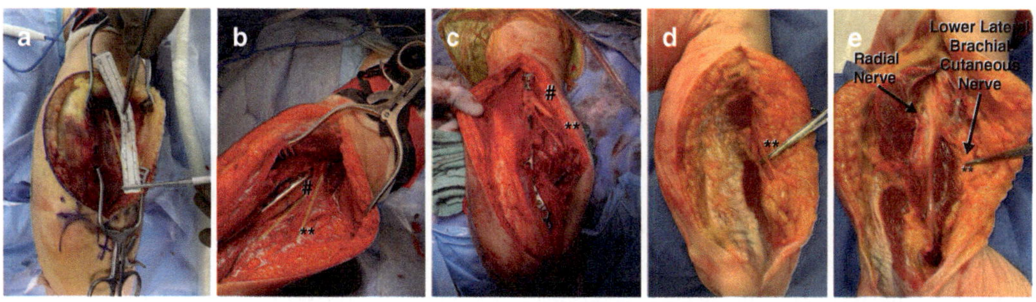

Fig. 5.2 Lower lateral brachial cutaneous nerve and its relation to the radial nerve in the brachium. Images depict a posterior approach to the brachium all oriented in right brachiums with top being proximal and bottom being distal. Radial is oriented to the right and ulnar to the left. Depicts the relative distance from the lateral epicondyle to the area where the cutaneous nerve is typically found exiting the triceps fascia. Same patient as (A) with a depiction of further development of the cutaneous nerve (**) to the brachium and the radial nerve proper (#). Depicts a similar approach to A & B but notice the orientation and location of the radial nerve proper (#) and cutaneous nerve to the brachium (**) which can vary depending on the triceps interval used. (D&E) Similar to A, B, & C

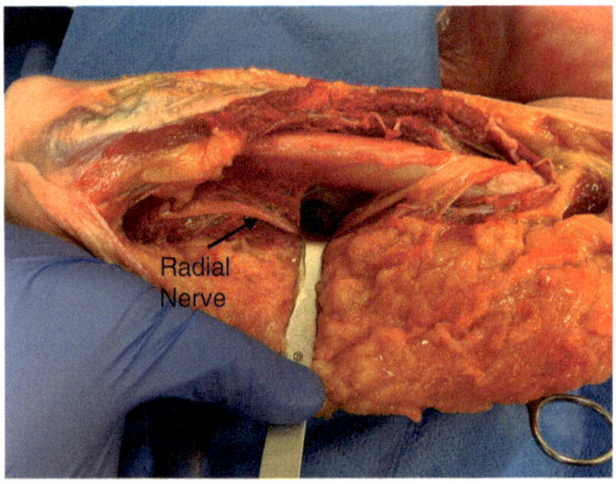

Fig. 5.3 Hohman retractor with pressure on radial nerve in the brachium

distal fractures and those distal fractures with midshaft extension. Furthermore, it is recommended to document the location of the nerve relative to the holes on the plate, should removal be required in the operative note. In addition, intraoperative photography can prove useful in documenting a nerve in continuity and that the plate has been placed below the nerve, given the high incidence of radial nerve palsy postoperatively.

5.2.2 Prevention of Radial Nerve Injury: Posterior Approach

- The lower lateral brachial cutaneous branch is easily identified and can be traced proximally to find the radial nerve proper to prevent injury [12].
- Bony landmarks such as the lateral epicondyle can identify a safe zone of dissection whereby the nerve may be located approximately 7.5 cm to 10 cm proximal [15].
- Lateral Hohman retractors should be avoided or used with extreme caution as they place compression directly on radial nerve (Fig. 5.3).
- Internal rotation of the distal fragment places increased tension on the radial nerve.

5.2.3 Prevention of Radial Nerve Injury: Anterolateral Approach

- Complete exposure of the entire brachialis will allow for the muscle to be split in half thus protecting the lateral third of the muscle and the radial nerve.
- The radial nerve is located directly posterior within the spiral groove, entering at the level of the deltoid insertion, 4 cm distal to the insertion of the latissimus dorsi tendon inferior aspect.
- The interval between the brachialis and brachioradialis may help identify the lateral antebrachial cutaneous nerve superficially and the radial nerve deep.

5.2.4 Natural History

Radial nerve palsy following nonoperative treatment of closed diaphyseal humerus fractures has been demonstrated to have a 70–77% rate of recovery with observation alone [5, 7]. Nonoperative management should be attempted for a minimum of 8–12 weeks with serial examinations. However, a recent systematic review demonstrates improved recovery of both primary and secondary radial nerve palsies with early exploration (within 3 weeks) [5, 7]. In this systematic review, the 638 nerve explorations resulted in neurolysis alone in 18.8%, extrication from fracture fragments in 10.5%, and repair laceration in 26.8% [7].

5.2.5 Initial Evaluation and Examination

Prior to any conservative or surgical intervention for humeral fractures, a thorough history and physical should be performed documenting any sensory or motor deficits, particularly of the radial nerve innervated musculature. Many authors have formalized an algorithm for treatment of the patient with a radial nerve palsy owing to the complex and controversial nature of the injury [16, 18].

Radial nerve palsy following closed treatment of diaphyseal humerus fractures has been demonstrated to have a 70–77% rate of recovery with observation [5, 7]. The algorithm for treatment for these injuries remains controversial with most authors waiting 3 months at a minimum with serial examinations prior to nerve exploration. However, as discussed previously, there is some emerging, but controversial, data that early exploration may improve recovery in these injuries [7].

Important prognostic indicators include spared sensory distribution of the nerve and recovery of proximal musculature. To that end, it is important to have a strong grasp on the anatomy and the pattern of reinnervation of the nerve. Abrams et al. studied the innervation pattern in cadaveric specimens suggesting that the mobile wad should recover first and the extensor indicis proprius last [19].

Physical examination alone is often reliable for the diagnosis of radial nerve palsy with the classic signs of:

- Diminished sensation over the first web space
- Lack of wrist extension
- Lack of finger extension
- Lack of thumb extension

A tenodesis effect of the wrist may help distinguish those injuries secondary to tendon involvement and those as a result of a nerve injury. In rare cases, it is possible to have both.

In cases where it is difficult to determine the continuity of the nerve, advanced imaging such as ultrasound or magnetic resonance neurography (MRN) should be obtained. Despite the improvement in MRN, hardware artifact if fractures were fixed with plates or intramedullary nails, and inflammation associated with acute injuries limit, the utility of MRN postoperatively [20]. Alternatively, ultrasound has shown promise in the setting of prior hardware, and even potentially having superior spatial resolution as compared to MRN [20] (Fig. 5.4).

5.2.6 Diagnostic Tests and Imaging

- Previous authors have recommended electrophysiologic studies at 6 weeks, with repeat studies at an additional 12 weeks [18]. It is often recommended that electrophysiologic studies are not performed prior to 6 weeks as this is the time required for Wallerian degeneration to occur [16, 18].
- Despite improvement in magnetic resonance neurography (MRN), hardware artifact and inflammation associated with acute injuries limit the utility of MRN in this setting [20].

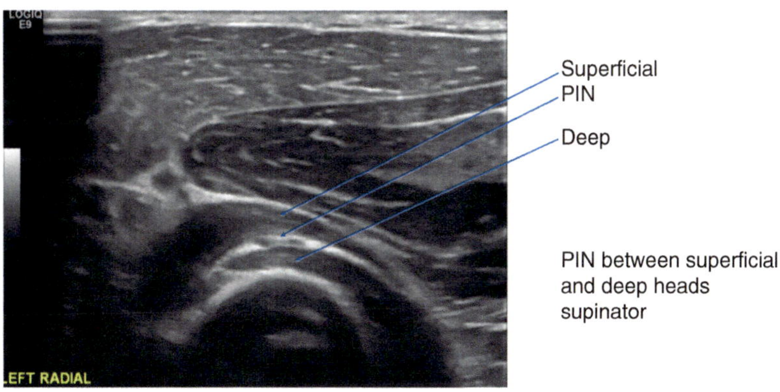

Fig. 5.4 Ultrasound demonstrating the sSuperficial radial nerve and the posterior interosseous nerve in the proximal forearm

For wrist extension, the most common transfers involve the PT to extensor carpi radialis brevis, which is chosen due to its more central insertion site on the long finger metacarpal to minimize radial deviation with wrist extension [26]. Although end-to-end is often performed in the chronic setting with no regenerative potential given its favorable direct line of pull, end-to-side transfer may be considered with the possibility of nerve recovery [26]. This procedure is performed via a curvilinear incision begun proximally over the radial aspect of the brachioradialis and sweeping dorsally over the wrist extensors. The superficial branch of the radial nerve is protected and the PT is identified deep to the brachioradial muscle and SBRN and radial to the radial artery inserting on the middle third of the radius. The pronator teres (PT) along with continuous periosteum of the distal radius is elevated to provide as much length as possible. The PT is then transferred subcutaneously superficial and radial to the brachioradialis and woven into the extensor carpi radialis brevis tendon, tensioned with the wrist in 45 degrees of extension [26, 27].

Thumb extension is restored most commonly by PL transfer to the extensor pollicis longus (EPL). However, the flexor digitorum superficialis (FDS) to the ring finger is another option with certain advantages over the PL. When the FDS is utilized it can be transferred to both the extensor indicis proprius (EIP) and EPL to allow for concomitant thumb and index finger extension as well as index extension independent of the other digits [27]. The PL is typically sectioned at the wrist crease through a small transverse incision using care to isolate and protect the palmar cutaneous branch of the median nerve. The EPL tendon is identified proximal to listers tubercle and sectioned as proximally as possible. The EPL tendon is typically subcutaneously transposed volarly to provide a more direct line of pull from the PL as well as accentuate abduction of the thumb along with IP joint extension. A third transverse incision at the base of the thumb metacarpal allows for adequate length to tension the tenorrhaphy with the thumb in full extension [26].

Finger extension is often targeted through transfer of FCR to extensor digitorum communis [26]. Other donor tendon possibilities include the flexor carpi ulnaris or flexor digitorum superficialis to the ring or long finger [27]. The authors prefer utilizing FCR as a donor as it allows for preservation of the flexor carpi ulnaris which is critical for grip and wrist strength and preservation of the dart-throwers motion [27]. This transfer is typically performed by transecting the FCR tendon distally at the wrist crease then transferring radially end-to-side into each of the EDC tendons, through a dorsal incision extending from proximal to the insertion of PT radially to end dorsally distal to the musculotendinous junction of the EDC tendons. This transfer is tensioned with the wrist in neutral, metacarpophalangeal joints in full extension, and the FCR tendon in 75% of maximal tension.

We prefer to perform the wrist extension transfer first and set tension at about 30 degrees of wrist extension; this then allows us to perform the other transfers in a length which will be under slight tension in neutral wrist position. Alternatively, others might prefer to perform the finger and thumb transfers first to enable motion in the wrist when tensioning the transfers. The wrist is then immobilized in pronation and wrist and metacarpophalangeal joint extension with a sugar tong for 4 weeks then in wrist extension splint for about 2 weeks thereafter. At 6 weeks postoperatively, we allow active ROM with strengthening at about 8 weeks.

5.2.10.1 Outcomes

In a study of nerve grafting proximal to the humerus in 13 patients with an average nerve graft of 12 cm, all regained elbow extension and 12 of 13 regained antigravity wrist extension. At 24 months, thumb and finger extension was M4 in 3 patients, M3 in 2, M2 in 2, and M0 in 6 [28]. A similar study defined outcomes of nerve repair versus grafting of the radial nerve based on location, defining zones: I – from the clavicle to the spiral groove, II – the spiral groove, III – the lateral arm, and IV – of the posterior interosseous nerve. In zones I, II, and III, antigravity wrist and elbow extension was achieved at or greater than 90% of cases. In zones II, III, and IV finger extension was achieved at rates greater than 75% as was thumb extension in zones III or IV [29].

Outcomes following tendon transfer procedures are uniformly good. A recent systematic review cites 96% recovery of antigravity wrist extension following tendon transfer [30]. Although not uniformly reported on, grip strength recovers to about 50% of the contralateral side and while wrist and finger active motion recovers to about 50% of the uninjured contralateral extremity [31]. The most commonly reported complication involves wrist flexion followed by radial deviation of the wrist, particularly when FCU is utilized and postoperative wrist stiffness, particularly limitations in flexion [31].

Nerve transfers for radial nerve palsy have less evidence supporting their use than nerve grafting, nerve repair, or tendon transfers. However, the evidence available is promising. Ray and McKinnon evaluated 19 patients who underwent median to radial nerve transfers for restoration of radial nerve function. All patients except one had 4/5 motor recovery of wrist extension and 12/15 patients had at least 4/5 recovery of finger and thumb extension, with an additional 2 patients recovering antigravity strength [32].

5.2.11 Technical Pearls and Pitfalls

- The lower lateral brachial cutaneous branch or the radial nerve between brachialis and brachioradialis are sites which are easily identified and can be traced proximally to find the radial nerve proper [12].
- Bony landmarks such as the lateral epicondyle can identify a safe zone of dissection whereby the nerve may be located approximately 7.5 cm to 10 cm proximal to the lateral epicondyle [15].
- Hohman retractors should be avoided or used with extreme caution as they place compression directly on radial nerve.
- Internal rotation of the distal fragment places increased tension on the radial nerve.
- One should record the location of the radial nerve on the plate in the operative report in case of the need for revision.

5.3 Periarticular Elbow – Ulnar Nerve

5.3.1 Risks/Incidence/Mechanism of Nerve Injury/Structures at Risk

Ulnar nerve injuries are the most commonly injured nerve to the upper extremity [33]. A previous study using the Nationwide Inpatient Sample demonstrated that most patients were male between the age of 18 and 44 years. Of these injuries, nearly 40% required early operative intervention [33]. The authors inferred that the mechanism of injury was likely related to trauma including motor vehicle/motorcycle accidents, sharp penetrating trauma (e.g., glass/ballistic injuries), or blunt trauma [34].

Iatrogenic injuries of the ulnar nerve can also occur during open and percutaneous interventions. For example, procedures that are at increased risk include flexion-type supracondylar humerus fractures, iatrogenic injury during fixation of pediatric supracondylar humerus fractures, or iatrogenic injury during elbow ulnar collateral ligament or ulna coronoid repair [35]. A recent systematic review demonstrated that the number needed to injure the ulnar nerve in pediatric patients with a supracondylar fracture treated with cross pinning was 1 in 28 patients [35].

5.3.2 Anatomic Considerations

The ulnar nerve represents the terminal branch of the medial cord of the brachial plexus arising from the C8 and T1 nerve roots. It begins medial to the axillary artery and travels toward the elbow just anterior to the triceps musculature. In the most superior aspect of the brachium, it courses within the anterior compartment and pierces the medial intermuscular septum about midway through the arm (Fig. 5.6). Distal to this transition to the posterior compartment represents an area of entrapment at the arcade of Struthers, a thickening of the deep investing fascia and muscle fibers from the medial head of the triceps [36]. In addition to the arcade, there are several other potential sites of compression that are important to consider in surgery, including the medial intermuscular septum [36]. As the nerve courses distally along the triceps it will enter the posterior aspect of the epicondylar groove, and into the cubital tunnel covered by Osborne's ligament between the two heads of the flexor carpi ulnaris. During surgery, these sites need to all be identified and addressed, particularly when performing a transposition of the nerve. There are no branches of the ulnar nerve proximal to the elbow [36–38]. At the level of the elbow, there is a dramatically increased amount of connective tissue within the substance of the ulnar nerve. The ulnar nerve enters the forearm between the two heads of flexor carpi ulnaris and continues on medial to the ulnar artery and deep to the flexor carpi ulnaris muscle. The first branch of the median nerve occurs about 1.6 cm distal to the medial epicondyle and innervates the flexor carpi ulnaris [39]. The next branches originate from the radial and ulnar aspect of the nerve and innervate the FCU and ulnarly innervated FDP muscles [39]. The dorsal ulnar cutaneous branch occurs about 9 cm proximal from the wrist crease and at that point the remaining two fascicles include the motor component ulnarly and the sensory component medially. Distally the nerve will then enter Guyon's canal ulnar to the hook for the hamate and divide to supply the hand via separate sensory and motor fibers.

5.3.3 Prevention Strategies

- Proper marking of the skin landmarks, including the medial and lateral epicondyle and olecranon so as to positively identify the cubital tunnel and medial aspect of the elbow throughout the procedure.
- The ulnar nerve should be identified and protected at the beginning of the procedure. We typically first identify the ulnar nerve between the humeral and ulnar heads of the FCU muscle belly and neurolyse it as far proximally or distally as required for exposure and completion of the index procedure. Furthermore, care should be taken as accidental traction on vessel loops can mitigate any advantages that they may provide. It is for this reason that we never place clamps on the vessel loops and instead tie them.

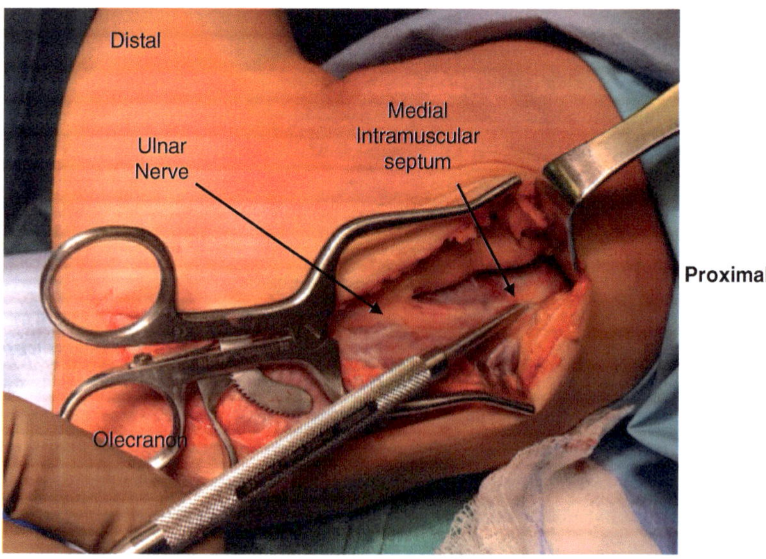

Fig. 5.6 Ulnar nerve piercing medial intramuscular septum. Figure depicting extensile release of the ulnar nerve about the proximal brachium with the elbow flexed to 90 degrees. The Freer elevator is underneath the fascial entrapment known as the arcade of Struthers

- Typically in our practice, the nerve is left in situ unless directly in contact with hardware or under undue tension in which cases typically a subcutaneous anterior transposition is performed.
- Avoidance of a medial pin during supracondylar humerus fractures unless completely necessary (use all lateral pins when possible) [40]. And when placing the medial pin, use a mini-open incision to safely protect the nerve.

5.3.4 Natural History

Ulnar nerve injuries have a significant effect on hand function as compared to other nerve injuries and the resultant detriment to patient's livelihoods [38, 41]. Given the long travel distance to reinnervate the intrinsic musculature of the hand, earlier repair as it may portend a better outcome. However, a course of nonoperative management of 6–9 months is warranted in patients without known lacerations, utilizing clinical judgment weighing the likelihood for recovery both with conservative management and with surgical intervention.

The intraneural topography of the ulnar nerve at the elbow has been shown to have an effect on which muscles and sensory deficits are encountered most commonly during ulnar nerve compression at the elbow [36]. However, in blunt contusions or frank injury, it may play less of a role. The ulnar paradox is a useful clinical evaluation whereby the patients clawing of the ulnar two digits will worsen as the FDP is reinnervated distally. It is therefore imperative to get patients into therapy and anti-claw splint immediately to prevent these and other contractures.

5.3.5 Initial Evaluation and Examination

A cervical spine evaluation for range of motion and cervical stenosis is paramount given the high rate of concomitant compression at multiple sites including the cervical spine. All motor groups should be tested including triceps strength, which along with distribution of pain and presence of cervical symptoms, may provide early clues as to the etiology and location of nerve compression. A critical evaluation of the posture of the hand and presence of clawing is critical as it dictates treatment options and is important for monitoring longitudinal progression of the disease. The ulnar innervated intrinsic musculature is responsible for flexion at the MP joints and extension at the PIP joints, as a result with ulnar motor weakness the hand posture becomes "ulnar minus" with the MP joints extended and the PIP joints flexed. The Bouvier technique is a technique by which the metacarpophalangeal joints are flexed and the response of PIP joints to attempts at active extension are monitored. With a positive Bouvier test, the PIP joints will be able to be fully extended actively with 90 degrees of MP flexion, which allows for tendon transfer options which are either static or dynamic and do not necessarily have to fully recapitulate intrinsic muscle function but instead may allow for MP flexion. Weakness of the FDP tendons, particularly to the ring and small fingers, as well as adductor pollicis is assessed. The Froments sign is present when the adductor pollicis muscle becomes weakened to the point where the FPL tendon is required for forceful key pinch. Sensory evaluation to the small finger and ulnar half of the ring finger is best evaluated by Semmes Weinstein monofilament testing, two-point discrimination, and moving two-point discrimination testing. The "Ulnar Paradox" is a described situation in which in a high ulnar nerve palsy, as the nerve reinnervates the FDP musculature, it causes increased finger flexion strength resulting in increased clawing despite recovery of the nerve.

5.3.6 Diagnostic Tests and Imaging

- Ulnar nerve injury is largely a clinical diagnosis, but diagnostic tests are often utilized for confirmation.
- One of the main values of electrodiagnostics is to provide baseline objective measures of ulnar nerve function and monitoring for recovery after nerve injury treated conservatively or with repair/reconstruction.

- MRN and US may provide useful data regarding extrinsic nerve compression and continuity, but particularly MRN may be less valuable in the acute setting or with hardware in place, and data regarding their utility in this setting are limited.

5.3.7 Nerve Surgical Techniques – Nerve Repair, Neurolysis, Nerve Grafting, Nerve Transfers

As with the radial nerve, we recommend repair or reconstruction of nearly all acute or painful chronic lesions of the ulnar nerve typically along with submuscular transposition. Intervention is typically pursued when there is no recovery within 6–9 months of trauma or clear evidence of nerve transection. Transposition of the ulnar nerve along with mobilization allows for about 5.3 cm of length gain [42]. It is our preference to perform submuscular transpositions as we feel this gains the most length and is the least likely to undergo reoperation, but there is certainly no definitive evidence against intramuscular or subcutaneous transpositions [43]. Again, if graft is required autograft versus allograft decisions are based on our subjective estimation of benefit of autograft versus morbidity of autograft harvest. There unfortunately is little unbiased high-quality evidence to guide the decision between autograft and allograft nerves for critical mixed motor-sensory nerves.

For ulnar nerve lesions above the elbow, we typically do not expect functional intrinsic function return after grafting in adults. We do often repair or reconstruct these nerves for neuroma prevention and possible potentiation of FCU and FDP strength often reserving autograft for those cases in which functional hand motor recovery is expected, such as children and young adults. For complete nerve transections in working-age, healthy individuals, we typically recommend concomitant anterior interosseous nerve (AIN) to ulnar motor (UM) nerve transfer (Fig. 5.7). We typically perform end-to-side transfer with lesions at or below the elbow and end-to-end

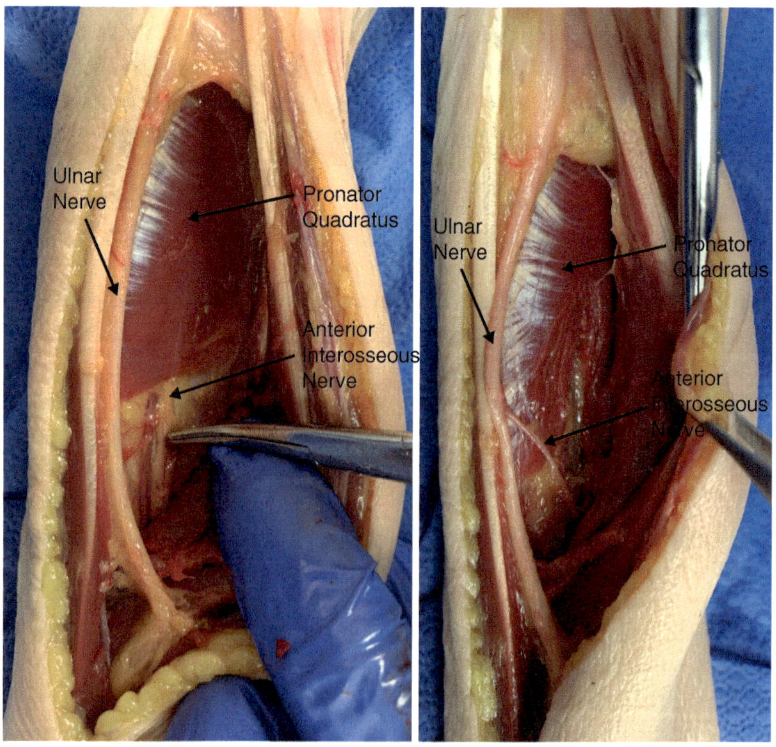

Fig. 5.7 Anterior interosseous to ulnar motor nerve transfer

transfer for lesions above the elbow. An incision just ulnar to the hook of the hamate is designed with Bruner style extensions over the wrist crease and extended proximally about 10 cm over the path of the flexor carpi ulnaris. Guyon's canal is completely released distally allowing visualization of the motor component deep and radial as it courses distal to the hook of the hamate. The FCU muscle is reflected ulnarly and the remainder of the flexor musculature radially exposing the radial artery and nerve. The ulnar nerve is carefully dissected free of surrounding tissue to allow for one to visually neurolyse it proximally to just proximal to the level of the dorsal ulnar sensory branch takeoff. The flexor tendons (with the exception of the flexor carpi ulnaris which is retracted ulnarly) are carefully swept off of the pronator quadratus, and the AIN is identified as it enters the proximal aspect of the muscle. The AIN is dissected into the pronator quadratus musculature until it begins to arborize to gain a few centimeters of additional length. It is then either coapted end-to-side in a tension-free manner to the ulnar motor component of the ulnar nerve or if end-to-end is planned, the ulnar motor component is transected sufficiently proximally such that a tension-free end-to-end coaptation can be performed [44].

5.3.8 Salvage Techniques

Unfortunately, ulnar nerve repair outcomes are imperfect, and late complications of ulnar nerve palsy can be devastating and difficult to treat. The primary functional deficit encountered is the ulnar claw hand posture for which multiple options have been described. The Bouviers test allows determination of options for restoration of function and insertion sites of tendon transfers. It is performed by passively flexing the MP joints, and the patient is asked to extend at the proximal interphalangeal (PIP) joints. Their ability to extend at the PIP joints demonstrates that either dynamic or static tendon transfer options to correct clawing may be utilized. With no ability to extend at the PIP joints, it is thought that dynamic options which insert into to the lateral bands may be best to assist in restoration of PIP extension.

5.3.9 Volar Capsulodesis

Volar metacarpophalangeal joint capsulodesis has been described. This procedure is relatively simple to perform and does not sacrifice a tendon for transfer. A single transverse incision is designed across the palm through which the A1 pulleys are identified. The A1 pulleys are divided and flexor tendons retracted and protected while a distally based flap of volar plate is freed from the metacarpal. The volar plate is advanced such that the MP joints are in about 30 degrees of flexion and a small trough can be made as a recipient site for the advanced volar plate. The volar plate is secured either with small suture anchors or placed through drill holes in bone [45]. There is concern that results following this procedure will decrease with time as the volar plate laxity recurs.

5.3.10 Tendon Transfers

Static and dynamic tenodeses have been described as have a number of tendon transfer procedures utilizing donors. Tendon transfers can be powered by flexor digitorum superficialis or wrist motors. Flexor digitorum superficialis transfers can include transfer into either only the ring and small finger or all four lesser digits. These tendon transfers can be inserted into the lateral band which may help to restore PIP extension, particularly in those with a Bouvier test suggestive of requiring such a transfer. There is concern regarding transfer into that lateral bands that it may also cause PIP hyperextension, due to the loss of the FDS and overpull of the lateral band. In an attempt to prevent PIP hyperextension, insertion into the proximal phalanx has been described [46]. A "Zancolli lasso" has been described in which the FDS tendon is passed through then over the A1 pulley and sutured to itself to correct claw posture without the risk of PIP hyperextension [47].

Unfortunately, flexor digitorum superficialis tendon transfers serve to improve claw posture but always weaken grip strength. Only those transfers which utilize wrist extensors and intercalary tendon graft are able to improve grip strength. Multiple transfers utilizing BR, ECRL, and ECRB have been described. These transfers utilize tendon graft, typically palmaris, split into two or four tails depending on degree of clawing of the index and long finger. The tendon grafts are passed through the intermetacarpal space and inserted into the proximal phalanx, lateral band, or proximal pulley system. This also allows for preservation of FDS limiting concern for PIP hyperextension.

Following clawing, weakness in thumb key pinch due to adductor pollicis wasting is likely the second most severe disability as a result of ulnar nerve palsy. In order to restore key pinch, a tendon transfer to recapitulate function of the adductor pollicis is designed. ECRB and BR are both utilized as donors. Due to limitations in length, tendon graft typically utilizing the palmaris longus is required. The graft is passed between the index and long finger metacarpals utilizing the second metacarpal as a pulley and the tendon inserted onto the adductor pollicis insertion. FDS to the ring or long finger can also be utilized to restore key pinch. The FDS tendon is divided into the digit and passed deep to the flexor tendons and inserted on the adductor pollicis insertion. This line of pull is extra-anatomic as compared to that of the ECRB or BR [48].

5.3.11 Outcomes for Nerve-Based Treatment and Outcomes for Salvage

Outcomes following nerve repair, grafting, and transfer for ulnar nerve lesions are poorly defined and highly variable in the literature. A recent systematic review analyzed four studies and a total of 78 patients who underwent supercharged end-to-side ulnar motor nerve transfer [49]. In this study, strength of grip and key pinch improved 202% and 179%, respectively; 91.9% of patients recovered intrinsic function at an average of 3.7 months [49]; and 8% of patients did not recover intrinsic strength [49]. Ulnar nerve repairs with and without AIN supercharge have been compared demonstrated improved intrinsic muscle reinnervation and clawing deformity correction after end-to-side nerve transfer than with repair alone [50].

Outcomes following soft tissue reconstruction including capsulodesis and tendon transfers for ulnar nerve palsy do not have the reliable rates of success seen in transfers for the radial nerve. Brown reported on 44 cases of MP capsulodesis with less than half having improvement in clawing and having 5 hands with near immediate failure of the ring and small fingers and 18 hands in which hyperextension recurred over the first year [45]. Due to this concern, a number of other options are often considered. Brandsma reported on 76 hands for which FDS was utilized for the restoration of intrinsic function with variable insertions utilized with clawing fully corrected in 21% of patients and improvement in 57% [51] In multiple studies, ECRB tendon transfer for improvement of pinch strength has improved up to 200% [52, 53]. Unfortunately, due to the complex nature of intrinsic hand function extra-anatomic reconstructions are less able to restore normal hand function as well as tendon transfers for extrinsic hand functions but can provide incremental improvement in function.

5.3.12 Technical Pearls and Pitfalls

- Prior to any procedure, mark the ulnar nerve and ulnar aspect of the elbow.
- Early during approach, find and protect the ulnar nerve.
- Transposition, particularly intramuscular, can provide significant excursion and should be considered in treatment of most ulnar nerve injuries about the elbow.
- With high ulnar nerve palsy, do not take FDS to ring or small as these are likely the only tendons powering the digit.

- When FDS is utilized, it should be divided just proximal to campers chiasm between the A1 and A1 pulleys to prevent PIP hyperextension [54, 55].

5.4 Radiocapitellar Joint and Proximal Radius – Posterior Interosseous Nerve

5.4.1 Risks/Incidence/Mechanism of Nerve Injury/Structures at Risk

As previously discussed, the radial nerve proper will cross from the posterior compartment of the arm to the anterior compartment. Once it travels between the brachialis and brachioradialis, it will give off a variable number of muscular branches to the extensors of the wrist (ECRB branch will sometimes come from the radial nerve proper and sometimes from the PIN). The preservation of active wrist extension is what differentiates a high radial nerve palsy from a low radial nerve palsy which affects only the PIN. After this point, there are several variations that can occur where the nerve will then branch giving off the PIN and the superficial branch of the radial nerve (SBRN). Injury to the radial nerve at this level or to the PIN at this level can have various presentations and effect on the wrist extensors, finger extensors, and thumb extensors.

The incidence of an isolated PIN palsy is relatively rare [56]. The true incidence is unknown and etiologies vary from nerve compression, fracture, tumor, parsonage turner syndrome, penetrating trauma/lacerations, and iatrogenic causes (e.g., elbow arthroscopy, surgical approach) [57]. In some recent reports, surgical exposures of the dorsal aspect of the forearm carried an 18% rate of nerve palsy with many recovering post surgery [58]. The posterior interosseous nerve has been shown to vary its proximity to the various structures of the proximal forearm based on the position of the forearm (e.g., supination/pronation) [59].

5.4.2 Anatomic Considerations

About 2–3 cm proximal to the lateral epicondyle between the brachialis and brachioradialis, the nerve branches to the brachioradialis and extensor carpi radialis brevis muscle branches exit the radial nerve. Immediately thereafter, the radial nerve proper splits into the posterior interosseous nerve and superficial branch of the radial nerve. The PIN travels just anterior to the radiocapitellar joint before passing dorsoradially around the radial head through substance of the supinator muscle to lie just dorsal to the interosseous membrane where it arborizes to innervate the majority of the extrinsic extensors. There is some variation in position of the posterior interosseous nerve in relation to the supinator including being very superficial (4%) and very deep and in direct contact with the periosteum of the radius (5%) [60]. The terminal branch of the radial nerve travels along the interosseous membrane at the floor of the fourth compartment to innervate the dorsal wrist capsule and intercarpal ligaments.

Patient history, surgical procedure performed, examination, as well as EMG/NCS and advanced imaging will likely provide adequate localization of possible lesions. In our experience, ECRB and ECRL are difficult to differentiate from ECRL alone by physical exam, EMG/NCS with possible ultrasound-guided needle localization can be beneficial if this information is likely to change surgical plan. The major approaches to the lateral aspect of the elbow, radial head/neck, and proximal radius include the Kocher, Kaplan, and Thompson approaches. The Kocher (anconeus/ECU interval) and Kaplan (ECRB/EDC) approaches allow access to the lateral aspect of the elbow joint in addition to the radial head and neck. The incisions are centered over the lateral epicondyle in a curvilinear fashion distally toward Lister's tubercle. The deep dissection is then carried through either the anconeus/ECU plane or the ECRB/EDC plane.

The Kaplan approach will allow for access to the anterior aspect of the joint if needed while the Kocher approach will provide more posterior access. Prior studies have demonstrated that the Kaplan approach allows for a larger viewable area with the capabilities of distal extension in to the Thompson approach [61]. The risk to the posterior interosseous nerve is anterior and distal to the dissection for both the Kocher and Kaplan approaches; however, the Kocher approach is more posterior the distance from the PIN is greater. Any straying from the interval poses significant risk to the nerve. As the plane is developed distally to the Thompson approach between the ECRB and EDC, the supinator should be located deep within the dissection. The location of the posterior interosseous nerve varies with forearm rotation and length of the radius. In relation to the radiocapitellar joint, the PIN lies a mean of 4.2 cm (range, 2.5 to 6.2 cm) in neutral rotation, 5.6 cm (range, 3.1 to 7.4 cm) in pronation, and (range, 1.7 to 4.5 cm) in supination [59]. The supinator may be elevated off of the radial aspect while placing the arm in supination. The nerve may rarely be in direct contact with the radius, and an elevator may be used to gently create distance to slide a plate subperiosteally (Fig. 5.8) [59, 62]. During these dissections, the muscular branches to the ECRB, supinator, and EDC may be at risk. Over tension and distraction may cause a temporary neuropraxia which should be monitored. The decision to deliberately expose the posterior interosseous nerve must be made by the surgeon intraoperatively requiring consideration size of the patient, length of proximal radius exposure required, and location of approach to the proximal radius along the volar-dorsal axis. The relationship of the nerve to any plate placed should be well documented.

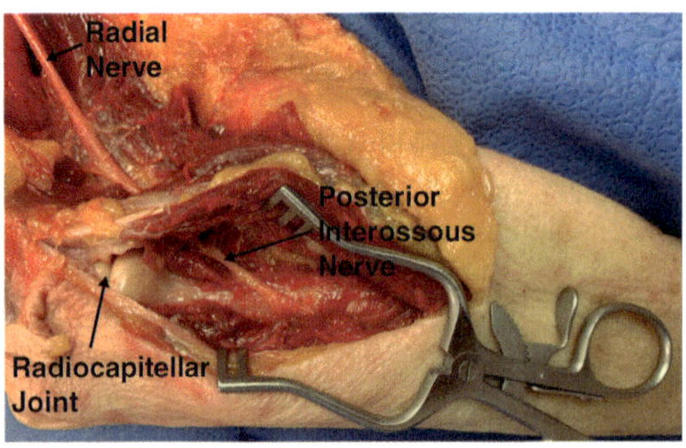

Fig. 5.8 Posterior interosseous nerve in relation to the radial neck

5.4.3 Prevention Strategies

- Pronation of the forearm is paramount to move the nerve further away from the operative technique when performing a Kocher/Kaplan approach or distal extension of one of these approaches [59].
- The average safe zone of proximal radial neck dissection is approximately 4 cm from the radiocapitellar joint in neutral rotation [59, 62].
- The supinator may be elevated off of the proximal radius protecting the nerve within the muscle utilizing care to prevent traction on the nerve and identify those patients in whom the nerve lies directly on the proximal radius.
- Document the relationship to the nerve to any implant placement should it need to be removed at a later time; take intraoperative photos to demonstrate the plate is deep to the nerve and that the nerve is in continuity.

5.4.4 Natural History

The PIN is a pure motor nerve and as such, the recovery can be predictably monitored with restoration of function in a predictable pattern with the more proximal musculature returning first. Abrams et al. have mapped out a predictable pattern of the muscular branches which may help inform the physician and the patient as to which muscles may return first, including wrist extensors, followed by finger extensors and finally thumb extensors [19]. Without any improvement in motor function, exploration of the nerve should be considered within 3 months [63]. A discussion of the risks and benefits of repairing/reconstructing the nerve versus tendon transfers or nerve transfers is necessary.

5.4.5 Initial Evaluation an Examination

In addition to those points for evaluation of a high radial nerve palsy, the following points should be included for a lower radial nerve palsy or PIN palsy:

- A tenodesis of the wrist should be performed to determine whether there is tendon involvement or if it is a nerve injury. Occasionally, both the nerve and tendons are injured.
- The resting posture of the wrist should be noted, including the presence of radial deviation with attempted active extension and strength and resistance testing.
- Recovery of the nerve should follow a predictable pattern as previously described.

5.4.6 Diagnostic Tests and Imaging

- Similar to the radial and ulnar nerve, clinical examination and patient history is more important than diagnostic tests and imaging for evaluation of the posterior interosseous nerve. Serial examinations remain the gold standard to monitor for recovery.
- Electromyography and nerve conduction studies are useful to confirm continuity of the nerve or provide a baseline from which to evaluate postoperative studies.
- MR neurography continues to be limited by metal artifact in many postoperative settings, but it along with ultrasound can provide invaluable imaging of the posterior interosseous nerve at the elbow and proximal forearm [50].

5.4.7 Nerve Surgical Techniques – Nerve Repair, Neurolysis, Nerve Grafting, Nerve Transfers

The discussion with patients is very similar for posterior interosseous nerve lesions as with radial nerve palsy as similar to high radial nerve palsies, tendon transfers do tend to function here very well. With true posterior interosseous nerve lesions, the sensory component is very small, and therefore we are less concerned with neuroma prevention, and if the possibility of nerve recovery is small due to patient age, comorbidities, or time course, we do not typically graft the posterior interosseous nerve for neuroma prevention purposes alone. Despite this fact, lesions of the posterior interosseous are closer to their motor endplates, and as a result the relative chance of motor recovery is increased and we are often recommending an attempt at grafting of these nerve injuries, always being left with the option for tendon transfers if unsuccessful. We typically do not feel as though nerve transfer provide significant benefits in these injuries as they typically do not move the nerve coaptation sites more distally than nerve grafting alone and may limit donors for tendon transfers if a nerve procedure is unsuccessful, but there are groups throughout the country who have successfully employed nerve transfers as described in the radial nerve section for these indications.

It is often appropriate to utilize or extend previous surgical approaches to identify the posterior interosseous nerve, but we often find that if previous incisions design allows for an appropriate skin bridge, often the most elegant approach is found by exploiting the interval between brachioradialis and extensor carpi radialis brevis. This interval is relatively easily identified as the brachioradialis appears darker and the ECRL lighter due to thicker fascia overlying the ECRL. The interval between these two muscles is then easily bluntly dissected, with any difficulty the surgeon should reassess that they are in the correct interval. The deep wound will demonstrate the fat surrounding the PIN, and the ECRB can be dissected off revealing the fascial edge of the superficial head of the supinator known as the arcade of Fröhse.

5.4.8 Salvage Techniques (Tendon Transfers, Joint Arthrodesis)

Options for treatment of posterior interosseous nerve injuries are very similar to that for radial nerve palsy as listed above with the noted exception of retained ability to achieve wrist extension. Occasionally, with wrist extension comes radial deviation for which tenodesis of extensor carpi radialis brevis to the functional extensor carpi radialis longus may provide benefit in better aligning the line of pull with the central axis of the wrist. It is also for this reason we prefer to utilize FCR as a donor to restore finger extension, as potentially sacrificing the function of FCR will also serve to rebalance the radial-sided overpull of the wrist extensors [26]. Other donor tendon possibilities include the flexor carpi ulnaris or flexor digitorum superficialis to the ring or long finger [27]. The authors prefer utilizing FCR as a donor as it allows for preservation of the flexor carpi ulnaris which is critical for grip strength and the dart-throwers motion [27]. This transfer is typically performed by transecting the FCR tendon distally at the wrist crease then transferring radially end-to-side into each of the finger extensors, tensioned with the wrist in neutral, metacarpophalangeal joints in full extension and the FCR tendon in 75% of maximal tension.

Thumb extension can be restored most commonly by PL transfer, although flexor digitorum superficialis to the ring finger is another viable option. When the FDS is utilized it can be transferred to both the EIP and EPL to allow for concomitant thumb and index finger extension as well as allow for index extension independent of the other digits [27]. The PL is typically sectioned at the wrist crease through a small transverse incision using care to isolate and protect the palmar cutaneous branch of the median nerve. The EPL tendon is identified proximal to Listers tubercle through a dorsal incision and sectioned as proximally as possible. The EPL tendon is typically subcutaneously transposed volarly to provide a more direct line of pull from the PL as well as accentuate abduction of the thumb along with IP joint extension. A third transverse incision at the base of the thumb metacarpal allows for adequate length to tension the tenorrhaphy with the thumb in full extension [26].

5.4.9 Outcomes for Nerve-Based Treatment and Outcomes for Salvage

Lesions of the PIN are typically unfortunate complications from otherwise simple procedures and therefore despite having reliable treatment options, they present diagnostic and management challenges. Outcomes of posterior interosseous nerve lesions are largely extrapolated from larger studies of radial nerve lesions, with some specific studies focusing solely on injuries to the posterior interosseous nerve alone. Similar to radial nerve palsy, the treatment of PIN palsy by tendon transfer is typically very successful, but nerve grafting and nerve transfer are certainly described options. In young, active patients who may benefit from independent finger motion either nerve grafting or nerve transfer could be considered. Typically nerve grafting is the treatment of choice for the PIN as the distance of nerve regeneration from the site of injury to the motor endplate is relatively short and not decreased by nerve transfer in this setting. In a study of 64 patients with posterior interosseous nerve lesions of whom 33 underwent nerve grafting, 95% recovered antigravity finger extension and 89% antigravity thumb extension within 24 months [29].

Tendon transfers for posterior interosseous nerve lesions benefit from the likely preservation of wrist extension typically allowing for two tendon transfers to adequately restore finger and thumb extension. There has not been significant study of tendon transfers for posterior interosseous nerve lesions alone, but much of the radial nerve tendon transfer data can likely be fairly extrapolated to posterior interosseous nerve lesions. Outcome measures described following tendon transfers are reported in a heterogeneous manner across the historical literature but as compared to the contralateral side, grip strength is commonly cited as recovering to about 50% of the contralateral side and while range of motion reporting is variable, it too likely recovers to about 50% of the uninjured contralateral extremity [31]. Many of the complications commonly noted following radial nerve tendon transfers are largely related to restoration of wrist extension (including limitations in wrist flexion and radial deviation of the wrist) which are unlikely to occur when wrist extension is preserved [31].

5.4.10 Technical Pearls and Pitfalls

- The radial nerve between brachialis and brachioradialis are sites which are easily identified and can be traced proximally to find the radial nerve proper [12].
- Anterior Hohman retractors on the radial neck should be avoided or used with extreme caution as they place compression directly on posterior interosseous nerve.
- Internal rotation of the distal fragment places increased tension on the radial nerve.

When closing incisions around the radial head and neck, care should be performed with depth of anterior suture throws as posterior interosseous nerve is very close as the distal portion of the incision is approached.

- When possible, the interval between brachioradialis and extensor carpi radialis brevis is the ideal interval for exploration of the posterior interosseous nerve as it offers the simplest dissection and direct access to the nerve.

5.5 Conclusion

The upper extremity, particularly the humerus and elbow are some of the more common sites of peripheral nerve injury, both posttraumatic and iatrogenic. The resultant deficits can represent profound functional losses, with variable expectations for functional recovery based on patient and injury factors. These nerve injuries are complicated both by the intricate anatomy and treatment algorithms as well as by the complicated cumbersome aspects of these injuries and their subsequent recovery. Generally peripheral nerve surgery options including nerve graft and nerve transfer can potentially offer a recovery that more closely recapitulates native function but suffers from patient and technical factors which may limit its success. Tendon transfers offer the allure of early, reliably recovery of function but certainly is extraphysiologic and necessitates strict adherence to therapy protocols and immobilization in the early postoperative period. Regardless, prevention and when necessary early identification, proper diagnosis, and timely referral and/or implementation of an appropriate treatment plan can significantly improve clinical outcomes, but care must be taken to carefully account for and manage the psychosocial aspects of these injuries to bring about the optimal care of the patient.

References

1. Ekholm R, et al. Fractures of the shaft of the humerus. An epidemiological study of 401 fractures. J Bone Joint Surg Br. 2006;88(11):1469–73.
2. Court-Brown CM, Caesar B. Epidemiology of adult fractures: a review. Injury. 2006;37(8):691–7.
3. Schoch BS, et al. Humeral shaft fractures: national trends in management. J Orthop Traumatol. 2017;18(3):259–63.
4. Gottschalk MB, et al. Humeral shaft fracture fixation: incidence rates and complications as reported by American Board of Orthopaedic Surgery Part II Candidates. J Bone Joint Surg Am. 2016;98(17):e71.
5. Shao YC, et al. Radial nerve palsy associated with fractures of the shaft of the humerus. J Bone Joint Surg. British volume. 2005;87-B(12):1647–52.
6. Schwab TR, et al. Radial nerve palsy in humeral shaft fractures with internal fixation: analysis of management and outcome. Eur J Trauma Emerg Surg. 2018;44(2):235–43.
7. Mangan JJ, Graham J, Ilyas AM. Radial nerve palsy recovery with fractures of the humerus: an updated systematic review. J Am Acad Orthop Surg. 2019;
8. Holstein A, Lewis GM. Fractures of the humerus with radial-nerve paralysis. J Bone Joint Surg Am. 1963;45:1382–8.
9. Bono CM, et al. Radial and axillary nerves. Anatomic considerations for humeral fixation Clin Orthop Relat Res. 2000;373:259–64.

10. Carlan D, et al. The radial nerve in the brachium: an anatomic study in human cadavers. J Hand Surg Am. 2007;32(8):1177–82.
11. Fleming P, et al. One-third, two-thirds: relationship of the radial nerve to the lateral intermuscular septum in the arm. Clin Anat. 2004;17(1):26–9.
12. Gerwin M, Hotchkiss RN, Weiland AJ. Alternative operative exposures of the posterior aspect of the humeral diaphysis with reference to the radial nerve. J Bone Joint Surg Am. 1996;78(11):1690–5.
13. Guse TR, Ostrum RF. The surgical anatomy of the radial nerve around the humerus. Clin Orthop Relat Res. 1995;320:149–53.
14. Shao YC, et al. Radial nerve palsy associated with fractures of the shaft of the humerus: a systematic review. J Bone Joint Surg Br. 2005;87(12):1647–52.
15. Zlotolow DA, et al. Surgical exposures of the humerus. J Am Acad Orthop Surg. 2006;14(13):754–65.
16. Ljungquist KL, Martineau P, Allan C. Radial nerve injuries. J Hand Surg Am. 2015;40(1):166–72.
17. Fu MC, et al. Surgical anatomy of the radial nerve in the deltopectoral approach for revision shoulder arthroplasty and periprosthetic fracture fixation: a cadaveric study. J Shoulder Elb Surg. 2017;26(12):2173–6.
18. Mohler LR, Hanel DP. Closed fractures complicated by peripheral nerve injury. J Am Acad Orthop Surg. 2006;14(1):32–7.
19. Abrams RA, et al. Anatomy of the radial nerve motor branches in the forearm. J Hand Surg Am. 1997;22(2):232–7.
20. Holzgrefe RE, et al. Imaging of the peripheral nerve: concepts and future direction of magnetic resonance neurography and ultrasound. J Hand Surg Am. 2019;44(12):1066–79.
21. Muzykewicz DA, Abrams RA. Transhumeral anterior radial nerve transposition to simplify anticipated future humeral reconstruction. J Hand Surg. 2017;42(7):578.e1–5.
22. Pet MA, Lipira AB, Ko JH. Nerve transfers for the restoration of wrist, finger, and thumb extension after high radial nerve injury. Hand Clin. 2016;32(2):191–207.
23. Dunnet W, Housden P, Birch R. Flexor to extensor tendon transfers in the hand. J Hand Surg Br. 1995;20(1):26–8.
24. Lowe JB 3rd, Tung TR, Mackinnon SE. New surgical option for radial nerve paralysis. Plast Reconstr Surg. 2002;110(3):836–43.
25. DP G. Radial nerve palsy. In: DP HRG, Pederson WC, et al., editors. Green's operative hand surgery. Philadelphia, PA: Elsevier; 2005. p. 113.
26. Sammer DM, Chung KC. Tendon transfers: Part I. Principles of transfer and transfers for radial nerve palsy. Plastic Reconstr Surg. 2009;123(5):169e–77e.
27. Seiler JG, Desai MJ, Payne HS. Tendon transfers for radial, median, and ulnar nerve palsy. J Am Acad Orthop Surg. 2013;21(11):675–84.
28. Bertelli JA, Ghizoni MF. Results of nerve grafting in radial nerve injuries occurring proximal to the humerus, including those within the posterior cord. J Neurosurg. 2016;2016(1):179–85.
29. Pan CH, Chuang DCC, Rodriguez-Lorenzo A. Outcomes of nerve reconstruction for radial nerve injuries based on the level of injury in 244 operative cases. J Hand Surg Eur Vol. 2010;35(5):385–91.
30. Compton J, et al. Systematic review of tendon transfer versus nerve transfer for the restoration of wrist extension in isolated traumatic radial nerve palsy. J Am Acad Orthop Surg Glob Res Rev. 2018;2(4):e001.
31. Cheah AE-J, Etcheson J, Yao J. Radial nerve tendon transfers. Hand Clin. 2016;32(3):323–38.
32. Ray WZ, Mackinnon SE. Clinical outcomes following median to radial nerve transfers. J Hand Surg Am. 2011;36(2):201–8.
33. Lad SP, et al. Trends in median, ulnar, radial, and brachioplexus nerve injuries in the United States. Neurosurgery. 2010;66(5):953–60.
34. Tapp M, et al. The epidemiology of upper extremity nerve injuries and associated cost in the US emergency departments. Ann Plast Surg. 2019;83(6):676–80.
35. Slobogean BL, et al. Iatrogenic ulnar nerve injury after the surgical treatment of displaced supracondylar fractures of the humerus: number needed to harm, a systematic review. J Pediatr Orthop. 2010;30(5):430–6.
36. Posner MA. Compressive ulnar neuropathies at the elbow: I. Etiology and diagnosis. J Am Acad Orthop Surg. 1998;6(5):282–8.
37. Posner MA. Compressive ulnar neuropathies at the elbow: II. Treatment. J Am Acad Orthop Surg. 1998;6(5):289–97.
38. Woo A, Bakri K, Moran SL. Management of ulnar nerve injuries. J Hand Surg Am. 2015;40(1):173–81.
39. Watchmaker GP, Lee G, Mackinnon SE. Intraneural topography of the ulnar nerve in the cubital tunnel facilitates anterior transposition. J Hand Surg Am. 1994;19(6):915–22.
40. Gottschalk HP, et al. Biomechanical analysis of pin placement for pediatric supracondylar humerus fractures: does starting point, pin size, and number matter? J Pediatr Orthop. 2012;32(5):445–51.
41. Rosberg HE, et al. Injury to the human median and ulnar nerves in the forearm--analysis of costs for treatment and rehabilitation of 69 patients in southern Sweden. J Hand Surg Br. 2005;30(1):35–9.
42. Smetana BS, et al. Submuscular versus subcutaneous ulnar nerve transposition: a cadaveric model evaluating their role in primary ulnar nerve repair at the elbow. J Hand Surg. 2017;42(7):571.e1–7.
43. Wade RG, et al. Safety and outcomes of different surgical techniques for cubital tunnel decompression: a systematic review and network meta-analysis. JAMA Netw Open. 2020;3(11):e2024352.
44. Brown JM, Yee A, Mackinnon SE. Distal median to ulnar nerve transfers to restore ulnar motor and sensory function within the hand. Neurosurgery. 2009;65(5):966–78.

45. Brown PW. Zancolli capsulorrhaphy for ulnar claw hand. Appraisal of forty-four cases. J Bone Joint Surg Am. 1970;52(5):868–77.
46. Burkhalter WE. Restoration of power grip in ulnar nerve paralysis. Orthop Clin North Am. 1974;5(2):289–303.
47. Hastings H, McCollam SM. Flexor digitorum superficialis lasso tendon transfer in isolated ulnar nerve palsy: a functional evaluation. J Hand Surg Am. 1994;19(2):275–80.
48. Hamlin C, Littler JW. Restoration of power pinch. J Hand Surg Am. 1980;5(4):396–401.
49. Dunn JC, et al. Supercharge end-to-side nerve transfer: systematic review. Hand. 2019:155894471983621.
50. Koriem E, et al. Comparison between supercharged ulnar nerve repair by anterior interosseous nerve transfer and isolated ulnar nerve repair in proximal ulnar nerve injuries. J Hand Surg Am. 2019;
51. Brandsma JW, Ottenhoff-De Jonge MW. Flexor digitorum superficialis tendon transfer for intrinsic replacement. Long-term results and the effect on donor fingers. J Hand Surg Br. 1992;17(6):625–8.
52. Hastings H 2nd, Davidson S. Tendon transfers for ulnar nerve palsy. Evaluation of results and practical treatment considerations. Hand Clin. 1988;4(2):167–78.
53. Smith RJ. Extensor carpi radialis brevis tendon transfer for thumb adduction—A study of power pinch. J Hand Surg Am. 1983;8(1):4–15.
54. Sammer DM, Chung KC. Tendon transfers: Part II. Transfers for ulnar nerve palsy and median nerve palsy. Plast Reconstr Surg. 2009;124(3):212e–21e.
55. Lee DH, Rodriguez JA. Tendon transfers for restoring hand intrinsic muscle function: a biomechanical study. J Hand Surg Am. 1999;24(3):609–13.
56. Cravens G, Kline DG. Posterior interosseous nerve palsies. Neurosurgery. 1990;27(3):397–402.
57. Kim DH, et al. Surgical treatment and outcomes in 45 cases of posterior interosseous nerve entrapments and injuries. J Neurosurg. 2006;104(5):766–77.
58. Perretta DJ, Brock KM, Tejwani NC. Early Complications Associated with the Thompson Approach to the Proximal Radius. Bull Hosp Jt Dis (2013). 2016;74(4):293–7.
59. Calfee RP, Wilson JM, Wong AH. Variations in the anatomic relations of the posterior interosseous nerve associated with proximal forearm trauma. J Bone Joint Surg Am. 2011;93(1):81–90.
60. Missankov AA, Sehgal AK, Mennen U. Variations of the posterior interosseous nerve. J Hand Surg. 2000;25(3):281–2.
61. Barnes LF, et al. Comparison of exposure in the Kaplan versus the Kocher approach in the treatment of radial head fractures. Hand (N Y). 2019;14(2):253–8.
62. Tornetta P 3rd, et al. Anatomy of the posterior interosseous nerve in relation to fixation of the radial head. Clin Orthop Relat Res. 1997;345:215–8.
63. Nigro PT, Cain R, Mighell MA. Prognosis for recovery of posterior interosseous nerve palsy after distal biceps repair. J Shoulder Elb Surg. 2013;22(1):70–3.

6 Nerve Injury Associated with Elbow Procedures

Lukas Pindur, Eduard Alentorn, and Andrés A. Maldonado

6.1 Elbow Arthroscopy: Ulnar, Median, and Radial Nerves

6.1.1 Incidence and Risk Factors for Nerve Injuries During Elbow Arthroscopy

Elbow arthroscopy can be a challenging procedure. The two main reasons are the reduced dimensions of this joint along with its usually complex pathology, and the close proximity of neurovascular structures. Nerve injuries during elbow arthroscopy have been reported to occur in about 2.5% of the cases in expert hands [1]. In the vast majority of cases, these injuries are transient and have a good prognosis. Because of the low incidence of nerve injuries, it is very difficult to conduct appropriate studies investigating the risk factors for nerve injury because of the risk of type II error. However, there are several factors that might increase the risk of nerve injuries: congenital elbow deformities, childhood post-traumatic developmental abnormalities, adulthood fracture sequelae, previous surgery (particularly if a nerve transposition has been performed), diabetes mellitus, heterotopic ossification, severe elbow stiffness, severe elbow osteoarthritis, not applying tips/tricks to prevent nerve injuries, and surgeries performed outside of the the surgeon's comfort zone. Most of these risk factors can be limited by a thorough clinical history, physical examination, and complementary studies. This information must be directed toward a deep understanding of the patient's anatomy and pathology, a precise and pertinent preoperative planning, and the use of a safety-driven strategy during surgery. It is also important for the surgeon to know when arthroscopy is or is not indicated under safe conditions for the given pathology and surgeon's experience. If these factors are taken into consideration altogether, elbow arthroscopy should be a safe and mostly effective procedure.

L. Pindur
Department of Plastic, Hand and Reconstructive Surgery, BG Trauma Center Frankfurt am Main, Academic Hospital of the Goethe University Frankfurt am Main, Frankfurt am Main, Germany

E. Alentorn
Instituto Cugat, Hospital Quirónsalud Barcelona, Barcelona, Spain

Mutualidad Española de Futbolistas, Delegación Cataluña, Federación Española de Fútbol, Barcelona, Spain

Fundación García-Cugat, Barcelona, Spain

A. A. Maldonado (✉)
Department of Plastic, Hand and Reconstructive Surgery, BG Trauma Center Frankfurt am Main, Academic Hospital of the Goethe University Frankfurt am Main, Frankfurt am Main, Germany

Department of Plastic Surgery, University Hospital Getafe, Madrid, Spain
e-mail: mail@andresmaldonado.es

C. J. Dy et al. (eds.), *Peripheral Nerve Issues after Orthopedic Surgery*,
https://doi.org/10.1007/978-3-030-84428-8_6

6.1.2 Mechanisms of Nerve Injuries

There are four main mechanisms of nerve injuries that can occur for several reasons: nerve compression, nerve traction, nerve laceration, and nerve transection. The most common mechanisms of nerve injury are compression and traction.

Nerve compression can occur when prophylactic nerve decompression of the ulnar nerve is not performed in cases with severe stiffness, particularly lack of elbow flexion. If elbow flexion is suddenly and completely restored, the ulnar nerve can suffer from a delayed-onset ulnar neuropathy by being compressed within the cubital tunnel. Nerve compression of the median or radial nerve is uncommon. The median nerve can sometimes be compressed by an inadequate patient positioning in which the elbow support is placed too distal and close to the elbow crease (Fig. 6.1). The radial nerve can be compressed by the inadequate use of retractors. Nerve traction can also occur because of the use of retractors but also because of manipulation under anesthesia.

Nerve laceration or complete transection occurs as a result of the surgical procedure, particularly during portal placement (proximal anterolateral portal, proximal anteromedial portal, anteromedial portal, or proximal posterolateral portal), work on the medial gutter, and anterior capsulectomy (See Anatomic Considerations section below).

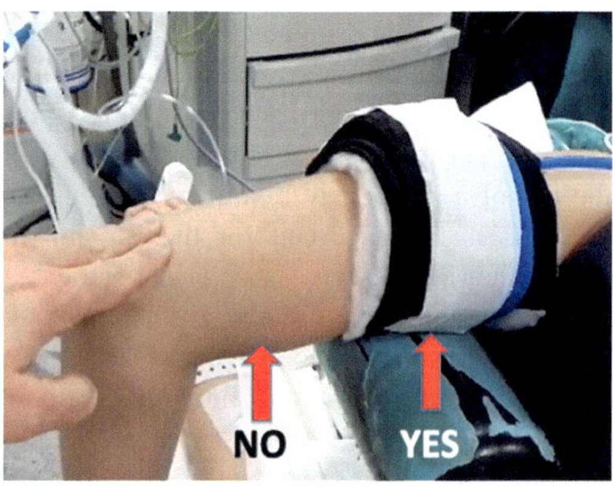

Fig. 6.1 Position of the arm holder proximal and away from the anterior elbow crease

6.1.3 Anatomic Considerations During Elbow Arthroscopy

This section reviews the nerves at risk for each portal for didactic reasons.

(a) Proximal anteromedial portal: created anterior to the intermuscular septum and 2 cm proximal to the medial epicondyle. With joint distension and elbow flexion, the ulnar nerve is about 7–18 mm from this portal, just posterior to the intermuscular septum, the medial antebrachial cutaneous nerve at 1–10 mm, and the median nerve at 7–22 mm.
(b) Anteromedial portal: placed 2 cm anterior and 2 cm distal to the medial epicondyle. This portal is about 1–5 mm from the medial antebrachial cutaneous nerve, and 14 mm from the median nerve.
(c) Proximal anterolateral portal: 1–2 cm proximal to the lateral epicondyle directly on the anterior humerus. The radial nerve is at risk for this portal, but the more the portal is moved proximally, the lower the risk of nerve injury. With joint distension and elbow flexion, this portal is at 10–15 mm from the radial nerve and 6–17 mm from the posterior antebrachial cutaneous nerve.
(d) Anterolateral portal: placed 3 cm distal and 2 cm anterior to the lateral epicondyle. The radial nerve is at 9–13 mm from this portal. It is important to note that this portal should not be placed distally to the radiocapitellar joint to avoid injury to the radial nerve. This portal is also at 22 mm from the posterior antebrachial cutaneous nerve and 16 mm from the lateral antebrachial cutaneous nerve.
(e) Soft-spot portal: placed at the center of the triangle between radial head, lateral epicondyle, and olecranon, at the soft spot. The posterior antebrachial cutaneous nerve is at 7 mm from this portal.
(f) Posterior portal: placed 3 cm proximal to the tip of the olecranon. The posterior antebrachial cutaneous nerve is at risk of injury (23 mm away from this portal). The ulnar nerve is about 15 mm from this portal.

(g) Proximal posterolateral portal: placed 2–3 cm proximal to the tip of the olecranon at the lateral border of the triceps tendon. Both the medial and posterior antebrachial cutaneous nerves are at risk as they are located about 25 mm away from this portal.

The risk of ulnar nerve laceration or transection is particularly true for the proximal anteromedial portal when previous anterior subcutaneous transposition of the ulnar nerve has been performed. In these circumstances, a precise location of the ulnar nerve is recommended preoperatively with the use of MRI or ultrasound. Also it is helpful to use intraoperative ultrasound imaging when establishing this portal so that the nerve can be avoided. If the location of the ulnar nerve cannot be clearly identified and protected, a mini-open approach when establishing the ulnar nerve is recommended (Fig. 6.2). Elbow swelling can dramatically increase the risk of ulnar, radial, or median nerve injuries, and must be avoided (see Prevention strategies section).

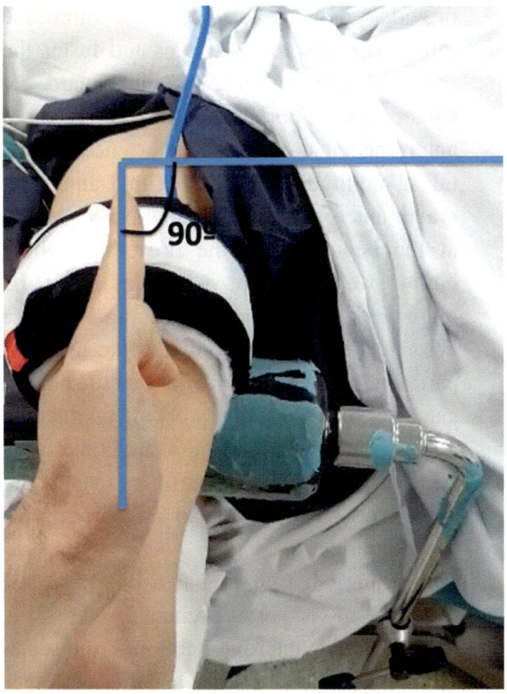

Fig. 6.2 Mini-open proximal anteromedial portal in a patient with previous anterior subcutaneous transposition of the ulnar nerve

Swelling not only puts the nerves close to the working space (joint) but also makes the surgeon lose anatomical references and get lost in the appropriate direction of the instruments.

In cases where the patients have loose bodies or osteophytes in the medial gutter, or tight posteromedial capsule (typically manifested by lack of elbow flexion), the ulnar nerve is at risk of laceration or transection while working in this area.

Anterior capsulectomy is a risky procedure for the radial nerve (deep branch) while working in front of the radial head, and for the median nerve while working in the anterior capsule more medially, especially in anatomical variants or loss of normal anatomy.

6.1.4 Prevention Strategies

The risk of nerve injuries can be significantly decreased by following several tips and tricks. Blonna et al. summarized these tips and tricks in 10 points [2]: (1) stay below your learning curve; (2) know where the nerves are; (3) use retractors; (4) avoid swelling (see recommendations below); (5) detach suction from the shaver; (6) don't use a burr near the ulnar nerve while working near the medial gutter; (7) shorten your grip on the burr for a better control of the instrument; (8) use a consistent step-wise technique; (9) have an experienced assistant; and (10) anticipate and limit adversity. To accomplish the first point, it is very important to know what surgical procedures usually imply a higher degree of difficulty, and when it is safe to progress to more difficult procedures. In patients without previous surgery, congenital or developmental abnormalities, or fracture sequalae, the estimated level of difficulty, from easier to more difficult are as follows: diagnostic arthroscopy, loose body removal, tennis elbow, local synovectomy or plica excision, radial head excision, cartilage procedures, ligament repair, and osteocapsular arthroplasty, particularly in cases with more severe osteoarthritis and joint stiffness. Although not validated, we do not recommend to perform cartilage, ligament, or osteocapsular arthroplasty procedures until a minimum of 50 previous arthroscopies in lower level procedures. These points summarize the general aspects than can be considered to minimize the risk of nerve injuries. Some specific aspects can be also mentioned for some of these general points:

(a) Patient positioning: adequate patient positioning is crucial to avoid nerve injuries and perform the surgical procedure successfully. For lateral decubitus, the arm should be placed above 90° for forward elevation (Fig. 6.3). This will avoid that the arthroscope or working instrument hits the patient or the arm holder so that the surgeon works comfortably without forced movements. The tourniquet should be placed as proximal as possible and the arm holder under the tourniquet. If the arm holder is placed to distal, the neurovascular structures may be pushed toward the joint.
(b) Landmark drawing: adequate drawing of the principal landmarks is helpful to prevent nerve injuries because it reminds you all the time what is medial and lateral, and helps in portal placement.
(c) Prophylactic ulnar nerve decompression: in cases where the elbow is stiff, particularly if there is a lack of elbow flexion, a 2-cm mini-open ulnar nerve decompression is recommended to avoid tardy ulnar neuropathy as a result of elbow motion. If the ulnar nerve is unstable after decompression, an anterior subcutaneous transposition of the ulnar nerve might be recommended.

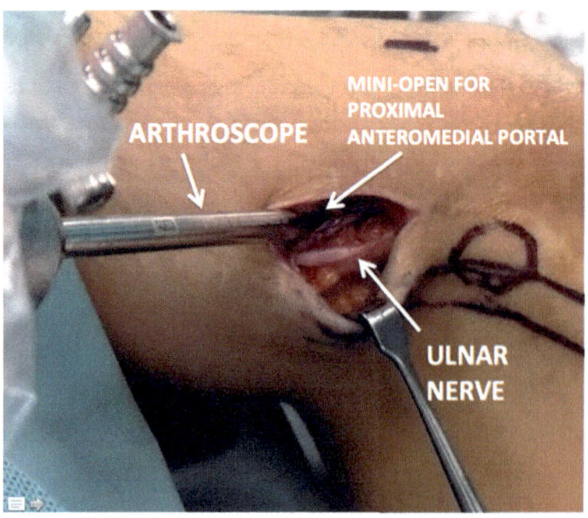

Fig. 6.3 Position of the arm holder so that at least 90° of forward flexion of the shoulder is left

(d) Capsule distention: fluid intraarticular infiltration is helpful because the capsule is distended so that the neurovascular structures are pushed apart from the joint.
(e) Portal placement: the use of the knife should be limited to the skin. Then, a hemostat can be used to spread the subcutaneous tissue longitudinally so that sensitive nerves are at lower risk of injury. For the proximal anteromedial portal, the ulnar nerve should be first palpated to ensure its posterior location. Then, a finger should be placed in the intermuscular septum while introducing the arthroscope, until the humerus is felt, and then the arthroscope is directed anteriorly and close to bone facing the center of the joint.
(f) Adequate fluid management: avoiding swelling is paramount. Fluid going inside the joint must go outside the joint. Inflow is regulated manually using a pulsatile lavage system that provides auditory feedback: the more the inflow is allowed, the louder and faster the sound from the pulsatile system is heard.
(g) Create risky portals first: the proximal anteromedial portal (and anteromedial portal, if required) and the proximal anterolateral or anterolateral portals should be created at the beginning of the procedure where elbow swelling is not present at all. If the main work is in the posterior compartment, a Wissinger rod can be left in the anterior compartment (or a PDS suture) so that the portals can be easily found after working on the posterior compartment. Some surgeons work first on the anterior compartment even if the main work is posterior, so as to minimize nerve injuries.
(h) In the anterior compartment, a Wissinger rod can be used for portal exchange. The rod is inserted in the anterolateral portal, the scope removed from the cannula, and the Wissinger rod introduced in the later until it exits the proximal anteromedial compartment. Then the same Wissinger rod is used to enter the

arthroscope in the anterolateral compartment while removing it medially until the scope is back into the joint.

(i) Use of retractors: accessory portals are recommended to use retractors (e.g., Wissinger rods) so that a space in which to work is created, and the neurovascular structures pushed away from the working area.

(j) The medial gutter: sometimes the medial gutter is involved in the main pathology: loose bodies, osteophytes, or tight posteromedial capsule preventing elbow flexion. The use of the mini-open medial incision to treat these conditions is highly recommended. The ulnar nerve is protected and the posteromedial capsule can be easily excised to gain elbow flexion. In addition, a portal through the mini-open can also be created to remove loose bodies or osteophytes, while protecting the ulnar nerve.

(k) Anterior capsulectomy: the use of the shaver should be limited. The "bite and peel" technique using a duckbill rongeur is recommended [2]. This instrument is first introduced through the proximal anteromedial portal while viewing from the anterolateral portal because the plane between the brachialis and the capsule is better identified. The duckbill is used using the bite and peel until the lateral edge of the brachialis is visualized. At this point, a fat strip is seen, which includes the radial nerve, and the instruments are switched around. The capsulectomy can be completed by first using fine dissecting scissors around this fat strip to decrease the risk of radial nerve injury, and the most lateral capsule released using a knife until just anterior to the lateral collateral ligament complex. Remnants of capsular tissue are removed using a shaver facing to the bone.

6.1.5 Natural History

Most injuries of nerves about the elbow tend to be grade I or II in the Sunderland classification (Table 6.1), with a good or excellent prognosis for spontaneous resolution. They often occur after transient stretching, compression from fracture fragments or displacement, tissue edema, or hematoma [3, 4]. Dislocations may lead to more severe nerve damage (grade III to V) [5].

Motor end plates become refractory to re-innervation between 15 and 18 months in adults [6]. Nerve regeneration after repair may proceed at a rate of about 1 mm/day [7, 8]. By using this equation, one may calculate the time frame in which nerve repair may re-innervate denervated muscles successfully. Because irreversible muscle atrophy probably occurs at about 18 months, this is the time by which the regenerated nerve must reach the target muscle [6, 9].

For the same degree of injury, the outcomes after repair are generally best for the radial nerve, followed by the median nerve and then the ulnar nerve. Outcomes after the repair of radial nerve injuries are relatively good because the radial nerve has a larger number of motor nerve fibers

Table 6.1 Classification of nerve injury according to Sunderland, modified by Mackinnon

Sunderland	Injured tissue	Degeneration	Regeneration
First degree	Myelin sheath	None, only demyelination	Complete, within 12 weeks
Second degree	Myelin sheath + axons	Wallerian degeneration	Complete, slow
Third degree	Myelin sheath + axons + endoneurium	Wallerian degeneration	Partial, slow
Fourth degree	Myelin sheath + axons + endoneurium + perineurium	Wallerian degeneration	None
Fifth degree	Myelin sheath + axons + endoneurium + perineurium + epineurium	Wallerian degeneration	None
Sixth degree	The fibers in one nerve show various degrees of injury	Combination of intact fascicles, demyelination, and Wallerian degeneration	Variable

and a shorter distance for nerve regeneration than the median and ulnar nerves. Outcomes after the repair of ulnar nerve injuries are the worst because the ulnar nerve innervates a small volume of muscle with a small muscle fiber size. After loss of innervation, the muscle fibers rapidly degenerate and atrophy [10].

6.1.6 Initial Evaluation and Examination

To confirm the nerve injury and potential for recovery, careful and complete clinical history and physical examination are essential [3, 7, 11, 12].

- The precise mechanism of injury: nerve injuries are accompanied by injuries of other structures which are essential for the functional outcome of nerve function. Where neurotmesis or high-grade nerve injury is likely, such as at sites of drilling during osteosynthesis, spontaneous regeneration cannot occur, and early surgical exploration is warranted. However, if low-grade injury, such as axonotmesis or neurapraxia, is suspected such as in mild to moderate fracture dislocations, spontaneous regeneration can occur and the patient is carefully followed up.
- Time of the injury. Upon planning the nerve repair/reconstruction, the time must be calculated by when the axons are to reach the motor end plates as these undergo irreversible damage after 18–24 months when denervated. After repair, the axons start to regenerate after about 1 month at a rate of 1–2 mm/day. For example in a lesion of the interosseus posterior nerve, if repaired early, complete reinnervation of the extensor muscles can be expected as the distance to the respective motor end plates and the reinnervation period are short. However, in a transection of the ulnar nerve around the elbow, the distance to the intrinsic hand muscles is relatively long, and complete reinnervation cannot be guaranteed even in timely repairs. Therefore, procedures shortening the reinnervation time, such as distal nerve transfer from anterior interosseous nerve to the motor branch of the ulnar nerve may be considered.
- Motor exam: muscle strength should be graded using the medical research council scale. The motor exam includes the following:
  - Ulnar nerve: FCU, FDP (fingers IV and V), lumbricals (III and IV), adductor pollicis, and interosseous and hypothenar muscles.
  - Median nerve and anterior interosseous nerve: FCR, PT, FDP (fingers II and III), FDS, FPL, lumbricals (I and II), and thenar muscles.
  - Radial nerve and posterior interosseous nerve: brachioradialis, ECRL, ECRB, supinator, ECU, EDC, EDM, APL, EPL, EIP.

Of note, there may be anatomical variations that make the clinical examination challenging. There may be various connections between two peripheral nerves that may lead to either worse or better clinical symptoms than expected after injury of a single nerve. The most common anatomical variation is the so-called Martin-Gruber anastomosis which is a connection between the motor and ulnar nerve in the forearm through which median nerve contributes motor axon to the ulnar nerve to innervate some or all of the intrinsic muscle normally innervated by the ulnar nerve [13]. Such anatomical variation may lead to intact intrinsic muscle function in high injuries (proximal to this connection) of the ulnar nerve. Another such anomaly is the Riche-Cannieu anastomosis which is a connection of the deep motor branch of the ulnar nerve in a hand to the thenar branch of the median nerve. Here the ulnar nerve contributes motor fibers to the thenar branch innervating thenar muscles [14]. In such an anomaly, injury to the ulnar nerve leads to paralysis of the intrinsic hand muscles including the thenar muscles. In injuries to the median nerve, on the other hand, the thenar muscles remain intact. These anatomical variations must be taken into account and can be confirmed via EDX.

- Sensory exam: hypoesthesia suggests there is incomplete nerve lesion caused by partial nerve transection, blunt injury, or compression of the nerve. Anesthesia of the skin region is a sign of complete nerve lesion, either transection of the nerve (Sunderland grade V) or blunt injury without nerve discontinuity involving all axons of the nerve (Sunderland grade I–IV). Hypoesthesia can be distinguished from the anesthesia by the ability of the patient to discriminate between the blunt and sharp object. The sensory exam includes the following:
  - Ulnar nerve: dorsal lateral surface of the hand; fingers IV and V.
  - Median nerve: palmar surface of fingers I to III; thenar and the proximal part of the palm.
  - Radial nerve or superficial radial nerve: dorsal medial surfaces of the hand.
  - Lateral antebrachial cutaneous nerve: anterolateral and posterolateral surfaces of the forearm.
  - Medial antebrachial cutaneous nerve: anteromedial and posteromedial surfaces of the forearm.
- Tinel's sign: an advancing Tinel's sign may be useful to monitor nerve recovery, although it does not correlate with the functional outcome [8].

6.1.7 Diagnostic Tests and Imaging

- Radiographic: evaluation of the bony structure should be carried out. If a fracture or dislocation is present, proper evaluation and treatment is critical for any nerve injury management [15, 16].
- Nerve imaging techniques: in closed injuries with compression or stretching component, ultrasonography (US) or magnetic resonance (MR) imaging may help provide information if the nerve was transected, remained in continuity, or if there is compression to the nerve as a result of swelling or hematoma. In open injuries, the nerve should be explored in the operating room, and imaging techniques are normally not needed.
- In the last few years, US has become a first-line modality for the evaluation of the peripheral nerves. The benefits of US over MR imaging include higher soft-tissue resolution, cost-effectiveness, portability, real-time and dynamic imaging, and the ability to scan an entire extremity quickly and efficiently. Moreover, US can be performed on patients who are not eligible for MR imaging, such as patients with a metallic implant (artifacts are usually not problematic with US) [17]. A recent study comparing US with MR imaging in the detection of peripheral nerve disease showed that although US and MR imaging had equal specificity (86%), US had greater sensitivity than MR imaging (93% vs. 67%) [18]. We believe these results are replicable when US is performed by an expert sonographer in multidisciplinary centers for peripheral nerve.
- Electrodiagnostic (EDX) studies: nerve injuries after elbow procedures, similar to nerve injuries after any other procedure, require nerve conduction studies (NCS) and needle-electromyography (EMG). In very early stages after the injury, the basic goal is to determine if the nerve remains in continuity [11]. Two weeks later, NCS and EMG may provide an idea about the overall damage to the nerve and its correlating prognosis due to the completion of the Wallerian degeneration [3, 15]. Electrophysiological indications of an axonal loss (e.g., reduced compound muscle action potential [cMAP], fibrillation potentials, and positive sharp waves) as seen in Sunderland II and III injuries are usually associated with a longer time for recovery, whereas an isolated conduction block (Sunderland I) is considered rather benign. Several months after the injury and/or after the surgical intervention, NCS and EMG may record reinnervation and the stage of recovery.

The above four elements (clinical history, physical exam, imaging techniques, and EDX studies) are critical and necessary to evaluate a potential nerve injury after an elbow procedure.

6.2 Surgical Therapy – Nerve Techniques, Salvage Procedures

6.2.1 Ulnar Nerve

These injuries are most often associated with maintained continuity of the nerve and various degrees of lesion of axons and endo- and perineurium (Sunderland I-IV). Generally, acute onset of sensory and/or motor deficit warrants close clinical attention and frequently surgical intervention. The treatment depends on the underlying cause. In dislocated fractures or elbow joint luxations, closed or open reduction is a first measure that needs to be performed without delay to prevent direct compression or traction exerted on the nerve by the dislocated bone structures. If satisfactory recovery occurs immediately, no other nerve procedures are needed initially. Nerve lesions may arise due to substantial swelling accompanying the original injury, most often in the typical sites of ulnar nerve entrapment such as cubital tunnel, the arcade of Struthers, or between the two heads of FCU. More often than not, it is very difficult if not impossible to tell if the neuropathy occurs due to an axonal lesion or mere compression of the nerve, typically within the cubital tunnel. In these situations, exploration and surgical decompression are indicated. If the bed of the ulnar nerve in the cubital tunnel is grossly injured with great potential for scarring, anterior transposition of the ulnar nerve in subcutaneous or intra-, sub-/ or transmuscular fashion may be considered. For exploration of the nerve around the elbow, a longitudinal skin incision is made between the medial epicondylus and olecranon going about 8–10 cm proximal along the medial intermuscular septum (IMS) and distally above the two heads of the flexor carpi ulnaris. During dissection in the subcutaneous tissue, care must be taken not to injury the branches of the medial antebrachial cutaneous nerve. Then, the IMS is incised and the ulnar nerve is decompressed proximally releasing the arcade of Struthers, followed be decompression in the cubital tunnel – incising the Osborne ligament and the fascial bands of the origin of the two heads of the FCU as well in the distal direction. Attention must be paid not to injure the motor branch to the FCU. After making sure the decompression is complete, evaluation of the indication of the anterior transposition is made. If the nerve is macroscopically intact and there is no concern of an excessive scarring due to the trauma, we prefer to do a simple decompression as described. If not, an anterior transposition is performed using any of its modifications. All of the modifications of the transposition (subcutaneous, intra-, sub-/ or transmuscular) have their advantages and disadvantages with none being clearly superior to the others. In a subcutaneous transposition, the proponents argue that by less dissection the potential for scarring is less while the proponents of the intra-, sub-/ or transmuscular transposition argue that under the flexor/pronator muscle mass, the nerve is better protected from further irritation. Irrespective of the particular procedures, the following principles should be applied: (1) release the nerve from all strictures and fascial bands, (2) after transposition avoid creating potentially new kinking sites. We prefer to perform the submuscular transposition of the nerve. The FCU muscle has to be released 1–2 cm distal to the medial epicondyle, and a periosteal elevator is used to reflect the muscle distally. The median nerve should be exposed, and the ulnar nerve has to be transposed anteriorly, adjacent, and parallel to the median nerve. Timely intervention with the elimination of compression of the ulnar nerve can prevent further progression of neuropathy as well as provide favorable conditions for the recovery of the axonal lesion that may have occurred during the initial trauma. In cases with an intact ulnar nerve whose primary pathology was from a traction or compression injury that was treated with decompression and a neurolysis, there has been recent traction in performing a supercharged end-to-side (SETS) transfer of the anterior interosseous nerve (AIN) to the motor branch of the ulnar nerve to help augment motor regeneration. A recent study by Power et al. [19] has described the more recent indications and appropriate patient selection for SETS in cubital tunnel syndrome. Based on this paper, patients with significantly decreased CMAP amplitude at the wrist pointing to an axonal loss and fibrillations or sharp waves in the intrinsic musculature should undergo this procedure (additionally to the ulnar nerve neurolysis and anterior transposition at the elbow). Of note, a prerequisite for SETS is a receptive muscle with still viable motor end plates. The receptiveness of the motor end plates to reinnervation is likely when the signs of spontaneous activity such as fibrillations and positive sharp waves are present in EMG. Another precondition for SETS is an intact anterior interosseous nerve. We believe this concept should be considered after an ulnar nerve injury associated with any elbow procedures.

If nerve transection is suspected based on the mechanism of injury, it is an absolute indication for the immediate surgical exploration (Fig. 6.4a–d), and primary nerve repair is performed if a tension-free end-to-end coaptation is possible after debridement of the nerve endings. If not, the nerve continuity is restored via nerve grafting. Most commonly, we use a sural nerve as a graft, but other nerves such as the medial brachial cutaneous nerve may be used. After harvesting the donor nerve, the diameter of both donor and recipient nerves are compared and a number of cables of the donor nerve is determined. The cables are glued together at the proximal and distal end using a fibrin sealant and the ends are cut precisely using a neurotome. The length of the graft must be set a little excessively so that it is little longer than the gap. In this way, tension-free

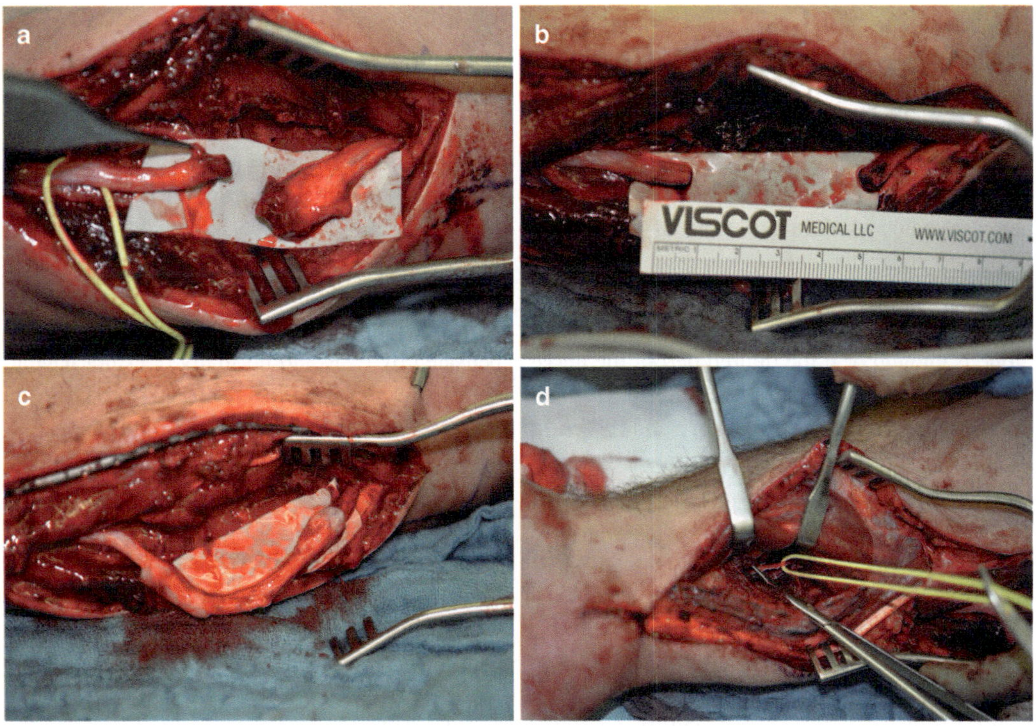

Fig. 6.4 A 50-year-old man with complete intrinsic muscle atrophy and elbow neuropathic pain 11 months after arthroscopic elbow surgery. (**a**) Intraoperative photograph after the ulnar nerve exploration. The nerve is in discontinuity with the typical neuroma in the proximal stump. (**b**) Photograph after neuroma resection. Note the 4 cm gap. (**c**) We decided to perform an ulnar nerve reconstruction using a 5 cm sural nerve graft for neuropathic pain and sensation recovery. (**d**) A distal anterior interosseous nerve transfer to the ulnar nerve (end-to-end) was performed

reconstruction is ensured. The nerve coaptation is performed epiperineurally with Nylon 9.0, and finally both coaptation sites are again secured with fibrin sealant. In transections of the ulnar nerve proximal to the elbow, the distance from the site of injury to the motor end plates of the intrinsic hand muscles is too far to ensure satisfactory reinnervation. Therefore, a nerve transfer from anterior interosseous nerve (AIN) to the motor branch of the ulnar nerve (MUN) in the distal part of the forearm is recommended early after the injury. While the gold standard is an end-to-end coaptation between the AIN and ulnar motor SETS coaptation has been described in the literature as an alternative [20].

6.3 Secondary Nerve Procedures

If the patient shows no or inadequate signs of regeneration (clinically and in the EDX study) after 4–6 months post-injury, surgical exploration should be considered. The cause of the absent regeneration may lie in chronic compression or scarring on and/or around the nerve or may be based on the more severe initial intraneural lesion (Sunderland IV). During the exploration, the nerve is neurolysed in the zone of the injury, inspected under the loupe or microscopic magnification for the presence of neuroma in continuity. Then, the decision has to be made if neurolysis alone is enough or if the injured part of the nerve corresponds to neuroma in-continuity with no potential for spontaneous recovery and resection with reconstruction must be performed. The surgeon may use visual clues such as the level of scarring of the injured nerve itself and its vascularity. However, this may be very subjective. In such situations, the use of intraoperative NAPs (nerve action potentials) or intraoperative EMG proved to be helpful. In evaluating NAP, the electrodes are placed proximal and distal to the nerve lesion and the response is recorded. If the NAPs are present, the neurolysis alone is performed, if not, the neuroma is excised, and the continuity is restored by nerve repair or grafting. Simultaneously during this procedure, the AIN to MUN transfer should be considered to ensure the reinnervation of the intrinsic hand muscles even though the initial injury was at the level of the elbow or even in the proximal forearm as the time with absent nerve regeneration has passed since the injury making the motor reinnervation of the intrinsic hand muscles through the repaired ulnar nerve unlikely. The AIN to MUN transfer is described on an example of a 25-year-old man with complete intrinsic muscle atrophy 3 months after a distal humerus fracture and ulnar nerve lesion and the elbow level (Fig. 6.5a–k). We prefer to perform AIN to MUN end-to-end nerve transfer if no sign of reinnervation is found in the intrinsic musculature. SETS coaptation is considered in situations where reinnervation is found in the EDX study without enough clinical improvement.

6.4 Salvage Procedures for the Ulnar Nerve

For chronic ulnar nerve injuries (more than 12 months), sensory and motor deficit are no longer treatable by nerve repair, transfers, or grafting procedures. Injuries around the elbow joint are mostly proximal to the motor branches to the FCU and FDP IV and V. Such condition is designated as "high ulnar nerve injury" while "low injury" is distal to these branches.

The loss of function of the FCU is well compensated by FCR and normally does not have to be addressed. In the hand, fine motor skills and strength are substantially impaired and claw deformity in the ring and little finger due to lost function of the intrinsic muscle may evolve. The index and middle finger are usually not or at least less affected, mostly by the action of the maintained function of the median-innervated lumbricals for these fingers.

6.4.1 Claw Deformity

The claw deformity contributes to the impaired function of the hand substantially and should, therefore, be treated. If the extent of the deformity is mild and a rest-function of the ulnar nerve

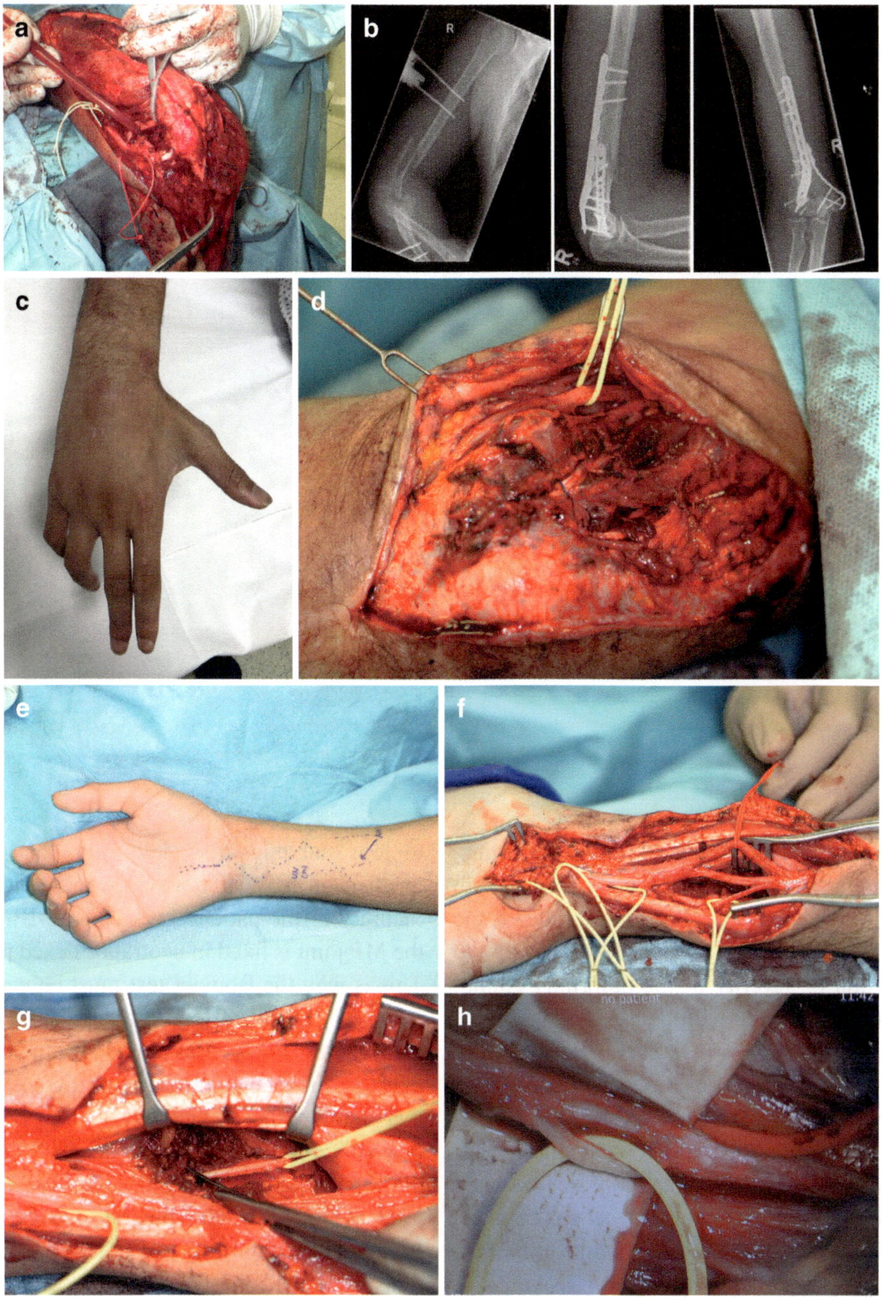

Fig. 6.5 A 25-year-old man with complete intrinsic muscle atrophy 3 months after a distal humerus fracture. (**a** and **b**) Closed reduction and external fixation were performed acutely, and the final osteosynthesis was performed 3 days after. (**c**) Note the atrophy of the intrinsic musculature 3 months after the injury. (**d**) During nerve exploration, the nerve was in continuity. NAPs were present, and reinnervation potentials were found at flexor carpi ulnaris but not at the hand intrinsic musculature. We decided to perform the ulnar nerve neurolysis and a distal anterior interosseous nerve to the ulnar motor nerve (end-to-end) transfer. (**e**) Plan for the nerve transfer. Note how we routinely perform the decompression of Guyon's canal. (**f**) The ulnar artery is protected with the red vessel-loop. The proximal yellow vessel-loop protects the dorsal branch of the ulnar nerve, and the distal one the ulnar nerve. (**g**) The anterior interosseous nerve is dissected into the muscular belly of the pronator quadratus and distally cut ("*d*onor – *d*istal"). (**h**) The motor fascicle of the ulnar nerve (the most ulnar one distal to the dorsal branch of the ulnar nerve) is dissected and cut proximally. (**i**) Note the coaptation of the motor branch of the ulnar nerve and the anterior interosseous nerve. (**j** and **k**) Follow-up 15 months after the nerve transfer

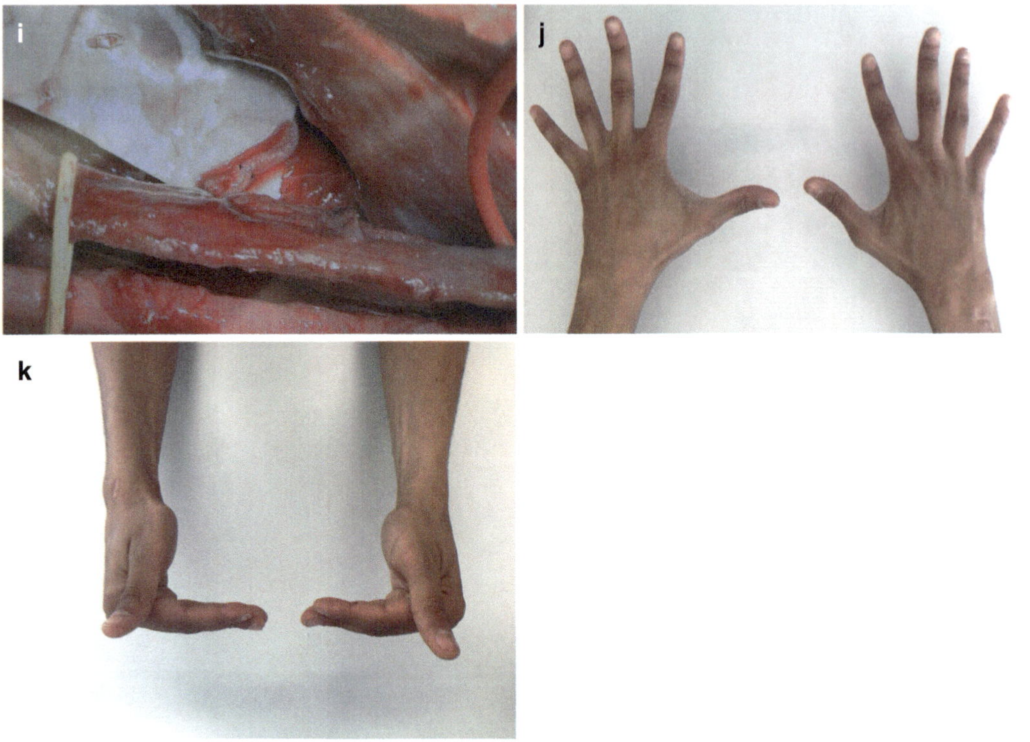

Fig. 6.5 (continued)

prevents the worst forms of claw deformity, physiotherapy sling with anti-claw splints with the MP joints flexed and IP joints extended is the preferred treatment of choice. However, if the progression or severity of the deformity cannot be treated effectively with conservative therapy, surgical intervention is necessary.

There are two types of procedures correcting the claw deformity: static and dynamic. Before the decision is made of which technique is suitable, careful clinical examination is necessary. The most critical questions are as follows: (1) Are the MP, PIP, and DIP joints supple or there is already joint contracture (reduced passive range of motion)? (2) Does passive flexion of the MP joint allow active extension of the PIP and DIP joint (Bouvier maneuver)? When the intrinsic muscles are paralyzed as is the case in a claw hand, the extension of the IP joints can still be possible by the action of the extrinsic extensors of the fingers (EDC, EIP, EDM). However, for the extension of the IP joints to occur, the hyperextension of the MP joint must be blocked. Due to long-standing claw deformity, the extensor mechanism may stretch which may lead to the inability of the patient to extend the IP joints if the MP joint is fixed in neutral or flexed position. This is why the Bouvier test must be performed to assess if clinically relevant stretching of the extensor mechanism has already occurred and so helps to select the appropriate surgical procedure that allows the extension of the IP joints. Formally, the Bouvier test is deemed positive if the patient can extend the IP joints when the MP joint is fixed in 40° flexion. (3) Is there a Boutonniere deformity as a result of palmar transposition of the lateral bands? If this is the case, the lateral bands must be relocated dorsally before the correction of the claw deformity is performed. The treatment algorithm is summarized in the Fig. 6.6. If the arthrolysis and/or relocation of the lateral bands is indicated, we recommend a staged reconstruction with the procedures correcting the claw deformity performed later when the passive ROM is certainly free and the lateral bands stable in their correct dorsal

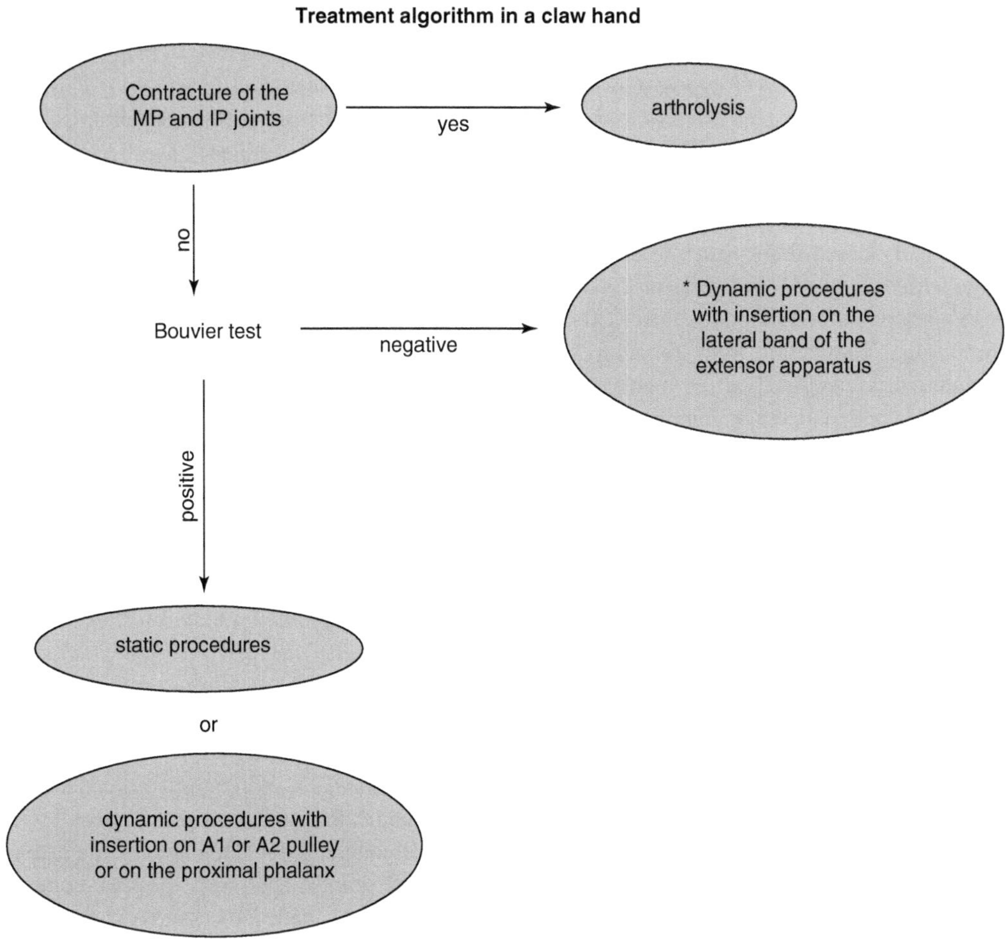

The Bouvier test is regarded positive if active extension in IP joints is possible when the MP joint is fixed 40° flexion.

* If there is a need or wish of the patient to increase the grip strength apart from correcting the claw deformity, dynamic procedures such as transfer of wrist extensors or flexors to the lateral bands are performed even though the Bouvier test is positive

Fig. 6.6 Treatment algorithm in a claw hand

location as opposed to do all procedures simultaneously. We believe there is too much risk jeopardizing the outcome with complete reconstruction in one session as the fixed flexion deformity may not be sufficiently improved or may recur ruining the demanding procedures correcting the claw hand. Performing the staged reconstruction also tests a patient's determination and motivation in postoperative engagement in physiotherapy after an arthrolysis helping the surgeon select appropriate candidates for the procedures involved in the reconstruction of the claw hand.

Static techniques: as stated above, prerequisites for the effectiveness of static procedures are positive Bouvier test and the absence of fixed joint contractures. Stated differently, the absence of an active extension of the IP joins after passive flexion of the MP joint is a contraindication for the static procedures (or dynamic procedures with insertion on the A1 or A2 pulley or proximal phalanx as opposed to the lateral bands of the extensor mechanism). The goal of static techniques is the correction of hyperextension of the MP joint with consequent correction of the flexion in the PIP and DIP joints. Palmar capsulodesis of the MP joint: first the A1 pulley is divided and the flexor tendon pulled away with a retractor. Distally based flap consisting of the palmar plate with the capsule of the MP joint is dissected with a scalpel. The MP joint is flexed 10–20°. In the original publication from Zancolli [21], the capsular flap was fixed to the metacarpal neck with a tension wire after creating a transverse tunnel. Today, fixation of the flap to the metacarpal neck with a bone anchor is possible. Roughening the palmar surface of the metacarpus with a bur may facilitate firm adhesion of the flap to the bone. Several modifications of this technique have been described [22, 23]. One such modification incorporates mobilization of the flexor tendon sheath over the MP joint and proximal part of the proximal phalanx. This modification should lead to more physiologic flexion beginning in the MP joint being followed by the IP joints. Postoperatively, the MP joint is immobilized in 20° flexion for 4 weeks. Hereafter, range-of-motion exercises are initiated under avoidance of forced passive extension of the MP joint.

Outcome of the palmar capsulodesis of the MP joint: according to literature, the recurrence of the clawing ranges between 5% and 52%. However, the exact percentage is difficult to assess due to differing and relatively short follow-ups [24, 25]. Modifications with fixed fixation of the palmar capsule such as the original one with tension wires or similarly robust fixation used nowadays with bone anchors are expected to have lower recurrence rate than methods using soft-tissue fixation.

In high ulnar nerve palsy, the FDP IV and V are paralyzed and thus flexion in the DIP joints of the ring and little finger are not possible. Additionally, the overall handgrip strength is diminished. In order to restore the function of these two muscles, the above-described procedures to correct the claw deformity can be combined with *side-to-side tenodesis of the FDP IV and V to FDP III* that is innervated by the median nerve. While the active flexion in the DIP joints is restored, the overall grip strength of the hand remains unaffected by this procedure.

Other static techniques have been described, such as using a strip of the ECRB, ECU [26], or free tendon grafts [27].

Dynamic techniques: as with static procedures, multiple techniques have been published in the literature, which use transfers of the FDS [28], ECRB or ECRL or FCR [29] tendons. In dynamic techniques, two groups of procedures must be distinguished: (1) dynamic techniques with insertion on A1 and or A2 pulley or on the proximal phalanx and (2) dynamic techniques with insertion on the lateral bands of the extensor mechanism:

1. *Dynamic techniques with insertion on A1 and or A2 pulley or on the proximal phalanx:*

The first group uses tendon transfers with insertion on A1 or A2 pulleys or insertion on the proximal phalanx. While these procedures count as dynamic, they only restore the active flexion in the MP joint and not automatically the extension in the IP joints. Therefore, they are contraindicated (just as static procedures) if the Bouvier test is negative. The most common representative of these procedures is the Zancolli-lasso procedure and its many modifications as described below.

Reliable results could be achieved with the Zancolli-lasso procedure (Fig. 6.7a–c), which is preferred at our institution. As opposed to static techniques, the active flexion of the MP joint is restored with simultaneous extension in PIP and DIP joints. Free passive range of motion of the MP and PIP joints must be present before this reconstruction; otherwise, teno-/arthrolysis is performed first. A skin incision is performed on the palmar side of the hand between 4 and 5 metacarpal, up to the DIP joints of the ring, and little finger in a zig-zag manner. The flexor sheaths 4 and 5 are exposed and the insertion of the FDS tendon on the basis of the middle phalanx is visualized after the A3 pulley is divided. Hereafter, the slips of the FDS tendons are

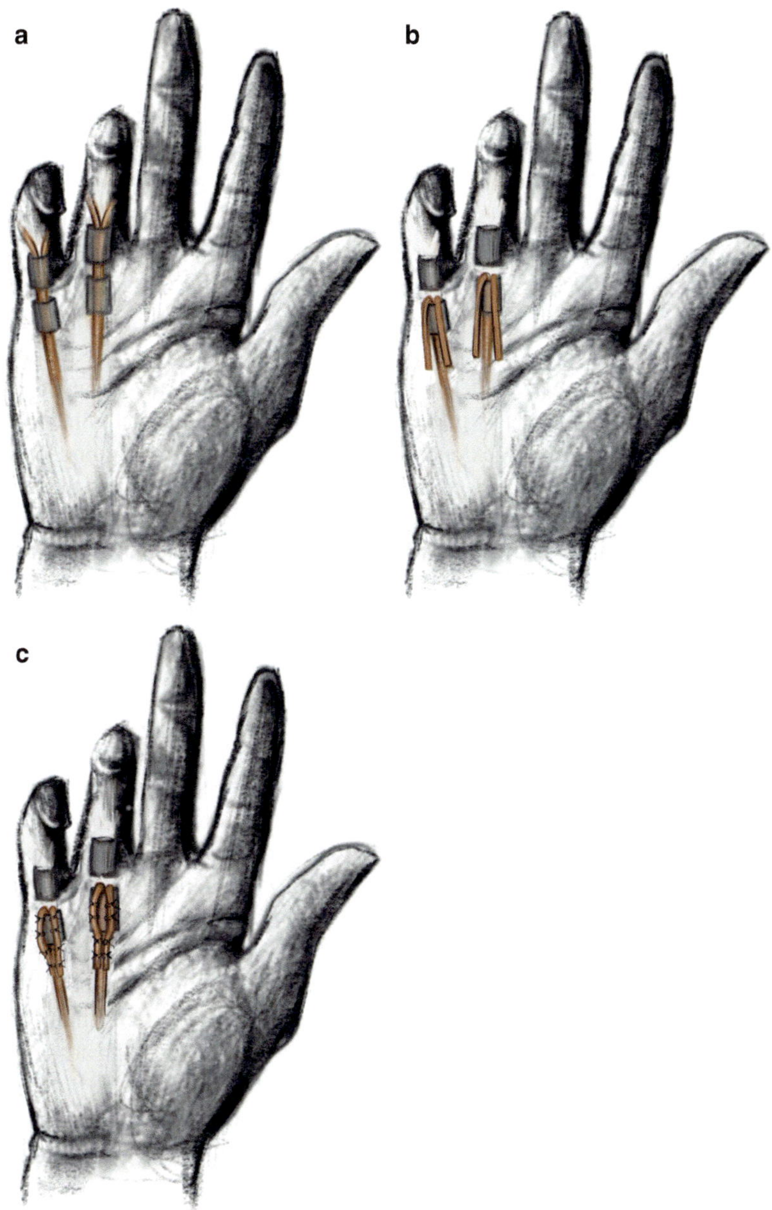

Fig. 6.7 Schematic diagram of Zancolli-lasso procedure. (**a**) Flexor tendons of the IV and V digits are exposed. (**b**) The FDS tendons are divided close to their insertions on the basis of the middle phalanx, transposed proximally, and pulled through an opening between the A1 and A2 pulley. (**c**) The FDS tendons are then wrapped around the A1 pulley and sutured to it and to themselves proximal to the A1 pulley

detached close to their bony insertion. An opening is made between the A1 and A2 pulley through which the FDS tendon is pulled. The MP joint is placed in 45–60° flexion and the FDS tendon is turned (lassoed) around the A1 pulley and sutured to itself as well as to the A1 pulley. Postoperatively, the patients are immobilized in a forearm splint with the wrist in a neutral position, the MP joints of the involved fingers in 60° flexion and IP joints in extension. A possible complication may be the development of swan neck deformity in up to 15% of cases, especially in patients with hypermobile joints [30]. The risk of developing swan neck deformity may be lowered by leaving one stump of FDS attached to the base of the middle phalanx with either leaving the proximal stump to scar to the head of the proximal phalanx or fix it there with a suture thus preventing the hyperextension in the PIP joint. Outcomes of the Zancolli-lasso procedure: the correction of the claw deformity can be achieved in up to 82% [31]. Worse results have frequently been attributed to not fully managed contractures of the MP and IP joints. Grip strength is not substantially increased. However, hand dexterity is subjectively improved.

2. *Dynamic techniques with insertion on the lateral bands of the extensor mechanism:*

If, however, the Bouvier test is negative, a new motor must be transferred that will both flex the MP joint and simultaneously prevent its hyperextension and also actively extends the IP joints. This effect can only be achieved if the new motor runs palmarly to the transverse metacarpal ligament (and so flexing the MP joint) and inserts to the lateral bands of the extensor mechanism through which it exerts a new active pulling force on these and thus extending the IP joints even in the presence of the slack of the extensor mechanism. Besides this effect, these types of transfers also increase the grip strength.

An example of several modifications of these procedures is the transfer of the ECRB prolonged with a free tendon graft that may be split to insert on several fingers as needed (so-called Brand I procedure) [32]. The tendon grafted is reputed in the intermetacarpal spaces palmar to the transverse metacarpal ligament and fixed to the lateral bands. The first incision is placed over the basis of the third metacarpal to release the ECRB tendon from its insertion. Next two incisions are placed over the intermetacarpal spaces and midaxial on the affected fingers to pass the tendon graft as described above. The suture is performed with the wrist in 30° extension, MP joint 45°flexion, and IP joints in extension. The immobilization of the wrist, MP, and IP joints in the set position is recommended for 1 month with following ROM exercises.

6.4.2 Impaired Thumb Adduction

Due to the insufficiency of the adductor pollicis (AdP), no thumb pinch can be achieved by the patient (the basis for the Froment sign). In patients with hypermobile joints, this may lead to hyperextension of the thumb MP joint and flexion of the IP joint. Restoration of thumb adduction and thus a power pinch can be achieved by the *transfer of the ECRB*. This technique was described by Smith [33]. A tendon graft, typically palmaris longus, is used to lengthen to ECRB tendon that is divided close to its insertion on the base of the third metacarpal. The ECRB tendon is pulled out of the extensor retinaculum through a proximal incision. Another incision is made over the interosseous space between the second and third metacarpal where a tunnel is made from dorsal to palmar. The last incision is made over the ulnar aspect of the thumb MP joint longitudinally. Through tunnel created deep to the transverse head of the AdP, the PL graft is passed and sutured to the insertion of the AdP on the thumb MP joint. The graft is passed back through space between metacarpal II and III and in the proximal wound, it is sutured to the ECRB. A key point for the correct tension of the suture, the thumb should passively abduct with the wrist in extension and adduct while it is flexed. Postoperatively, the thumb is immobilized in a neutral position with the wrist in 40° extension for 4 weeks after which ROM exercises are initiated.

Outcomes: the vast majority of the patients are satisfied with the results of the procedure and report significant improvement in pinching and grasping of the thumb and index finger. The pinch strength is expected to double after the reconstruction of thumb adduction via the ECRB transfer being around half of its healthy contralateral thumb [33].

In failed attempts to restore the thumb adduction with a tendon transfer or deformities of the thumb MP (hyperextension) and IP joint (flexion), arthrodesis of either of the two joins may improve the pinch grip. It is preferred to fuse the MP joint and maintain motion in the IP joint if possible so the patient can control small objects in the pinch grip between the thumb and the index finger.

Concluding remarks: in ulnar nerve palsy, the lost sensation in the little and part of the ring finger and on the ulnar side of the dorsum of the hand has no significant clinical implications and does not contribute substantially to impaired hand function. Regarding the above-described motor impairments in ulnar nerve palsy, thorough and honest discussion of the condition and the expected results with the patient are mandatory. Significant parts of important hand function are preserved through the innervation by the median nerve. In many patients, the deformities may not be so severe as to warrant surgical therapy, especially in those who do not feel comfortable with long postoperative physiotherapy that is essential for good outcomes. The ulnar-innervated intrinsic muscles and their interplay provide the basis for the very complex fine motions, and dexterity of the hand and surgical corrections with all their technical refinements and innovation cannot restore all these fine motions to the original state. Rather, they may correct particular deficits and deformities. It is, therefore, imperative to explain these factors to the patients so that they have realistic expectations on what can and what cannot be achieved with surgical interventions. Last but not least, some deformities have a serious impact not only on the function of the hand but also on the aesthetic aspect, for example in patients with severe claw deformity. A correction for this indication may be justifiable.

6.4.3 Median Nerve

The same principles apply for the decision-making in surgical therapy for the median nerve as for the above-described ulnar nerve. Acute posttraumatic entrapment may occur in predilection sites, such as between the two heads of pronator teres or in the region of the fibrous arch of FDS muscle. Sometimes, isolated lesion to the AIN due to hematoma or swelling may develop and manifest clinically similar to anterior interosseous syndrome with a motor deficit of FPL, FDP to index and long finger and pronator quadratus. Decompression of the median nerve is the appropriate therapy in an acute setting. The skin incision in the form of lazy S is located in the proximal forearm up to the elbow crease. Then lacertus fibrosus is divided and the tendinous part of the humeral head of PT is lengthened via proximal and distal incision decreasing the pressure on the median nerve. The median nerve is identified and any compression sites are eliminated (Fig. 6.8a–b). Typically, the leading tendinous edge of the FDS origin has to be excised. The indication for decompression in the acute setting is to be made cautiously and individually based on the clinical findings and the dynamic of neurological deficits as the median nerve in this location has a very good capacity for spontaneous recovery. However, if there is no recovery after 6–9 months, the exploration and neurolysis should be performed.

6.5 Salvage Procedures for the Median Nerve

Chronic palsy of the median may result from inadequate or delayed initial therapy or is a consequence of the severity of the injury and devel-

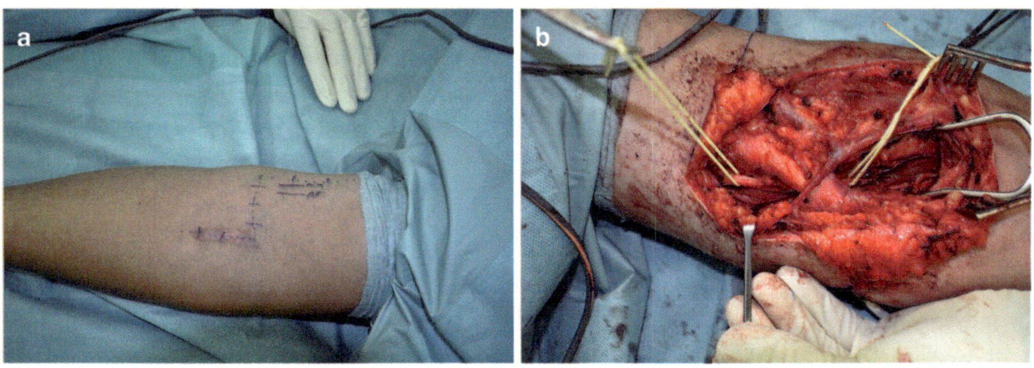

Fig. 6.8 A 50-year-old man with dysesthesia in thumb and index finger 5 months after a distal biceps refixation. (**a**) Incisions to perform a median nerve exploration. (**b**) The nerve was in continuity but scarred

ops in spite of correct therapy. The functional deficit depends on the level of injury. In injuries around the elbow high injury (proximal to the branching of AIN), low injury (distal to the branching of AIN), or injury to the AIN alone may occur with a corresponding motor and sensory deficit. In high median nerve palsy, the following motor functions are impaired or absent: forearm pronation, wrist flexion, finger flexion – especially that of the index and middle finger and thumb opposition. The extent of the functional deficit of each depends on anatomic variations between the ulnar and median nerve, most common of which is the Martin-Gruber anastomosis [34]. Also, intact ulnar nerve maintains satisfactory flexion (FCU) of wrist and ring and little finger (FDP IV and V).

- *Pronation*: the necessity to restore active pronation has been debated in the literature with some promoting its importance [35] and others arguing that pronation is maintained by brachialis, FDP, and ECU [36]. Thus, it seems to be reasonable to individualize the indication for the restoration of pronation based on the concrete strength of pronation in each patient as well as their wishes, occupation, and leisure activities. The restoration of pronation is typically ensured through *rerouting of biceps brachii tendon* [37]. First, lazy S incision is made over the ventral part of the elbow. The insertion of the biceps tendon is visualized. Care must be exercised to avoid injury to the radial artery and nerve. The biceps tendon is mobilized from its insertion to the musculocutaneous junction. The tendon is then divided in a z-fashion, thus lengthening the tendon with one part of the tendon left attached to the radius and the other to the muscle belly. The distal part of the tendon is passed around the radial neck from the ulnar side and the two tendon parts are sutured together side-to-side in full pronation. Postoperatively, the elbow is immobilized for 4 weeks in full pronation with subsequent range-of-motion exercises.
- *Flexion of the thumb and index finger*: the function of the paralyzed FPL muscle is restored by the transfer of brachioradialis that is innervated by the radial nerve. For the flexion of the index and long finger either the transfer from ECRL tendon to FDP II and III is performed or side-to-side tenodesis from the ulnar-innervated FDP IV and V to FDP II and III.
- *Thumb opposition*: thorough clinical examination and patient counseling must precede the indication for the opponensplasty as some degree of thumb opposition may be present in spite of complete median nerve palsy. This is most likely due to preserved ulnar nerve innervation. Apart from that, even the inability to oppose the thumb must not necessarily be associated with diminished hand function to such a degree as to warrant the opponensplasty [38], especially when the non-dominant hand is affected.
- Multiple techniques of opponensplasty have been described in the literature of which the following four are performed most commonly: (1) FDS opponensplasty [39], (2) EIP opponensplasty [40], (3) ADM opponensplasty [41, 42], and (4) PL opponensplasty [43].
- Several principles must be followed to achieve a successful result for any tendon transfer: (1) the excursion and strength of the donor muscle must be similar to that of abductor pollicis brevis (APB) and opponens pollicis (OP); (2) the line of pull of the donor tendon must be similar to those of APB and OP – this may be achieved naturally by the course of the donor tendon or by creating a pulley, mostly in the region of os pisiforme. Here, we describe some of the most commonly performed techniques of the opponensplasty.
- At our institution, the EIP opponensplasty (Figs. 6.9a–c and 6.10a–d) is the preferred technique to restore the thumb opposition for its minimal donor site morbidity, avoiding the need to create a pulley and reliable functional results. Typically, at least four skin incisions are necessary: The first incision is made over the MCP-II-joint to harvest the EIP tendon. The EIP tendon lies usually ulnarly to the EDC-II. Another hint for identification of the EIP is the fact that its muscle belly is the most

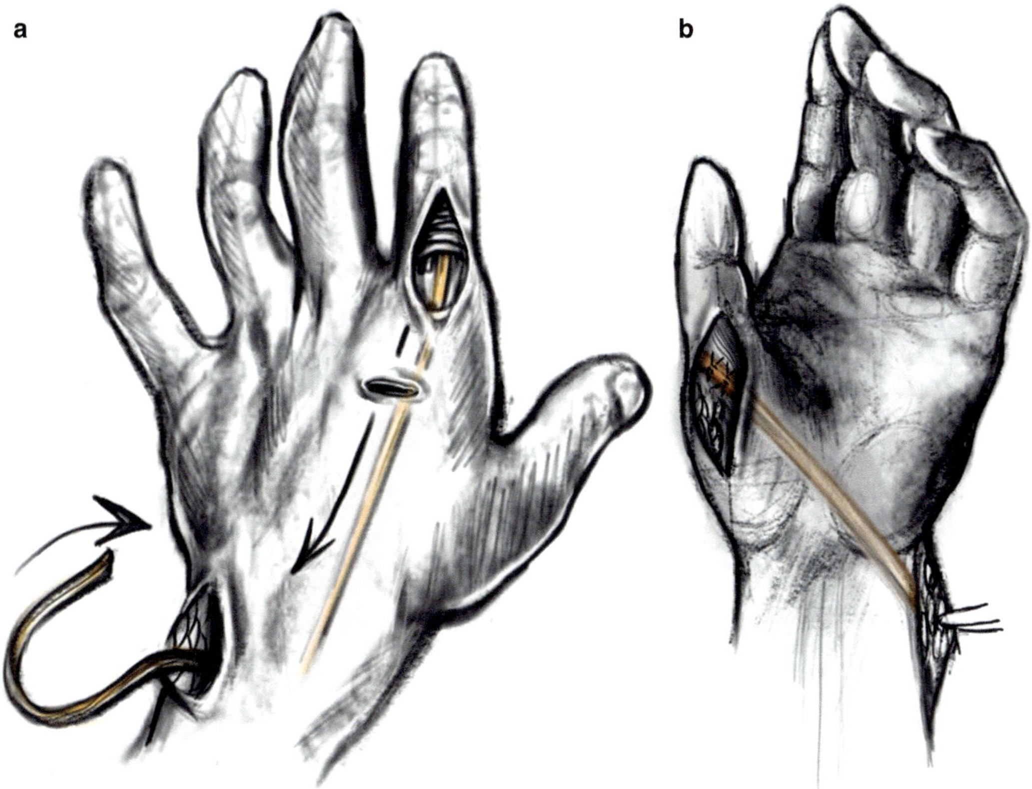

Fig. 6.9 Schematic diagram of extensor indicis proprius (EIP) opponensplasty. (**a**) EIP tendon is divided through the distal incision at the level of MP joint. Then, it is pulled through the subcutaneous tunnel to the distal ulnodorsal aspect of the forearm in order to be wrapped around the neck of the ulna to the palmar side. Sometimes, an additional incision is needed to free the EIP tendon from the attachments with EDC-II tendon. (**b**) The tendon is transposed subcutaneously to the radiopalmar side of the MP joint of the thumb where it is attached to the fascia of the (abductor pollicis brevis) ABP, alternatively also to the capsule of the MP joint and extensor pollicis longus (EPL) tendon

distally placed of all extensor tendons. It is useful to sling the distal part of the tendon on a suture to avoid squeezing it with the forceps. The second incision is made over the 4th extensor compartment that is opened and the EIP tendon pulled in this wound. Sometimes, an additional incision is needed between the two to release the EIP tendon from attachments with the EDC-II tendon. Then, the third incision is made longitudinally on the ulnar side of the wrist at the level of the pisiform. Here care must be taken to avoid injury to the dorsal branch of the ulnar nerve. The EIP tendon is retrieved through a subcutaneous tunnel that may be created by a hemostat. It is important to make sure it is deep to the dorsal branch of the ulnar nerve. Hereafter, the last incision is made over the dorsoradial aspect of the MP joint of the thumb, and using a tendon passer a tunnel is created subcutaneously palmar to the flexor retinaculum and the tendon pulled toward the thumb. The tendon is sutured to the APB tendon either side-to-side or weaving through it. Alternatively, an additional suture (FiberWire or Ethibond 4.0) may be made to the capsule of the MP joint and EPL tendon. For the good functional result, the tension of the suture is crucial. It is recommended that suture be tight with the wrist in a neutral position and the thumb in maximal opposition. In

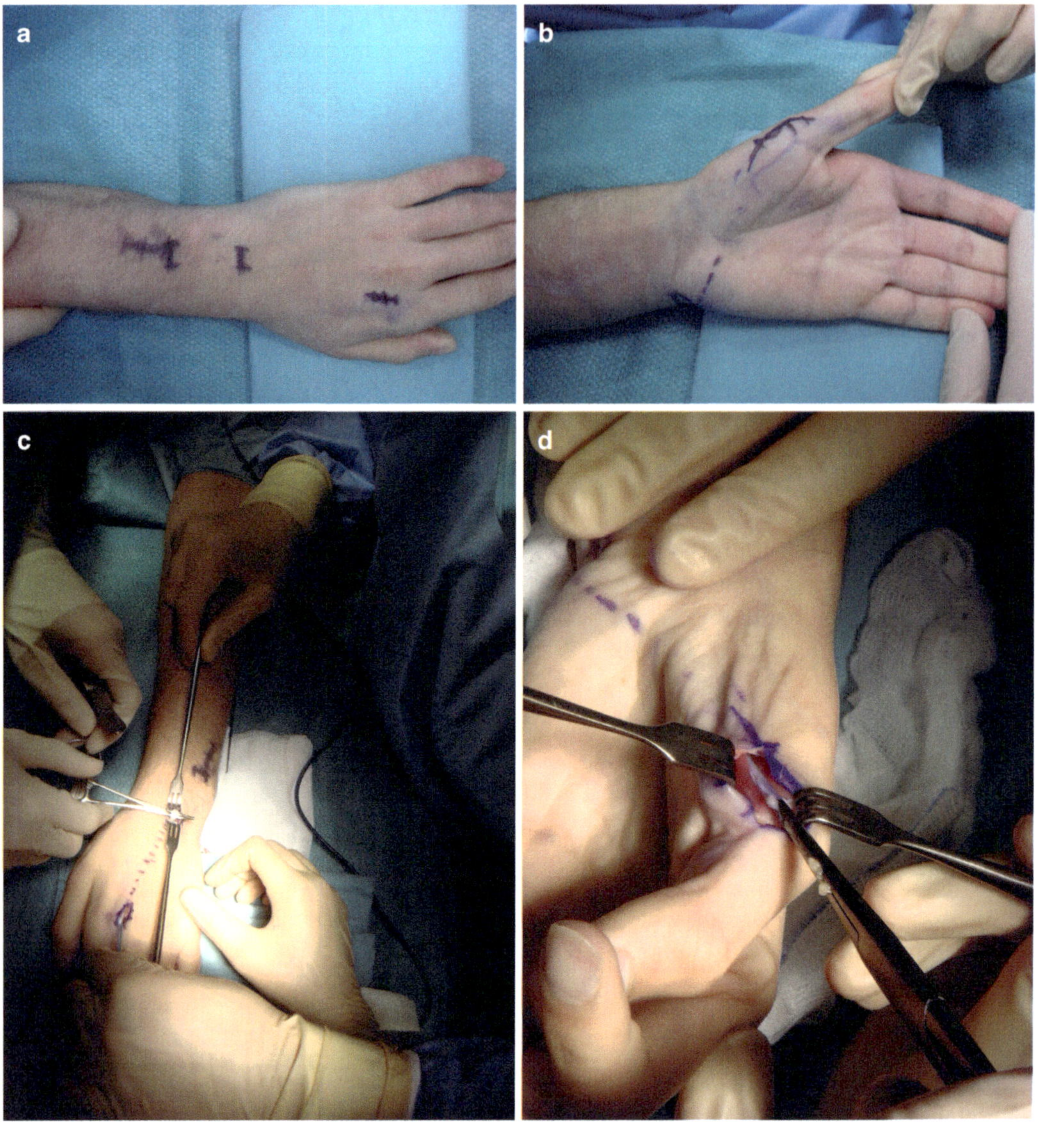

Fig. 6.10 Extensor indicis proprius (EIP) to abductor pollicis brevis (APB) transfer after a chronic median nerve injury at the elbow. (**a** and **b**) Skin incisions for the tendon transfer. The first incision is made over the MCP-II-joint to harvest the EIP tendon. The second incision is made over the 4th extensor compartment that is opened and the EIP tendon pulled in this wound. The third incision is made longitudinally on the ulnar side of the wrist at the level of pisiform. The last incision is made over the dorsoradial aspect of the MP joint of the thumb (**c**) EIP before the distal cut. (**d**) The tendon is sutured to the APB tendon side-to-side

this position, the wrist and thumb are immobilized for 4 weeks after which ROM exercises are initiated.

A persistent sensory deficit of the thumb and the fingers may lead to skin injuries and/or burns as well as to impairment of fine motor skills in the hand, mainly grasp between the thumb and the index finger. In situations where reinnervation is not expected, a distal nerve transfer may be considered. A simple method with reproducible results is a nerve transfer of the branches of the superficial branch of the radial nerve (SBRN) to the digital nerves of the thumb and the index finger [44]. The V-skin incisions are made over the proximal phalanx of the thumb on the ulnar side and of the index finger on the radial side, and the SBRN are sutured end-to-end on the digital nerve II and III, respectively. It can be expected that the protective sensation be restored by 6 months postoperatively.

6.5.1 Radial Nerve

Due to traction and compression, lesions of the radial nerve around the elbow can develop either from trauma or postoperatively. Hematoma or swelling may exacerbate the injury. While acute compression of the nerve is possible anywhere along the course of the nerve in the elbow region, it is most likely that it occurs at sites of naturally confined spaces. The radial nerve emerges in the elbow region after exiting the spiral groove about 10 cm proximal to the lateral epicondyle. Then it pierces the lateral intermuscular septum to enter the ventral compartment. During fractures of the distal humerus or surgical approach to treat these fractures, the nerve is susceptible to injury in this region due to relative fixation to the intermuscular septum and tethering while under traction. The nerve runs further distally along the lateral border of the brachialis muscles, deep to brachioradialis, and on the annular ligament. In the region of the radial head, there are also fibrous bands with a tethering effect rendering the nerve susceptible to injury. The radial nerve bifurcates here giving off the superficial sensory branch that runs further under the brachioradialis and the deep, predominantly motor branch that enters the arcade of Frohse, formed by a fibrous arch of the origin of the supinator muscle. The nerve descends distally between the two heads of the supinator and exits the muscle as posterior interosseous nerve (PIN) that gives motor branches to the extrinsic extensors and abductors. It is obvious that because of numerous fibrous attachments, the radial nerve may be injured at different levels by the injury itself, accompanying compression due to hematoma or during the surgical therapy of the original bony or joint injury. Here like for any other peripheral nerve, precise clinical evaluation is mandatory. If an acute neurologic deficit is present, especially with imminent compartment syndrome, surgical exploration, decompression, and neurolysis are indicated. In the rare cases of avulsion, a nerve repair or grafting is performed in a standard manner.

An ultrasound is performed routinely as soon as the patient comes to our clinic by a specially trained neurologist. If the nerve is not in-continuity, immediate surgery is planned. If the nerve is in-continuity, reinnervation signs should be observed via serial physical and EDX examinations in the first 4 months; otherwise, surgical exploration is performed (Fig. 6.11). In low-grade nerve injury (Sunderland II, III), the reinnervation process begins several months after an injury and can carry on for 1–2 years. EMG signs of nerve regeneration are reduction in the numbers of fibrillation potentials and emergence of polyphasic motor unit potentials (MUPs). Polyphasic MUP has five or more phases as opposed to normal MUPs that have two or three. Later on, if the reinnervation occurs successfully, the MUPs become wide in duration and high in amplitude.

In lesions Sunderland grade I-III, the recovery is usually complete within 4–9 months. During this period, physiotherapy with range-of-motion exercises for the wrist and finger and splinting to prevent joint contractures are of great importance. In more severe lesions (Sunderland grade IV) or those lesions that show no sign of regeneration after 4 months, surgical exploration and neurolysis are indicated (Fig. 6.11). If a neuroma-in-continuity is found, intraoperative electrodiagnostic studies will help to decide if neurolysis alone is sufficient or excision of the neuroma in continuity and reconstruction with a nerve graft needs to be performed.

6.5.2 Nerve Transfers

Injuries around the elbow are usually managed by nerve repair or autologous nerve graft with good prospects of reinnervation. However, if there is no reinnervation of the radial-innervated wrist extensors and finger and thumb

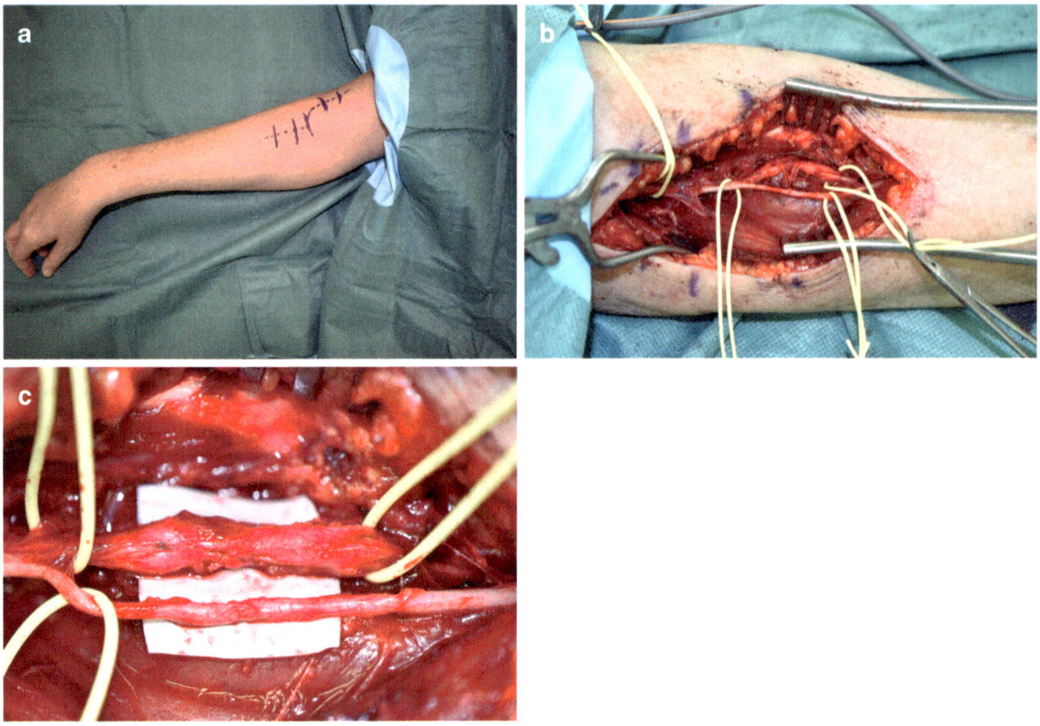

Fig. 6.11 A 40-year-old woman presented with a complete posterior interosseous nerve (PIN) palsy without recovery signs 4 months after an elbow arthroscopy. (**a**) Skin incisions for the exploration. (**b**) A neuroma-in-continuity was found in the PIN. The PIN presented NAPs during the intraoperative electrodiagnostic study. (**c**) Only careful neurolysis under the microscope was performed. The patient recovered full range of motion 8 weeks after the neurolysis

extensors by 6-month post-injury, or if the patient presents delayed with a radial nerve injury that has not been treated primarily, restoration of muscle function by nerve transfers may be considered. The absence of a suitable proximal stump to which the nerve graft is supposed to be coapted may be another indication for nerve transfer. This may occur when the consequence of the injury is the destruction of the nerve with scarring over a long distance. A more obvious indication for nerve transfers are injuries to the radial nerve more proximally, such as around the axilla for which no sufficient reinnervation is expected. Mackinnon reported on the good restoration of wrist and finger extension as well as grip strength with the transfer of *the motor branch to the FDS to ECRB* and of *the FCR to the posterior interosseous nerve* [45]. We routinely combine these nerve transfers with the pronator teres to ECRB tendon transfer, so that the patient does not have to wait for nerve regeneration to gain wrist extension.

6.6 Salvage Procedures for the Radial Nerve

If for any reason no or insufficient reinnervation of the radialis-innervated muscles occurs with persistent wrist drop, inability to extend the thumb and the fingers in MP joints, tendon transfers are indicated. Although multiple various options exist as to which donor muscles to choose, several very reliable reconstructions evolved that can be seen as equivalent:

1. Pronator teres (PT) to extensor carpi radialis brevis (ECRB); flexor carpi radialis (FCR) to extensor digitorum communis (EDC) (Brand

transfer); palmaris longus (PL) to extensor pollicis longus (EPL) [Brand].
2. PT to ECRB and ECRL; FCU to EDC (jones transfer) and EPL; PL to EPB and APL [Merle d´Aubigné (46)].
3. PT to ECRB; FDS III and IV to EDC and EIP (modified Boyes transfer); PL to EPL [Boyes (47)].

All techniques use the PT-to-ECRB transfers for wrist extension while differing in the way the finger and thumb extension is restored. The transfers using the FCU should not be the first choice as the FCU tendon is an important stabilizer at the ulnar side of the wrist, with twice the strength as FCR and plays an important role in dart thrower's motion. Apart from that, in the lower radial nerve palsy, a lack of action of the FCU leads to the radial deviation of the wrist due to the intact ECRL. At our institution, the Brand-reconstruction as described above is used primarily. However, in specific situations, such as in patients with wrist arthrodesis, the Boyes procedure may be a more suitable choice as the FDS tendons possess better excursion and allow complete extension in the MP joints while the wrist is fused in slight extension. In contrast, for the complete finger extension with the FCR or FCU transfers, full extension is achieved with the help of the tenodesis effect when the wrist is slightly flexed [48]. The disadvantage of the FDS transfer is the more difficult reeducation as the action of FDS is not synergistic for the extension in the finger MP joints.

Steps of the tendon transfers (PT to ECRB, FCR to EDC, PL to EPL) (Fig. 6.12): long lazy S incision on the palmar side of the forearm from the wrist crease up to the proximal third of the forearm and the FCR and PL tendons are identified and mobilized. Then, the fascia over the BR is cautiously incised and the radial sensory nerve (RSN) lying under is visualized and protected. BR muscle is pulled radially with a retractor. Radial vessels are located deeper and medially to the RSN. The PT muscle and its tendon can be easily found between the radial vessels and RSN. Hereafter, the PT tendon is mobilized with a scalpel down to the radius. In order to maximize the length of the PT tendon, several centimeters long strip of periosteum is harvested off the radius with an elevator extending PT tendon. Fascial attachments in the distal part of the PT muscle are divided to provide better excursion of the transferred muscle. The second incision is made in the distal third of the forearm dorsally in a lazy S fashion. The dissection occurs proximal to the extensor retinaculum. The four tendons of the EDC, ECRB, and EPL are dissected free. Here the EPL tendon is divided as proximally as possible close to the musculocutaneous junction. The third short incision is made at the base of the thumb. The EPL tendon is identified and the free proximal end is pulled in this wound to be then subcutaneously rerouted into the palmar wound where it is sutured to the PL tendon. The PT and FCR tendons are rerouted into the dorsal wound over the BR muscle. Before suturing the tendons, an unhindered line of pull without any kinking must be secured. The FCR is weaved through the four EDC tendons, while the tension is set with wrist and finger MP joints in neutral position allowing clenching the fist passively. The PL is sutured with EPL with the wrist in neutral position and thumb in maximal extension. Finally, the PT to ECRB tendon is sutured using a Pulvertaft weaving technique without dividing the ECRB. This is especially useful if some degree of reinnervation of the ECRB is thinkable. The tension of the suture should be tight with the wrist at 45° extension while allowing full passive flexion of the wrist. As suture material, FiberWire or Ethibon 3.0 can be used. Postoperatively, wrist, thumb, and MP joints of the fingers are immobilized for 4 weeks with a splint and another 4 weeks at nights. The active range-of-motion exercises are commenced in the fifth postoperative week.

6.6.1 Sensory Nerves Around the Elbow

- *The lateral antebrachial cutaneous nerve (LACN)*

LACN is the terminal purely sensory branch of the musculocutaneous nerve. Roughly 3 cm

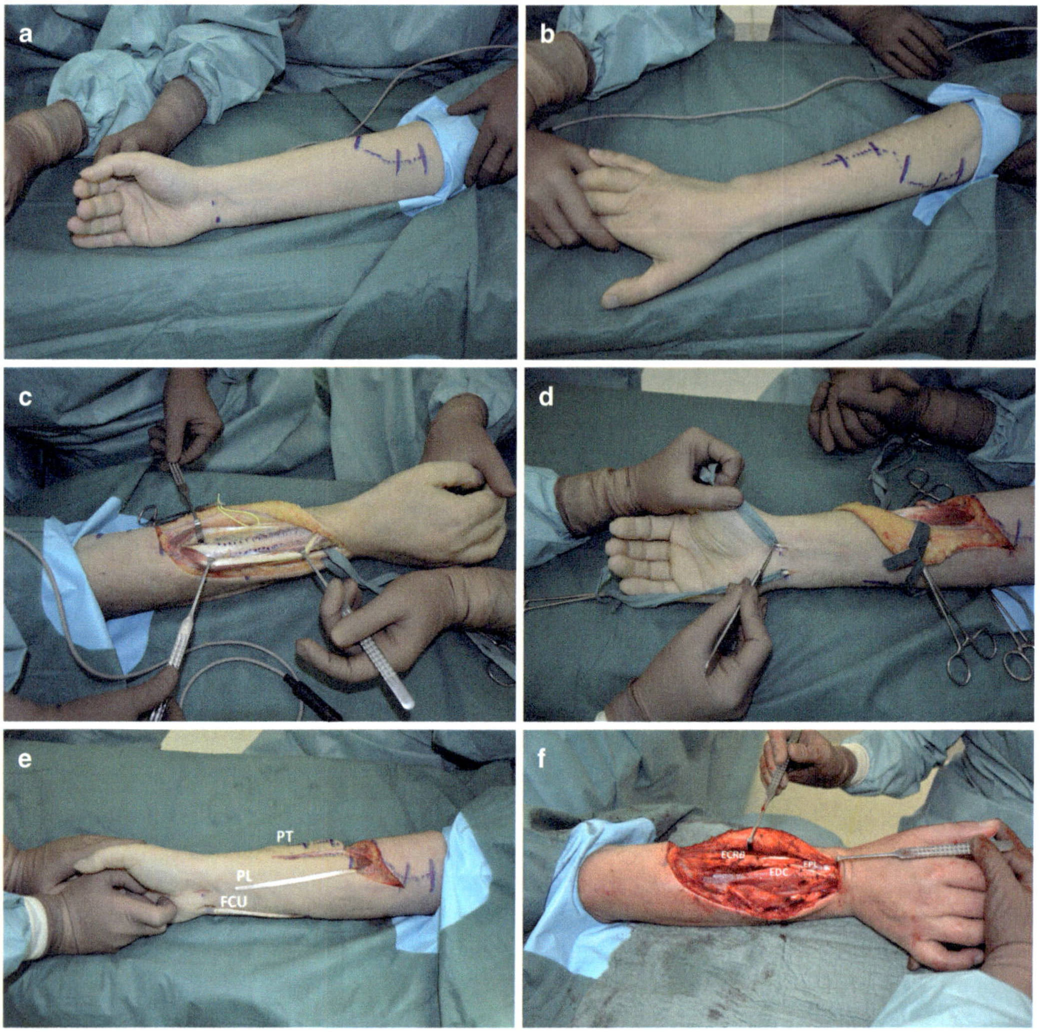

Fig. 6.12 A 54-year-old patient presented with a chronic radial nerve injury and a weak FCR muscle (M3). Pronator teres (PT) to extensor carpi radialis brevis (ECRB), flexor carpi ulnaris (FCU) to extensor digitorum communis (EDC), palmaris longus (PL) to extensor pollicis longus (EPL) tendon transfer were performed. (**a** and **b**) Skin incisions for the tendon transfer. (**c**) The PT muscle and its tendon can be easily found between the radial vessels and RSN. In order to maximize the length of the PT, several centimeters long strip of periosteum is harvested off the radius with an elevatorium. (**d**) PL and FCU are cut distally. (**e**) PL, FCU, and PT are dissected free. (**f**) EPL, EDC, and ECRB are dissected and sutured to the PL, FCU, and PT tendons, respectively

proximal to the lateral epicondyle it pierces the brachial fascia. It can be found between biceps brachii and brachialis muscle. Then it crosses the elbow in the subcutaneous tissue approximately 4 cm medial to the lateral epicondyle and branches in the anterior and posterior branch that innervate the anterolateral and posterolateral skin of the forearm, respectively. The nerve is especially prone to injury during the approach to the distal humerus. If the nerve is accidentally transected, the primary repair is the treatment of choice. In case the nerve lesion is detected postoperatively, the patient should be informed that recovery may occur spontaneously. The sensory deficit is usually not substantially disturbing to the patient. As a late complication of the injury, a painful neuroma can develop. A typical neuroma is diagnosed clinically with sharply limited area of pain to light touch (allodynia) and positive (painful) Tinel sign with a distribution of the paraesthesias/dysesthesias in the sensory distribution of the nerve. A test infiltration with local anesthetic may be applied to rule out centralization of the pain. MRI may be used to confirm the diagnosis and help localize it exactly as part of the planning before surgery. This can be treated with neuromodulation. If the pain does not improve, surgical exploration and neuroma excision are indicated. The proximal nerve stump is then buried in muscle tissue.

- *The medial antebrachial cutaneous nerve (MACN)*

The MACN runs on the medial side of the arm, a branch of the medial cord of the brachial plexus. It pierces the muscle fascia in the middle or distal third of the arm and runs distally in the subcutaneous tissue. Proximal to the medial epicondyle, it branches in the anterior and posterior branch. While the anterior branch runs lateral to the medial epicondyle, usually 2–3 cm lateral to the medial epicondyle, the posterior branch has usually another 1–4 branches that cross posteriorly to the medial epicondyle proximally or at the level of medial epicondyle in about 90% of cases [49]. The nerve or its branches may be injured during the fracture reposition and osteosynthesis as well as in cubital tunnel release. The principles of the therapy are similar to those of the LACN. The sensory deficit on the medial side of the forearm is usually not disturbing.

6.7 Technical Pearls and Pitfalls

- The majority of iatrogenic nerve lesions around the elbow recover without intervention.
- Clinical history, physical exam, imaging techniques, and EDX studies are critical and necessary to select the patients in which spontaneous recovery is unlikely.
- In order to avoid joint contractures, physiotherapy with range-of-motion exercises and splinting are essential before regenerations occur.
- If nerve transection is suspected, exploration and nerve repair are indicated as soon as possible.
- Primary nerve repair remains the gold standard for the treatment of a complete nerve transection. Tension must be avoided in any nerve repair in any position of the surrounding joints. Autologous nerve grafts should be used if tension cannot be avoided.
- In specific situations, nerve transfers may be the best option to achieve reinnervation. Type of injury and patient expectations should be considered to choose the right reconstructive option.
- Chronic injuries (>12 months) can be treated with tendon transfers. They may restore the most important motor functions of the hand, thumb, and fingers. Free passive range of motion of the joints and intact donor muscles are a prerequisite for tendon transfers.

Acknowledgment We thank Jana Pindur for the illustrations.

References

1. Kelly EW, Morrey BF, O'Driscoll SW. Complications of elbow arthroscopy. J Bone Joint Surg Am. 2001;83(1):25–34. https://doi.org/10.2106/00004623-200101000-00004.
2. Blonna D, Wolf JM, Fitzsimmons JS, O'Driscoll SW. Prevention of nerve injury during arthroscopic capsulectomy of the elbow utilizing a safety-driven strategy. J Bone Joint Surg Am. 2013;95(15):1373–81. https://doi.org/10.2106/JBJS.K.00972.
3. Ristic S, Strauch RJ, Rosenwasser MP. The assessment and treatment of nerve dysfunction after trauma around the elbow. Clin Orthop Relat Res. 2000;370:138–53. https://doi.org/10.1097/00003086-200001000-00013.
4. Samardzić M, Grujicić D, Milinković ZB. Radial nerve lesions associated with fractures of the humeral shaft. Injury. 1990;21(4):220–2. https://doi.org/10.1016/0020-1383(90)90006-g.
5. Nelson AJ, Izzi JA, Green A, Weiss AP, Akelman E. Traumatic nerve injuries about the elbow. Orthop Clin North Am. 1999;30(1):91–4. https://doi.org/10.1016/s0030-5898(05)70063-8.
6. Nath RK, Mackinnon SE. Nerve transfers in the upper extremity. Hand Clin. 2000;16(1):131–9,

ix. Available from: https://www.ncbi.nlm.nih.gov/pubmed/10696582
7. Chiu DT, Ishii C. Management of peripheral nerve injuries. Orthop Clin North Am. 1986;17(3):365–73. Available from: https://www.ncbi.nlm.nih.gov/pubmed/3737134
8. Lovett WL, McCalla MA. Nerve injuries: management and rehabilitation. Orthop Clin North Am. 1983;14(4):767–78. Available from: https://www.ncbi.nlm.nih.gov/pubmed/6355959
9. Adams JE, Steinmann SP. Nerve injuries about the elbow. J Hand Surg Am. 2006;31(2):303–13. https://doi.org/10.1016/j.jhsa.2005.12.006.
10. He B, Zhu Z, Zhu Q, Zhou X, Zheng C, Li P, et al. Factors predicting sensory and motor recovery after the repair of upper limb peripheral nerve injuries. Neural Regen Res. 2014;9(6):661–72. https://doi.org/10.4103/1673-5374.130094.
11. Gruen P. Evaluation and surgical management of peripheral nerve problems. Neurosurgery. 1999;44:839–40. https://doi.org/10.1097/00006123-199904000-00078.
12. Hirachi K, Kato H, Minami A, Kasashima T, Kaneda K. Clinical features and management of traumatic posterior interosseous nerve palsy. J Hand Surg Br. 1998;23(3):413–7. https://doi.org/10.1016/s0266-7681(98)80071-5.
13. Srinivasan R, Rhodes J. The median-ulnar anastomosis (Martin-Gruber) in normal and congenitally abnormal fetuses. Arch Neurol. 1981;38(7):418–9. https://doi.org/10.1001/archneur.1981.00510070052007.
14. Dumitru D, Walsh NE, Weber CF. Electrophysiologic study of the Riche-Cannieu anomaly. Electromyogr Clin Neurophysiol. 1988;28(1):27–31. Available from: https://www.ncbi.nlm.nih.gov/pubmed/3168913
15. Thoder JJ, Kozin SH. Management principles to treat nerve loss after violent trauma to the upper extremity. Hand Clin. 1999;15(2):289–98, ix. Available from: https://www.ncbi.nlm.nih.gov/pubmed/10361639
16. Amillo S, Mora G. Surgical management of neural injuries associated with elbow fractures in children. J Pediatr Orthop. 1999;19(5):573–7. Available from: https://www.ncbi.nlm.nih.gov/pubmed/10488853
17. Brown JM, Yablon CM, Morag Y, Brandon CJ, Jacobson JA. US of the peripheral nerves of the upper extremity: a landmark approach. Radiographics. 2016;36(2):452–63. https://doi.org/10.1148/rg.2016150088.
18. Zaidman CM, Seelig MJ, Baker JC, Mackinnon SE, Pestronk A. Detection of peripheral nerve pathology: comparison of ultrasound and MRI. Neurology. 2013;80(18):1634–40. https://doi.org/10.1212/WNL.0b013e3182904f3f.
19. Power HA, Kahn LC, Patterson MM, Yee A, Moore AM, Mackinnon SE. Refining indications for the supercharge end-to-side anterior interosseous to ulnar motor nerve transfer in cubital tunnel syndrome. Plast Reconstr Surg. 2020;145(1):106e–16e. https://doi.org/10.1097/PRS.0000000000006399.
20. Barbour J, Yee A, Kahn LC, Mackinnon SE. Supercharged end-to-side anterior interosseous to ulnar motor nerve transfer for intrinsic musculature reinnervation. J Hand Surg Am. 2012;37(10):2150–9. https://doi.org/10.1016/j.jhsa.2012.07.022.
21. Zancolli EA. Claw-hand caused by paralysis of the intrinsic muscles: a simple surgical procedure for its correction. J Bone Joint Surg Am. 1957;39-A(5):1076–80. Available from: https://www.ncbi.nlm.nih.gov/pubmed/13475406
22. Sapienza A, Green S. Correction of the claw hand. Hand Clin. 2012;28(1):53–66. https://doi.org/10.1016/j.hcl.2011.09.009.
23. Zancolli EA. Intrinsic paralysis of the ulnar nerve—physiopathology of the claw hand. In: Structural and dynamic bases of hand surgery. Philadelphia: JB Lippincott; 1979. p. 159–206.
24. Brown PW. Zancolli capsulorrhaphy for ulnar claw hand. Appraisal of forty-four cases. J Bone Joint Surg Am. 1970;52(5):868–77. Available from: https://www.ncbi.nlm.nih.gov/pubmed/5479477
25. Leddy JP, Stark HH, Ashworth CR, Boyes JH. Capsulodesis and pulley advancement for the correction of claw-finger deformity. Plast Reconstr Surg. 1973;51:477. https://doi.org/10.1097/00006534-197304000-00044.
26. Riordan DC. Tendon transfers in hand surgery. J Hand Surg Am. 1983;8(5 Pt 2):748–53. https://doi.org/10.1016/s0363-5023(83)80264-0.
27. Parkes A. Paralytic claw fingers–a graft tenodesis operation. Hand. 1973;5(3):192–9. https://doi.org/10.1016/0072-968x(73)90028-4.
28. Littler JW. Tendon transfers and arthrodeses in combined median and ulnar nerve paralysis. J Bone Joint Surg Am. 1949;31A(2):225–34. Available from: https://www.ncbi.nlm.nih.gov/pubmed/18116560
29. Brand PW. Tendon grafting: illustrated by a new operation for intrinsic paralysis of the fingers. J Bone Joint Surg Br. 1961;43-B(3):444–53. https://doi.org/10.1302/0301-620X.43B3.444.
30. Brandsma JW, Ottenhoff-de Jonge MW. Flexor digitorum superficialis tendon transfer for intrinsic replacement: long-term results and the effect on donor fingers. J Hand Surg Am. 1992;17(6):625–8. https://doi.org/10.1016/0266-7681%2892%2990187-7.
31. Hastings H 2nd, McCollam SM. Flexor digitorum superficialis lasso tendon transfer in isolated ulnar nerve palsy: a functional evaluation. J Hand Surg Am. 1994;19(2):275–80. https://doi.org/10.1016/0363-5023(94)90019-1.
32. Brand PW. Paralytic claw hand; with special reference to paralysis in leprosy and treatment by the sublimis transfer of Stiles and Bunnell. J Bone Joint Surg Br. 1958;40-B(4):618–32. https://doi.org/10.1302/0301-620X.40B4.618.
33. Smith RJ. Extensor carpi radialis brevis tendon transfer for thumb adduction–a study of power pinch. J Hand Surg Am. 1983;8(1):4–15. https://doi.org/10.1016/s0363-5023(83)80044-6.
34. Roy J, Henry BM, PĘkala PA, Vikse J, Saganiak K, Walocha JA, et al. Median and ulnar nerve anastomoses in the upper limb: a meta-analysis. Muscle

Nerve. 2016;54(1):36–47. https://doi.org/10.1002/mus.24993.
35. Hsiao EC, Fox IK, Tung TH, Mackinnon SE. Motor nerve transfers to restore extrinsic median nerve function: case report. Hand. 2009;4(1):92–7. https://doi.org/10.1007/s11552-008-9128-9.
36. Bertelli JA, Soldado F, Lehn VLM, Ghizoni MF. Reappraisal of clinical deficits following high median nerve injuries. J Hand Surg Am. 2016;41(1):13–9. https://doi.org/10.1016/j.jhsa.2015.10.022.
37. Owings R, Wickstrom J, Perry J, Nickel VL. Biceps Brachii rerouting in treatment of paralytic supination contracture of the forearm. J Bone Jt Surg. 1971;53:137–42. https://doi.org/10.2106/00004623-197153010-00013.
38. Jensen EG, Gert JE. Restoration of opposition of the thumb. Hand. 1978;10:161–7. https://doi.org/10.1016/s0072-968x(78)80007-2.
39. Royle ND. An operation for paralysis of the intrinsic muscles of the thumb. J Am Med Assoc. 1938;111:612. https://doi.org/10.1001/jama.1938.72790330003006a.
40. Burkhalter W, Christensen RC, Brown P. Extensor indicis proprius opponensplasty. J Bone Joint Surg Am. 1973;55(4):725–32. Available from: https://www.ncbi.nlm.nih.gov/pubmed/4283744
41. Huber E. Relief operation in the case of paralysis of the median nerve. J Hand Surg Br. 2004;29(1):35–7. https://doi.org/10.1016/j.jhsb.2003.10.003.
42. Nicolaysen J. Transplantation of the M. abductor dig. V. Where there is no ability to oppose the thumb. J Hand Surg Br. 2004;29(1):38–9. https://doi.org/10.1016/j.jhsb.2003.10.002.
43. Camitz H. Uber die behandlung der oppositionslahmung. Acta Chir Scand. 1929;65:77–81.
44. Bertelli JA, Ghizoni MF. Very distal sensory nerve transfers in high median nerve lesions. J Hand Surg Am. 2011;36(3):387–93. https://doi.org/10.1016/j.jhsa.2010.11.049.
45. Mackinnon SE, Roque B, Tung TH. Median to radial nerve transfer for treatment of radial nerve palsy. Case report. J Neurosurg. 2007;107(3):666–71. https://doi.org/10.3171/JNS-07/09/0666.
46. Merle d'Aubigné R, Lance P. Tendon transplantation in treatment of posttraumatic radial paralysis. Sem Hop. 1946;22:1666.
47. Chuinard RG, Boyes JH, Stark HH, Ashworth CR. Tendon transfers for radial nerve palsy: use of superficialis tendons for digital extension. J Hand Surg Am. 1978;3(6):560–70. https://doi.org/10.1016/s0363-5023(78)80007-0.
48. Sammer DM, Chung KC. Tendon transfers: part I. Principles of transfer and transfers for radial nerve palsy. Plast Reconstr Surg. 2009;123(5):169e–77e. https://doi.org/10.1097/PRS.0b013e3181a20526.
49. Masear VR, Meyer RD, Pichora DR. Surgical anatomy of the medial antebrachial cutaneous nerve. J Hand Surg Am. 1989;14(2 Pt 1):267–71. https://doi.org/10.1016/0363-5023(89)90019-1.

Nerve Injury After Distal Radius, Metacarpal, and Finger Fractures

7

Travis J. Miller, Robin N. Kamal, and Paige M. Fox

7.1 Risks/Incidence/Mechanism of Injury

Fractures of the upper extremity place peripheral nerves at significant risk. Peripheral nerve injury is estimated to occur in 3.3% of all traumas that involve the upper extremity [1]. The risk of nerve injury is higher for patients who require open interventions for extremity conditions due to the potential for iatrogenic injuries [2]. The goal of this chapter is to provide anatomic review of relevant neuroanatomy for distal radius, metacarpal, and phalangeal fractures and to provide guidance for avoiding iatrogenic nerve injury. Diagnosis and techniques of nerve repair and salvage are discussed.

T. J. Miller
Division of Plastic and Reconstructive Surgery, Stanford University, Stanford, CA, USA
e-mail: travismi@stanford.edu

R. N. Kamal
Chase Hand and Upper Limb Center, Department of Orthopaedic Surgery, Stanford University School of Medicine, Stanford, CA, USA
e-mail: rnkamal@stanford.edu

P. M. Fox (✉)
Chase Hand and Upper Limb Center, Division of Plastic and Reconstructive Surgery, Stanford University School of Medicine, Stanford, CA, USA
e-mail: pfox@stanford.edu

7.1.1 Distal Radius

Median nerve injury has been described in many series of distal radius fractures and has even been reported to be the most common complication in some reports, occurring in up to 30% of patients [3]. These injuries may be due to direct compression from fracture fragments and associated edema or, less commonly, from laceration from fracture fragments or median artery thrombosis [4–6]. Risk of median nerve injury with fracture type is unclear. Bieneck et al. did not find a correlation of carpal tunnel syndrome with different fracture patterns [4]. Other groups have found a correlation of median nerve compression with higher degrees of comminution and higher grade AO fracture pattern [7, 8]. Gelberman et al. demonstrated that carpal canal pressures beyond 40–50 mmHg lead to progressive sensory and motor dysfunction [9]. However, when Fuller et al. examined carpal tunnel pressures for 24 h after volar plating of a distal radius fracture, they showed that while pressures may reach up to 65 mmHg, these decreased to 31 mmHg or less within 24 h after surgery. No patients had long-term median nerve symptoms despite transient rises in carpal tunnel pressures [10].

Radial and ulnar nerve injuries have also been reported but occur much less frequently due to the anatomic distance between the radius and these nerves; most injuries to ulnar and radial

C. J. Dy et al. (eds.), *Peripheral Nerve Issues after Orthopedic Surgery*,
https://doi.org/10.1007/978-3-030-84428-8_7

nerves from distal radius fractures are from pressure points during casting [3].

Palmar cutaneous nerve (PCN) injury, while rare, is also possible with distal radius fracture treatment. Samson et al. found that after reviewing 1280 patients who underwent distal radius fixation, 7 patients (0.5%) suffered iatrogenic palmar cutaneous nerve injury [11]. No patients had PCN injury preoperatively; thus, PCN injury from a closed distal radius fracture in isolation appears rare.

7.1.2 Metacarpal Fractures

Risk of nerve injury during the treatment of metacarpal fractures correlates to the metacarpals involved. Injury to the ulnar nerve, specifically the deep motor branch, has been reported in many series on fractures of the ring or small finger metacarpal bases near the carpometacarpal (CMC) joint [12–14]. Case reports have also documented injury to the deep motor branch from index and middle finger metacarpal fractures, though this appears to be comparatively rare [15]. The sensory branch of the radial nerve (SBRN) and dorsal sensory branch of the ulnar nerve (DSBUN) can also be injured by metacarpal fractures during the surgical approach, though there is little discussed in the literature on its incidence.

7.1.3 Phalangeal Fractures

For phalangeal fractures, the volar and dorsal digital nerves are at risk, especially during open injury. Vascular compromise for closed injuries has been reported, and injury to the nerves is also possible [16]. Digital nerve entrapment during callus formation after a closed reduction has been reported [17]. Open treatment of phalangeal fractures places the digital nerves at risk, though the incidence of iatrogenic injury is unknown [18].

7.2 Pertinent Anatomy

7.2.1 Distal Radius

Laceration of the median nerve from distal radius fracture fragments is rare, likely due to the interposing tissue of the pronator quadratus (PQ), flexor pollicis longus (FPL), the flexor digitorum profundus (FDP), and the flexor digitorum superficialis (FDS) [6]. During surgical exposure for the distal radius volarly, the Henry or modified Henry approaches are most commonly used. Both approaches use an 8–10 cm incision directly over the FCR tendon. In the original Henry approach, the radial artery is identified and preserved, and the deep compartment is exposed between the radial artery and FCR sheath. In the modified Henry approach, the FCR sheath is incised [19]. One disadvantage to the modified Henry approach is that the PCN can run within the FCR sheath and may be injured in the approach. Anatomic studies suggest that the PCN runs within the ulnar edge of the sheath but does not cross the FCR tendon [19].

At the level of the distal radius, the median nerve may not be directly visualized during a volar approach. The median nerve may be as close as 0.1 mm to the FCR at 10 cm proximal to the wrist crease, but the FCR and median nerve diverge distally and lie about 2 cm apart at the wrist crease [19]. However, even without direct trauma, retraction during exposure may lead to nerve injury, including branches of the median nerve to surrounding flexor tendons. In particular, weakness of the flexor pollicis longus (FPL) has been reported in the immediate postoperative period [20]. The proximity of the median nerve and PCN to the FCR can be seen in Fig. 7.1.

If a distal radius repair is combined with an open carpal tunnel release, some surgeons have advocated for two separate incisions. The rationale is that an incision traversing over the FCR to the carpal tunnel will place the PCN at risk [21, 22]. A single-incision approach has been advo-

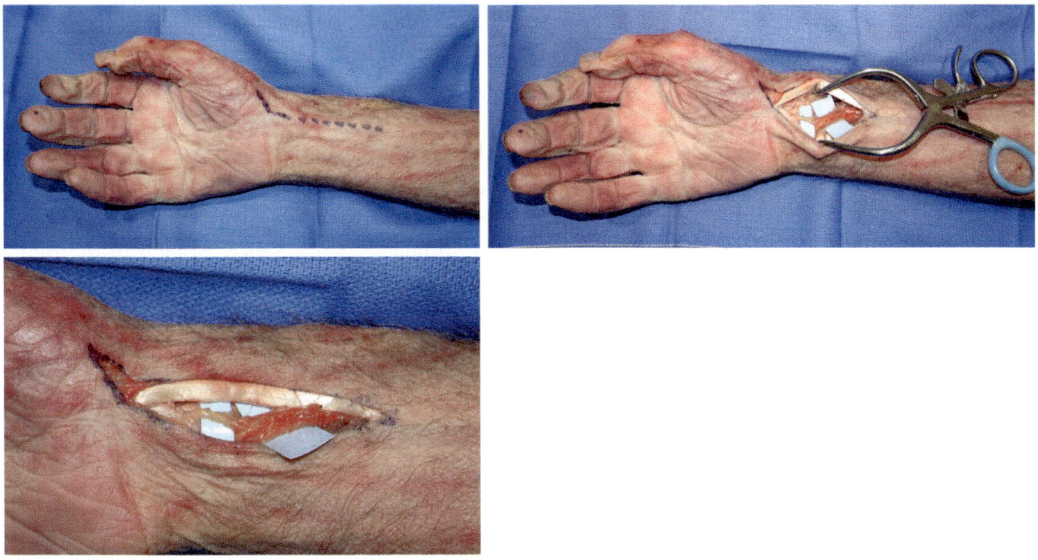

Fig. 7.1 The palmar cutaneous nerve (PCN) is at risk for injury during a modified Henry approach. Top panel: Markings for modified Henry approach over the flexor carpi radialis (FCR) to approach the distal radius. Middle panel: Retraction of FCR radially showing the path of the median nerve. The PCN can be seen distally, which lies on the ulnar side of the FCR subsheath. Bottom panel: Magnified view demonstrating the takeoff of the PCN from the median nerve with the FCR in situ. Note the intimate relationship between the PCN and FCR

cated from cadaveric studies demonstrating PCN sparing, but the PCN is at risk with any approach to the distal radius or carpal tunnel [23].

7.2.2 Metacarpal Fractures

The ulnar nerve passes through Guyon's canal, and the deep branch of the ulnar nerve passes deep to a tendinous arch formed by the flexor digitorum minimi brevis spanning the pisiform and hook of the hamate. As the nerve proceeds deeper into the palm, it lies deep to the interossei fascia and enters between the two heads of the adductor pollicis. The nerve runs intimately with the metacarpal bases and CMC joints in its course and is at risk with volarly subluxated fractures or dislocations near these points [24]. Figure 7.2 demonstrates the branches of the ulnar nerve within Guyon's canal.

The DSBUN has significant variation in its anatomy with up to three branches arborizing around the level of the wrist. On average, these branches arborize between 2 cm proximal and 3.15 cm distal to the ulnar styloid [25]. An example can be seen in Fig. 7.3. After crossing the wrist, branches will course radially on the dorsum of the hand, and incisions on the dorsum of the ulnar metacarpals may risk injury to the branches of the DSBUN. Injury to the DSBUN has been demonstrated with percutaneous pinning of the 5th metacarpal base [25].

The SBRN emerges from the undersurface of the brachioradialis (BR) approximately 8.5 cm proximal to the radial styloid, pierces the deep fascia, and splits into a medial and lateral branch [26]. The lateral branch supplies the radial side of the thumb, while the medial branch will supply the ulnar thumb and send proximal dorsal digital nerves to the index, middle, and radial

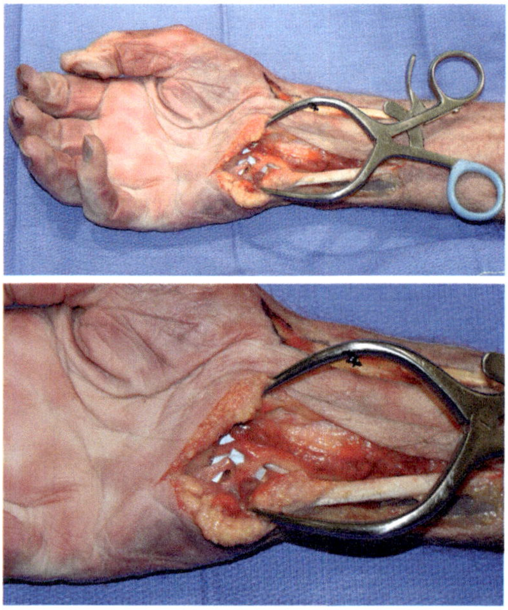

Fig. 7.2 Terminal branches of the ulnar nerve. Top panel: Dissection of the ulnar nerve just radial to the flexor carpi ulnaris (FCU) with exposure of the ulnar nerve in Guyon's canal. Bottom panel: Magnified view of the distal ulnar nerve branches. Two sensory branches can be seen as the distal branches innervating the hypothenar skin and continuing to the ulnar aspect of the small finger and the common digital nerve to the ulnar aspect of the ring finger and the radial aspect of the small finger. The motor branch, which is the most proximal branch in the photo, can be seen diving deep to the hypothenar musculature

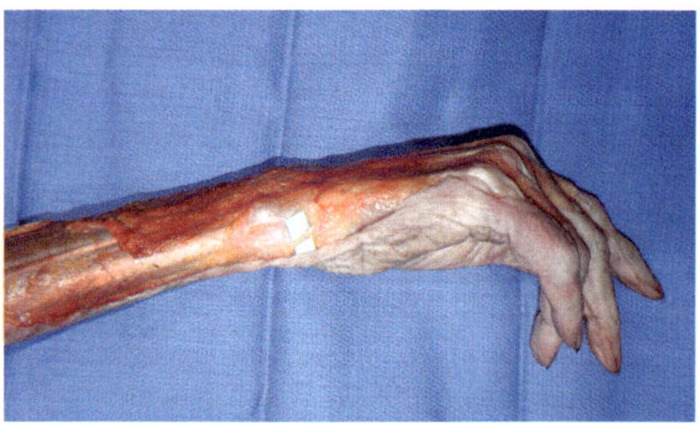

Fig. 7.3 Dorsal sensory branch of the ulnar nerve (DSBUN). In this specimen, the DSBUN is crossing to the dorsal hand distal to the ulnar styloid, though its course can be more proximal and dependent on wrist position

ring finger. Similar to the DSBUN, dorsal approaches to the thumb, index, or middle finger may place the SBRN at risk. Figure 7.4 demonstrates the proximity of branches of the SBRN to metacarpal approaches. Figure 7.5 demonstrates branches of both the SBRN and DSBUN to the dorsal hand. Figure 7.6 shows the intimacy of the SBRN branch to the radial styloid and thumb metacarpal, which may be at risk during exposure of a metacarpal base or radial styloid fracture.

7.2.3 Phalangeal Fractures

As noted above, the SBRN and DSBUN will provide some proximal sensation to the dorsal digits. A large portion of finger sensation comes from dorsal branches of the proper digital nerves. Common digital nerves from the median and ulnar nerves will travel deep to the superficial palmar arch and branch into proper digital nerves proximal to the finger web spaces. These nerves will enter the digits and travel lateral to the flexor tendon sheaths, about 2 mm volar to the midaxial line. Dorsal branches will typically arise from the digital nerves at the base of the proximal phalanx, pierce Cleland's ligament, and become more superficial as they progress distally [27]. Figure 7.7 demonstrates the relationship between the digital nerve and its dorsal branch.

Midaxial incision are designed to avoid injury to the digital nerves but straying of the incision or variability of the nerve course (which is often seen after prior surgeries or in fibrosing conditions such as Dupuytren disease) can lead to either volar or dorsal nerve injury. Volar Bruner incisions are designed to leave neurovascular bundles deep during skin elevation, but inadvertent nerve transection may occur especially at the point of the incisions at the edges of flexor creases.

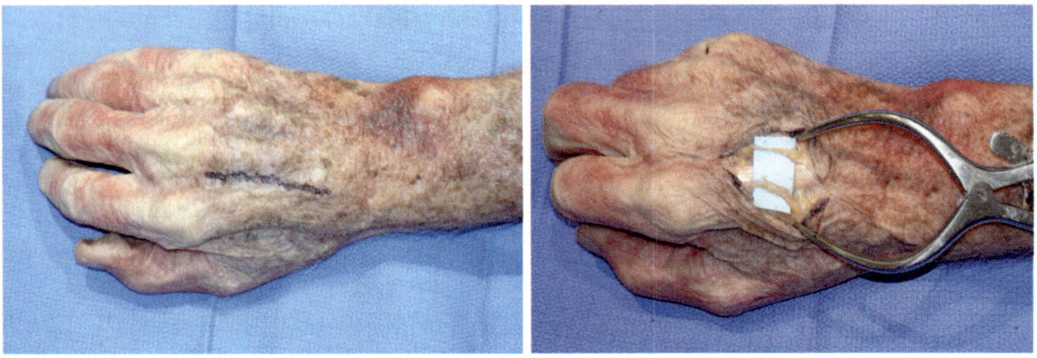

Fig. 7.4 Dorsal approaches to the metacarpals place dorsal sensory nerves at risk. Top Panel: A dorsal approach to the index or middle finger metacarpal is demonstrated. Bottom Panel: Branches of the sensory branch of the radial nerve (SBRN) are at risk with this approach. Two branches of the SBRN can be seen in proximity to this incision

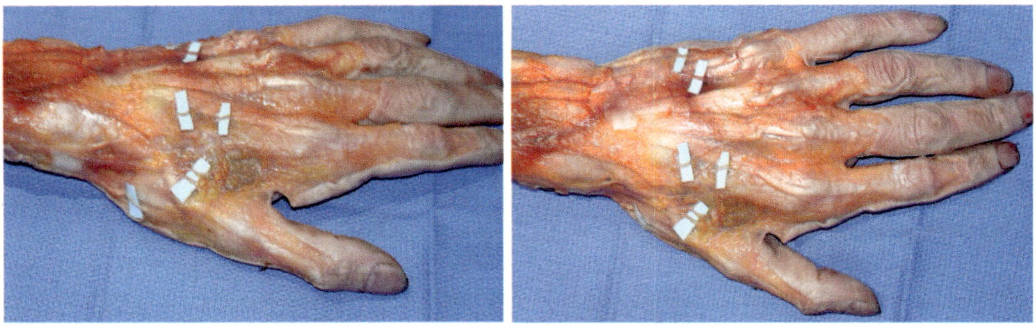

Fig. 7.5 Branching patterns of the sensory branch of the radial nerve (SBRN) and dorsal sensory branch of the ulnar nerve (DSBUN). Top panel: Branches of the SBRN in the dorsal hand are seen with branches overlying the dorsal thumb, index, and middle finger metacarpals. Bottom panel: Branches of the DSBUN can also be viewed on the ulnar side of the hand with branches over the small and ring finger metacarpals

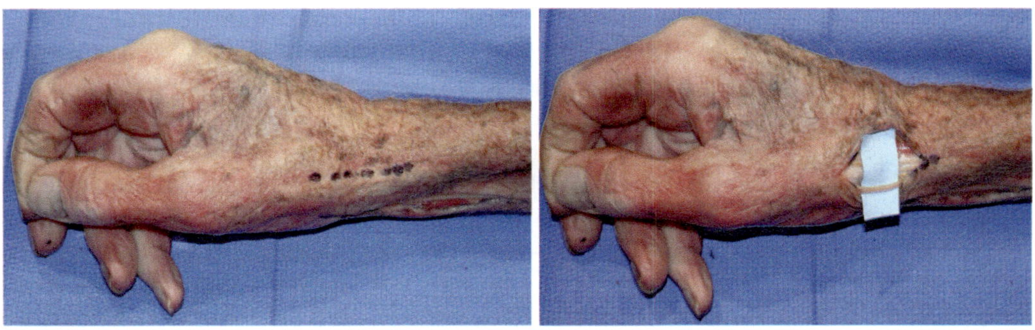

Fig. 7.6 Sensory branch of the radial nerve (SBRN) to the thumb. Top panel: Potential incision for exposure of thumb metacarpal base, trapezium, or radial styloid. Bottom panel: Note the proximity of the SBRN from the radial styloid to the thumb metacarpal base

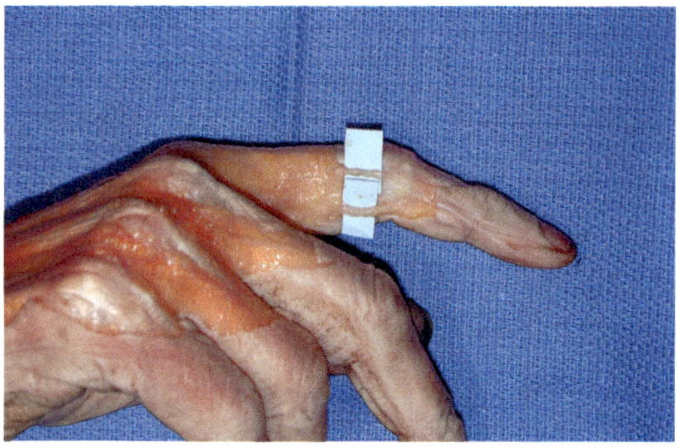

Fig. 7.7 Nerves to the finger. The ulnar digital nerve to the index finger can be seen volarly. The dorsal branch of the ulnar digital nerve, which arises at the base of the proximal phalanx, can be seen dorsally

7.3 Prevention Strategies

7.3.1 General

- Blunt retractors should be used when possible to avoid inadvertent nerve puncture.
- Dissection should be performed in the plane of the nerve (rather than perpendicular) to decrease risk of laceration or traction injury.
- Superficial nerves should be elevated and protected within skin flaps and not skeletonized when possible.

7.3.2 Distal Radius

- Serial examination should be performed before and after closed reduction. Neurapraxia is common, but if symptoms are severe (dense numbness, motor dysfunction, severe pain) or worsen after reduction, urgent carpal tunnel release is indicated.
- Consider carpal tunnel release early if neuropraxia is present at time of injury.
- Refrain from median nerve blocks intraoperatively to allow for postoperative assessment
- Incising through the radial FCR sheath during the modified Henry approach will help avoid PCN injury [19].
- Consider direct identification of the median nerve for open distal radius fractures and hardware removal.

7.3.3 Metacarpals

- Assess intrinsic motor function at time of injury; the first dorsal interosseous and adductor pollicis are the most distal muscles innervated by the deep ulnar motor branch.
- For dorsal fracture exposure, dissect longitudinally along the bone to stay in line with the course of the SBRN or DSBUN.
- For percutaneous pin placement at the base of the small finger metacarpal, consider a mini incision to avoid blind pin placement through the DSBUN [25].

7.3.4 Phalanges

- When using a midaxial approach, perform dissection longitudinally in line with neurovascular bundles.
- Dorsal approaches should be straight midline to avoid injury to dorsal sensory nerves.
- When raising volar Bruner flaps, the neurovascular bundles must be identified and excluded from the skin flap.
- Ischemia time with digital tourniquets should be minimized. Use of commercial devices or a 1 inch length of a Penrose drain will limit risk of excessive occlusion pressure [28, 29].

7.4 Typical Course/Natural History

For any nerve injury, early recognition is critical. It is particularly important to establish the timing of injury and a baseline physical exam since any changes in the exam will aid in determining severity. Early intervention and/or referral to therapy will also often lead to improved outcomes. It is thus important to understand the symptomatology and natural course of injured nerves.

After injury to the PCN, its territory of sensation at the base of the thenar eminence is sacrificed. However, morbidity from PCN injury manifests as nerve irritation and/or neuroma [30]. Symptoms range from light irritation to severe hand deficiency. Chronic wrist pain (pillar pain) has also been attributed to PCN injury. Scarring over an intact nerve may be sufficient to cause a painful scar and paresthesia [31]. Such symptoms are unlikely to resolve on their own without operative intervention.

The median nerve is subject to traction injury during distal radius exposure – cases of neurapraxia should improve in days to weeks. Dense numbness in the median nerve distribution or motor findings (thenar muscular palsy) would be concerning for a more severe injury. In cases of nerve transection (neurotmesis), recovery will not occur spontaneously [32]. Untreated acute carpal tunnel syndrome will also likely result in permanent median nerve dysfunction [33].

For injuries to the SBRN and DSBUN, numbness to the dorsal hand is well tolerated. However, these nerves are susceptible to neuroma formation and painful paresthesia when injured. Resolution of these symptoms after a direct injury often does not resolve without surgical management [34]. For injuries to the deep ulnar nerve, loss of the lumbricals will lead to development of an ulnar claw deformity, the severity of which correlates with the severity of the nerve injury.

Injuries to the digital nerves will also lead to numbness in their cutaneous distribution. Patients may find numbness in the tips of the fingers bothersome, especially in the working surfaces of their hand. For unilateral digital nerve injuries, it is possible that cross-innervation may substitute over time from the intact side, but it is controversial whether this crossover innervation is clinically meaningful [35–37]. Patients may note numbness in the ipsilateral side of the injury years later. Neuroma formation is also possible for both unrepaired and repaired nerves with an incidence of around 5% [36].

7.5 Initial Evaluation/Exam

- Time of suspected injury is crucial; neurapraxia may not show signs of improvement for 2–3 weeks [32].
- Static two-point discrimination and Semmes Weinstein testing provide objective measures of sensory nerve impairment. These can be compared to the uninjured side to test for injury and tracked over time for recovery [38].
- The Ten Test (asking the patient to grade sensation in the injured area as a number between 0 and 10 where 0 is no sensation and 10 is normal sensation) has also been shown to have excellent interrater reliability and reproducibility [39].
- A positive Tinel test points toward a nerve injury, and an advancing Tinel test provides evidence that a peripheral nerve is regenerating [40].
- Vasomotor changes (lack of sweating, flattening of skin folds/fingerprints, cold intolerance) may be subtle signs of nerve injury [41].
- For deep branch of ulnar nerve injuries:
  - Intrinsic-minus position/clawing of ring and small fingers with hyperextension of metacarpophalangeal (MP) joints and flexion at the proximal interphalangeal (PIP) and distal interphalangeal (DIP) joints (Duchenne sign).
  - Clawing is more profound than in high ulnar nerve injuries due to unopposed force of extrinsic flexors.
  - Normal sequence of finger flexion is impaired; IP joints contract prior to MP joints, causing fingertips to push objects away from patient grasp [42].
  - Paralysis of adductor pollicis, deep head of flexor pollicis brevis (FPB), and first dorsal interosseous causes 80% loss of pinch strength [43].
  - FPL overuse to compensate for pinch leads to IP flexion with thumb pinch (Froment's sign) and thumb MP hyperextension (Jeanne's sign) with MP laxity [44]
  - Active abduction and adduction of fingers is absent.
  - Unopposed action of extensor digiti minimi will lead to static abduction of small finger (Wartenburg's sign) [45].
- For median nerve injuries:
  - Sensory deficit will involve the volar thumb, index, middle, and radial half of ring finger.

- Proximal injury will cause weakness of pronation, FCR, and extrinsic finger flexors.
- Thenar weakness will be present with inability of the patient to abduct and oppose the thumb.
- Mixed examination may be present with partial nerve injury or with Martin-Gruber connections (17% of patients) [46, 47].

7.6 Diagnostic Tests/Imaging

- Adjunctive tests are supplemental, not replacements, for thorough history and physical exam.
- For motor nerves, timing of examination is crucial. Once nerve disruption has been established, nerve repair should be performed as soon as possible; however, electrodiagnostic findings will not be definitive until >4 weeks after injury.

7.6.1 Electrodiagnostic Tests

- Nerve conduction studies (NCS) and electromyogram (EMG) are commonly used to quantify injury and/or recovery.
- Typically not utilized sooner than 3 weeks after injury:
  - If laceration is suspected, conduction block can be seen at transection site before Wallerian degeneration occurs [48]:
    - If desired for this indication, NCS must be done in first week after injury as degeneration will be complete by 1–2 weeks [49].
  - Inching studies may also be useful in determining localization of block.
  - Fibrillation potentials on EMG will not be seen until after 3 weeks.
- Most patients with suspected nerve injury should have studies at least 4–8 weeks after injury:
  - Recovery of segmental demyelination requires this time frame [50].
  - Improvement of neurapraxic injury may obviate need for NCS/EMG.
- With neurapraxic injury, compound muscle action potential (CMAP) and nerve action potential (NAP) distal to lesion are maintained with stimulus. Proximal stimulation will show partial or complete conduction block with loss of CMAP amplitude and slowed conduction velocity:
  - Some conduction slowing may be permanent due to shorter internodes after recovery, but this is not clinically significant [49].
  - F-waves and H-waves may be useful for proximally injured nerves but not at level of forearm, wrist, and hand [49, 51].
- With partial neurapraxia, abnormal recruitment of muscle fibers will be seen with a decreased number of motor unit action potentials (MUAPs) with normal amplitude and rapid firing.
- In severe neurapraxia, there will be no voluntary MUAPs, but fibrillations will not be present.
- For axonotmesis and neurotmesis, CMAP and NAP distal to lesion will decrease with degree of axon loss:
  - CMAPs are lost by day 9 after injury, NAPs by day 11.
  - Fibrillation potentials will be seen in even moderate axon loss.
  - No voluntary MUAPs are present in complete lesions.
  - In partial lesions, collateral sprouting occurs, and MUAPs will appear polyphasic and with long duration.
  - As sprouts mature, MUAPs become less jittery and more stable.
  - Stable MUAPs indicate limits of reinnervation; unsatisfactory clinical recovery may be an indication for surgical intervention.

7.6.2 Diagnostic Blocks

- In cases of symptomatic neuroma, injection around nerve of interest may be helpful in selecting patients who may benefit from nerve exploration:
  - Placebo effect may be confounding in patient affirmation of block efficacy [52].
- 1% lidocaine is used in most practices, should provide relief for 2–6 h.
- Ultrasound-guided nerve injection may increase precision and accuracy of nerve targeting, though this has not been compared to visual landmarks only in a controlled setting [53].

7.6.3 Imaging

- MR Neurogram (MRN) is a relatively new technique:
  - Resolution high enough to detect epineurium as distinct layer.
  - For nerves over 3 mm, individual fascicles may be visualized [54].
  - For moderate neurapraxia, MR will show edema and increase in nerve volume.
  - Neuroma-in-continuity may be visible for axonotmetic injuries [48].
  - 3D reconstructions may aid with visualizing compression site.
  - Denervated muscle fibers will show edema-like changes acutely, fatty infiltration chronically.
  - 3 T magnet preferred, gadolinium not necessary, radiologist familiar with reading MRNs is mandatory [55].
- Ultrasound may help identify neuromas or nerve compression through changes in nerve diameter.

7.7 Surgical Techniques

If a nerve injury is identified, how the injury is to be approached needs to be carefully weighed. The benefits of exploration should be weighed against potential risks. For patients who present with pain due to a focally identified neuroma, patients may experience great relief after exploration, neuroma excision, and nerve repair. Patients who have less focal neuropathic symptoms, such as in complex regional pain syndrome (CRPS), may not have such success [56]. The expectations of the patient must be tempered as well; for sensory nerves, satisfactory repairs are considered those that provide S3+ or higher on the Mackinnon–Dellon scale, which equates to a static two-point discrimination less than 15 mm and a moving two-point discrimination less than 7 mm [57]. Up to 69% of cases may demonstrate meaningful recovery with proper technique, though it should be explained to patients that sensation will likely never return to pre-injury levels [58].

For motor nerves, special consideration must be taken with regard to the timing of repair. Motor endplates degenerate 12–18 months after injury, and nerves only regrow at 1 mm/day; thus, there is a time limit to when nerve repair will have meaningful results for motor reinnervation. When a motor nerve laceration is identified, patients will have the best results when the repair is performed early. For patients who have had a motor nerve injury beyond the 1-year window, they are often best served by salvage techniques.

7.7.1 Primary Nerve Repair

Primary nerve repair, when feasible, is the gold standard for severe axonotmesis and neurotmesis injuries. Primary coaptation of nerves outperforms those performed with grafts for sensory and motor outcomes, and primary nerve repair has proven effective for neuroma prevention. Repair with epineural microsutures with gross fascicular matching in a well-vascularized bed is the goal. Group fascicular repair (repairing intraneural fascicles) has not been shown to be superior to standard epineural repair [59].

It should be noted however that primary repair should be performed only if nerve coaptation can be performed tension free. Studies in animal models have demonstrated an 8% nerve elongation will significantly impair blood flow within the nerve, and this is worsened with further strain on the nerve [60]. Thus, to maximize nerve recovery, coaptation should be performed without tension. Positioning of the limb joints must also be taken into consideration; for instance, for a median nerve laceration, the nerve should be repaired with the wrist extended rather than in flexion, otherwise the required nerve gap may be underestimated. Prior to repair, nerves must be debrided to healthy-appearing fascicles, and necrotic or scarred nerve must be excised. Debriding the nerve to viable ends will increase the gap size.

- Primary repair should be performed when feasible for severe axonotmesis or neurotmesis.
- Primary repair should be performed with epineural microsutures (8-0 or 9-0 in most cases).
- Nerve repair must be tension free in all positions of the operated limb; if tension exists nerve grafting should be considered.
- Quality/quantity of nerve debridement should not be sacrificed to maintain length.

7.7.2 Neurolysis

The term neurolysis in surgical vernacular may refer to external neurolysis (dissecting a nerve in its entirety away from surrounding tissue) or internal neurolysis (dissecting individual fascicles within the nerve). In cases of suspected compression or surrounding scarring after a traumatic injury, external neurolysis may play a therapeutic role. Dissection of the nerve away from a scarred area and transposition into a well-vascularized bed may alleviate neuropathic pain. In some cases, scarring may cause extrinsic compression and neurolysis can help relieve this compression. Often, nerve compressions can be visualized with an "hour-glass" shape of the nerve caused by the extrinsic compression. In some cases where there is suspected tethering of the nerve to surrounding tissue, encasing the nerve in tissue or products that aid in gliding may be useful. Wrapping scarred nerves in autogenous veins has shown improved outcomes in some studies [61, 62]. Additionally there are many commercial anti-adhesion and nerve wrapping products that may improve nerve gliding, though long-term studies are lacking.

Internal neurolysis may play a role for patients where intraneural scarring is suspected or identified. Internal neurolysis requires opening of the perineurium and dissecting between fascicles. In cases of severe nerve compression, perineural scarring may develop and lysis of constrictive bands on fascicles may be beneficial. Another indication for internal neurolysis is neuroma-in-continuity. These cases can be challenging as the surgeon should strive to maintain intact fascicles while at the same time resecting all embedded scar tissue. Intraoperative nerve stimulation or EMG can be very helpful in these cases that involve motor nerves as viable fascicles can be identified and preserved. Scarred fascicles can be excised, and nerve grafts used for repair.

- In general, nerves should be freed from scarred beds and placed into well-vascularized tissue.
- Consider intraoperative nerve stimulation for neuroma-in-continuity to help preserve intact fascicles.

7.7.3 Nerve Grafting

When a tension-free primary repair is not possible, nerve grafts are required for repair. The need for nerve grafts will be more likely in high-energy traumatic injuries or in repair of delayed injuries. The peripheral nerve surgeon should be judicious about using grafts as more nerve coaptations may decrease the number of axons that ultimately reach the end target, but the surgeon should not be hesitant to use a graft when required. In delayed cases or when a large gap is expected, use of either nerve autografts or allografts should be discussed with the patient preoperatively [63].

Historically, interposition autologous nerve grafts were the only graft material available, and they remain the gold standard for nerve grafting today. Grafts may be used within their own epineurium or they can be separated into fascicles to form a cable graft. The latter is useful for nerve mismatch where the donor nerve is significantly smaller in size than the recipient. Donor nerve grafts are harvested from expendable sensory nerves such as the sural or medial antebrachial nerve. Traditionally, the nerve graft is placed in reversed orientation to prevent theoretical loss of axons down side branches of the donor graft. The axons within the graft undergo Wallerian degeneration and the graft merely acts to provide mechanical and chemotactic guidance for regenerating axons [64]. One downside to the use of nerve autografts is that they sacrifice sensory innervation to the territory provided by the donor nerve.

Processed nerve allograft, which are decellularized but provide the biomechanical scaffold for nerve ingrowth, are also options for nerve repair. Functional recovery for injuries with gaps between 5 and 50 mm has been demonstrated with outcomes equivalent to autografts [65]. Early data shows promise of processed nerve allografts in mixed and motor nerve repair, though use of allograft for motor nerves is not yet widespread [66]. Manufactured nerve conduits or use of autogenous vein as a conduit are also options for short gap lengths less than 3 cm, but these modalities compare less favorably to autografts or allografts at longer gap lengths [67, 68]. In our practice, allografts are used for repair of pure sensory nerves, while mixed and motor nerves will receive autologous grafts.

Most commonly, the sural nerve is used for autogenous grafting. For the sural nerve, the patient should be informed that a sensory defect on the lateral aspect of the leg and lateral foot should be expected. The leg should be prepped circumferentially. The nerve is most easily identified 2 cm posterior to the lateral malleolus and 1–2 cm proximal. The first incision should be made here, and then as the nerve is traced proximally, stair step incisions may be made vs. a single longitudinal incision. A tendon stripper may facilitate isolating the nerve when stair step incisions are used. Up to 30 cm or more of nerve graft may be obtained [69]. The sural nerve will be about 3 mm in diameter [70]. If a thicker nerve is required, a cable graft can be constructed by cutting the sural nerve into segments of the required length and creating a composite nerve of appropriate thickness with fibrin glue.

- Use of a nerve graft should be considered preoperatively for cases with a wide zone of injury or for delayed cases where scarring and neuroma formation has occurred.
- Autologous nerve graft is the gold standard for nerve repair:
  - Nerves can be used as whole grafts or split into smaller fascicles.
  - Nerves can also be bundled into cable grafts using fibrin glue to match diameter of a larger recipient nerve.
  - Sural nerve is a common choice for autogenous donor.
- Processed nerve allograft should be considered for sensory nerves with gaps 5–50 mm, with no donor site morbidity:
  - Less convincing data exists for use in mixed and motor nerves.

7.8 Salvage Techniques

When nerve repair is not possible, or symptoms persist despite attempts at repair, alternative treatments must be considered. For motor nerve injuries, nerve repair may not lead to clinically meaningful outcomes with delayed (>12–18 months) presentation. For these injuries, tendon transfers must be considered to replace lost motion.

For painful neuromas or nerve injuries that continue to generate neuropathic symptoms despite repair attempts, there are numerous options for salvage.

7.8.1 Motor Nerve Injuries

7.8.1.1 Median Nerve Tendon Transfers

For injury to the median nerve at the level of the distal forearm and wrist, the most notable deficit will be due to denervation of the thenar musculature with resultant loss of thumb abduction, opposition, and pronation with loss of pinch. With weakness of the FPB (which also has innervation from the ulnar nerve to the deep head), MP hyperextension may be seen with IP joint flexion. The suppleness of these joints must be assessed before performing a transfer; if contractures are present, correction of these should also be considered preoperatively or at the time of transfer [71]. Adequacy of the thumb webspace must also be assessed as this may be contracted with a chronic injury. Webspace deepening and adductor release may be necessary before opponensplasty in these cases.

Motors that are commonly used are the FDS of the ring finger, the extensor indicis proprius (EIP), the palmaris longus (PL) with a palmar aponeurosis extension (Camitz), or the abductor digiti minimi (ADM). It is debatable which transfers lead to best replication of thumb motion, and each transfer is sufficient to restore function when applied to patients with adequate donors [72]. For each type of transfer, an adequate pulley must be selected to optimize the line of pull for opposition. In general, one point of insertion is desirable.

The FDS ring transfer is straightforward and has adequate length and power to replace opposition function. Ideally patients do not have baseline hyperextension of the ring finger PIP joint, otherwise a postoperative swan neck may develop.

- FDS transfer (Fig. 7.8):
  - A Bruner incision is made over the PIP joint and the two slips of the FDS are identified.
  - In the Royle–Thompson technique, a counter incision is made radially to the thenar eminence. The FDS is identified leaving the carpal tunnel and then passed over the ulnar palmar aponeurosis to form a pulley [73, 74].
  - Alternatively in the Bunnell technique, a loop of distal FCU is used as a pulley [75].
  - Insertion point made at the distal APB tendon with a Pulvertaft weave.
  - Thumb should be fully opposed with the wrist in neutral.
- EIP transfer:
  - Utilizes the pisiform as a pulley:
  - Advantages over FDS transfer: no weakening of power grip and very little functional disability [76].
  - A short incision is made over the index MP joint with the EIP divided just proximal to extensor hood. If the hood is taken and not repaired, extensor lag may develop [77].

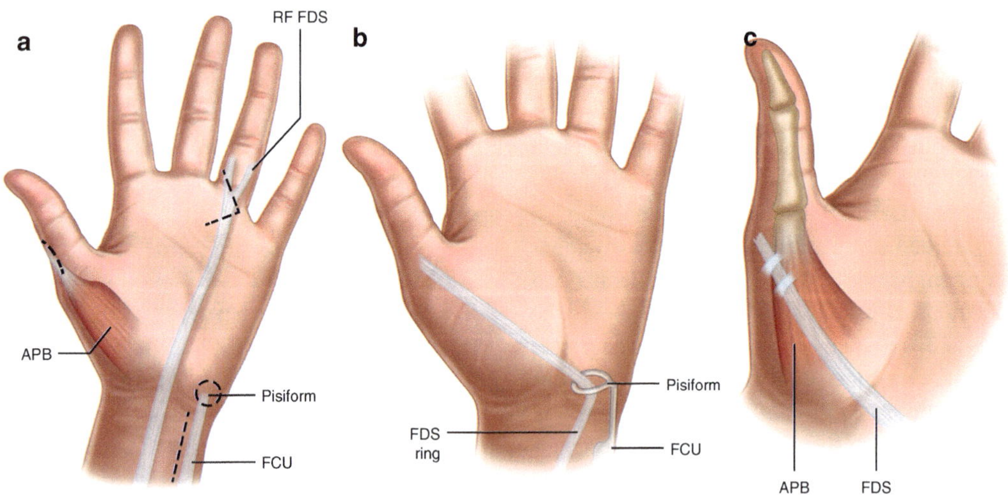

Fig. 7.8 Flexor digitorum superficialis (FDS) transfer for opposition. (**a**) The three planned incisions over the ring finger proximal phalanx, distal wrist, and abductor pollicis brevis (APB) insertion are shown. (**b**) The FDS is divided just proximal to its insertion on the proximal phalanx and passed through a distally based loop of flexor carpi ulnaris. (**c**) The FDS is weaved into the APB insertion with the thumb in opposition and the wrist in neutral

  - A counter incision is made to deliver the EIP proximal to the extensor retinaculum. An additional incision may be required in the dorsal hand to free the EIP tendon from soft tissue attachments.
  - An incision is made on the ulnar wrist near the pisiform. The EIP tendon is delivered around the pisiform. Care should be taken to ensure the path of the EIP is superficial to the FCU to avoid ulnar nerve compression.
  - Insertion point made at the APB tendon.
  - Thumb should be in full opposition with wrist in 30 degrees of flexion.
- Palmaris longus opponensplasty (Camitz):
  - May not be suitable for some traumatic or iatrogenic injuries to the median nerve as palmaris may be scarred [78].
  - PL presence must be confirmed by physical exam prior to surgery.
  - A longitudinal incision is made 2 cm proximal to the wrist crease over the PL with extension into the palm in line with the ring finger and extending to the mid palmar crease. Care is made to preserve the palmar cutaneous nerve, which will lie radial to the PL.
  - The PL is freed into the forearm and into the palm and kept in continuity with a 1-cm-wide strip of palmar fascia.
  - The carpal tunnel is released, and a counter incision is made over the abductor pollicis brevis (APB) insertion.
  - The palmar fascial strip is then delivered to the thumb wound and secured to the APB insertion. The thumb should be in full opposition with the wrist neutral.
- ADM opponensplasty (Huber):
  - This transfer may also improve the palm's appearance by increasing the bulk of the thenar eminence with the ADM muscle belly [72, 79].
  - A midlateral incision is made on the ulnar border of the little finger proximal phalanx and extended proximally to the distal palmar crease to the radial side of the hypothenar eminence.
  - The two ADM insertions (at the base of the proximal phalanx at the extensor apparatus) are freed, and the muscle is released from soft tissue attachments toward its origin at the pisiform
  - Care must be taken not to damage the neurovascular pedicle on the proximal radiodorsal aspect. The pedicle can also be identified proximally and traced distally.
  - The origin of the ADM on the flexor carpi ulnaris (FCU) tendon must be preserved. This and the neurovascular pedicle limit the reach of the transfer.
  - A counter incision is made at the thumb APB insertion. The ADM must be flipped 180° (like turning a book page) to reach the APB insertion. An additional incision in the thenar crease may assist in tunneling.
  - The thumb should be placed in full opposition (and this likely will be necessary at the time of inset based on the length of the ADM muscle). Wrist position is not critical.

7.8.1.2 Ulnar Nerve Transfers

Clawing of the fingers in ulnar nerve palsy is due to paralysis of the interossei muscles of the fingers and the lumbricals of the ring and small fingers. The loss of MP flexion and extension of the PIP and DIP joints results in an "intrinsic minus" posture. Clawing is more apparent during use of the hand than at rest and is more apparent in individuals with lax finger joints. When assessing a claw hand, it is important to ascertain whether all involved joints are supple and if correction of the hyperextension at the MP will result in full extension of the IP joints (Bouvier maneuver). If this is the case, operations that target only MP joint hyperextension (MP capsulodesis or Zancolli lasso) will correct the deformity. If the PIP joints remain flexed when the MP joints are corrected, an extension transfer at the IP joints will also be needed. For chronic deformities, lateral band migration volarly may occur due to stretch of the transverse retinacular fibers of the extensor mechanism; in these cases, lateral band vectors need to be corrected, or a tendon transfer may worsen rather than correct the deformity. Additionally, the MP, PIP, and DIP joints should be supple prior to performing transfers.

7.8.2 Static Procedures

- Only appropriate if MP flexion corrects the deformity of the IP joints

Palmar capsulodesis of the MP joint [80] (Fig. 7.9):

- A transverse incision is made over the A1 pulleys of the affected fingers.
- The A1 pulley of each finger is divided as in a trigger finger, and the flexor tendons are retracted to expose the volar plate.
- Two longitudinal incisions are made in the volar plate.
- The proximal volar plate is released from the metacarpal neck resulting in a distally based flap of volar plate.
- The flap is advanced proximally onto the metacarpal using a bone tunnel or a bone anchor to keep the MP joint in 20 degrees of flexion.

Riordan Static Tenodesis: ECU (and can use ECRL if more than ring and small finger involved)

- ECU is split longitudinally with proximal division of one-half of the tendon bulk off of the musculotendinous junction and the distal insertion kept intact.
- The radial lateral band of the extensor apparatus is exposed at the proximal phalanx of each finger and a tendon slip is passed through the interosseous space and lumbrical canal and sutured to the radial lateral band.
- The tenodesis is sutured with the wrist in 30 degrees of extension, MP joints in 80 degrees of flexion, and IP joints extended.
- Alternatively, free tendon grafts can be used and looped through the extensor retinaculum

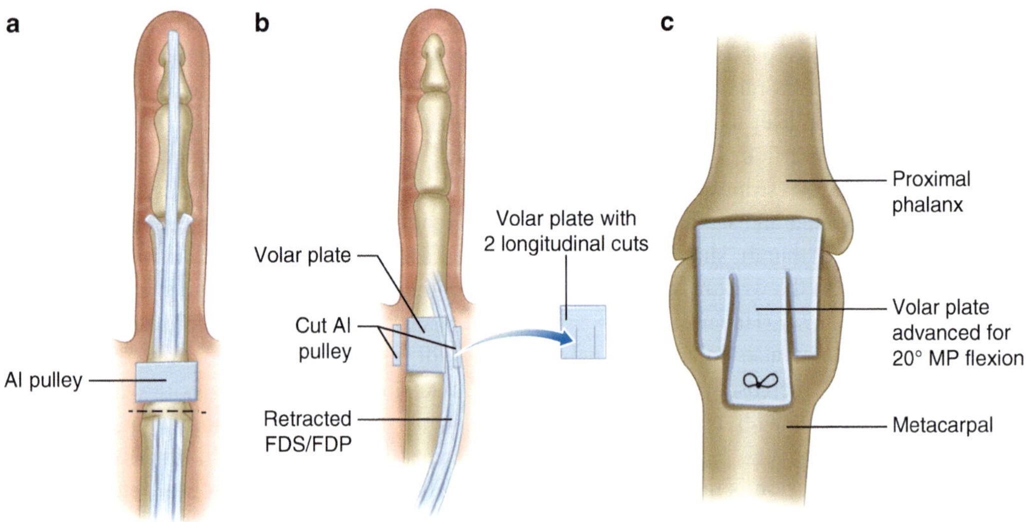

Fig. 7.9 Metacarpophalangeal (MP) capsulodesis. (**a**) An incision is designed just proximal to the A1 pulley. (**b**) The A1 pulley is divided and the flexor tendons are retracted so the volar plate can be visualized. Two longitudinal incisions are made in the volar plate to create a proximally based flap. (**c**) The flap is advanced on the metacarpal to create 20° of flexion of the MP joint. The flap is secured in place via bone tunnels or a bone anchor

as the proximal anchor, which provides a theoretical wrist-powered tenodesis (Fowler's technique) [81].

7.8.3 Dynamic Transfers

Many techniques have been described. One common theme is that whichever muscle is selected to power the transfer, it must pass palmar to the axis of rotation of the MP joint to achieve flexion (i.e. palmar to the transverse metacarpal ligament).

Superficialis transfer:

- Most commonly utilized FDS of middle finger.
- FDS middle is detached from its insertion and split into slips (up to four for a total claw hand).
- Each slip is passed through the lumbrical canal of each finger, palmar to the deep transverse metacarpal ligament and sutured to the radial lateral band of each finger (Stiles–Bunnell procedure) [82].
- Each slip sutured with wrist in 30 degrees flexion, MP joints in 80–90 degrees flexion, and IP joints in full extension.
- Many modifications, including the Zancolli lasso, which use a proximally based FDS slip from each finger sutured onto itself after passing over the A1 pulley [83].

EIP, ERCB/ECRL, FCR, and PL can all serve as transfers to correct clawing deformity. However, these motors have insufficient tendon length to reach to target of the lateral bands, and free tendons grafts must be obtained. Again, it is key that each transfer pass volar to the MP joint to provide the correct vector of pull.

7.8.4 Adductorplasty

Another deficit that patients may notice with ulnar motor nerve injury is loss of thumb adduction force due to loss of adductor pollicis, the first dorsal interosseous, and the deep head of FPB. It is estimated that up to 80% of power pinch is lost with low ulnar palsy [84]. Without the ulnar innervated intrinsic muscles, EPL and FPL are the only remaining adductors of the thumb, and over time the thumb can collapse into a "Z"-deformity with hyperextension of the MP joint and flexion of the IP joint. Goals of adductorplasty are to restore adduction force to the thumb, provide active flexion of the MP joint, and regain extension of the IP joint.

ECRB as motor (Smith) [85]:

- The ECRB is divided at its insertion at the MF metacarpal base through a transverse dorsal wrist incision.
- A second more proximal transverse dorsal wrist incision is made to retrieve the tendon proximal to the extensor retinaculum.
- A third incision is made in the dorsal hand in the second intermetacarpal space. A window is formed through the interosseous muscles into the palmar space.
- A fourth incision is made on the ulnar side of the MP joint of the thumb. A blunt hemostat is then used to make a volar subcutaneous tunnel to the interosseous window.
- A tendon graft (usually PL) is secured to the adductor pollicis tendon, and the other end is passed through the volar subcutaneous tunnel and through the interosseous window into the hand dorsum.
- The graft is then secured proximally to the ECRB tendon.
- Tension is set such that the thumb lies just palmar to the index finger with the wrist neutral.
- BR, ECU, ECRL, and EIP can also be used as motors with similar technique.

FDS as motor (Edgerton and Brand) [86]:

- The ring FDS is released at its insertion on the proximal phalanx and withdrawn into a palmar incision.
- The FDS is passed around a pulley, such as the fascia of the middle finger metacarpal.
- The FDS vector should follow the transverse vector of the adductor pollicis. The tendon is inserted into the adductor tubercle.

7.9 Treatment of Symptomatic Neuromas

Persistent painful nerve injuries may require salvage procedures even in the absence of motor deficits. Simple excision of the neuroma is usually ineffective. Nerve repair, either with primary repair or with an interposition graft, should be considered as a primary treatment for a lacerated nerve but often the distal target cannot be located. For these patients, numerous options exist to attempt to "quiet" overactive, painful nerves. It is valuable to demonstrate improvement of neuroma pain by blocking the nerve in question prior to embarking on surgical intervention. If a diagnostic block does not provide relief, it is unlikely that surgery performed on the nerve will lead to a positive result for the patient. Blocking the nerve in question will also demonstrate potential areas of skin innervation that will be lost after neuroma resection. Potential for persistent pain, even after surgery, must be discussed with the patient preoperatively.

7.9.1 Burying Nerve in Bone, Muscle, or Veins

Implantation of the proximal nerve stump into surrounding tissues is the most commonly performed technique for terminal neuromas [87–89]. In principle, burying the nerve in deep tissues increases the distance required for axonal sprouts to reach the cutaneous surface, thereby providing cushion and protection for the nerve and reducing painful aberrant firing. The advantages of this procedure include its simplicity and limited morbidity.

- An adequate recipient site should be selected prior to surgery. Pronator quadratus, thenar musculature, or hypothenar musculature can be considered in the wrist and proximal hand.
- For digital nerves, neurolysis can be performed proximally to allow burying into muscle.
- The identified neuroma should be excised.
- For muscle or vein burying, the nerve end should be secured within the tissue (and intraluminal in the case of veins) with 8-0 epineurial stitches.
- For bone implantation, a cortical window can be made with a burr to fit the nerve and the nerve can be sutured in place with sutures through drilled bone tunnels.

7.9.2 Nerve-to-Nerve Transfer

This technique is designed to provide a pathway for regenerating axons using an undamaged nerve's support structure and has demonstrated promise in animal models and clinically [90, 91]. For this technique to be employed, a healthy nerve must be close to the damaged nerve to allow for coaptation – possible injury to the recipient nerve must be considered.

- The damaged nerve is resected to a healthy end.
- An epineural window of the appropriate size is microsurgically dissected in the recipient nerve.
- An epineural-to-epineural repair is performed with the nerve stump of the injured nerve invaginated in the epineurium of the recipient in an end-to-side fashion.

7.9.3 Centro-central Neurorrhaphy

Attempts to control growth of a painful terminal nerve end through intraneural fascicular coaptation or coaptation to the end of a nearby nerve (centro-central neurorrhaphy) has been performed in animals and in the upper extremity [92, 93]. Coaptation to a nearby nerve end is ideally performed if there are two neuromas present in nearby nerves, and coaptation is similar as in a primary repair. For intraneural coaptation, the nerve must have at least two fascicles, and intraneural dissection must be performed to dissect each fascicle to an unscarred end and the perineurium coapted end to end.

7.9.4 Allograft Use

Use of allograft to direct nerve growth away from cutaneous innervation is one strategy for management of neuroma (relocation nerve grafting). The neuroma is resected to a healthy end and a nerve repair is performed to an appropriately sized allograft. The blind end of the allograft can then be directed to a vascularized bed, as noted above. Another alternative is to split the allograft distally and perform an end-to-end coaptation with the two free ends, creating a "nerve to nowhere."

7.9.5 Nerve Caps

Placing a cap on the terminal ends of nerves has been attempted to prevent painful regrowth of the nerve end. Both synthetic materials and autologous tissues such as free vein grafts have been used [94–97] to prevent axonal escape.

7.9.6 Regenerative Peripheral Nerve Interfaces (RPNIs)

Originally designed for prosthetic control, RPNIs prevent neuroma formation by providing targets for peripheral nerve ingrowth with free muscle grafts. The muscle becomes reinnervated by the nerve, reducing ectopic nerve activity and mechanical and chemical sensitivity [98].

- The neuroma bulb is excised in its entirety to healthy-appearing nerve. For larger nerves (median, ulnar), interfascicular dissection can be performed to make subsequent wrapping of the nerve more facile.
- Free muscle grafts (approximately 3 × 1 × 1.5 cm) are harvested from local or distal tissue. In the forearm, volar forearm muscular provides numerous potential donors without functional deficit. In the distal forearm or hand, distant donor sites may be considered.
- Muscle should be harvested longitudinally in the muscle bulk to reduce local tissue trauma.
- The nerve is placed into the center of the graft and the epineurium of the nerve end is secured to the epimysium with 6-0 nonabsorbable stitches. The remainder of the muscle is closed around the nerve as a wrap with 6-0 nonabsorbable stitches.
- The constructed RPNIs should be placed away from the closure site if possible to prevent potential tethering to the incision scar.
- All dissection and suturing can easily be performed under loupe magnification.

7.9.7 Targeted Muscle Reinnervation (TMR)

Similar to RPNI and also initially described as a technique to improve precision for myoelectric prostheses, TMR has also been demonstrated as a treatment for neuroma pain [99]. In this technique, cut ends of peripheral nerves are coapted to smaller adjacent motor nerve branches which provides an end function for the painful, aberrantly firing nerve. However, successful application of this technique requires expendable recipient muscles that may receive the aberrant nerve. There are limited sites to perform TMR in the distal forearm and hand, and thus while TMR may be considered for select cases, its scope is limited for distal upper extremity nerve injuries.

7.10 Outcomes for Nerve-Based Treatment and Salvage

7.10.1 Nerve Repair after Injury

Compared with high nerve injuries, outcomes for low median and ulnar nerve injuries fare better; return of intrinsic function is much more attainable with a nerve repair distally than after a high nerve injury. In a meta-analysis which included 23 studies of median and ulnar nerve injuries, Ruijs et al. found that median nerve recovery tended to be superior to ulnar nerve recovery after repair. Additional variables for favorable recovery included younger age and early repair. Notably, use of nerve grafts did not appear detrimental for recovery [100]. Gaul et al. studied intrinsic motor recovery after ulnar nerve laceration; key pinch strength returned to 86% of prior strength in younger patients under 18 years of age and to 82% in older patients with low ulnar nerve injuries [101]. For digital nerve repair, a meta-analysis by Jain et al. found only 24% of patients achieve sensation that matched pre-injury levels, though a separate meta-analysis by He et al. reported that satisfactory (2PD better than 15 mm) was recovered in 80% of patients [36, 57].

7.10.2 Tendon Transfers

It is interesting to note that while there are multiple methods of tendon transfers for specific functions, there are few, if any, studies comparing outcomes between techniques. The selections of specific techniques is dictated by surgeon preference and available donors in specific patients [72]. There are also very few studies examining tendon transfers after distal nerve trauma or iatrogenic injury. However, multiple studies for opponensplasty have reported good or excellent functional results in excess of 85% despite different techniques [102–105]. It is notable that patient perception of outcome does not always correlate with functional outcome [106]. Similarly, there are numerous techniques to restore function for ulnar nerve palsy and there are few trials that compare methods or long-term outcomes. However, results are meaningful to patients in restoring activities of daily living and occupational abilities [42, 107].

7.10.3 Neuroma Repair Techniques

There are no well-controlled trials comparing different types of neuroma salvage operations. The highest quality studies consist of large case series. Implantation of the proximal nerve stump into vascularized tissue has been shown to decrease neuropathic pain and improve hand function. Dellon and Mackinnon studied nerve burying in a series of 60 patients and found that >80% of patients had good to excellent results. Factors that were predictive of a poor outcome included digital neuromas, patients on Workmen's compensation, and patients who had three or more previous nerve pain operations [108]. Of the techniques discussed above, nerve implantation into vascularized tissue has the longest track record [87].

For the remaining techniques for neuroma repair, sample sizes are relatively small and reports on long-term outcomes are variable. Kon and Bloem described outcomes for centro-central neurorrhaphy in the hand for 18 patients with an average 18-month follow-up and reported only one of their 18 patients had a recurrent neuroma. Swanson et al. described use of silicone nerve caps in 18 patients with 15 being relieved of neuroma symptoms. In contrast, Tupper and Booth reported the use of silicone caps in 32 patients and noted no improvement compared to neurectomy alone [94, 95]. Al-Qattan reported the use of end-to-side neurorrhaphy in three patients with painful neuromas after trauma and reported no recurrence of pain after a 20 month period [91]. Similarly, the use of relocation nerve grafting has been reported in small series only [109].

The formation of RPNIs is a relatively new technique and outcome studies to date are relatively small. An outcome study by Woo et al. in 16 amputees reported 71% of patients experienced a decrease in neuroma pain [110]. Kubiak et al. compared 45 patients undergoing prophylactic RPNIs at the time of limb amputation versus 45 controls. Patients who received RPNIs had a lower rate of symptomatic neuromas (0% vs. 13.3%) and a lower rate of phantom limb pain (51.1% vs. 91.1%) [111]. Similarly, TMR has demonstrated promise in reducing phantom limb pain for amputees [112]. However, it is important to recognize that these studies are performed in patients undergoing neuroma repair after major amputations, and it is untested whether these results are generalizable to neuromas from isolated nerve injury.

7.11 Technical Pearls and Pitfalls

- Distal radius fractures
  - Initial exam should include evaluation of the median nerve before and after closed reduction.
  - If median nerve exam is worsening, urgent carpal tunnel release is indicated.
  - Avoid median nerve or regional blocks intraoperatively so that nerve can be assessed postoperatively if concerns exist.
  - Incise through radial side of FCR when performing a volar approach to avoid injury to the PCN.
  - For suspected nerve injuries, identify nerve proximally outside of the zone of injury where anatomy is not distorted.
  - PCN injuries have low morbidity from sensory deficit but may cause painful neuromas. If injury is recognized, repair vs. burying the nerve in attempt to avoid neuropathic pain is indicated.
  - Median nerve injuries must be recognized and repaired early to maximize motor outcomes.
  - Carpal tunnel release should also be considered in the setting of postoperative complex regional pain syndrome (CRPS).
- Metacarpal fractures
  - Assess intrinsic muscle function at the time of injury.
  - Injuries with an ulnar nerve palsy are an indication for early repair and nerve exploration.
  - Early repair of a motor branch injury is critical to optimize outcomes.
  - For exposure of metacarpal fractures, dissect longitudinally to prevent SBRN and DSBUN injuries. Iatrogenic injuries noted at the time of fracture fixation should be repaired.
  - Consider potential nerve injuries with K wire placement for closed approaches (i.e. DSBUN around the ulnar styloid).
- Phalangeal fractures
  - Dorsal approaches allow significant protection of the neurovascular bundles unless extensive dissection is performed.
  - Care must be taken to preserve neurovascular bundles in midaxial and volar approaches.
  - Avoid excessive use of finger tourniquet to prevent pressure injuries to neurovascular bundles.
  - Loss of sensation to dorsal surfaces of the fingers may be tolerated and cross-innervation may play a role over time, though painful neuromas should be addressed.

References

1. Huckhagel T, Nüchtern J, Regelsberger J, Lefering R, TraumaRegister DGU. Nerve injury in severe trauma with upper extremity involvement: evaluation of 49,382 patients from the TraumaRegister DGU® between 2002 and 2015. Scand J Trauma Resusc Emerg Med. 2018;26(1):76.
2. Zimmermann MS, Abzug JM, Chang J, Stern PJ, Osterman AL. Iatrogenic nerve injuries in common upper extremity procedures. Instr Course Lect. 2014;63:105–11.
3. Cooney WP, Dobyns JH, Linscheid RL. Complications of Colles' fractures. J Bone Joint Surg Am. 1980;62(4):613–9.
4. Bienek T, Kusz D, Cielinski L. Peripheral nerve compression neuropathy after fractures of the distal radius. J Hand Surg Br. 2006;31(3):256–60.
5. Chu CH, Chih CJ, Wei KY, Tsuang YH. Entrapment of index flexor digitorum profundus and median nerve: an unusual complication of distal radial fracture--a case report. Kaohsiung J Med Sci. 1998;14(5):303–7.
6. Dennison DG. Median nerve injuries associated with distal radius fractures. Tech Orthop. 2006;21(1):48.
7. Dresing K, Peterson T, Schmit-Neuerburg KP. Compartment pressure in the carpal tunnel in distal fractures of the radius. A prospective study. Arch Orthop Trauma Surg. 1994;113(5):285–9.
8. Brüske J, Niedźwiedź Z, Bednarski M, Zyluk A. Acute carpal tunnel syndrome after distal radius fractures–long term results of surgical treatment with decompression and external fixator application. Chir Narzadow Ruchu Ortop Pol. 2002;67(1):47–53.

9. Gelberman RH, Szabo RM, Williamson RV, Hargens AR, Yaru NC, Minteer-Convery MA. Tissue pressure threshold for peripheral nerve viability. Clin Orthop Relat Res. 1983;178:285–91.
10. Fuller DA, Barrett M, Marburger RK, Hirsch R. Carpal canal pressures after volar plating of distal radius fractures. J Hand Surg Br. 2006;31(2):236–9.
11. Samson D, Power DM. Iatrogenic injuries of the palmar branch of the median nerve following volar plate fixation of the distal radius. J Hand Surg Asian Pac Vol. 2017;22(03):343–9.
12. Gore DR. Carpometacarpal dislocation producing compression of the deep branch of the ulnar nerve. J Bone. 1971;53(7):1387–90.
13. Guimaraes RM, Benaïssa S, Moughabghab M, Dunaud JL. Carpometacarpal dislocations of the long fingers. Apropos of 26 cases with review of 20 cases. Rev Chir Orthop Reparatrice Appar Mot. 1996;82(7):598–607.
14. Peterson P, Sacks S. Fracture-dislocation of the base of the fifth metacarpal associated with injury to the deep motor branch of the ulnar nerve: a case report. J Hand Surg Am. 1986;11(4):525–8.
15. Dahlin L, Palffy L, Widerberg A. Injury to the deep branch of the ulnar nerve in association with dislocated fractures of metacarpals II–IV. Scand J Plast Reconstr Surg Hand Surg. 2004;38(4):250–2.
16. Lim J-S, Han K-T, Ko J-G, Kim M-C. Jeopardized digital circulation from a closed phalangeal fracture. Plast Surg Case Stud. 2016;2(2):31–2.
17. Maurya S, Bhandari P. Post traumatic entrapment neuropathy of digital nerve — a case report and review of literature. Indian J Neurotrauma. 2011;8(1):57–8.
18. Carpenter S, Rohde RS. Treatment of phalangeal fractures. Hand Clin. 2013;29(4):519–34.
19. Conti Mica MA, Bindra R, Moran SL. Anatomic considerations when performing the modified Henry approach for exposure of distal radius fractures. J Orthop. 2016;14(1):104–7.
20. Chilelli BJ, Patel RM, Kalainov DM, Peng J, Zhang L-Q. Flexor pollicis longus dysfunction after volar plate fixation of distal radius fractures. J Hand Surg Am. 2013;38(9):1691–7.
21. Orbay JL, Badia A, Indriago IR, et al. The extended flexor carpi radialis approach: a new perspective for the distal radius fracture. Tech Hand Up Extrem Surg. 2001;5(4):204–11.
22. Ilyas AM. Surgical approaches to the distal radius. Hand. 2011;6(1):8–17.
23. Gaspar MP, Sessions BA, Dudoussat BS, Kane PM. Single-incision carpal tunnel release and distal radius open reduction and internal fixation: a cadaveric study. J Wrist Surg. 2016;5(3):241–6.
24. Atkins SE, Logan B, Mcgrouther DA. The deep (motor) branch of the ulnar nerve: a detailed examination of its course and the clinical significance of its damage. J Hand Surg Eur Vol. 2009;34(1):47–57.
25. Naik AA, Hinds RM, Paksima N, Capo JT. Risk of injury to the dorsal sensory branch of the ulnar nerve with percutaneous pinning of ulnar-sided structures. J Hand Surg Am. 2016;41(7):e159–63.
26. Samarakoon LB, Lakmal KC, Thillainathan S, Bataduwaarachchi VR, Anthony DJ, Jayasekara RW. Anatomical relations of the superficial sensory branches of the radial nerve: a cadaveric study with clinical implications. Patient Saf Surg. 2011;5:28.
27. Tellioglu AT, Sensoz O. The dorsal branch of the digital nerve: an anatomic study and clinical applications. Ann Plast Surg. 1998;40(2):145–8.
28. Lahham S, Tu K, Ni M, et al. Comparison of pressures applied by digital tourniquets in the emergency department. West J Emerg Med. 2011;12(2):242–9.
29. Lubahn JD, Koeneman J, Kosar K. The digital tourniquet: how safe is it? J Hand Surg Am. 1985;10(5):664–9.
30. MacDonald RI, Lichtman DM, Hanlon JJ, Wilson JN. Complications of surgical release for carpal tunnel syndrome. J Hand Surg Am. 1978;3(1):70–6.
31. Carroll REMD, Green DPMD. The significance of the palmar cutaneous nerve at the wrist. Clin Orthop Relat Res. 1972;83:24–8.
32. Menorca RMG, Fussell TS, Elfar JC. Peripheral nerve trauma: mechanisms of injury and recovery. Hand Clin. 2013;29(3):317–30.
33. Tosti R, Ilyas AM. Acute carpal tunnel syndrome. Orthop Clin N Am. 2012;43(4):459–65.
34. Laing T, Siddiqui A, Sood M. The management of neuropathic pain from neuromas in the upper limb: surgical techniques and future directions. Plast Aesthet Res. 2015;2(4):165.
35. Weinzweig N. Crossover innervation after digital nerve injury: myth or reality? Ann Plast Surg. 2000;45(5):509–14.
36. Jain A, Dunlop R, Hems T, Tang JB. Outcomes of surgical repair of a single digital nerve in adults. J Hand Surg Eur Vol. 2019;44(6):560–5.
37. Tadjalli HE, McIntyre FHB, Dolynchuk KN, Murray KAM. Importance of crossover innervation in digital nerve repair demonstrated by nerve isolation technique. Ann Plast Surg. 1995;35(1):32–5.
38. Jerosch-Herold C. Assessment of sensibility after nerve injury and repair: a systematic review of evidence for validity, reliability and responsiveness of tests. J Hand Surg Br. 2005;30(3):252–64.
39. Uddin Z. The power function of the ten test for measuring neural sensitivity in clinical pain or sensory abnormalities. Proc Singapore Healthcare. 2017;26(1):62–5.
40. Davis EN, Chung KC. The Tinel sign: a historical perspective. Plast Reconstr Surg. 2004;114(2):494–9.
41. Efstathopoulos D, Gerostathopoufos N, Misitzis D, Bouchlis G, Anagnostou S, Daoutis NK. Clinical assessment of primary digital nerve repair. Acta Orthop Scand. 1995;66(sup264):45–7.
42. Woo A, Bakri K, Moran SL. Management of Ulnar Nerve Injuries. J Hand Surg Am. 2015;40(1):173–81.
43. Burkhalter WE. Restoration of power grip in ulnar nerve paralysis. Orthop Clin North Am. 1974;5(2):289–303.

44. Drury W, Stern PJ. Froment's paper sign and Jeanne's sign—unusual etiology. J Hand Surg Am. 1982;7(4):404–6.
45. Wartenberg R. Nerves of the arm: some of their affections; their diagnosis. Cal West Med. 1943;59(1):22–4.
46. Leibovic SJ, Hastings H. Martin-Gruber revisited. J Hand Surg Am. 1992;17(1):47–53.
47. Cavalheiro CS, Filho MR, Pedro G, Caetano MF, Vieira LA, Caetano EB. Clinical repercussions of Martin-Gruber anastomosis: anatomical study. Rev Bras Ortop. 2016;51(2):214–23.
48. Pederson WC. Median nerve injury and repair. J Hand Surg Am. 2014;39(6):1216–22.
49. Campbell WW. Evaluation and management of peripheral nerve injury. Clin Neurophysiol. 2008;119(9):1951–65.
50. Gilliatt RW, Ochoa J, Rudge P, Neary D. The cause of nerve damage in acute compression. Trans Am Neurol Assoc. 1974;99:71–4.
51. Sathya GR, Krishnamurthy N, Veliath S, Arulneyam J, Venkatachalam J. F wave index: a diagnostic tool for peripheral neuropathy. Indian J Med Res. 2017;145(3):353–7.
52. Malessy MJA, de Boer R, Romero IM, et al. Predictive value of a diagnostic block in focal nerve injury with neuropathic pain when surgery is considered. PLoS One. 2018;13(9):e0203345.
53. Nwawka OK, Miller TT. Ultrasound-guided peripheral nerve injection techniques. Am J Roentgenol. 2016;207(3):507–16.
54. Chhabra A. Peripheral MR neurography: approach to interpretation. Neuroimaging Clin N Am. 2014;24(1):79–89.
55. Chhabra A, Zhao L, Carrino JA, et al. MR neurography: advances. Radiol Res Pract. 2013;2013:809568. Available from: https://www.ncbi.nlm.nih.gov/pmc/articles/PMC3622412/
56. Sebastin SJ. Complex regional pain syndrome. Indian J Plast Surg. 2011;44(2):298–307.
57. He B, Zhu Z, Zhu Q, et al. Factors predicting sensory and motor recovery after the repair of upper limb peripheral nerve injuries. Neural Regen Res. 2014;9(6):661–72.
58. Grinsell D, Keating CP. Peripheral nerve reconstruction after injury: a review of clinical and experimental therapies. Biomed Res Int. 2014;2014:698256. Available from: https://www.hindawi.com/journals/bmri/2014/698256/
59. Lundborg G. A 25-year perspective of peripheral nerve surgery: evolving neuroscientific concepts and clinical significance. J Hand Surg Am. 2000;25(3):391–414.
60. Clark WL, Trumble TE, Swiontkowski MF, Tencer AF. Nerve tension and blood flow in a rat model of immediate and delayed repairs. J Hand Surg Am. 1992;17(4):677–87.
61. Sadek AF, Fouly EH, Hamdy M. Functional and electrophysiological outcome after autogenous vein wrapping of primary repaired ulnar nerves. Microsurgery. 2014;34(5):361–6.
62. Sotereanos DG, Giannakopoulos PN, Mitsionis GI, Xu J, Herndon JH. Vein-graft wrapping for the treatment of recurrent compression of the median nerve. Microsurgery. 1995;16(11):752–6.
63. Sunderland SS. The anatomy and physiology of nerve injury. Muscle Nerve. 1990;13(9):771–84.
64. Millesi H. Progress in peripheral nerve reconstruction. World J Surg. 1990;14(6):733–47.
65. Cho MS, Rinker BD, Weber RV, et al. Functional outcome following nerve repair in the upper extremity using processed nerve allograft. J Hand Surg Am. 2012;37(11):2340–9.
66. Safa B, Shores JT, Ingari JV, et al. Recovery of motor function after mixed and motor nerve repair with processed nerve allograft. Plast Reconstr Surg Glob Open. 2019;7(3):e2163.
67. Colen K, Choi M, Chiu D. Nerve grafts and conduits. Plast Reconstr Surg. 2009;124(6S):e386–94. Available from: insights.ovid.com
68. Konofaos P, Halen JPV. Nerve repair by means of tubulization: past, present, future. J Reconstr Microsurg. 2013;29(03):149–64.
69. Strauch B, Goldberg N, Herman CK. Sural nerve harvest: anatomy and technique. J Reconstr Microsurg. 2005;21(2):133–6.
70. Mahakkanukrauh P, Chomsung R. Anatomical variations of the sural nerve. Clin Anat. 2002;15(4):263–6.
71. Sridhar K. Tendon transfer for median nerve palsy. Indian J Plast Surg. 2011;44(2):357–61.
72. Wolfe SW, Hotchkiss RN, Pederson WC, Kozin SH, Cohen MS, Green DP. Green's operative hand surgery 2017 [cited 2019 Feb 10]. Available from: https://www.clinicalkey.com/dura/browse/bookChapter/3-s2.0-C20121066969
73. Royle ND. An operation for paralysis of the intrinsic muscles of the thumb. JAMA. 1938;111(7):612–3.
74. Thompson TC. A modified operation for opponens paralysis. JBJS. 1942;24(3):632.
75. Bunnell S. Surgery of the intrinsic muscles of the hand other than those producing opposition of the thumb. JBJS. 1942;24(1):1.
76. Burkhalter W, Christensen RC, Brown P. Extensor indicis proprius opponensplasty. J Bone Joint Surg Am. 1973;55(4):725–32.
77. Browne EZ, Teague MA, Snyder CC. Prevention of extensor lag after indicis proprius tendon transfer. J Hand Surg Am. 1979;4(2):168–72.
78. Terrono AL, Rose JH, Mulroy J, Millender LH. Camitz palmaris longus abductorplasty for severe thenar atrophy secondary to carpal tunnel syndrome. J Hand Surg Am. 1993;18(2):204–6.
79. Huber E. Relief operation in the case of paralysis of the median nerve. J Hand Surg Br. 2004;29(1):35–7.
80. Zancolli EA. Claw-hand caused by paralysis of the intrinsic muscles: a simple surgical procedure for its correction. JBJS. 1957;39(5):1076.

81. Riordan DC. Tendon transplantations in median-nerve and ulnar-nerve paralysis. J Bone Joint Surg Am. 1953;35-A(2):312–20.
82. Littler JW. Tendon transfers and arthrodeses in combined median and ulnar nerve paralysis. J Bone Joint Surg Am. 1949;31A(2):225–34.
83. Durdzinska A, Gjika E, Durand S. Correction of Z-deformity of the thumb after trapeziectomy by modified Zancolli lasso procedure. J Hand Surg Eur Vol. 2019;44(7):749–50.
84. Goldner JL. Tendon transfers for irreparable peripheral nerve injuries of the upper extremity. Orthop Clin North Am. 1974;5(2):343–75.
85. Smith RJ. Extensor carpi radialis brevis tendon transfer for thumb adduction–a study of power pinch. J Hand Surg Am. 1983;8(1):4–15.
86. Edgerton MT, Brand PW. Restoration of abduction and adduction to the unstable thumb in median and ulnar paralysis. Plast Reconstr Surg. 1965;36:150–64.
87. Eberlin KR, Ducic I. Surgical algorithm for neuroma management: a changing treatment paradigm. Plast Reconstr Surg Glob Open. 2018;6(10):e1952.
88. Mass DPMD, Ciano MCMD, Tortosa RMD, Newmeyer WLMD, Kilgore ESJ. Treatment of painful hand neuromas by their transfer into bone. Plast Reconstr Surg. 1984;74(2):182–5.
89. Herbert TJ, Filan SL. Vein implantation for treatment of painful cutaneous neuromas. A preliminary report. J Hand Surg Br. 1998;23(2):220–4.
90. Aszmann OC, Korak KJ, Rab M, Grünbeck M, Lassmann H, Frey M. Neuroma prevention by end-to-side neurorraphy: an experimental study in rats. J Hand Surg Am. 2003;28(6):1022–8.
91. Al-Qattan MM. Prevention and treatment of painful neuromas of the superficial radial nerve by the end-to-side nerve repair concept: an experimental study and preliminary clinical experience. Microsurgery. 2000;20(3):99–104.
92. Kon M, Bloem JJ. The treatment of amputation neuromas in fingers with a centrocentral nerve union. Ann Plast Surg. 1987;18(6):506–10.
93. Low CK, Chew SH, Song IC, Ng TH, Low YP. End-to-side anastomosis of transected nerves to prevent neuroma formation. Clin Orthop Relat Res. 1999;369:327–32.
94. Tupper JW, Booth DM. Treatment of painful neuromas of sensory nerves in the hand: a comparison of traditional and newer methods. J Hand Surg Am. 1976;1(2):144–51.
95. Swanson AB, Boeve NR, Lumsden RM. The prevention and treatment of amputation neuromata by silicone capping. J Hand Surg Am. 1977;2(1):70–8.
96. Edds MV. Prevention of nerve regeneration and neuroma formation by caps of synthetic resin. J Neurosurg. 1945;2(6):507–9.
97. Galeano M, Manasseri B, Risitano G, et al. A free vein graft cap influences neuroma formation after nerve transection. Microsurgery. 2009;29(7):568–72.
98. Hsu E, Cohen SP. Postamputation pain: epidemiology, mechanisms, and treatment. J Pain Res. 2013;6:121–36.
99. Kuiken TA, Li G, Lock BA, et al. Targeted muscle reinnervation for real-time myoelectric control of multifunction artificial arms. JAMA. 2009;301(6):619–28.
100. Ruijs ACJ, Jaquet J-B, Kalmijn S, Giele H, Hovius SER. Median and ulnar nerve injuries: a meta-analysis of predictors of motor and sensory recovery after modern microsurgical nerve repair. Plast Reconstr Surg. 2005;116(2):484–94.
101. Gaul JS. Intrinsic motor recovery--a long-term study of ulnar nerve repair. J Hand Surg Am. 1982;7(5):502–8.
102. Anderson GA, Lee V, Sundararaj GD. Extensor indicis proprius opponensplasty. J Hand Surg. 1991;16(3):334–8.
103. Anderson GA, Lee V, Sundararaj GD. Opponensplasty by extensor indicis and flexor digitorum superficialis tendon transfer. J Hand Surg. 1992;17(6):611–4.
104. Patond KR, Betal BD, Gautam V. Results of thumb correction in leprosy using different techniques. Indian J Lepr. 1999;71(2):155–66.
105. Palande DD. Opponensplasty in intrinsic-muscle paralysis of the thumb in leprosy. J Bone Joint Surg Am. 1975;57(4):489–93.
106. Schwarz RJ, Macdonald M. Assessment of results of opponensplasty. J Hand Surg Br. 2003;28(6):593–6.
107. Hastings H, McCollam SM. Flexor digitorum superficialis lasso tendon transfer in isolated ulnar nerve palsy: a functional evaluation. J Hand Surg. 1994;19(2):275–80.
108. Dellon AL, Mackinnon SE. Treatment of the painful neuroma by neuroma resection and muscle implantation. Plast Reconstr Surg. 1986;77(3):427–38.
109. Freniere BB, Wenzinger E, Lans J, Eberlin KR. Relocation nerve grafting: a technique for management of symptomatic digital neuromas. J Hand Microsurg. 2019;11(Suppl 1):S50–2.
110. Woo SL, Kung TA, Brown DL, Leonard JA, Kelly BM, Cederna PS. Regenerative peripheral nerve interfaces for the treatment of postamputation neuroma pain: a pilot study. Plast Reconstr Surg Glob Open. 2016;4(12):e1038.
111. Kubiak CA, Kemp SWP, Cederna PS, Kung TA. Prophylactic regenerative peripheral nerve interfaces to prevent postamputation pain. Plast Reconstr Surg. 2019;144(3):421e–30e.
112. Dumanian GA, Potter BK, Mioton LM, et al. Targeted muscle reinnervation treats neuroma and phantom pain in major limb amputees: a randomized clinical trial. Ann Surg. 2019;270(2):238–46.

Median and Ulnar Nerve Injury at the Elbow and Wrist

8

Callie Jewett and Mihir Desai

8.1 Ulnar Nerve Injury at the Elbow

8.1.1 Risks/Incidence/Mechanism of Injury

Entrapment of the ulnar nerve is the second most common compressive neuropathy behind carpal tunnel and can happen along any length of the nerve but is most common in the cubital tunnel [27]. Subsequently, cubital tunnel release is a common orthopedic procedure. The goal of the procedure is to relieve compression on the ulnar nerve, thus relieving patients' ulnar neuropathy; however, there is a risk of recurrent compression or iatrogenic injury to the ulnar nerve. Seventeen percent of traumatic nerve injuries occur secondary to iatrogenic damage [34]. Injury is due to direct or indirect mechanisms and can occur due from both intrinsic and extrinsic etiologies. Intraoperatively, the ulnar nerve may be injured from complete or partial dissection. Intrinsic pathology due to fracture fragments, fracture malunion, or excess callus formation can cause ulnar compression within the cubital tunnel [27]. Extrinsic injury may occur from iatrogenic compression from placement of surgical retractors, implants, positioning or even prolonged upper arm tourniquet use [49, 69].

In addition to injury during cubital tunnel release, the ulnar nerve is at risk from trauma. Approximately 2% of all adult fractures involve the elbow [3] in a bimodal distribution with peak incidences between 12 and 19 years and in those over 80 years of age [51]. As the humeral shaft approaches the distal humerus, it bifurcates into the medial and lateral columns. Mouchet first described ulnar nerve palsies from distal humerus fractures in 1914 [48]. When evaluating patients with periarticular fractures, it is important to perform a thorough neurovascular exam and document any preexisting nerve injuries. Traumatic ulnar nerve injuries occur equally at the arm and elbow, less commonly in the forearm and wrist [42]. Iatrogenic ulnar nerve injury following surgical fixation of periarticular elbow fractures results from surgical manipulation of the ulnar nerve, inadequate release, and postoperative immobilization resulting in fibrosis. For all medial and posterior approaches to the elbow, the ulnar nerve should be identified and tagged to prevent iatrogenic injury.

C. Jewett (✉)
Department of Orthopaedic Surgery at Vanderbilt University Medical Center, Nashville, TN, USA
e-mail: callie.jewett@vumc.org

M. Desai
Division of Hand and Upper Extremity, Department of Orthopaedic Surgery at Vanderbilt University Medical Center, Nashville, TN, USA
e-mail: mihir.j.desai@vumc.org

C. J. Dy et al. (eds.), *Peripheral Nerve Issues after Orthopedic Surgery*,
https://doi.org/10.1007/978-3-030-84428-8_8

8.1.1.1 Pertinent Anatomy

The ulnar nerve arises from the C8 and T1 nerve roots and the medial cord of the brachial plexus. It travels with the brachial artery at the level of the upper arm until the insertion of coracobrachialis where it separates and travels posteriorly with the ulnar collateral artery within the anterior compartment. It then pierces the medial intermuscular septum, traveling from the anterior compartment to the posterior compartment. It travels under the arcade of Struthers, lying on top of the medial head of the triceps. At the level of the elbow, the ulnar nerve lies posterior to the medial epicondyle between the olecranon and the medial epicondyle within the cubital tunnel. The floor of the cubital tunnel is formed by the medial collateral ligament and elbow joint capsule and the roof is formed by the arcuate ligament. Distal to the cubital tunnel, the ulnar nerve then travels between the two heads of FCU and lies between FCU and FDS as it moves distally into the anterior compartment of the forearm.

There are several sites of compression of the ulnar nerve at the elbow including the medial intramuscular septum, the arcuate ligament at the cubital tunnel, and the two heads of FCU. Less commonly nerve compression can happen due to rare anatomic variants: proximally at the arcade of Struthers or distally due to an anomalous anconeus epitrochlearis [38, 58].

8.1.2 Prevention Strategies

In a systematic review, 75% of patient who underwent cubital tunnel release reported some residual symptoms [26]. Persistent symptoms after cubital tunnel release are typically due to scarring, incomplete decompression, missed diagnosis, iatrogenic injury, or ulnar nerve instability at the elbow [52, 54]. Adequate proximal and distal dissection can help surgeons ensure sufficient release. The nerve should be followed proximally, and the point where the nerve crosses from the anterior to the posterior compartment should be identified. Typically, there is a band of fascia at the septum that needs to be released and less commonly found, the arcade of Struthers [58]. To ensure adequate exposure, place the tourniquet high when positioning and prepping the patient so this proximal dissection can be performed. Distally, the nerve should be followed into the muscle of FCU to ensure complete release of the FCU fascia encasing the nerve. Additionally, if the patient has an anconeus epitrochlearis, a myotomy is necessary to ensure complete decompression of the nerve [47].

There is not a consensus on whether a transposition should be performed at the time of primary cubital tunnel release. The authors prefer to transpose when there is documented instability of the ulnar nerve preoperatively or intraoperatively. If there is documented electrodiagnostic denervation of the intrinsic muscles, then we would also recommend transposition.

During primary cubital tunnel release, the surgeon must take care as the median antebrachial cutaneous nerve often crosses the surgical field [36]. The medial antebrachial cutaneous nerve originates from the medial cord of the brachial plexus. Transection of the MABCN during cubital tunnel release can result in a painful neuroma that can be misdiagnosed as recurrent disease and may ultimately require neuroma excision [55]. Typically, the MABCN is deeper than expected and lies along the triceps fascia and crosses the surgical field at or below the medial epicondyle [24, 36].

Several techniques can be employed to help prevent iatrogenic ulnar nerve injury during the approach to and fixation of distal humerus fractures. When identifying the nerve, it is important to adequately liberate the nerve proximally and distally. This will prevent unnecessary traction and compression on the nerve during retraction. Additionally, this will help prevent postoperative compression within the cubital tunnel from local tissue swelling related to the trauma and surgery. We have found that securing a penrose drain with a suture as opposed to a hemostat around the nerve to be a superior method of retraction to avoid unnecessary traction on the ulnar nerve from surgeons, first assists and scrub techs.

There is not a clear consensus on whether or not the ulnar nerve should be transposed at the conclusion of the procedure. The soft tissue damage associated with distal humerus fractures is severe and postoperative scar formation around the ulnar nerve can be expected. Some argue that the soft tissue dissection required for a transposition at the end of the procedure is substantially more than that required for the primary procedure [19]. Wiggers has demonstrated that the incidence of ulnar neuropathy after surgical treatment of the distal humerus is independent of transposition [70], whereas Wang transposed 20 patients at the time of open reduction and internal fixation and had no incidence of postoperative neurapraxia [68]. Conversely, Chen demonstrated in a retrospective study that patients who underwent anterior transposition were four times more likely to have ulnar nerve symptoms postoperatively [20]. Unfortunately, there is no level 1 evidence for or against transposition. We prefer anterior transposition of the ulnar nerve into the subcutaneous tissues at the conclusion of the procedure.

8.1.2.1 Typical Course/Natural History

Without intervention, about half of ulnar neuropathies due to compressive pathology resolve without intervention [45]. There has not been much clinical research on the long-term outcomes of severe ulnar nerve injuries. Most patients with early compressive disease have intermittent numbness and parasthesias in the ring and small fingers that is worse at night; however, as the disease progresses this becomes more constant. Patients with closed untreated ulnar nerve injuries risk losing hand intrinsic function [71]. Patients will often complain of clumsiness and loss of dexterity. It is important for the clinician to obtain a complete history as to not miss concurrent cervical myelopathy.

8.1.2.2 Initial Evaluation/Exam

Many patients with cubital tunnel syndrome will have tenderness to palpation over the ulnar nerve at the medial elbow. This point of tenderness may be at the level of the cubital tunnel or distally as the nerve travels underneath the FCU fascia. Additionally, special attention should be paid to whether the nerve is hypermobile or subluxating over the medial epicondyle.

Patients with ulnar nerve injuries will have numbness and/or paresthesias within the ulnar half of the ring and the entire small finger. The distribution of numbness and parasthesias can differentiate between high and low ulnar nerve injuries. The dorsal cutaneous branch of the ulnar nerve, which branches from the common ulnar nerve proximal to Guyon's canal, supplies the sensation to the dorsal ulnar half of the hand. Patients with high ulnar nerve pathology will have numbness over the dorsum of their hand as well as in their ring and small fingers; as opposed to patients with low ulnar nerve pathology who will retain the sensation to the dorsum of their hand.

Hand weakness is also a typical presentation as the ulnar nerve innervates the hand intrinsics. Patients with high ulnar nerve injuries are unable to fire flexor carpi ulnaris and flexor digitorum profundus of the ring and small finger in addition to intrinsic muscle paralysis. This results in a claw deformity as well as weakness with pinch and grip. The motor exam in patients with ulnar nerve injuries should test the function of FDP to the ring and small fingers as well as to the palmar and dorsal interossei and the two most ulnar lumbricals.

Below are some specific exam techniques that can be used to isolate ulnar nerve function.

- Froment's sign – thumb IP hyperflexion with pinch
- Jeanne's sign – thumb MCP hyperextension and abduction with pinch
- Wartenberg's sign – small finger abduction with finger extension

When testing intrinsic muscle function, the examiner must be aware of potential anatomic variations in which the interossei or lumbricals are innervated by the median nerve. For example, 7% of the population have an anomaly known as the Martin–Gruber communication, in which the anterior interosseus nerve communicates with the ulnar nerve in the proximal forearm, thus providing a dual innervation to flexor digitorum profundus and the intrinsics [28, 43]. There is also an analogous connection in the hand known as the Riche–Cannieu interconnection, which is a connection between the recurrent branch of the median nerve and the ulnar nerve that allows the median nerve to innervate all the lumbricals [27].

One must differentiate ulnar nerve palsies from brachial plexus and cervical spine pathology. Spurling's test for cervical nerve compression and Allen's test for thoracic outlet syndrome can help in differentiating between these pathologies. Sensory assessment in the distributions of the medial antebrachial cutaneous nerve and medial brachial cutaneous nerve are also useful in localizing the lesion.

8.1.3 Diagnostic Tests/Imaging

Several diagnostic tests can be useful when diagnosing ulnar nerve injury. We recommend obtaining plain radiographs of the elbow to identify any posttraumatic deformity or soft tissue calcifications that may be causing compression and symptoms.

EMG can be helpful in diagnosis as it can help delineate the location of nerve pathology [71]. EMG is limited with severe axonal injury and in acute injury. It also does not take into account anatomic variants [71]. It is also important to note that EMG is highly operator-dependent, and results vary from patient to patient due to comorbidities or age [62]. They can be very helpful if the surgeon is trending an exam as they can document nerve recovery or worsening neuropathy [62].

Ultrasound may provide a benefit over MRI or CT. In addition to being relatively easy to perform and cheap, it can show the topography of the nerve as well as changes in the muscles due to denervation [12]. CT or MRI may be helpful to identify soft tissue or bony variants as possible areas of compression.

8.1.4 Surgical Techniques

8.1.4.1 Revision Cubital Tunnel

In patients who have failed cubital tunnel release, a revision cubital tunnel release may be required. Several options are available for revision surgery including neurolysis, transposition, and nerve wrapping with biologic materials such as fat, vein, or implants like collagen or porcine submucosal nerve wraps. Please refer to Example 8.1 for intraoperative photographs of a revision carpal tunnel with external neurolysis.

Historically, the most popular revision technique is submuscular transposition in which the nerve is fully released and placed in the plane below the flexor pronator mass [67]. Unfortunately, this technique requires the release of the flexor pronator mass from the medial epicondyle and requires 2–3 weeks of postop immobilization. As expected, the success rate of revision cubital tunnel release and submuscular transposition is less than that of patients undergoing primary cubital tunnel release [67]. It remains a useful surgical technique; however, it has not been shown to be superior to simpler techniques such as a subcutaneous transposition. In a systematic review, a combined analysis of all revision cubital tunnel release techniques had a 78% success rate, with a 71% success rate with submuscular transposition [60].

More recently, many surgeons opt to use nerve wraps in revision cubital tunnel surgery. Unfortunately, there is not an abundance of literature on the use of nerve wrapping in the treatment of nerve compression; however, the safety of nerve wraps in patients with neuropathy secondary to scarring has been shown [30]. Several biomaterials are available for nerve wraps: collagen, porcine extracellular matrix, and amniotic membranes. The authors prefer semi-transparent products because this allows visualization of the underlying nerve. In a review of 15 patients who underwent revision cubital tunnel surgery with collagen wrapping of the ulnar nerve, 83% reported improvement of symptoms [60]. In another review of 12 patients treated with porcine extracellular nerve wrapping at the time of revision cubital tunnel release, patients had significant decrease in preoperative pain levels as well as improved grip and pinch strength [46]. We have found several techniques that are useful when using nerve wraps to minimize complications. It is important to not "overwrap" the nerve thus causing a potential site of compression. Furthermore, it is helpful to release the tourniquet and obtain hemostasis before applying and securing the nerve wrap. Lastly, the surgeon should be cautious of placing the wrap directly subcutaneously, as it can cause a foreign body reaction; we prefer to avoid the use of wraps where this may occur.

Example 8.1 Revision cubital tunnel with external neurolysis (Figs. 8.1, 8.2, and 8.3).

When performing revision cubital tunnel surgery, the authors prefer to perform a neurolysis, anterior transposition, and the use of a pedicled adipose flap, as seen in Example 8.2. Rosenwasser initially described this technique in 2014. In this procedure, a well-vascularized adipose flap is created and the nerve is subsequently wrapped creating a similar environment to that of peripheral nerves. This technique reduces postoperative perineural scarring [25].

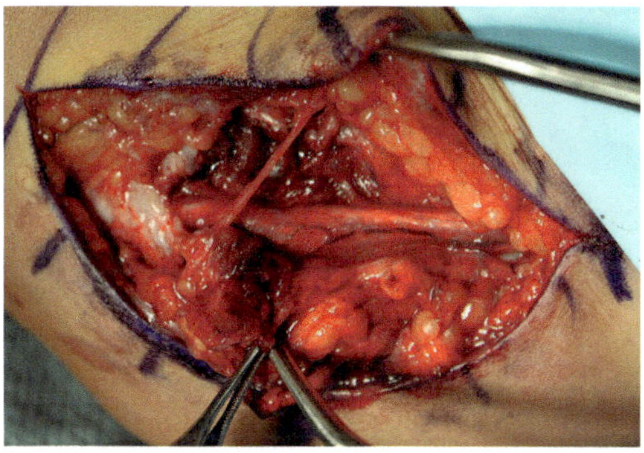

Fig. 8.1 Intraoperative photograph of scar around an ulnar nerve following cubital tunnel release with subcutaneous transposition

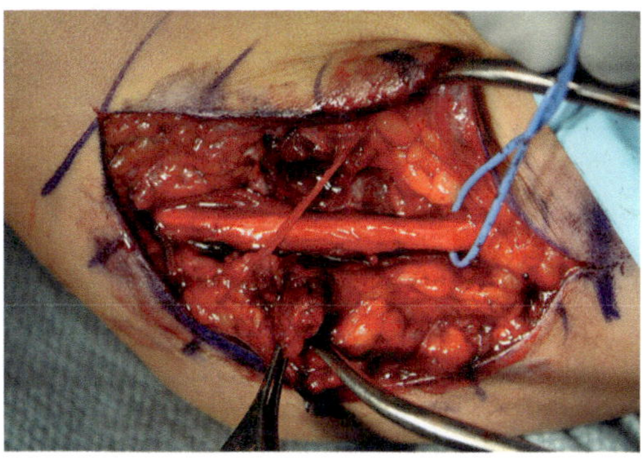

Fig. 8.2 External neurolysis is performed so that the ulnar nerve can be mobilized

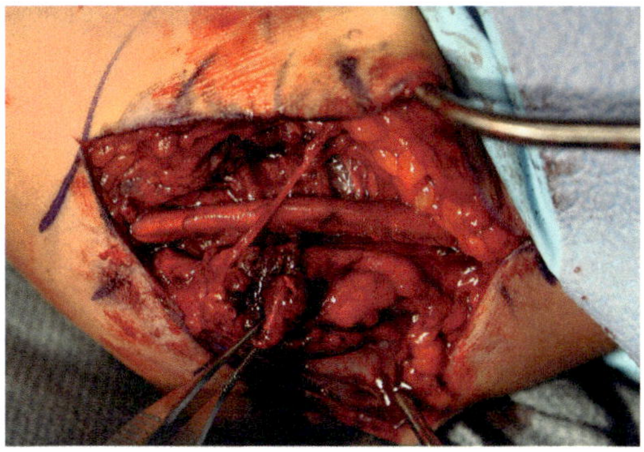

Fig. 8.3 The nerve is transposed anteriorly with a fascial sling to prevent future subluxation

Technique

- The ulnar nerve is exposed and decompressed using a classic cubital tunnel approach.
- In revisions, neurolysis is performed; the ulnar nerve is freed from any scar tissue and mobilized.
- A vascularized adipose flap is then created from the anterior subcutaneous tissue overlying the nerve.
- A central cutaneous artery from the brachial artery is identified supplying the flap. Care must be taken to maintain this vascular supply to the flap.
- The fat is then elevated using sharp dissection from the subcutaneous tissue while visualizing the vascular pedicle.
- The ulnar nerve is transposed anteriorly and completely wrapped by the pedicle in a posterior to superior fashion.
- The pedicle is sutured to the subcutaneous tissue, thus completely encompassing the ulnar nerve.
- Once wrapping is complete, the elbow is taken through normal range of motion to ensure nerve gliding through the adipose tissue.

Example 8.2 Vascularized adipose flap (Figs. 8.4, 8.5, 8.6, 8.7, 8.8, and 8.9).

The surgical approach to ulnar nerve neuropathy following surgical fixation of the distal

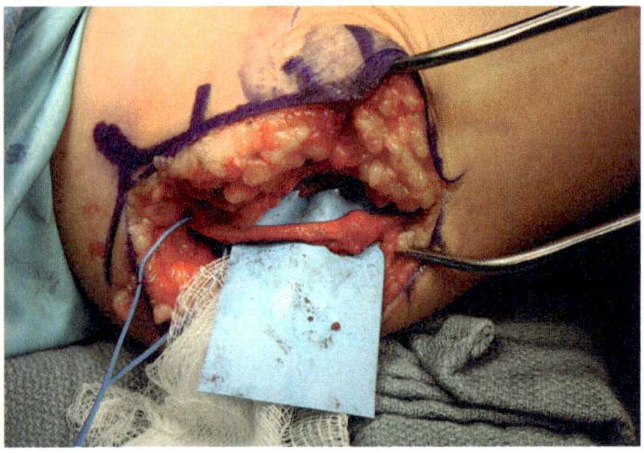

Fig. 8.4 Intraoperative photo of an ulnar nerve neuroma following a missed ulnar nerve injury

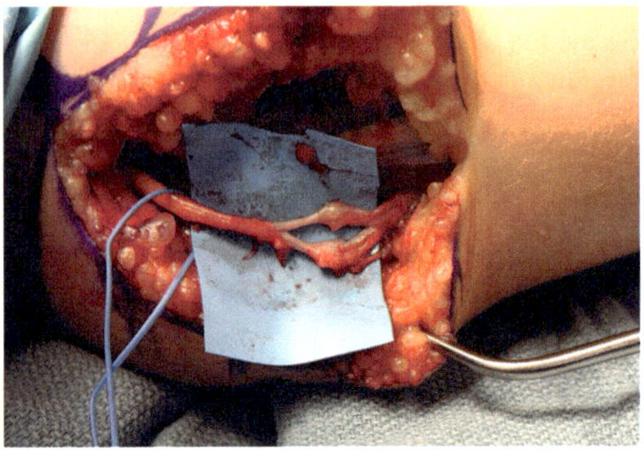

Fig. 8.5 Internal neurolysis is performed after the completion of external neurolysis

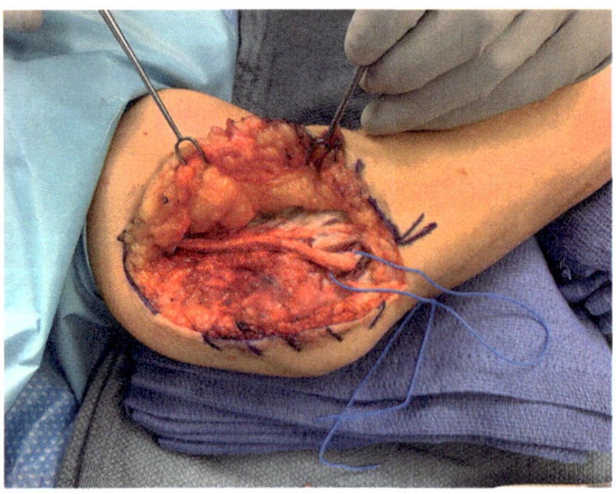

Fig. 8.6 A vascularized adipose flap is then created from the anterior subcutaneous tissue overlying the nerve

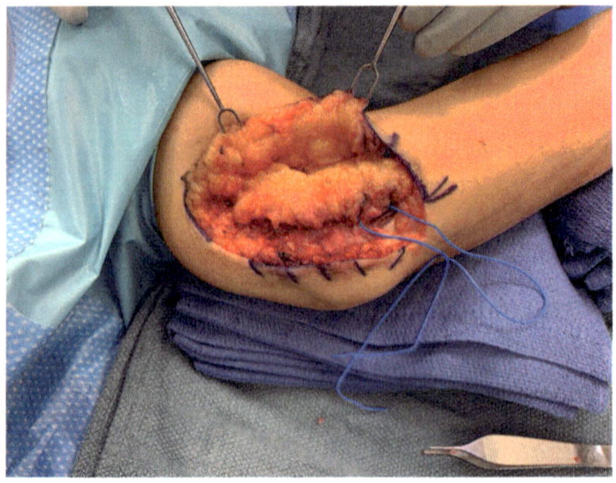

Fig. 8.7 A central cutaneous artery from the brachial artery is identified supplying the flap. The fat is then elevated using sharp dissection from the subcutaneous tissue while visualizing the vascular pedicle

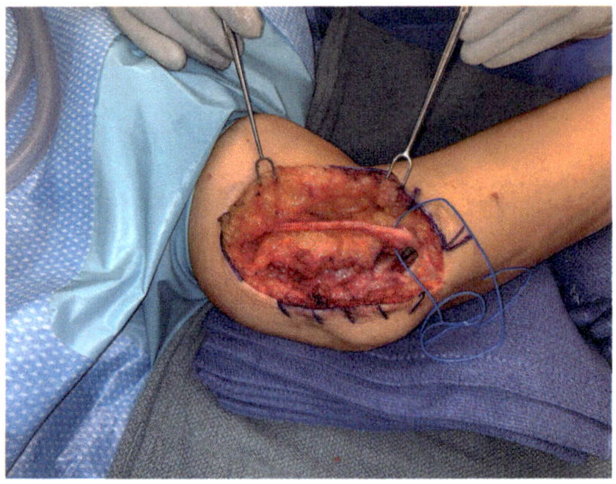

Fig. 8.8 The ulnar nerve is transposed anteriorly and completely wrapped by the pedicle in a posterior to superior fashion

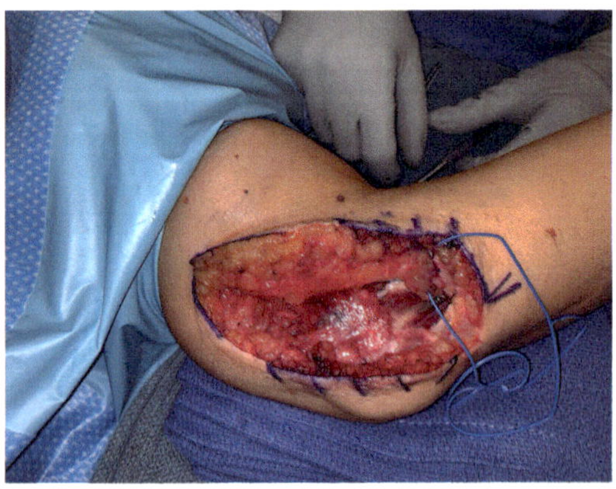

Fig. 8.9 The pedicle is sutured to the subcutaneous tissue, thus completely encompassing the ulnar nerve

humerus is similar to that of revision cubital tunnel. If patients present with postoperative ulnar neuropathy, ulnar nerve neurolysis has good reported outcomes. In 20 patients with ulnar neuropathy following the surgical treatment of elbow fractures treated with ulnar neurolysis and transposition, 17 patients reported good-to-excellent improvement in function and symptoms [39].

8.1.4.2 Nerve Transfer Techniques

The anterior interosseous nerve can be transferred to the ulnar nerve transfer to preserve the motor endplates to the distal muscles innervated by the ulnar nerve. In this procedure, detailed in Example 8.3, the terminal branch of AIN to pronator quadratus is transferred in a reverse end-to-side manner to an ulnar nerve motor branch in the forearm [8]. In a retrospective study, 85% of patients who underwent the reverse end-to-side AIN to ulnar nerve transfer had improvement of hand intrinsic function [7].

Technique

- An incision is made that extends from ulnar to the thenar crease to about 8–12 cm proximal above the ulnocarpal joint.
- Distally, the palmar carpal ligament is identified and Guyon's canal is released.
  - This allows for better visualization of the deep motor branches of the ulnar nerve, which is ulnar to the hook of the hamate and deep to the hypothenar muscles.
- Proximally, the dorsal sensory branch of the ulnar nerve arises from the ulnar nerve proper approximately 8 cm above the ulnocarpal joint and is identified.
  - The topography of the nerve fascicles is consistent at this level such that from ulnar to radial, the fascicles are arranged as sensory–motor–sensory.
  - The most ulnar sensory fascicles make up the dorsal sensory branch, which have divided from the ulnar nerve proper.
  - The most ulnar fascicles within the ulnar nerve proper are the motor fascicles to the intrinsic muscles.
- At the most proximal aspect of the incision, the flexor muscles are retracted radially and the pronator quadratus (PQ) is identified.
- AIN is found entering the PQ. The muscle is divided to trace the AIN distally to divide the nerve with as much length as possible.
- AIN is then divided distally and then transposed toward the ulnar nerve.
- Flexor digitorum profundus can be released proximally to prevent tension on AIN.
- Under the microscope, the motor fascicular bundle of the ulnar nerve is identified through an epineural window and separated from its neighboring sensory bundles.
- Once the motor fascicle has been identified, a tension-free coaptation is performed in an end-to-side fashion with 9.0 nylon epineural suture. We have found that a large (~5 mm) epineural window is necessary to properly perform the end-to-side transfer.
- The wrist should be taken through full pass ROM to ensure that the repair is tension free.

Example 8.3 AIN to ulnar nerve transfer (Figs. 8.10, 8.11, 8.12, 8.13, 8.14, 8.15, 8.16, 8.17, and 8.18).

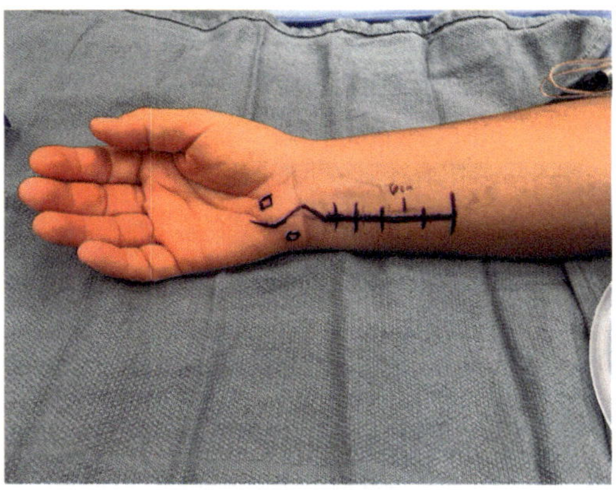

Fig. 8.10 A Brunner-type incision across the wrist just ulnar to the thenar crease that extends 8–10 cm above the ulnocapital joint

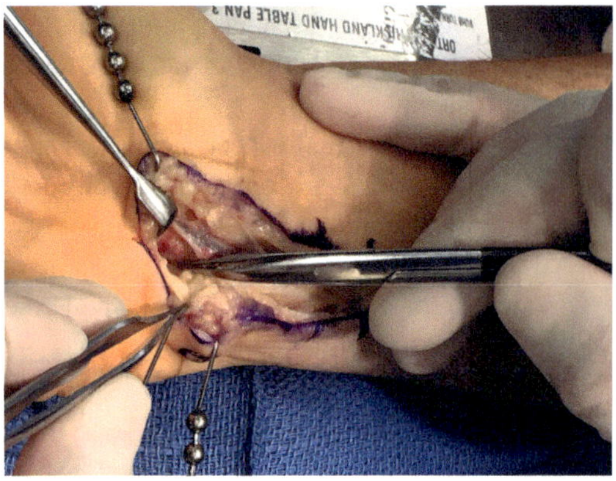

Fig. 8.11 The palmar carpal ligament is identified and Guyon's canal is released

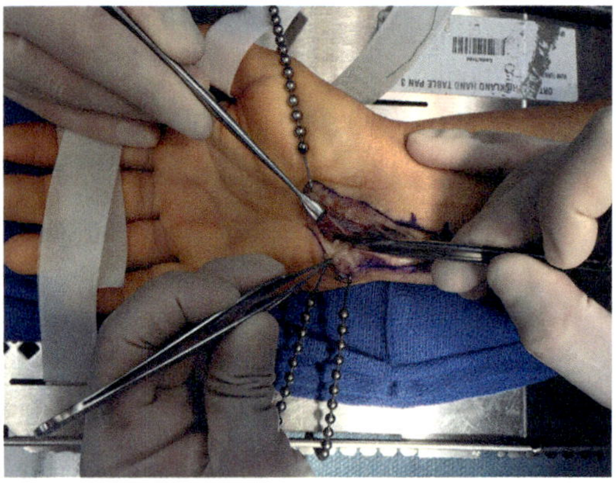

Fig. 8.12 The deep motor branches of the ulnar nerve is identified ulnar to the hook of the hamate and deep to the hypothenar muscles. These fascicles can be followed proximally to better visualize the branch of the dorsal sensory nerve fascicles from ulnar nerve proper

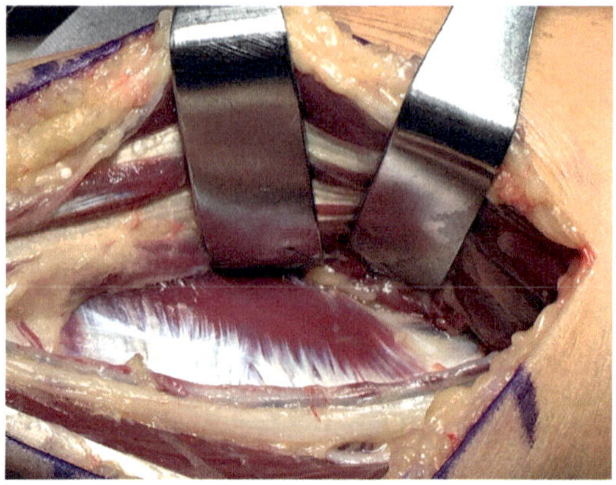

Fig. 8.14 At the most proximal aspect of the incision, the flexor muscles are retracted radially and the pronator quadratus (PQ) is identified

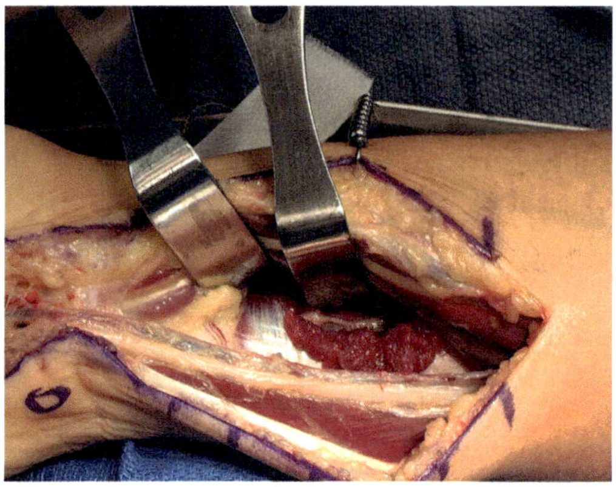

Fig. 8.15 AIN is found entering the PQ. The muscle is divided to trace the AIN distally to divide the nerve with as much length as possible

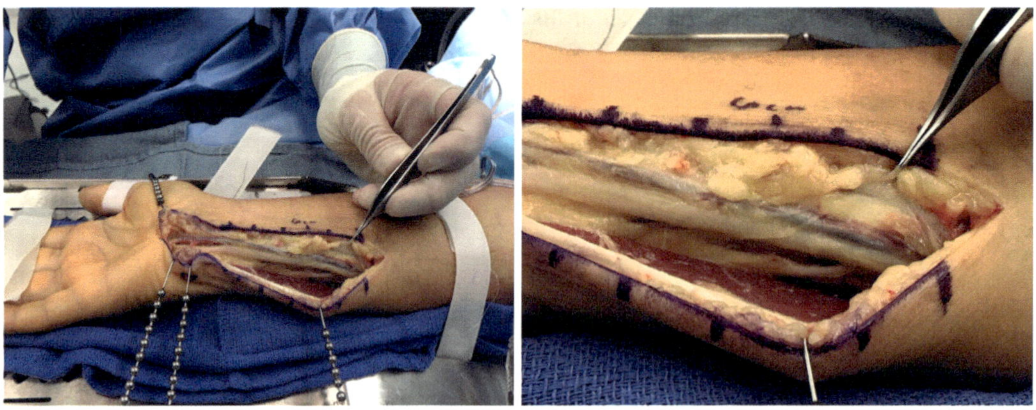

Fig. 8.13 The dorsal sensory branch of the ulnar nerve branches at about 6–10 cm proximal to the ulnocarpal joint

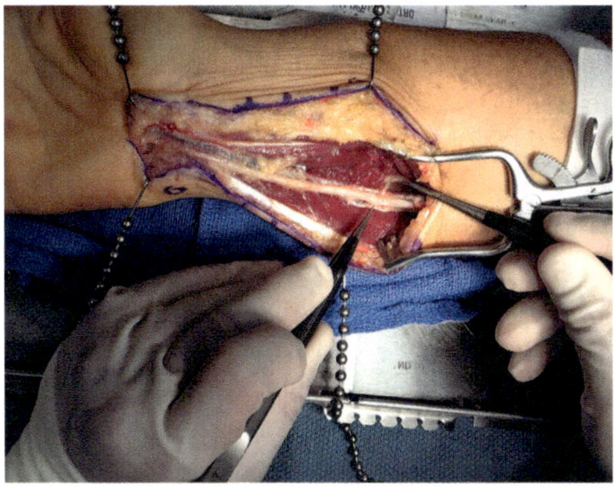

Fig. 8.16 AIN is then divided distally and then transposed toward the ulnar nerve

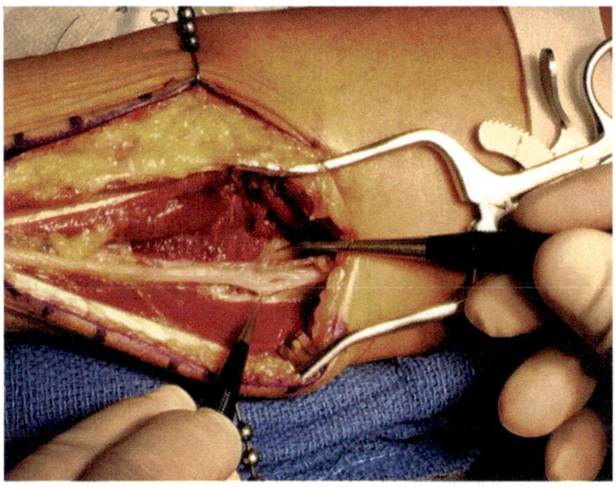

Fig. 8.17 Under the microscope, the motor fascicular bundle of the ulnar nerve is identified through an epineural window and separated from its neighboring sensory bundles

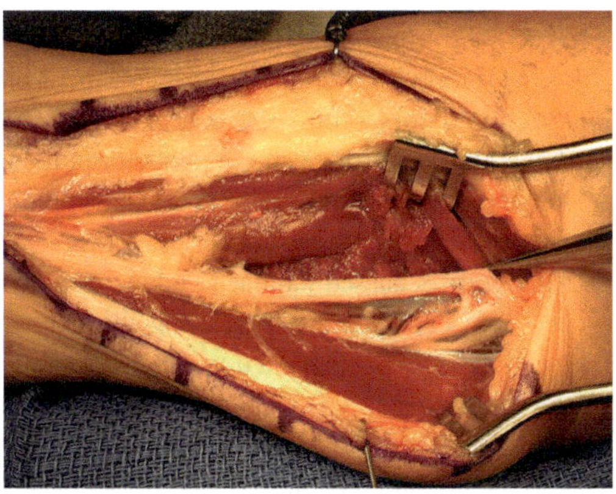

Fig. 8.18 A tension-free coaptation is performed in an end-to-side fashion with 9.0 nylon epineural suture

8.1.5 Salvage Techniques

8.1.5.1 Tendon Transfer Techniques

Clawing deformity in ulnar nerve injury is due to loss of intrinsic muscle function. Without the intrinsic function, unopposed extensor digitorum communis function causes hyperextension at the MCP joint. The claw deformity in the ring and small finger results from reciprocal flexion at the PIP and DIP. Thus, to correct the claw deformity, several tendon transfers can be performed to prevent MCP hyperextension.

The most common tendon transfers used to correct the clawing deformity are the Zancolli lasso or the modified Stiles–Bunnell transfer. When deciding between these two procedures, one must evaluate the integrity of the PIP central slip. This can be determined by the Bouvier maneuver. With claw deformity, patients are unable to actively extend the PIP joint when the MCP is hyperextended. Patients with a positive Bouvier's maneuver are able to actively extend PIP with MCP extension blocked, indicating that the central slip remains competent [10].

The Zancolli lasso uses flexor digitorum superficialis (FDS) of the affected finger to restore MCP flexion. It is indicated when patients have a positive Bouvier maneuver or central slip compensation [10]. In a retrospective study by Hastings and McCollum, 19 out of 23 digits treated with the Zancolli lasso reported successful correction of the claw deformity at their 5-year follow-up [29]. The procedure originally described by Zancolli recommends using FDS to each individual finger [72]. Alternatively, Anderson suggests using the middle finger FDS tendon and splitting it into four to symmetrically control MCP flexion of all fingers [2]. The procedure corrects clawing by setting the hand in an intrinsic plus position. Unfortunately, this technique can create an iatrogenic swan neck deformity from PIP hyperextension from the loss of FDS influence on PIP flexion. Transecting the FDS tendon proximal to the bifurcation helps to prevent this [10].

Technique

- A zigzag Bruner's incision is made midpalm and the tendon sheath between the A1 and A2 pulleys is identified and incised.
- The FDS tendon is then transected about 2 cm proximal to its bifurcation, pulled from the tendon sheath and out of the A1 pulley.
- Using 3-0 suture, the tendon is then repaired to itself superficial to the A1 pulley.
- The tendon repair should be performed with the wrist in neutral and the MCP in about 50° of flexion.

The Stiles–Bunnell transfer technique is used when the patient does not have a compensatory central slip, that is, they are unable to actively extend PIP during both MCP hyperextension and when the MCP joints are blocked [10]. In this procedure, the FDS tendon of the long finger is used to create MCP flexion and IP extension [16]. Excessive tension during insertion can result in PIP hyperextension and a swan neck deformity [57].

Technique

- Similar to the Zancolli procedure, a midpalm incision is made to retrieve the FDS tendon and the FDS tendon is transected just proximal to its bifurcation between the A1 and A2 pulleys.
- The tendon is then split longitudinally and retracted from the tendon sheath proximally.
- Two radial incisions are made over the proximal phalanx of the ring and small fingers to expose the radial lateral bands of each finger.
- The ends of the tendon are then tunneled through the lumbrical canal which places the tendon graft palmar to the MCP axis of rotation.
- The tendon grafts are inserted into the lateral bands of the small and ring fingers with the wrist in neutral, the MCP joints in about 60° of flexion, and the PIP joints in full extension.

To restore thumb adduction and power pinch the extensor carpi radialis brevis (ECRB) is commonly used [57]. Patients with impaired power pinch who underwent an ECRB adductorplasty had a two-fold increase in pinch force postoperatively [59].

Technique

- A dorsal incision is made in the fourth web space and the ECRB tendon is detached from its insertion at the fourth metacarpal base.
- The tendon is retracted proximally beneath the extensor retinaculum. It is routed dorsal to palmar between the second and third metacarpals to allow the third metacarpal to act as a pulley.
- A small incision is made over the thumb MCP joint to expose the adductor pollicis insertion and the graft is secured to the insertion. A free tendon graft can be used to obtain the appropriate length and tension.

The use of brachioradialis tendon extended with a tendon graft has also been described to restore thumb adduction and power pinch. After the transfer is complete, there should be strong thumb adduction with the wrist in neutral and moderate tension on the brachioradialis tendon.

Technique

- An incision is made between FCR and the radial artery and the brachioradialis tendon is freed from overlying fascia. The tendon can be extended with a tendon graft, typically a palmaris longis graft.
- Three additional incisions are made over the radial thumb MCP joint, the palmar third web space, and dorsal third web space.
- A tendon graft from a slip of abductor pollicis longus is then sewn into abductor pollicis brevis.
- This graft is passed palmar to adductor pollicis. This can be visualized using the palmar incision. It is then passed dorsally through the third web space.
- The brachioradialis tendon graft is then passed into the dorsal incision.
- The two grafts are sewn together with the wrist in neutral and the thumb fully extended. There should be no tension on the graft.

8.1.6 Outcomes

Postoperative outcomes of primary cubtial tunnel release are related to pre-operative disease severity. Overall, the primary cubital tunnel release has about a 90% success rate for mild cases. However, the total relief rate decreases for more severe cases [24]. The success following revision cubital tunnel is less reliable. Nonetheless, revision cubital tunnel with neurolysis and nerve wrapping has been shown to be effective in reducing pre-operative pain and improvement in grip strength [46]. Outcomes following nerve transfer for ulnar nerve injuries are variable. Following supercharge end-to-end procedures, instrinsic function is more likely to return following nerve transection and less reliably returns following compression injuries [7]. In the setting of ulnar nerve injuries, tendon transfers that restore thumb adduction typically restore pinch strength to about 50% of normal [10]. Tendon transfers that improve instrinic function like the Zancolli lasso and Stiles-Bunnell transfer tend to maintain excellent correction of claw deformities [72]. Additionally, ERCB transfer offers improved grip strength [59].

8.2 Wrist

8.2.1 Carpal Tunnel Release

8.2.1.1 Risks/Incidence/Mechanism of Injury

Carpal tunnel is one of the most frequently performed orthopedic procedures likely due to the increase in ambulatory surgery centers and the use of local anesthesia. Iatrogenic median nerve injury secondary to carpal tunnel release occurs in about 0.06% of cases. A large retrospective review from 2014 on iatrogenic nerve injuries found that the median nerve was the most commonly iatrogenically damaged nerve, and the majority of iatrogenic median nerve injuries occur during carpal tunnel surgery [4, 49]. Whether or not the operative surgeon is trained in hand surgery is one of the most significant factors contributing to median nerve injury during carpal tunnel release [6].

In primary carpal tunnel surgery, there remains a choice between open versus endoscopic carpal tunnel release. Open carpal tunnel release remains the gold standard for carpal tunnel surgery; however, as minimally invasive surgery gains popularity, endoscopic release is gaining popularity. In open release, the transverse carpal tunnel ligament is visualized and transected to release compression within the carpal tunnel. In endoscopic release, a single incision and portal is made to transect the retinaculum. The outcomes of endoscopic release are encouraging with some authors reporting a 93% success rate [41]. In a randomized control trial, Kang et al. found that patients prefer endoscopic over mini-open carpal tunnel release, mainly because of scar formation and pain with the open technique [31]. However, the risk of nerve injury is higher in patients undergoing endoscopic CTR when compared to open CTR [13]. With lack of complete visualization, patients may experience a devastating transection of the median nerve during ECTR [40]. As seen in Example 8.4, median nerve repair after injury following ECTR can involve an extensive incision, a large nerve gap, and subsequent nerve grafting. Early reports of the outcome of ECTR reported frequent major neurovascular injury; however, more recent studies suggest that these findings may have been due to surgeon inexperience with endoscopic surgery, rather than the endoscopic technique itself [65]. Although more recent studies have suggested similar patient outcomes and relief of symptoms with open and endoscopic techniques, the authors prefer open carpal release as we believe good visualization reduces the possibility of median nerve injury.

Example 8.4 Median nerve injury after endoscopic CTR (Figs. 8.19, 8.20, and 8.21).

The median nerve is also at risk during the treatment of distal radius fractures or as a result of the initial trauma. In a survey conducted in 2001, radius fractures accounted for 44% of all emergency room visits for hand and wrist fractures [21]. In a prospective study, traumatic median nerve injury occurred primarily in the

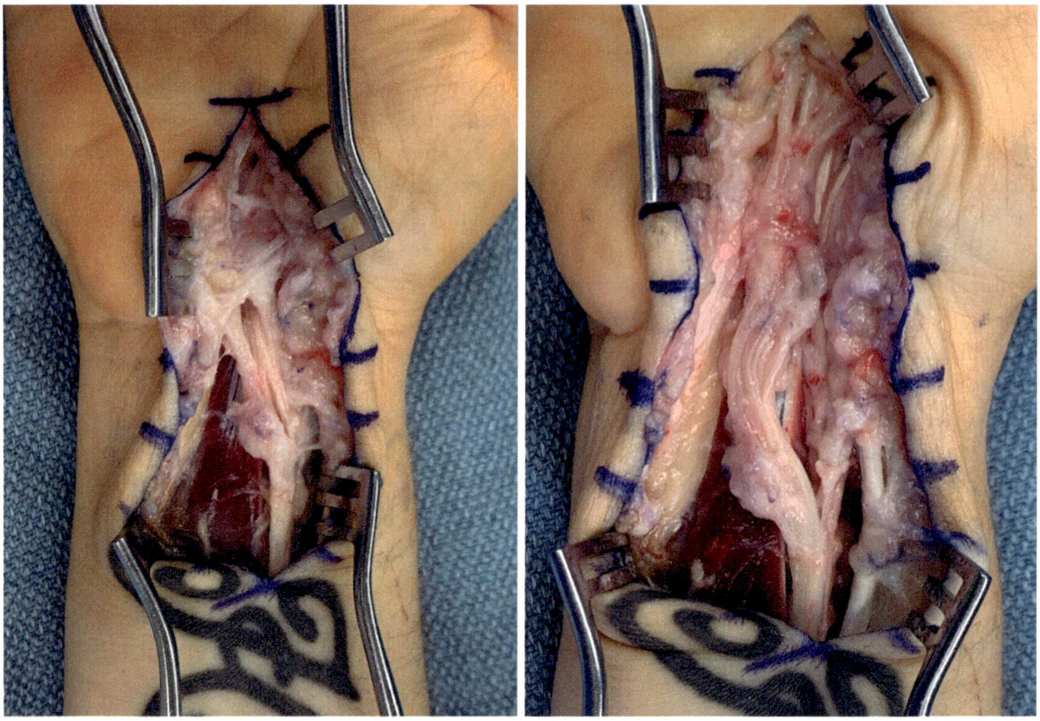

Fig. 8.19 Intraoperative photograph of an exploration of median nerve injury following endoscopic carpal tunnel release

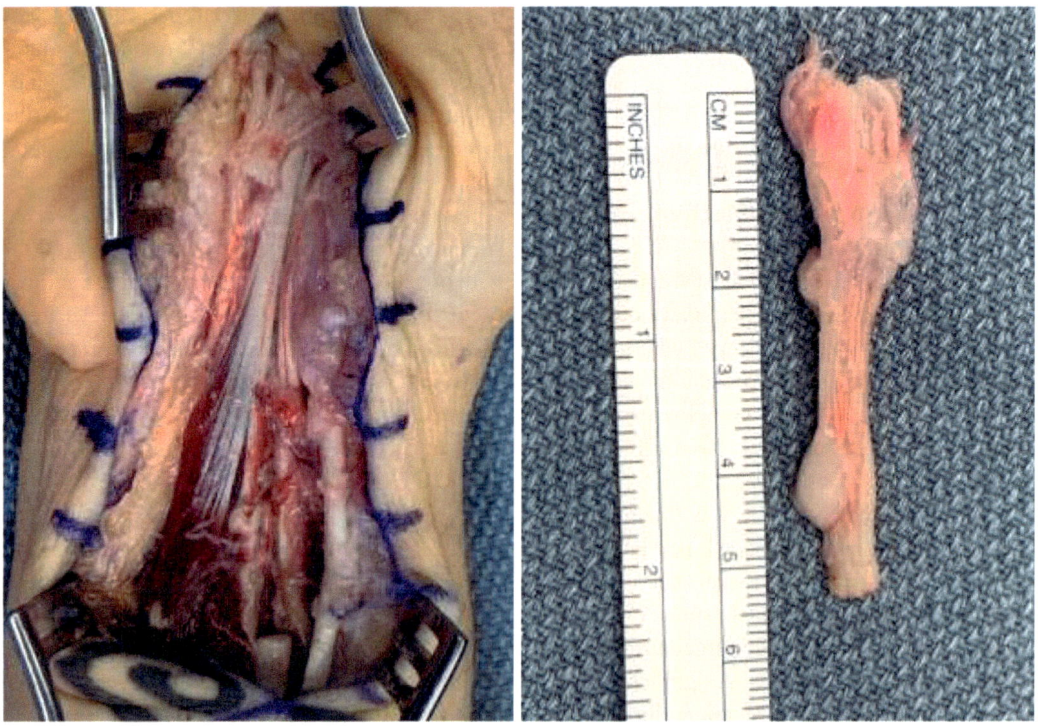

Fig. 8.20 A 5.5-cm nerve gap (left) following the resection of an injured median nerve (right) following endoscopic carpal tunnel release

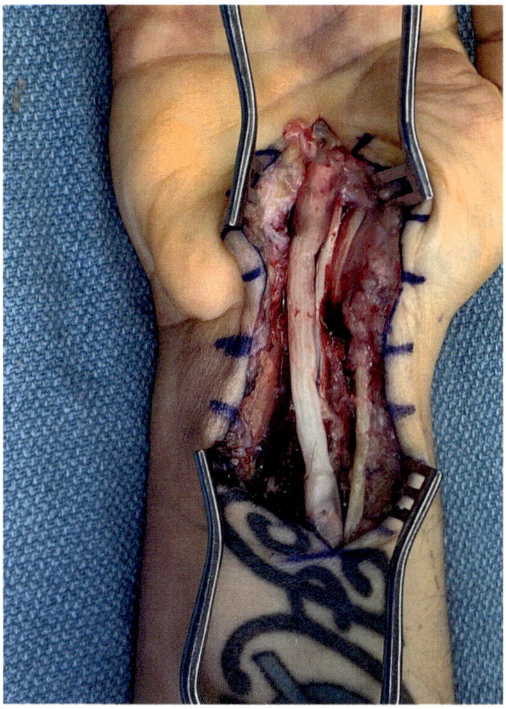

Fig. 8.21 Successful median nerve repair following grafting with nerve allograft

forearm and in the wrist [42]. Complication rates from volar locking plating of a distal radius fracture have been reported from 3% to 36% [64]. Carpal tunnel syndrome is the most common nerve-related complication from operative fixation of distal radius fractures. The rate of carpal tunnel syndrome from use of volar locking plate fixation of distal radius fractures has been reported from 2% to 8% [1, 64], although similar rates have been described for nonoperative treatment of distal radius fractures [1]. Carpal tunnel syndrome following distal radius fractures is thought to be a product of the nerve damage from the fracture, surrounding soft tissue fibrosis or scarring following healing from the trauma, or from prominent callus from fracture healing. The approach to carpal tunnel syndrome after distal radius fracture is similar to that of revision carpal tunnel release.

Median nerve injury following distal radius fracture can also result from the surgical approach itself. Common approaches for volar locking plating of a distal radius fracture include the classic volar Henry approach through the interval between the flexor carpi radialis and radial artery or modified Henry approach through the FCR tendon sheath. The median nerve is located deep and ulnar to the FCR tendon. Surgeons must be cautious of identifying and protecting the nerve during this approach to avoid iatrogenic compression or transection.

8.2.1.2 Pertinent Anatomy

The carpal tunnel is a canal that is enclosed by the carpal bones and the transverse carpal ligament through which the median nerve, the eight tendons from the flexor digitorum superficialis and flexor digitorum profundus, and the tendon of flexor pollicis longus traverse. The median nerve typically is found just deep to the transverse carpal ligament and slightly radially from the center. The median nerve is the most superficial structure within the carpal tunnel. As such, injury to the median nerve may occur during incision of the transverse carpal ligament resulting in a mixed sensory and motor median nerve palsy.

The recurrent branch of the median nerve is a motor branch of the median nerve that innervates abductor pollicis brevis, opponens pollicis, and the superficial head of the flexor pollicis brevis. Its branch point varies, putting it at risk during CTR. The most common take off described is a radial-volar subligamentous take off; however, Lanz has described ulnar, transligamentous and extraligamentous take offs [56]. The thenar branch may be injured by surgical dissection distal to the carpal tunnel or if it is encountered beneath the transverse carpal ligament. This results in a purely motor nerve palsy and paralysis of the thenar muscles.

8.2.1.3 Prevention Strategies

Careful attention to anatomy and methodical surgical technique is of utmost importance during primary carpal tunnel release to prevent injury to the median nerve. The incision should be made in line with the radial border of the index finger. To avoid damage to the palmar cutaneous branch of the median nerve, the incision should not extend proximally past the proximal border of the transverse carpal ligament. Similarly, the distal incision should not pass the Kaplan's cardinal line to protect the third digital nerve as well as the superficial palmar arch.

8.2.1.4 Typical Course/Natural History

The early stages of compressive damage to the median nerve may be reversible with proper treatment, however the late stages may not be [50]. Patients with long-standing median nerve injuries or severe median nerve compression will have thenar weakness and visible atrophy of thenar muscles. Additionally, patient have constant, as opposed to intermittent, numbness in the thumb, index, and radial half of the long finger. Interestingly, patients with long-standing low median nerve injury or compression will have more neuropathic pain than their counterparts with earlier staged disease [73].

8.2.1.5 Initial Evaluation/Exam

Injury to the median nerve at the level of the wrist will result in a low median nerve palsy. Patients will have both motor and sensory symptoms. If the nerve injury is secondary to a compressive etiology, patients will complain of pain and parasthesias over the palmar-radial aspect of the hand [62]. On motor exam, the examiner will find that the patient will be unable to abduct and oppose the thumb secondary to loss of innervation of the thenar muscles [35]. In low median nerve injuries, the ability to fire flexor pollicis longus and flexor digitorum profundus to the index finger may be preserved because the anterior interosseous branch of the median nerve branches proximal to the wrist.

8.2.1.6 Diagnostic Tests/Imaging

As with ulnar nerve pathology, a variety of testing can be used to diagnosis median nerve pathology and palsies. Plain radiographs should be taken to evaluate for any posttraumatic deformity causing compression, soft tissue calcifications, tumor, or Keinbock's disease [62]. Carpal tunnel view is rarely helpful. EMG can be helpful in determining the level of median nerve injury or compression. In low median nerve injuries, patients will have denervation of their thenar muscles [62]. Whereas, in high median nerve injuries there will also be denervation of proximal forearm muscles such as flexor carpi radialis, flexor digitorum to the index finger, and flexor pollicis longus [62]. As mentioned previously in the discussion about ulnar nerve injuries, ultrasound, CT, and MRI can be performed to help delineate soft tissue abnormalities or variations that may be causing nerve compression or injury.

8.2.1.7 Surgical Techniques Revision Carpal Tunnel

Many patients feel immediate relief after carpal tunnel release. However, failure of primary CTR has been reported in 7–25%, with reports of 5–12% requiring revision surgery [32]. Persistent carpal tunnel syndrome refers to the recurrence of preoperative symptoms after carpal tunnel release [73]. Treatment failure may be due to incomplete release, recurrent compression, or incorrect diagnosis. Incomplete release is the most common need for revision surgery. As opposed to patients with primary CTS, patients with recurrent or persistent carpal tunnel syndrome following CTR tend to present with neurogenic pain as opposed to numbness [73]. Recurrent compression occurs more frequently in patients with comorbidities such as diabetes and hypertension [44].

Strickland described a technique in which the median nerve is protected in a vascularized hypothenar fat pad [61]. The fat pad receives it blood supply from a branch of the ulnar artery within Guyon's canal. The hypothenar fat pad is dissected from the subcutaneous tissue and the ulnar nerve and artery are identified proximally near Guyon's canal. The canal is released and the flap is mobilized radially while maintaining the ulnar arterial supply to cover the median nerve. This provides the nerve with a protected, enriched trophic environment. Patients who underwent revision carpal tunnel release with a hypothenar fat flap have been shown to have reported improvement in nighttime parasthesias, neuropathic pain, as well as grip strength [5, 61].

As with revision cubital tunnel release, nerve wrapping has been described with revision carpal tunnel. In a review of ten patients who underwent revision carpal tunnel with nerve wrapping, at 3-year follow–up, all patients had improvement of clinical symptoms, improved two-point discrimination, and median nerve conduction tests [33].

Excision and nerve grafting is indicated in when there is clear median nerve injury, the nerve is injured in multiple areas or the nerve is damaged beyond repair. We recommend a combination of neurolysis and nerve grafting in clinical situations where there is partial injury and a demarcated zone of injury.

Example 8.5 Revision carpal tunnel (Figs. 8.22 and 8.23).

8.2.1.8 Salvage Techniques

To restore thumb opposition, several tendon transfers can be performed. Most commonly used techniques are the Burkhalter, Royle-Thompson, or Camitz.

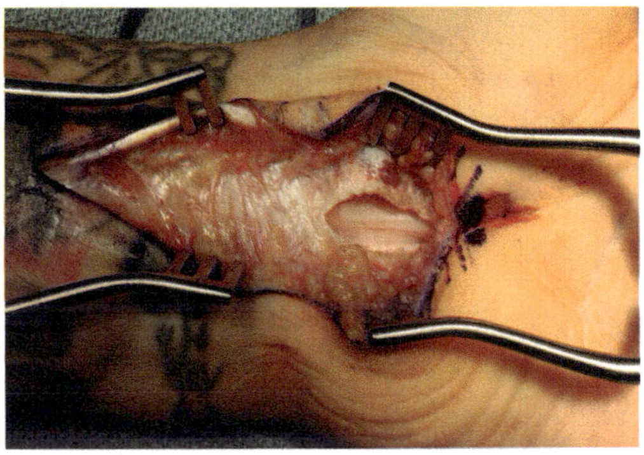

Fig. 8.22 Intraoperative photograph of an incompletely released carpal tunnel

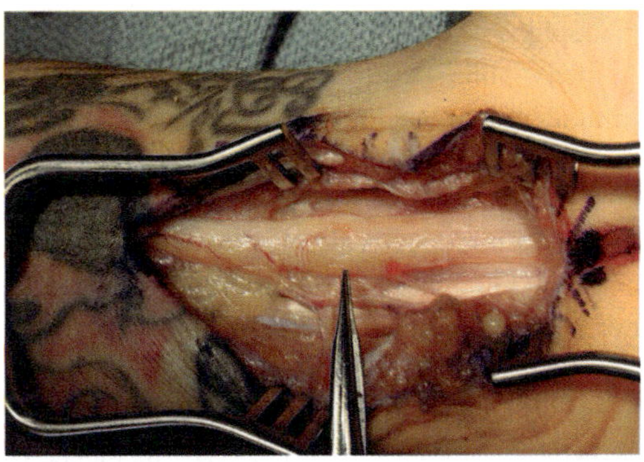

Fig. 8.23 After external neurolysis is performed, the median nerve is found to have the classic "hourglass" sign

Burkhalter first described the transfer of extensor indicis proprius to abductor pollicis brevis to restore thumb opposition [17]. The EIP tendon is passed along this same route and then attached to the APB insertion. Anderson et al. reported that 87% of patients treated with this technique had a good or excellent result [2].

Technique

- A longitudinal incision is made over the dorsal index finger MCP joint.
- EIP is identified palmar and ulnar to the extensor digitorum comminus tendon and divided on the proximal edge of the extensor hood. If necessary, the tendon can be elongated by taking a slip of the extensor mechanism. The extensor hood should be repaired with braided suture.
- A second incision is made on the ulnar aspect of the dorsal wrist just proximal to the ulnar styloid. When making this incision it is important to keep in mind where the dorsal sensory branch of the ulnar nerve crosses the wrist.
- The EIP is identified in the 4th extensor compartment. The extensor retinaculum over the 4th compartment is released and the tendon is mobilized through the dorsal incision.
- Two additional incisions are made on the radial side of pisiform and on the radial border of the thumb MCP joint.
- Using blunt dissection, a subcutaneous tunnel is made from the dorsal wrist incision to the pisiform incision and then to the thumb MCP incision.
- The tendon graft is passed through this tunnel and repaired to the APB insertion.

Royle-Thompson refers to the transfer of FDS of the ring finger to APB insertion with the use of a Bunnell pulley to redirect the vector of pull [15]. Cooney et al. showed a 40% restoration of thenar strength following this transfer in a biomechanical study [22].

Technique

- A transverse palmar skin incision is made over the A1 pulley of the ring finger. The A1 pulley

is identified and incised longitudinally as in a trigger finger release.
- The FDS and FDP tendons to the ring finger are identified and separated. Traction is applied to the FDS tendon and then it is transected transversely proximal to the bifurcation. During this step, the surgeon must protect the FDP tendon.
- A second incision is made along the volar ulnar forearm over the flexor carpi ulnaris (FCU) insertion on the pisiform. Through this incision, FCU, FDS to the ring finger, and the ulnar neurovascular bundle are identified.
- While protecting the neurovascular bundle, the radial half of FCU is transversely divided just proximal to the insertion on the pisiform. The radial half of FCU is separated from the ulnar half of FCU.
- The radial tendon graft is looped through the ulnar half of FCU and secured near the pisiform to create a pulley.
- The ring finger FDS graft is then retracted through the volar incision and passed through the pulley.
- A third incision over the radial thumb MCP joint is made and the FDS graft is passed subcutaneously to this incision.
- One slip of the graft is secured to the distal radial aspect of the APB tendon and the other slip is attached to the extensor hood.

Camitz initially described the transfer of palmaris longis to APB in 1929 [18]. Today it is typically reserved for patients with long-standing carpal tunnel syndrome [57]. Terrono et al. showed that 94% of patients underwent the Camitz procedure with regard to improvement of thumb dexterity [63]. Patients must have a palmaris longus to properly perform the procedure.

Technique
- A longitudinal incision is made from the wrist crease and extended distally to the proximal palmar crease.
- The palmaris longus tendon is identified and harvested. The length can be extended by also harvesting the palmar fascia.
- A second incision is made over the dorsum of the thumb MCP joint and the harvested tendon is passed subcutaneously from the palmar incision to the thumb incision.
- The palmaris longus tendon is then attached to the insertion of APB. The restoration of thumb abduction results from the vector of pull of the PL [14].

8.2.1.9 Outcomes

Outcomes following secondary carpal tunnel syndrome are worse than primary carpal tunnel syndrome and patients typically experience less relief in their symptoms [9]. As with revision cubital tunnel, revision carpal tunnel involves neurolysis with a possible hypothenar flap or nerve wrapping. As detailed in Example 8.5, when performing revision carpal tunnel surgery, a longer more ulnar incision that extends to the wrist crease is made to allow for visualization of the median nerve proximal and distal to the prior scaring [73]. Approaching the prior scarring from the ulnar border allows for identification of normal anatomical landmarks and facilitates safe dissection [66, 73]. Surgeons may have to also release Guyon's canal to protect the ulnar neurovascular bundle during this approach [66]. The median nerve is followed proximally and distally into the carpal tunnel and external, and/or internal neurolysis is performed per the surgeon's discretion.

Complex regional pain syndrome includes a constellation of symptoms such as sensory and motor abnormalities as well as pain that results in dysfunction, disability, and chronic pain. The pathophysiology of CRPS is thought to be heterogeneous. Three major physiologic pathways have been identified that contribute to the development of CRPS: maladaptive neuroplasticity, vasomotor dysfunction, and aberrant inflammatory mechanisms [37]. Complex regional pain syndrome is common following upper extremity fracture; however, the incidence varies greatly on the diagnostic criterion that is used [11]. These patients experienced more pain after injury and were unlikely to be symptom free at 1 year [11]. The incidence of CRPS following surgical fixation of distal radius fractures is 8.8% [53]. Female gender, more communited fracture patterns or open fractures, high-energy mechanisms, and comorbid fibromyalgia are predictive of the development of CRPS [23, 53]. It has been suggested that surgeons should assess patients for these potential risk factors before fixation of distal radius fractures and treat with prophylactic ascorbic acid preoperatively or with corticosteroids postoperatively to reduce inflammation and free radical formation [53]. There is little evidence supporting effective interventions for the prevention of CRPS.

References

1. Alter TH, Sandrowski K, Gallant G, Kwok M, Ilyas AM. Complications of volar plating of distal radius fractures: a systematic review. J Wrist Surg. 2019;8:255–62.
2. Anderson GA. Ulnar nerve palsy. In: Green DP, Hotchkiss RN, Pederson WC, et al., editors. Green's operative hand surgery. 5th ed. Philadelphia: Elsevier; 2005. p. 1161–96.
3. Anglen J. Distal humerus fractures. J Am Acad Orthop Surg. 2005;13(5):291–7.
4. Antoniadis G, Kretschmer T, Pedro MT, Konig RW, Heinen CPG, Richter HP. Iatrogenic nerve injuries. Dtsch Arztebl Int. 2014;111(16):273–9.
5. Athlani L, Haloua JP. Strickland's hypothenar fat pad flap for revision surgery in carpal tunnel surgery. Prospective study of 34 cases. Hand Surg Rehabil. 2017;36(3):202–7.
6. Azari KK, Speiss AM, Buterbaugh GA, Imbriglia JE. Major nerve injuries associated with carpal tunnel release. Plast Reconstruc. 2007;119:1977–8.
7. Baltzer H, Woo A, Oh C, Moran S. Comparison of ulnar intrinsic function following supercharge end-to-side anterior Interossesous-to-ulnar motor nerve transfer: a matched cohort study of proximal ulnar nerve injury patients. J Plas Recon Surg. 2016;138(6):1264–72.
8. Barbour J, Yee A, Kahn LC, Mackinnon SE. Supercharged end-to-side anterior interosseous to ulnar motor nerve transfer for intrinsic musculature Reinnervation. J Hand Surg. 2012;37(10):2150–9.
9. Beck JD, Brothers JG, Maloney PJ, Deegan JH, Tang X, Klena JC. Predicting the outcome of revision carpal tunnel release. J Hand Surg Am. 2012;37(2):282–7.
10. Bednar MS. Tendon transfers for ulnar nerve Palsy. In: Weisel SW, editor. Operative techniques in orthopedic surgery. 2nd ed. Philadelphia: Wolters Kluwer; 2016. p. 3201–7.
11. Beerthuizen A, Stronks DL, Van't Spijker A, Yaksh A, Haraets BM, Klein J, Huygen FJ. Demographic and medical parameters in the development of complex regional pain syndrome type 1 (CRPS): Prospective study on 596 patients with a fracture. Pain. 2012; 153:1187–92.
12. Bodner G, Harpt C, Gardetto A, et al. Ultrasonography of the accessory nerve: Normal and pathologic findings in cadavers and patients with iatrogenic accessory nerve palsy. J Ultrasound Med. 2002;21:1159–63.
13. Boeckstyns ME, Sorensen AI. Does endoscopic carpal tunnel release have a higher rate of complications than open carpal tunnel release? An analysis of published series. J Hand Surg Br. 1999;24(1):9–15.
14. Braun RM. Palmaris longus tendon transfer for augmentation of the thenar musculature in low median palsy. J Hand Surg Am. 1978;3(5):488–91.
15. Bunnell S. Opposition of the thumb. J Bone Joint Surg Am. 1938;20(2):269–84.
16. Bunnell S. Tendon transfers in the hand and forearm. Instr Course Lect. 1949;6:106–10.
17. Burkhalter W, Christensen RC, Brown P. Extensor indicis proprius opponensplasty. J Bone Joint Surg Am. 1973;55(4):725–32.
18. Camitz H. Surgical treatment of paralysis of opponens muscle of thumbs. Acta Chir Scand. 1929;65:77–83.
19. Cannada LK. Distal humerus fractures. In: Stannard JP, Schmidt AH, editors. Surgical treatment of orthopaedic trauma. 2nd ed. New York: Thieme; 2016. p. 398–421.
20. Chen RC, Harris DJ, Leduc S, Borrelli JJ Jr, Tornetta P III, Ricci WM. Is ulnar nerve transposition beneficial during open reduction and internal fixation of distal humerus fractures? J Orthop Trauma. 2010;24:391–4.
21. Cheng KC, Spilson SV. The frequency and epidemiology of hand and forearm fractures in the United States. J Hand Surg. 2001;26A(5):908–15.
22. Cooney WP, Linscheid RL, An KN. Opposition of the thumb: An anatomic and biomechanical study of tendon transfers. J Hand Surg. 1984;9(6):777–86.
23. Crijns TJ, van der Gronde B, Ring D, Leung N. Complex regional pain syndrome after distal radius fractures is uncommon and is often associated with fibromyalgia. Clin Orthop Relat Res. 2018;476:744–50.
24. Curtin CM, Ladd AL. Surgical treatment of cubital tunnel syndrome. In: Weisel SW, editor. Operative techniques in orthopedic surgery. 2nd ed. Philadelphia: Wolters Kluwer; 2016. p. 3161–8.
25. Danoff JR, Lombardi JM, Rosenwasser MP. Use of pedicled adipose flap as a sling for anterior subcutaneous transposition of the ulnar nerve. J Hand Surg. 2014;39(3):552–5.
26. Delton AL. Review of treatment results for ulnar nerve entrapment at the elbow. J Hand Surg [Am]. 1989;14:688–700.
27. Elhassen B, Steinmann SP. Entrapment neuropathy of the ulnar nerve. J Am Acad Orthop Surg. 2007;15(11):672–81.
28. Eversmann WW Jr. Entrapment and compression neuropathies. In: Green DP, editor. Operative hand surgery. 3rd ed. New York: Churchill Livingstone; 1993. p. 1341–9.

29. Hastings H II, McCollam SM. Flexor digitorum superficialis lasso tendon transfer in isolated ulnar nerve palsy: a functional evaluation. J Hand Surg Am. 1994;19(2):275–80.
30. Jordaan PW, Uhiara O, Power D. Management of the scarred nerve using porcine submucosa extracellular matrix nerve wraps. J Musculoskelet Surg Res. 2019;3:128–33.
31. Kang HJ, Koh H, Lee TJ, Choi YR. Endoscopic carpal tunnel release is preferred over Mini-open despite similar outcome: a randomized trial. Clin Orthop Relat Res. 2013;471:1548–54.
32. Karl JW, Gancarczyk SM, Strauch RJ. Complications of carpal tunnel release. Orthop Clin N Am. 2016;47:425–33.
33. Kokkalis ST, Mavrogenis AF, Vottis C, Paptheodorou L, Papagelopoulos PJ, Soucacos PN, Soterano DG. Median nerve biodegradeable wrapping; clinical outcome of 10 patients. Acta Orthop Belg. 2016;82(2):351–7.
34. Krestchmer T, Antoniadis G, Braun V, Rath SA, Richter HP. Evaluation of iatrogenic lesions in 722 surgically treated cases of peripheral nerve trauma. J Neurosurg. 2001;94:905–12.
35. Leit ME, Weiser RW, Tomaino MM. Patient-reported outcome after carpal tunnel release for advanced disease: a prospective and longitudinal assessment in patients older than age 70. J Hand Surg Am. 2004;29(3):379–83.
36. Lowe JB III, Maggi SP, Mackinnon SE. The position of crossing branches of the medial antebrachial cutaneous nerve during cubital tunnel surgery in humans. Plast Reconstr Surg. 2004;114:692–6.
37. Marinus J, Moseley GL, Birklein F, Baron R, Maihofner C, Kingery WS, van Hilten JJ. Clinical features and pathophysiology of complex regional pain syndrome. J Neurol. 2011;10(7):637–48.
38. Maslow JI, Johnson DJ, Block JJ, Lee DH, Desai MJ. Prevalence and clinical manifestations of the anconeus epitrochlearis and cubital tunnel syndrome. Hand (N Y). 2018;15(1):69–74.
39. McKee MD, Jupiter JB, Bosse G, Goodman L. Outcome of ulnar neurolysis during post-traumatic reconstruction of the elbow. J Bone Joint Surg Br. 1998;80(1):100–5.
40. Murphy RX Jr, Jennings JF, Wukich DK. Major neurovascular complications of endoscopic carpal tunnel release. J Hand Surg Am. 1994;19(1):114–8.
41. Nazerani S, Motamedi MHK, Nazerani T, Saraii A, Keremati MR. Endoscopic carpal tunnel release: A5-Year Experience. J Trauma. 2014;19(4):15–9.
42. Nobel J, Munro CA, Prasad VS, Midha R. Analysis of upper and lower extremity peripheral nerve injuries in population of patients with multiple injuries. J Trauma. 1998;45:116–2.
43. Norkus SA, Meyers MC. Ulnar neuropathy of the elbow. Sports Med. 1994;17:189–99.
44. O'Malley MJ, Evanoff M, Terrono AL, Millender LH. Factors that determine reexploration treatment of carpal tunnel syndrome. J Hand Surg Am. 1992;17(4):638–41.
45. Padua L, Aprile I, Caliandro P, Foschini M, Mazza S, Tonali P. Natural history of ulnar entrapment at elbow. Clin Neurophysiol. 2002;113(12):1980–4.
46. Paptheodorou LK, Willams BG, Sotereanos DG. Preliminary results of recurrent cubital tunnel syndrome treated with neurolysis and porcine extracellular matrix nerve wrapping. J Hand Surg Am. 2015;40(5):987–92.
47. Park IJ, Kim HM, Lee JY, Jeong C, Kang Y, Hwang S, Sung BY, Kang SH. Cubital tunnel syndrome caused by Aconeous Epitrochlearis muscle. J Korean Neurosurg Soc. 2018;61(5):618–24.
48. Posner MA. Compression ulnar neuropathies at the elbow: I. Etiology and diagnosis. J Am Acad Orthop Surg. 1998;6(5):282–8.
49. Pulos N, Shin EH, Spinner RJ, Shin AY. Management of Iatrogenic Nerve Injuries. J Am Acad Orthop Surg. 2019;27:e838–48.
50. Rizzo. Carpal tunnel release: endoscopic, open and revision. In: Weisel SW, editor. Operative techniques. 2nd ed. Philadelphia: Wolters Kluwer; 2016. p. 3139–48.
51. Robinson CM, Hill RM, Jacobs N, Dall G, Court-Brown CM. Adult distal humeral metaphyseal fractures: epidemiology and results of treatment. J Orthop Trauma. 2003;17(1):38–47.
52. Rogers MR, Bergfield TG, Aulicino PL. The failed ulnar nerve transposition: Etiliogy and treatment. Clin Orthop Relat Res. 1991;269:193–200.
53. Roh YH, Lee BM, Noh JH, Baek JR, Oh JH, Gong HS, Baek GH. Factors associated with complex regional pain syndrome type I in pateitns with surgical treated distal radius fracture. Arch Orthop Trauma Surg. 2014;134:1775–81.
54. Ruchelsman DE, Lee SK, Posner MA. Failed surgery for ulnar nerve compression at the elbow. Hand Clin. 2007;23:359–71.
55. Sarris I, Gobel F, Gainer M, et al. Medial brachial and antebrachial cutaneous nerve injuries: effect on outcome in revision cubital tunnel surgery. J Reconstr Microsurg. 2002;18:665–70.
56. Seiler JG, Daruwalla JH, Payne SH, Faucher GK. Normal palmar variant anatomy and variations that impact median nerve decompression. J Am Acad Orthop Surg. 2017;25:e194–203.
57. Seiler JG, Desai MJ, Payne SH. Tendon transfers for radial, median and ulnar nerve Palsy. J Am Acad Orthop Surg. 2013;21(11):675–84.
58. Siqueria MG, Martins RS. The controversial arcade of Struthers. Surg Neurol. 2005;64(suppl 1):S17–20.
59. Smith RJ. Extensor carpi radialis brevis tendon transfer for thumb adduction: a study of power pinch. J Hand Surg Am. 1983;8(1):4–15.

60. Soltani AM, Bassan JA, Best MJ, Mir HS, Panthaki Z. Revision decompression and collagen nerve wrap for recurrent and persistent compression neuropathies of the upper extremity. Annu Plast Surg. 2013;72(5):572–8.
61. Strickland JW, Idler RS, Lourie GM, Plancher KD. The hypothenar fat pad flap for management of recurrent carpal tunnel syndrome. J Hand Surg. 1996;21(5):840–8.
62. Szabo RM, Steinberg DR. Nerve entrapment syndromes in the wrist. J Am Acad Orthop Surg. 1994;2(2):115–23.
63. Terrono AL, Rose JH, Mulroy J, Millender LH. Camitz palmaris longus abductorplasty for severe thenar atrophy secondary to carpal tunnel syndrome. J Hand Surg Am. 1993;18(2):204–6.
64. Thorninger R, Madsen ML, Waever D, Borris LC, Rolfing JHD. Complications of volar locking plating of distal radius fractures in 576 patients with 3.2 years follow up. Inj Int J Care Inj. 2017;48:1104–9.
65. Tse RW, Hurst LN, Al-Yafi TA. Early major complications of endoscopic tunnel release: a review of 1200 cases. Can J Plast Surg. 2003;11(3):131–4.
66. Tung TH, Mackinnon SE. Secondary carpal tunnel surgery. Plast Reconstr Surg. 2001;107(7):1830–43.
67. Vogel BR, Nossaman BC, Rayan GM. Revision anterior submuscular transposition of the ulnar nerve for failed subcutaneous transposition. Br J Plast Surg. 2004;57:311–6.
68. Wang KC, Shih HN, Hsu KY, Shih CH. Intercondylar fractures of the distal humerus: routine anterior subcutaneous transposition of the ulnar nerve in a posterior approach. J Trauma. 1994;36:770–3.
69. Warner MA. Perioperative neuropathies. Mayo Clin Proc. 1998;73:567–74.
70. Wiggers JK, Brouwer KM, Helmerhorst GT, Ring D. Predictors of diagnosis of ulnar neuropathy after surgically treated distal humerus fractures. J Hand Surg Am. 2012;37:1168–72.
71. Woo A, Bakri K, Moran S. Management of ulnar nerve injuries. J Hand Surg. 2015;40:173–81.
72. Zancolli E. Tendon transfers. In: Structural and dynamic bases of hand surgery. 2nd ed. Philadelphia: JB Lippincott Co; 1979. p. 159–206.
73. Zieske L, Ebersole GC, Davidge K, Fox I, Mackinnon S. Revision carpal tunnel surgery: a 10-year review of intraoperative findings and outcomes. J Hand Surg Am. 2013;38(8):139–49.

Part III

Nerve Injuries after Orthopedic Surgery of the Pelvis, Lower Extremity and Spine

9 Pelvic, Acetabular, Hip, and Proximal Femur Fractures: Intrapelvic and Extra-pelvic Neuroanatomy

Kitty Wu and Christopher J. Dy

9.1 'Border Nerves': Ilioinguinal, Iliohypogastric, and Genitofemoral

9.1.1 Iliohypogastric Nerve

In 1893, Ruge used the term 'Grenznerven' to describe the iliohypogastric, ilioinguinal, and genitofemoral nerves. This translates to 'border nerves' as all three nerves provide sensation to the skin 'bordering' the abdomen and thigh [1].

The iliohypogastric nerve is the highest somatic nerve from the lumbar plexus and provides motor innervation to the transversus abdominus and internal oblique muscles and sensation to the upper buttock and pubis. Arising from the ventral rami of the T12–L1 roots, it shares dorsal horn cells with the ovary and distal fallopian tube and can result in referred pain to these areas [2]. From there, the iliohypogastric nerve pierces the psoas muscle laterally and courses anteriorly along the surface of the quadratus lumborum. It pierces the abdominal fascia midway between the anterior superior iliac spine (ASIS) and iliac crest and courses between the transversus abdominis and internal oblique, heading towards the iliac crest. After a short course, the iliohypogastric nerve pierces the internal oblique and traverses between the internal and external oblique, in a similar course to the ilioinguinal nerve. Approaching the ASIS, the iliohypogastric nerve divides into the lateral cutaneous branch, providing sensation to a superolateral quadrant of the buttock and the anterior branch which provides motor innervation to the transversus abdominis and internal oblique muscles. The anterior branch travels with the ilioinguinal nerve and becomes subcutaneous 1 cm superior to the inguinal ligament and 2 cm medial the ASIS, giving sensation to the superior mons.

9.1.2 Ilioinguinal Nerve

The ilioinguinal nerve arises from ventral rami of the L1–L2 roots and shares dorsal horn cells with the fallopian tube and uterus. Similar to the iliohypogastric nerve, it pierces the psoas muscle and courses along the surface of the quadratum lumborum muscle towards the ASIS (Fig. 9.1). Just medial to the ASIS, the ilioinguinal nerve gives a recurrent branch providing sensation to small longitudinal area over the iliac crest [3]. The nerve pierces the transversalis fascia and transversus abdominis to travel between the transversus abdominis and internal oblique. After

K. Wu
Department of Plastic and Reconstructive Surgery, Western University, London, ON, Canada
e-mail: kwu92@uwo.ca

C. J. Dy (✉)
Department of Orthopedic Surgery, Washington University, St. Louis, MO, USA
e-mail: dyc@wustl.edu

C. J. Dy et al. (eds.), *Peripheral Nerve Issues after Orthopedic Surgery*, https://doi.org/10.1007/978-3-030-84428-8_9

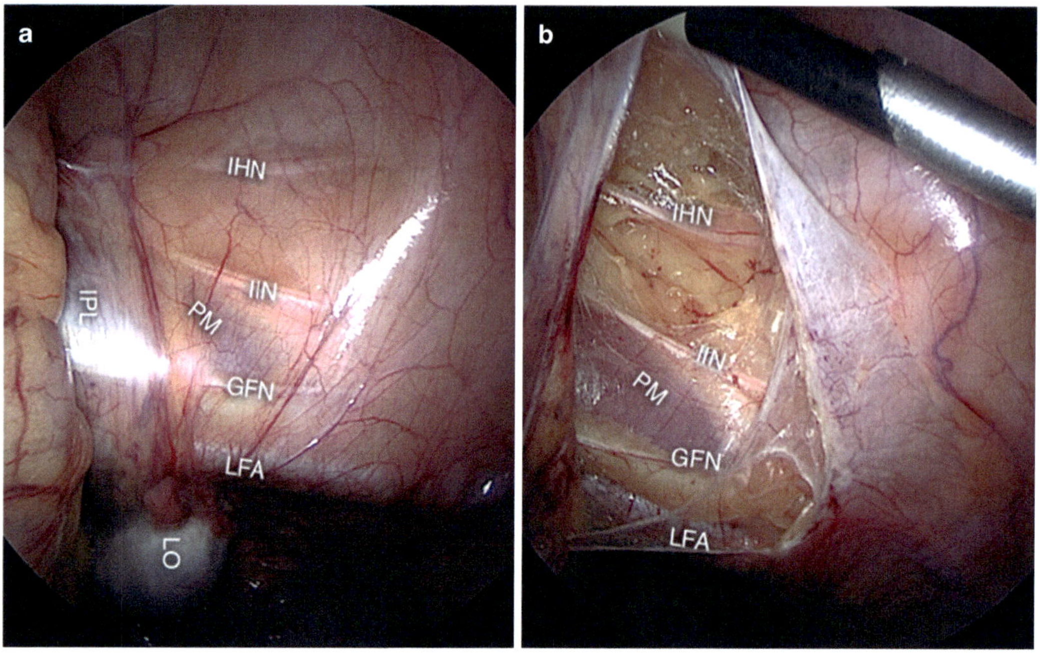

Fig. 9.1 Laparoscopic dissection of iliohypogastric (IHN), ilioinguinal (IIN), and genitofemoral nerve (GFN) with overlying peritoneal intact (**a**) and after exposure (**b**). PM – piriformis muscle, IPL – infundibulopelvic ligament, LFA – left femoral artery, LO – left ovary. (Image copyright Dr. Nucelio Lemos, used with permission)

a short course, it then pierces the internal oblique to the run between the internal and external oblique, providing motor innervation to both. The step-wise passage through the transversus abdominus and internal oblique creates two tether points that renders it vulnerable to entrapment by fibrotic muscle fibres and fascia [3], especially at the second passage point through the internal oblique. It then passes through the inguinal canal with the spermatic cord and provides sensation to the medial femoral triangle, mons, and labia majora or scrotum.

9.1.3 Genitofemoral Nerve

The genitofemoral nerve arises from the ventral rami of the L1–L2 roots. The nerve pierces the psoas muscle 4–12 cm from the sacral prominence, emerges at its medial border at the level of the third and fourth lumbar vertebrae, and descends behind the ureters [1]. This is in contrast to the ilioinguinal and iliohypogastric nerves which emerge from the lateral border of the psoas (Fig. 9.1). After a mean distance of 7 cm, the nerve then branches into its genital and femoral divisions. The genital branch passes medial to the external iliac artery, courses with the ilioinguinal nerve through the inguinal canal, along the posteromedial surface of the spermatic cord. The terminal branches then provide sensation to the mons, labial majora, or anterior scrotum. The femoral branch passes 3–10 cm medial to the ASIS under the inguinal ligament to enter the femoral sheath. It then pierces the anterior femoral sheath to provide sensation to the skin overlying the lateral femoral triangle [2]. Proximal bifurcation of the genital and femoral branches has been described in 42% of patients, with both branches piercing the psoas muscle separately [4]. In men, the genitofemoral nerve also provides motor innervation for the cremasteric reflex.

The terminal genital branches often interconnect with the sensory branches of the ilioinguinal nerve, and they are often difficult to clinically differentiate from each other [5]. Four distinct patterns are described: Type A (43.7%) sensory dominance of the genitofemoral nerve after the ilioinguinal nerve provides motor branches to the abdominal wall; Type B (28.1%) sensory dominance of the ilioinguinal nerve, with the genitofemoral nerve providing only motor innervation to the cremasteric muscle; Type C (20.3%) dominance of genitofemoral nerve; however, ilioinguinal nerve provides some sensation to the mons and inguinal crease; Type D (7.8%) sensory co-dominance of ilioinguinal and genitofemoral nerve [1].

9.2 Femoral Nerve

The femoral nerve is formed from the posterior divisions of the L2, L3, and L4 lumbar roots with variable contributions from L1 and L5. Within its intrapelvic course, the nerve provides branches to the iliacus and psoas muscles prior to emerging from the lateral border of the psoas. Variations have been described with muscular slips of the iliacus or psoas either piercing the femoral nerve (7%) or running over and covering nerve (0.8%), contributing to possible intrapelvic compression points [6]. The femoral nerve then runs between the iliacus and psoas muscles, deep to the iliacus fascia, towards the inguinal ligament (Fig. 9.2).

The femoral nerve enters the femoral triangle deep to the inguinal ligament and lateral to the femoral artery. The femoral nerve divides into two branches, 4 cm distal to the inguinal ligament. The anterior branch provides motor innervation to the sartorius and sensation to the medial thigh. The lateral branch provides motor innervation to the rectus femoris, vastus medialis, vastus intermedius, and vastus lateralis muscles. Motor nerve entry points to the rectus femoris and vastus intermedius were in the proximal muscle bellies at 4.94 cm and 6.7 cm from the common femoral nerve branch point [7]. The vastus medialis and lateralis motor branches enter within the midportion of the muscle at 11.3 cm and 10.3 cm, respectively [7]. The posterior branch continues as the saphenous nerve and provides sensation to the medial thigh, lower leg, and foot (see Chap. 12: Distal femur, tibial plateau, and tibial shaft fractures).

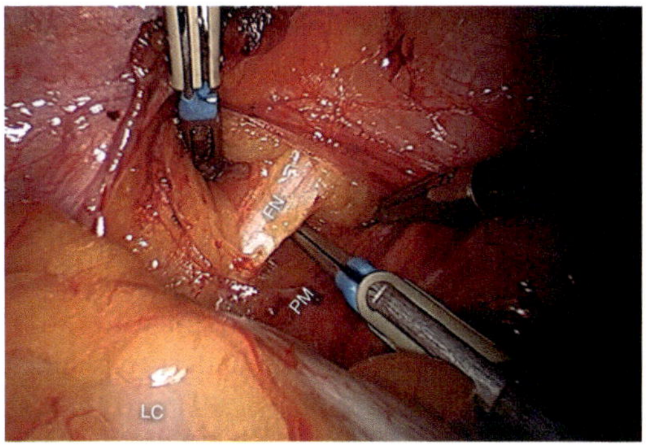

Fig. 9.2 Laparoscopic view of left femoral nerve (FN). The FN enters the retroperitoneal space on the posterolateral aspect of the psoas muscle (PM). LC – left colon. (Image copyright Dr. Nucelio Lemos, used with permission)

9.3 Lateral Femoral Cutaneous Nerve

The lateral femoral cutaneous nerve (LFCN) is a predominantly sensory nerve, most commonly arising from the dorsal division of the ventral rami of the L2–L3 lumbar roots, providing sensation to the anterolateral thigh and efferent sympathetic vasomotor and pilomotor responses [8]. The LFCN is found arising from the L2–L3 roots most commonly (58.75%), but can also derive from the L1–L2 roots (15%), L2 root (11.25%), and femoral nerve (7.5%) [9]. Further variations include origin from the genitofemoral nerves or for the LFCN to be replaced by a branch of the ilioinguinal nerve [10–12].

The LFCN traverses through the psoas muscle and after emerging from its lateral border, courses obliquely in the pelvis towards the ASIS [9]. Classically, the LFCN exits the lesser pelvis, piercing the tensor fascia lata (TFL), beneath the inguinal ligament, before dividing into the anterior femoral and posterior gluteal branches in the deep subcutaneous tissue of the anterolateral thigh [13]. The exit point of the LFCN from the pelvis and its branching pattern in the proximal thigh is highly variable. The LFCN classically exits the pelvis medial to the ASIS (62%), but can also be found exiting just above (27%) or lateral (11%) to the ASIS within a groove in the iliac crest [13, 14]. Based on a meta-analysis of 1720 subjects, the most common exit point is 1.9 cm medial to the ASIS as a single branch [15] (Fig. 9.3). In 38–50% of cases, the LFCN divides proximal to the inguinal ligament [13, 16]. When the LFCN divides distal to the inguinal ligament, the mean distance from the ASIS to the point of division was 34.5 mm (10–72 mm) [16].

The LFCN can be sheathed within its own fascial canal from its exit point from the pelvis until it arborizes into its distal branches [14] (Fig. 9.4). This fascial canal is contiguous with the posterior lamina of the iliac fascia and the deep fascia of the thigh and can act as a point of compression [14].

Rudin describes three major branching patterns of the LFCN in the proximal thigh: sartorius type (36%) with a dominant anterior branch coursing along the lateral border of sartorius and an absent or small posterior branch; posterior type (32%) with posterior branch equal or thicker than the anterior branch crossing the medial border of the TFL, and fan type (32%) with multiple branches crossing over the TFL and lateral border of sartorius (Fig. 9.5).

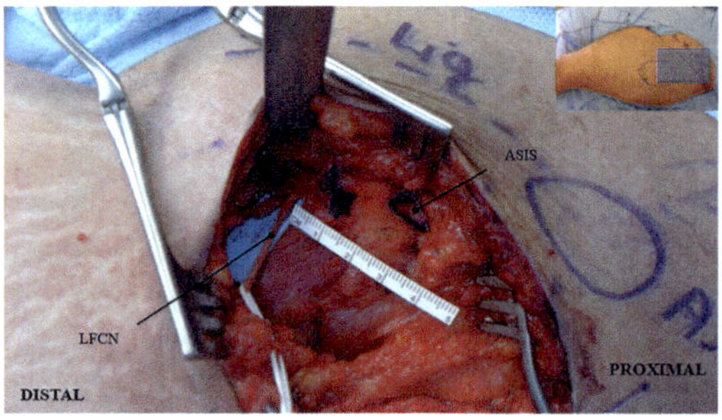

Fig. 9.3 Lateral femoral cutaneous nerve (LFCN) decompression of the left leg. LFCN nerve emerges beneath the inguinal ligament, through the tensor fascia lata, 2 cm medial to the anterior superior iliac spine (ASIS). (Image copyright Dr. Christopher Dy, used with permission)

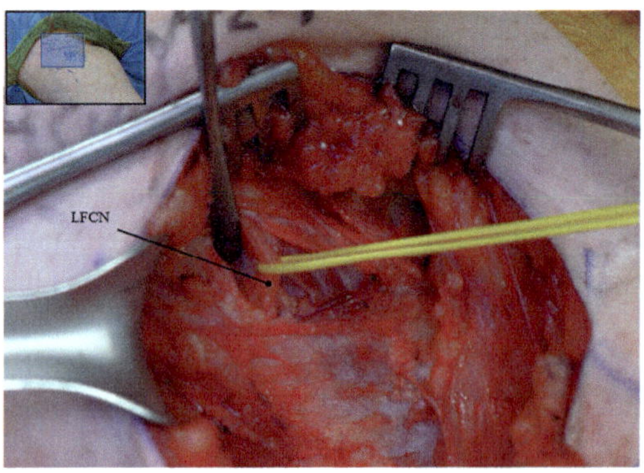

Fig. 9.4 Lateral femoral nerve decompression of right leg showing LFCN traversing within its own fascial canal lateral to the sartorius muscle and fascia. (Image copyright Dr. Christopher Dy, used with permission)

In a study of 45 cadaver dissections, the LFCN branches crossed the skin incision for the direct anterior approach for total hip arthroplasty (THA) in 42% of cases [17]. In sartorius-type branching patterns, the anterior LFCN branch was protected in all cases by the superficial aponeurosis of the TFL [13, 17]. The anterior femoral branch either lies within the intermuscular space between the TFL and sartorius (53%) or crosses the anterior margin of the TFL 46 mm (range 27–92 mm) distal to the ASIS [16]. In contrast, in 68% of cases with posterior-type branching patterns, the posterior branch crosses the line of the skin incision. Furthermore, the posterior branch diverges laterally just distal to the ASIS, crossing the anterior border of the TFL 44.5 mm (range 24–92 mm) distal to the ASIS [16]. With its more proximal location, this posterior branch is at increased risk with proximal extensions during the direct anterior approach to the hip. In patients with the 'fan-type' injury, Rudin concludes that injury is unavoidable during the anterior approach to the hip joint [13].

9.4 Obturator

The obturator nerve is formed from the anterior divisions of the L2, L3, and L4 lumbar roots and emerges from the medial border of the psoas. The nerve then travels over the sacral ala into the lesser pelvis and follows the lateral pelvic wall to exit the pelvis through the obturator canal (Fig. 9.6). This canal is formed by the bony obturator foramen, obturator internus muscle, and obturator membrane. The nerve enters the canal coursing above the obturator artery and exits the canal lateral to the artery. The obturator nerve exits the obturator canal 11.4 cm from the ASIS and 3 cm from the pubic tubercle [18]. Within this canal, the obturator nerve divides into an

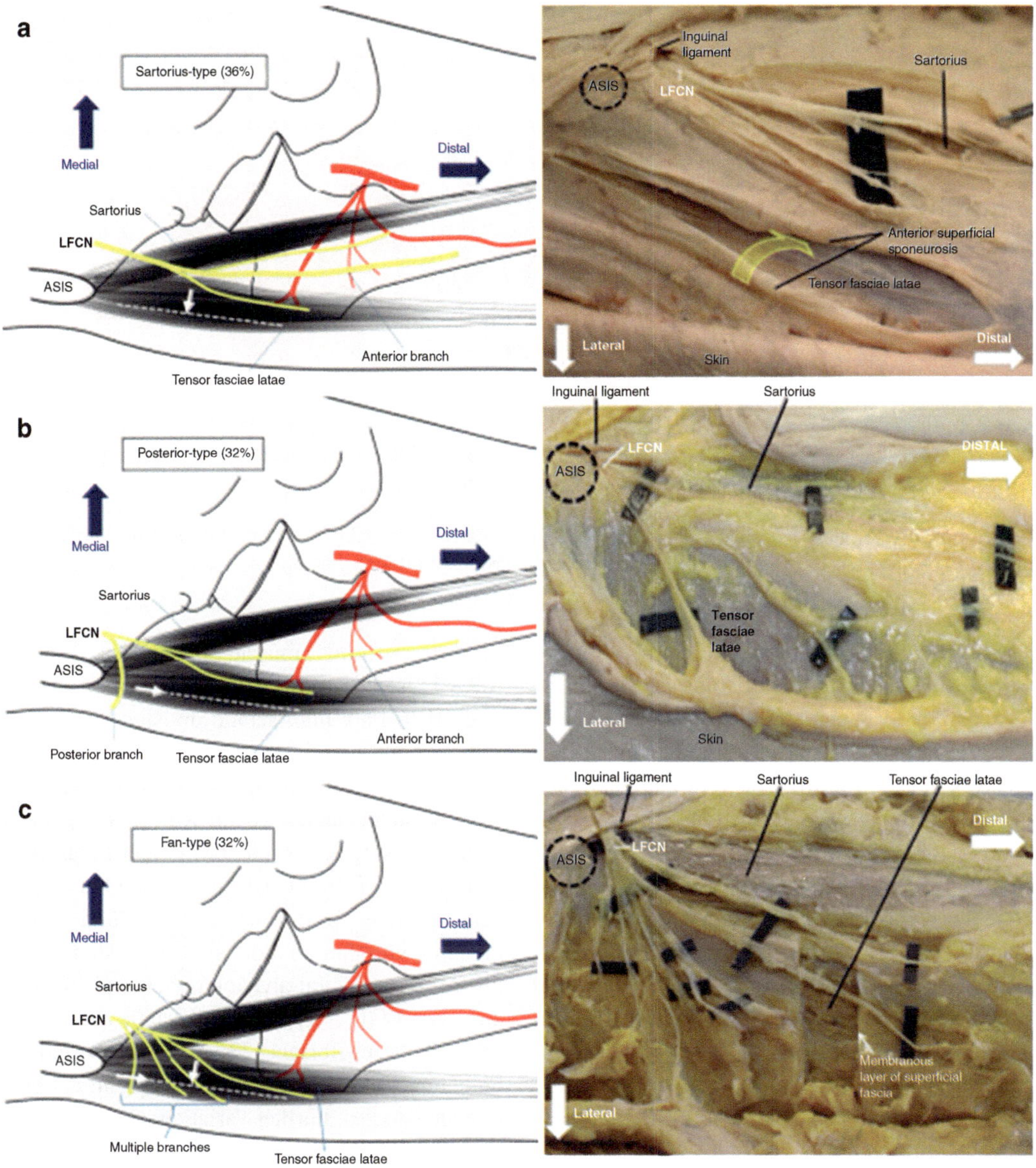

Fig. 9.5 Three major ranching patterns of the lateral femoral cutaneous nerve. (**a**) Sartorius type (36%) with a dominant anterior branch and an absent or small posterior branch; (**b**) posterior type (32%) with posterior branch equal or thicker than the anterior branch crossing the medial border of the TFL, and (**c**) fan type (32%) with multiple branches crossing over the TFL and lateral border of sartorius. (Permission for reprint from Rudin et al. [13])

anterior division, which courses anterior to the obturator externus and adductor brevis, and a posterior division, which pierces the obturator externus to descend deep to the adductor brevis. The anterior division provides an articular branch to the hip, sensation to the medial thigh, and motor innervation to the adductor longus, adductor brevis, gracilis, and pectineus. Anatomic variations have been described with a cutaneous sensory branch from the anterior division of the obturator nerve extending into the lower leg and foot [19]. This branch coursed posterior to the great saphenous vein and terminated in the medial ankle and foot.

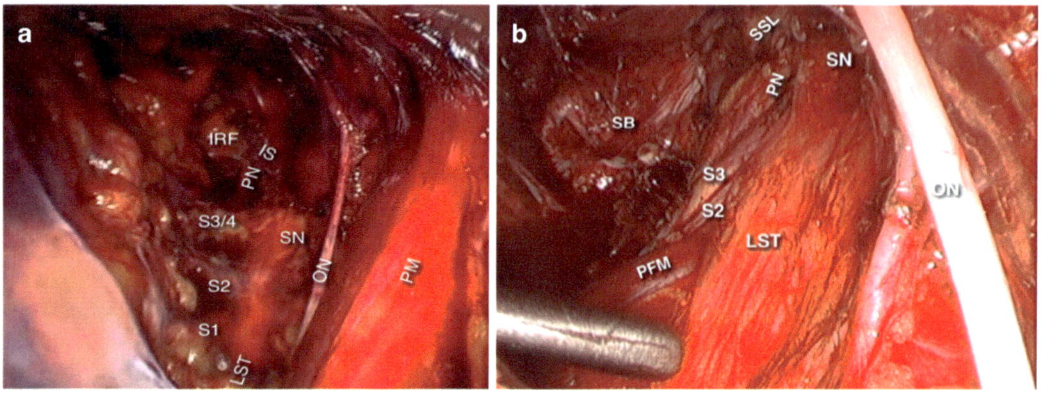

Fig. 9.6 Nerves of the obturator space (right side). Picture (**a**) is the final aspect of a laparoscopic approach to Alcock's Canal Syndrome, where the sacrospinous ligament has been transected to expose the pudendal nerve (PN). In picture (**b**), the sacrospinous ligament (SSL) is intact. In both pictures, the internal and external iliac vessels are retracted medially. (ON – obturator nerve; PM – psoas muscle; SN – sciatic nerve; LST – lumbosacral trunk; PN – pudendal nerve; IRF – ischiorectal fossa; IS – ischial spine; SB – sacral bone; PFM – piriformis muscle). (Image copyright Dr. Nucelio Lemos, used with permission)

The posterior division of the obturator nerve provides sensation to the articular capsule of the knee and motor innervation to the adductor magnus and obturator externus. The pectineus also receives innervation from the femoral nerve, and the adductor magnus is also supplied by the tibial component of the sciatic nerve [20]. An accessory obturator nerve is reported in 13.2% of patients originating from the anterior divisions of the L3 and L4 roots, coursing over the sacral ala, and then passing deep to the pectineus muscle before communication with the anterior branch of the proper obturator nerve [21].

9.5 Sciatic

The sciatic nerve is the largest peripheral nerve in terms of length and cross-sectional area and is formed from the L4 to S3 lumbosacral roots. The anterior L4 to S3 roots contribute to the tibial component and the posterior L4 to S2 roots contribute to the peroneal component of the sciatic nerve. The nerve then exits the pelvis through the greater sciatic foramen and classically descends deep to the piriformis muscle, although anatomic variations are described in 6–16.9% of limbs [22, 23]. Beaton and Anson described six configurations of the course of the sciatic nerve in relation to the piriformis muscle (Fig. 9.7): Type 1 (89.8%), sciatic nerve travels deep to piriformis; Type II (6.1%), high sciatic division with peroneal division piercing the piriformis muscle and tibial division travelling deep to it; Type III (0.7%), high sciatic division with peroneal division traversing above piriformis and tibial division below; Type IV (0.7%), undivided sciatic nerve piercing piriformis; Type V, high sciatic division with peroneal division traversing above piriformis and tibial division piercing piriformis; and Type VI (0.7%), undivided sciatic nerve traveling above piriformis [23, 24]. Type V and VI branching patterns are rare and frequently absent in many studies. Further variations not described in Beaton and Anson's classification include the presence of supernumerary piriformis muscle bellies with separate tendinous insertions into the greater trochanter [23].

In the upper thigh, the tibial component provides motor innervation to the long head of biceps femoris, semi-tendinosis, semimembranosus, and adductor magnus, while the peroneal component provides innervation to the short head of biceps femoris. The sciatic nerve then bifurcates into the common peroneal and tibial nerve 8–10 cm proximal to the knee joint [24, 25]. (See Chap. 12 for more detailed anatomic description of the distal common peroneal and tibial nerves.)

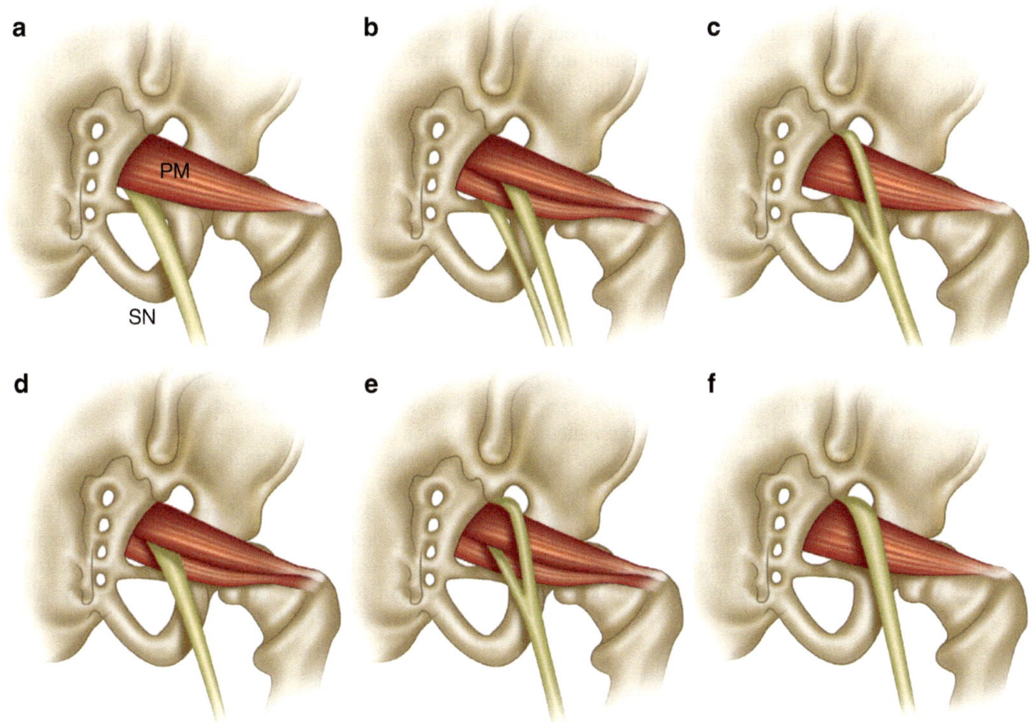

Fig. 9.7 Variations in the course of the sciatic nerve in relation to the piriformis muscle as described by Beaton and Anson. (**a**) Type 1 – sciatic nerve travels deep to piriformis; (**b**) Type II – high sciatic division with peroneal division piercing the piriformis muscle and tibial division travelling deep; (**c**) Type III – high sciatic division with peroneal division traversing above piriformis and tibial division below; (**d**) Type IV – undivided sciatic nerve piercing piriformis; (**e**) Type V – high sciatic division with peroneal division traversing above piriformis and tibial division piercing piriformis; (**f**) Type VI – undivided sciatic nerve traveling above piriformis

References

1. Mackinnon SE (2015) The "border nerves": iliohypogastric, ilioinguinal, and genitofemoral. In: Nerve Surgery, 1st edn. Thieme Publishers, New York, pp 345–354
2. Perry CP. Peripheral neuropathies and pelvic pain: diagnosis and management. Clin Obstet Gynecol. 2003;46(4):789–96.
3. Kopell HP, Thompson WA, Postel A. Entrapment neuropathy of the ilioinguinal nerve. N Engl J Med. 1962;266:16–9.
4. Lyon EK. Genitofemoral causalgia. Can Med Assoc J. 1945;53(3):213–6.
5. Kim DH, Murovic JA, Tiel RL, Kline D. Surgical management of 33 ilioinguinal and iliohypogastric neuralgias. J Neurosurg. 2005;56(5):1013–20. https://doi.org/10.1227/01.NEU.0000158320.64387.F8.
6. Vasquez MT, Murillo J, Maranillo E, Parkin IG, Sanudo J. Femoral nerve entrapment: a new insight. Clin Anat. 2007;20(2):175–9.
7. Tung T, Chao A, Moore A. Obturator nerve transfer for femoral nerve reconstruction: anatomic study and clinical application. Plast Reconstr Surg. 2012;130(5):1066–74.
8. Reichert F. Meralgia paresthetica; a form of causalgia relieved by interruption of the sympathetic fibers. Surg Clin North Am. 1933;13:1443.
9. Topol M. Anatomic variations of the lateral femoral cutaneous nerve: remnants of atypical nerve growth pathways revisited by intraneural fascicular dissection and a proposed classification. World Neurosurg. 2018;118:e687–98. https://doi.org/10.1016/j.wneu.2018.07.021.
10. Sunderland S. *Nerves and nerve injuries*. Edinburgh: Livingstone Ltd; 1981.
11. Piersol GA. Human anatomy. Philadelphia: JB Lippincott; 1930.
12. Keegan JJ, Holyoke E. Meralgia paresthetica—an anatomical and surgical study. J Neurosurg. 1962;19:341–5.
13. Rudin D, Manester M, Ullrich O, Erhardt J, Grob K. The anatomical course of the lateral femoral cutaneous nerve with special attention to the anterior approach to the hip joint. J Bone Joint Surg Am. 2016;98(7):561–7.
14. Hanna A. The lateral femoral cutaneous nerve canal. J Neurosurg. 2017;126:972–8. https://doi.org/10.3171/2016.1.JNS152262.972.

15. Ramakrishnan PK, Henry BM, Vikse J, et al. Anatomical variations of the formation and course of the sural nerve: a systematic review and meta-analysis. Ann Anat. 2015;202:36–44. https://doi.org/10.1016/j.aanat.2015.08.002.
16. Ropars M, Morandi X, Huten D, Thomazeau H, Berton E, Darnault P. Anatomical study of the lateral femoral cutaneous nerve with special reference to minimally invasive anterior approach for total hip replacement. Surg Radiol Anat. 2009;31:199–204. https://doi.org/10.1007/s00276-008-0433-3.
17. Sugano M, Nakamura J, Hagiwara S, et al. Anatomical course of the lateral femoral cutaneous nerve with special reference to the direct anterior approach to total hip arthroplasty. Mod Rheumatol. 2019;30(4):752–7. https://doi.org/10.1080/14397595.2019.1637992.
18. Jo SY, Chang JC, Bae HG, et al. A morphometric study of the obturator nerve around the obturator foramen. J Korean Neurosurg Soc. 2016;59(3):282–6.
19. Staples B, Ennedy E, Kim T, et al. Cutaneous branch of the obturator nerve extending to the medial ankle and foot: a report of two cadaveric cases. J Foot Ankle Surg. 2019;58(6):1267–72. https://doi.org/10.1053/j.jfas.2019.03.007.
20. Vasilev SA. Obturator nerve injury: a review of management options. Gynecol Oncol. 1994;53(2):152–5. https://doi.org/10.1006/gyno.1994.1108. PMID: 8188073.
21. Katritsis E, Anagnostopoulou S, Papadopoulos N. Anatomical observations on the accessory obturator nerve (based on 1000 specimens). Anat Anz. 1980;148:440–5.
22. Smoll NR. Variations of the piriformis and sciatic nerve with clinical consequence: a review. Clin Anat. 2010;23:8–17.
23. Natsis K, Totlis T, Konstantinidis GA, Paraskevas G, Piagkou M, Koebke J. Anatomical variations between the sciatic nerve and the piriformis muscle: a contribution to surgical anatomy in piriformis syndrome. Surg Radiol Anat. 2014;36:273–80.
24. Beaton LE, Anson BJ. The relation of the sciatic nerve and of its subdivisions to the piriformis muscle. Anat Rec. 1937;70:1–5.
25. Gustafson KJ, Grinberg Y, Joseph S, Triolo RJ. Human distal sciatic nerve fascicular anatomy: implications for ankle control using nerve-cuff electrodes. J Rehabil Res Dev. 2012;49(2):309–22. https://doi.org/10.1682/JRRD.2010.10.0201.

Pelvic, Acetabular, Hip, and Proximal Femur Fractures: Surgical Exposures and Treatment of Nerve Injury

10

Mitchel R. Obey, Kitty Wu, Christopher J. Dy, and Milton T. Little

10.1 Surgical Approaches to the Pelvis, Acetabulum, and Proximal Femur

10.1.1 Ilioinguinal Approach

The ilioinguinal approach permits visualization of the anterior wall and anterior column of the acetabulum. Through this approach, one can perform both direct and indirect reduction of anterior fracture moieties including both column, anterior column posterior hemi-transverse, transverse, and the abovementioned acetabular fractures. The approach was originally described and reported by Robert Judet and Emile Letournel in 1964 through cadaveric studies [1]. The approach utilizes three separate windows through which acetabular fracture care can be performed and the superficial dissection and each individual window is associated with its own risk of injury to neurovascular structures.

M. R. Obey (✉)
Department of Orthopedic Surgery, Washington University School of Medicine, St. Louis, MO, USA
e-mail: obeym@wustl.edu

K. Wu
Department of Plastic and Reconstructive Surgery, Western University, London, MO, USA

C. J. Dy
Department of Orthopedic Surgery, Washington University, St. Louis, MO, USA

M. T. Little
Cedars-Sinai Medical Center, Los Angeles, CA, USA

10.1.1.1 Superficial Dissection

The skin incision is started midline approximately 1–3 cm superior to the pubic tubercle, and then extended laterally across the lower abdomen and curving proximally to the anterior superior iliac spine (ASIS). It is continued posteriorly along the iliac crest to the junction of the center and posterior third of the iliac crest. Sharp dissection is taken down through the subcutaneous tissue to expose the aponeurosis of the external oblique muscle. There are no internervous planes during this stage of the approach; however, the most common neurological injury during this approach is to the lateral femoral cutaneous nerve (LFCN) [2, 3]. Visualization of the lateral femoral cutaneous nerve medial to the ASIS is an important aspect of the exposure (Fig. 10.1).

Tips to Avoid Injury: Lateral Femoral Cutaneous Nerve

Injury to the LFCN has been reported between 12% and 57% in previous studies [4, 5], and injury risk can be decreased by flexing the hip joint during the surgery to alleviate tension on the nerve [6]. The anatomical variations of the LFCN have been documented in studies dating as early as 1885 [7], and becoming familiar with the most common branching patterns will decrease risk of iatrogenic injury [3, 8, 9]. The LFCN commonly is a distal branch of the posterior divisions of the L2–L3 spinal nerve roots, and after exiting the lesser pelvis underneath the inguinal ligament, it bifurcates distally to form the anterior and posterior cutaneous branches [10]. Previous authors have identified up to seven different variations in the point of exit of the LFCN from the pelvis [7],

C. J. Dy et al. (eds.), *Peripheral Nerve Issues after Orthopedic Surgery*,
https://doi.org/10.1007/978-3-030-84428-8_10

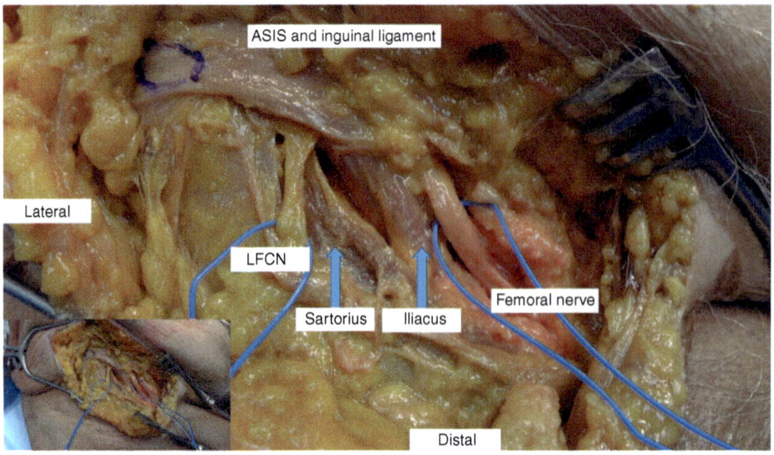

Fig. 10.1 Superficial cadaveric dissection displaying the relationship of the LFCN to the ASIS, inguinal ligament, and surrounding neurovascular structures as it passes distally into the thigh. (Image copyright Dr. Christopher Dy, used with permission)

and furthermore, five different branching patterns [11]. A recent meta-analysis of 24 studies (n = 1720 subjects) reported the most common exit point from the pelvis to be medial to the sartorius muscle (86.8%) as a single branch (79.1%) on an average 1.9 (1.65–2.14) cm medial to the ASIS. It is also important to be aware that the nerve can be found exiting above or below the inguinal ligament, through the ASIS, through the sartorius muscle, and lateral to the ASIS. Additionally, a branching pattern in which the nerve bifurcates proximal to the inguinal ligament within the pelvis has been previously described [11], and it can easily be unrecognized during the approach. Given the significant variation in both branching and exit patterns, care must to be taken during the superficial dissection portion of this approach to avoid injury to the LFCN.

10.1.1.2 Lateral Window

The lateral window is the space along the false pelvis extending from the posterior sacroiliac joint to the iliopsoas anteriorly. When developing the lateral window, one should identify the fascia/tendinous junction between the hip abductors and abdominal muscles which is identified as a shiny white line along the iliac crest. Once the fascia is incised, the iliacus muscle can then be elevated off the internal iliac fossa with blunt dissection. For iliacus retraction, pelvic ring fractures or fractures which involve the sacroiliac joint, the dissection may be taken more posteriorly across the sacroiliac joint for exposure and visualization. This more midline posterior approach places the fifth lumbar (L5) nerve root at risk.

Tips to Avoid Injury: Fifth Lumbar (L5) Nerve Root

The L5 nerve root is at risk of injury during the more medial subperiosteal elevation of the iliacus muscle as you cross the sacroiliac joint. The L5 nerve root runs along the sacral ala, and it is critical to identify and protect the nerve root laying on the anterior surface of the lateral aspect of the sacrum (Fig. 10.2).

10.1.1.3 Middle Window

The middle window is formed by dissection of the iliopectineal fascia from the iliopectineal eminence. This allows the creation of a window between the medial border of the iliopsoas and the femoral nerve and lateral border of the femoral vessels and lymphatics. This space is commonly utilized for reduction, clamp, and hardware placement during fixation of acetabular fractures. As your superficial dissection extends medially from the ASIS, the external oblique aponeurosis is divided 1.5–2 cm proximal to the inguinal liga-

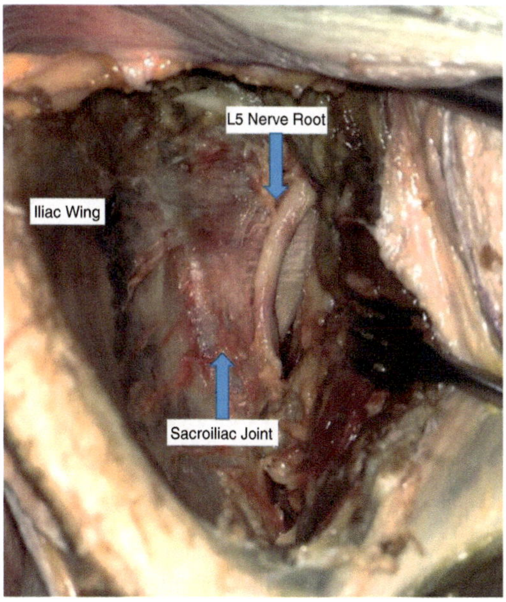

Fig. 10.2 Deep cadaveric dissection through lateral window displaying the L5 nerve root running over the sacral ala. (Image copyright Dr. Milton Little, used with permission)

ment extending it from the ASIS to just medial to the lateral edge of the rectus abdominis muscle. As stated above, the LFCN medial to the ASIS should be protected as you dissect down through the external oblique aponeurosis. In taking the dissection medially, the external inguinal ring can be identified, and the dissection should be taken proximal to the ring to avoid overtightening during closure. From there, the spermatic cord or round ligament and the inguinal nerve will be visible in a male or female patient, respectively. Reflecting the external oblique fascia distally will allow for visualization of the internal inguinal ring and unroof the inguinal canal to allow isolation and mobilization of its contents (i.e., spermatic cord/round ligament, ilioinguinal nerve). The LFCN should again be identified and protected at this point.

Tips to Avoid Injury: Ilioinguinal Nerve
The ilioinguinal nerve will be located within the contents of the inguinal canal running along side the spermatic cord/round ligament, and injury is often caused by excessive retraction during the case. A wide penrose drain can be placed around these structures to keep them together and can be sutured rather clamped for gentle retraction.

The floor of the inguinal canal, the inguinal ligament, can be then be identified running from the ASIS to the pubic tubercle. Incise the ligament, releasing the common origin of the internal oblique, transversus abdominis muscles and fascia. This will expose the underlying psoas sheath and iliopsoas muscle fibers just medial to the ASIS. You must identify and protect the femoral nerve, which is found medial to the iliopsoas muscle often lying on or deep to the muscle at this location.

Tips to Avoid Injury: Femoral Nerve
The femoral nerve is the largest branch of the lumbar plexus, commonly arising from the dorsal branches of the second through fourth ventral rami, and it is most commonly found passing underneath the inguinal ligament medial to the iliopsoas and medial to the femoral artery (Fig. 10.3). It continues distally to divide into the anterior and posterior branches within the thigh. However, anatomical variations in the femoral nerve occur in 25% of patients [12], and may include early division of the femoral nerve within the pelvis, origin of LFCN, and also splitting of the femoral nerve into two slips by psoas major or accessory slips of iliacus muscle [12]. When incising the inguinal ligament to expose the underlying psoas sheath, it is important to identify and protect this structure. This structure is primarily at risk with the dissection of the iliopectineal fascia from the iliopsoas.

10.1.1.4 Medial Window

The medial window provides access to the superior pubic ramus and quadrilateral plate and is located between the ipsilateral rectus and the spermatic cord/round ligament. As the exposure is carried medially, one must be careful to visualize and protect the inferior epigastric artery and vein which will be found at this point and often requires ligation. The conjoint tendon of the internal oblique and transversus abdominis and tendon of the rectus abdominis must be divided from the pubic insertions. This will expose extraperitoneal adipose tissue, and with blunt dissec-

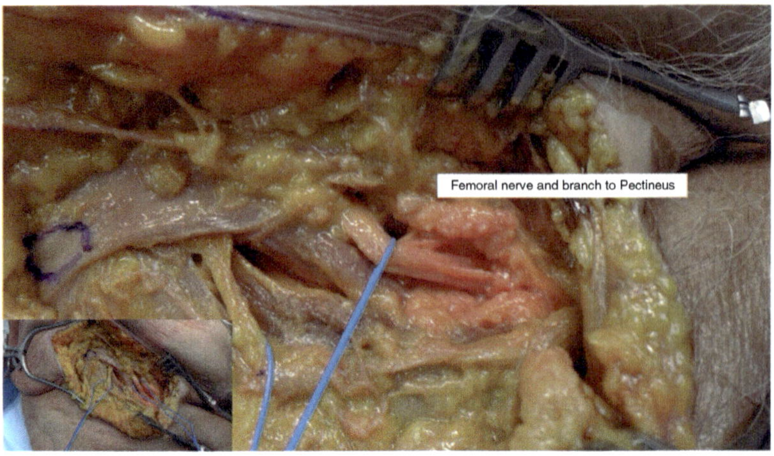

Fig. 10.3 Deep cadaveric dissection through the middle window displaying the relationship of the femoral nerve to the ASIS, inguinal ligament, and surrounding neurovascular structures. (Image copyright Dr. Christopher Dy, used with permission)

tion the retropubic space (i.e., "Cave of Retzius") can be developed. Just medial to the femoral nerve will be the iliopectineal fascia (IPF) which has already been removed from the iliopectineal eminence when the middle window is dissected. As the dissection is carried into the true pelvis medial to the spermatic cord/round ligament, one must identify the obturator artery and nerve medial and posterior to the external iliac vessels.

Tips to Avoid Injury: Obturator Nerve

The obturator nerve commonly arises from the ventral divisions of the second, third, and fourth lumbar nerves, and is commonly found descending through the muscle fibers of the psoas major muscle and emerging from its medial border. It then continues along the lateral wall of the lesser pelvis, above and in front of the obturator vessels, to the upper part of the obturator foramen as it passes through a small hiatus in the obturator foramen to enter the thigh and subsequently divide into anterior and posterior branches (Fig. 10.4) [13]. It is important to be aware that anatomical variations in branching patterns of the common obturator nerve exist, and there are three primary variations that have been recognized. These include division into the anterior and posterior branches before entering the obturator canal (i.e., intrapelvic, 23.2%), within the obturator canal (51.8%), and after the obturator canal (i.e., extrapelvic, 25%) [13]. When performing the deep dissection medially, and during fracture reduction, it is important to identify and protect this structure. Additionally, this nerve may be entrapped in the anterior column fracture along the pubic root/obturator ring (Fig. 10.5). Care must be taken to identify the nerve and free the nerve from the fracture fragments to avoid further injury.

In a portion of patients, the obturator artery or vein will have an anomalous anastomosis between the external iliac or inferior epigastric artery known as the corona mortis. Darmanis et al. found the corona mortis in 83% of cadaveric specimens. The anastomosis may be arterial (36%), venous (60%), or mixed [14]. If present, the vessel(s) may be clamped, ligated, and divided to avoid an avulsive traction injury. Once the corona mortis has been controlled, exposure to the true and false pelvis has been completed and fracture reduction and fixation can be performed through all three surgical "windows."

10.1.2 Anterior Intrapelvic Approach (AIP)

The AIP (often called the Modified Stoppa Approach) was first described in the context of repairing inguinal hernias in the works of Rives et al. [15] and Stoppa et al. [16]. Several years later, modifications to the surgical approach were made so that it may serve as an anterior intrapelvic extraperitoneal approach through the rectus abdominis muscle for fixation of acetabular fractures such as T-type patterns (Fig. 10.6) [17, 18]. Through the approach, the surgeon can access the pubis, quadrilateral surface, sciatic buttress, and anterior sacroiliac joint marking up to 79% of the inner true pelvis. It provides an alternate approach to some anterior fracture moieties while avoiding

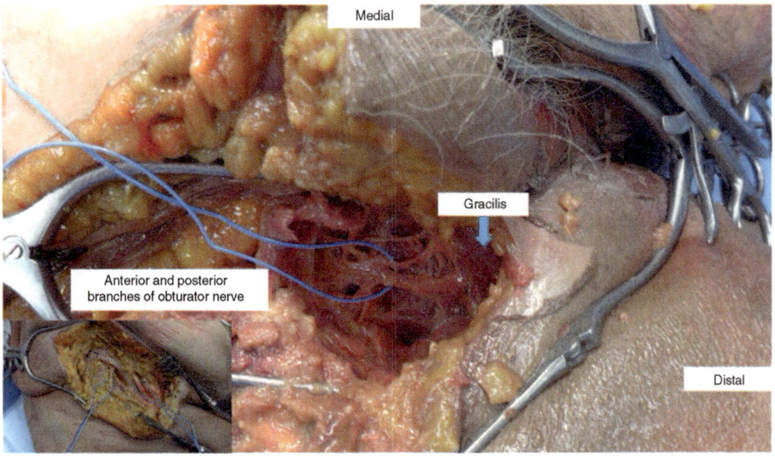

Fig. 10.4 Deep cadaveric dissection through the medial window displaying the anterior and posterior branches of the obturator nerve as it emerges from the obturator foramen. (Image copyright Dr. Christopher Dy, used with permission)

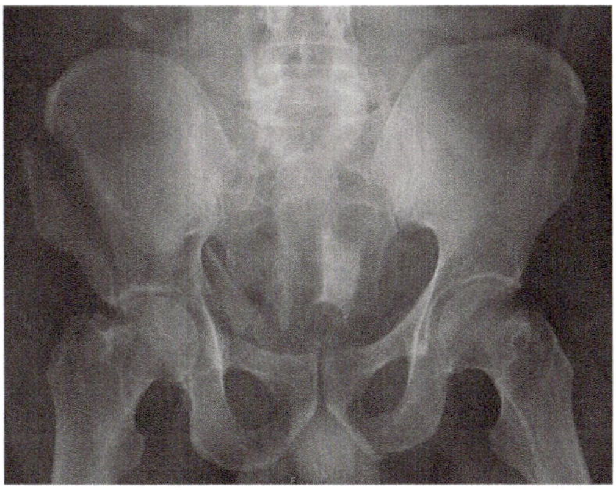

Fig. 10.5 Anterior column posterior hemi-transverse acetabulum fracture

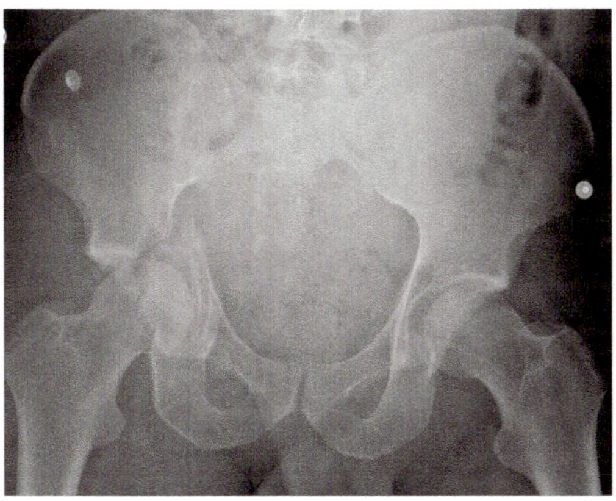

Fig. 10.6 T-type acetabular fracture

the middle window of the ilioinguinal approach by working from the opposite side of the pectineal eminence. The approach can also be combined with the lateral and middle window of the ilioinguinal approach to avoid the deep and superficial inguinal rings [19]. Utilization of the AIP while avoiding the middle window allows the surgeon to avoid prolonged retraction and manipulation of the femoral nerve, and external iliac vessels. The approach can be taken through a vertical midline incision or a Pfannenstiel incision made from approximately 1–2 cm proximal to the pubic symphysis and extended 5–10 cm lateral in each direction from the midline. The dissection is taken sharply down to the level of the rectus fascia, which is then split in the midline in line with its fibers. The amount of vertical dissection of the rectus muscle is the limiting factor in the exposure rather than the width of Pfannensteil incision. Next, the transversalis fascia is incised just superior to the pubic symphysis, and the retropubic space (i.e., Retzius space) can be entered by blunt dissection. At this point, it is important to protect the urinary bladder from injury, and sponges can be packed into this space to accomplish the task along with a malleable retractor. The pubis is now accessible, and careful subperiosteal dissection can be performed along the superior pubic ramus to the internal iliac fossa. As the dissection is carried laterally toward the acetabulum, you must identify and protect the external iliac vessels, femoral nerve, and iliopsoas muscle. This can be accomplished by placement of a retractor underneath these structures to retract them laterally and anteriorly away from the surgical field. It is also at this point when you may encounter the vascular anastomosis between the external iliac vessels and obturator vessels (i.e., corona mortis). If present, this anastomosis will be located on the posterior surface of the superior pubic ramus and must be ligated to allow further exposure and dissection along the pelvic brim. The iliopectineal fascia is elevated from the anterior column and pectineal eminence, and this dissection is extended anteriorly over the pectineal eminence and posteriorly toward the anterior surface of the sacroiliac joint. Finally, the dissection is taken down along the quadrilateral surface and medial aspect of the posterior column. During this point of the dissection, you must identify the obturator internus muscle, and just next to it will be an area of fat which contains the obturator neurovascular bundle. Care must be taken to free the neurovascular bundle from the anterior column or pubic root fracture if present. The obturator nerve must be protected, and gently retracted away from the surgical field. You will now have access to the anterior column, acetabulum, and anterior sacroiliac joint.

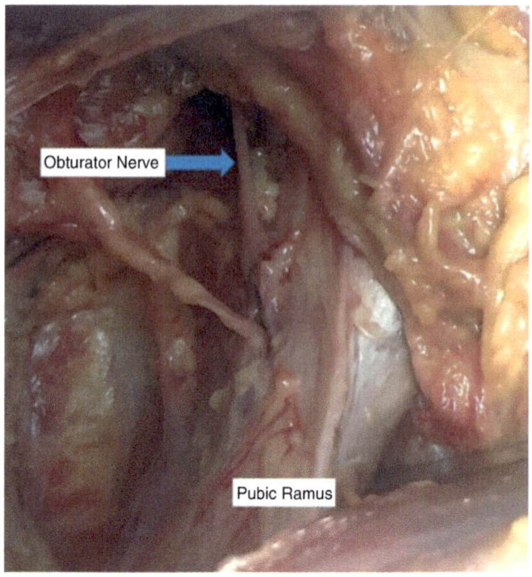

Fig. 10.7 Cadaveric dissection showing obturator nerve entering small hiatus in the obturator foramen to enter the thigh. (Image copyright Dr. Milton Little, used with permission)

Tips to Avoid Injury: Obturator Nerve

The obturator nerve commonly arises from the ventral divisions of the second, third, and fourth lumbar nerves, and is commonly found descending through the muscle fibers of the psoas major muscle and emerging from its medial border. It then continues along the lateral wall of the lesser pelvis, above and in front of the obturator vessels, to the upper part of the obturator foramen as it passes through a small hiatus in the obturator foramen to enter the thigh and subsequently divide into anterior and posterior branches [13] (Fig. 10.7). When carrying the final dissection down along the quadrilateral surface, identify the area of fat medial to the obturator internus where this nerve is running.

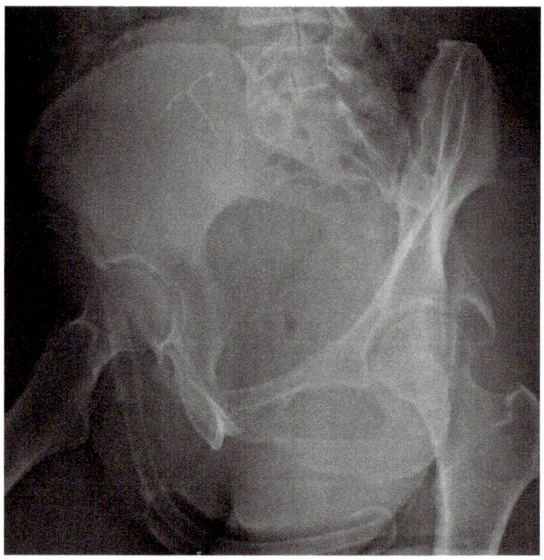

Fig. 10.8 Posterior wall acetabulum fracture

10.1.3 Kocher-Langenbeck Approach

The combination of the Kocher and Langenbeck approaches to the posterior acetabulum was initially described by Letournel and Judet [1]. It is a common approach for access to the posterior wall and posterior column (Fig. 10.8). The skin incision is centered over the greater trochanter, and the Langenbeck limb extends proximally from the tip of the greater trochanter to within 6 cm of the posterior superior iliac spine (PSIS). The Kocher limb extends from the greater trochanter distally along the shaft of the femur. Sharp dissection is taken down through the subcutaneous tissue to the level of iliotibial band. After incising the tensor fasciae lata fascia, the gluteus maximus muscle belly is split in line with this raphe. Care is taken not to disrupt the gluteus maximus tendinous insertion while splitting the gluteus fibers. The intervascular interval of the gluteus maximus muscle is identifiable by a raphe located at the junction of the upper one-third (supplied by superior gluteal artery) and lower two-thirds (supplied by inferior gluteal artery) of the muscle. The tissues can now be retracted posteriorly to expose the short external rotators, sciatic nerve, and superior gluteal vessels. The sciatic nerve will be found overlying the quadratus femoris muscle, and it is critical to identify and protect it during the approach (Fig. 10.9). The short external rotators (piriformis and conjoint tendon) can then be released with a 1 cm cuff of tissue near the tendinous insertions on the greater trochanter and reflected medially to further protect the sciatic nerve. The obturator internus tendon can be followed medially into the lesser sciatic notch, and the tendon can be utilized to protect the sciatic nerve.

Tips to Avoid Injury: Sciatic Nerve

The sciatic nerve is commonly formed by the convergence of the anterior divisions of the L4–S3 spinal nerve roots within the pelvis [20]. It can be as wide as 2 cm at its origin and separates into two common nerves: tibial nerve and common peroneal nerve. The sciatic nerve is commonly found exiting the pelvis through the greater sciatic notch. However, there have been as many as six anatomic variations in the relationship between the sciatic nerve and piriformis muscle [20–23]. Thus, it is important for the surgeon to be aware of these variations in order to avoid accidental injury to the nerve during the surgical approach. It should also be remembered that when performing the case prone, the leg should be kept with the knee flexed and hip extended as much as possible throughout the case to avoid traction injury.

The quadratus femoris and obturator externus muscles should be left intact to protect the underlying ascending branch of the medial circumflex femoral artery. If further exposure is required, the tendinous insertion of the gluteus maximus can be incised but doing so may remove the check reign on retractors and place the sciatic nerve at increased risk of a traction injury. Finally, identify the gluteus medius and minimus muscles of the posterior and lateral aspects of the ilium. These can be released and elevated subperiosteally and retracted to expose the underlying ilium. The superior gluteal nerve and vessels may now be visible exiting the greater sciatic notch with the piriformis muscle. Proximal and medial elevation of the gluteus minimus places the superior gluteal nerve and vessels at risk of injury. If further exposure of the posterior column and acetabulum is needed, a trochanteric osteotomy can be made. You will now have access to the posterior column and wall of the acetabulum.

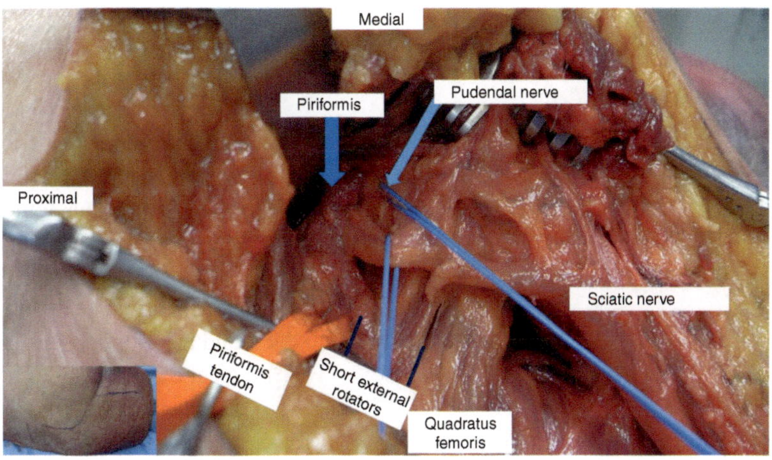

Fig. 10.9 Deep cadaveric dissection exposing the sciatic nerve, and its relationship to the underlying quadratus femoris muscle, short external rotator muscles, and piriformis tendon. (Image copyright Dr. Christopher Dy, used with permission)

10.1.4 Hueter/Smith Peterson Approach

The anterior approach to the hip was first described by the German surgeon Carl Hueter in 1881 [24]. It was later popularized in the early 1900s after modifications were made by Dr. Smith-Petersen to improve the traditional anterior iliofemoral approach (i.e., Hueter, or Smith-Petersen) [25, 26]. It was again modified by the French Surgeon Emile Letournel who described an extension of the anterior approach to the hip, known as the extended iliofemoral approach, for the treatment of acetabular and proximal femur injuries such as femoral neck fractures (Fig. 10.10). In this approach, an 8–10 cm incision is made approximately 2–3 cm lateral and 1 cm distal to the ASIS and extended distally toward the lateral edge of the patella. The incision is made parallel to the fibers of the tensor fasciae lata (TFL). Sharp dissection is taken down through the subcutaneous tissue to expose the fascia overlying the TFL. An incision in the fascia is made at the junction of the anterior two-thirds and posterior two-thirds of the TFL muscle belly. At this level the first internervous plane is reached, which is between the sartorius muscle (femoral nerve) and TFL (superior gluteal nerve). It is important to be aware that when developing the interval between the TFL and sartorius muscles, the LFCN is at risk of injury.

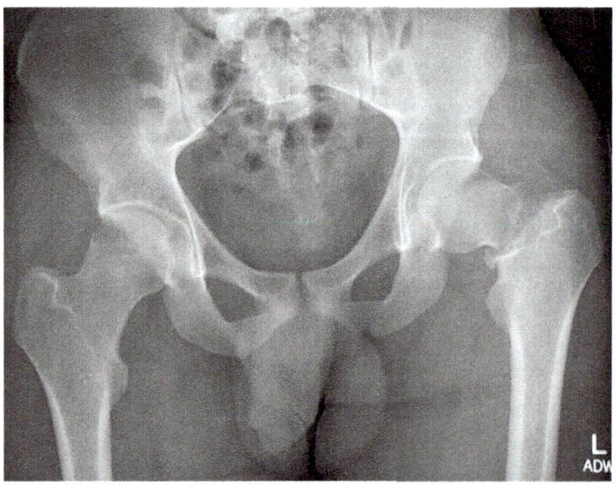

Fig. 10.10 Transcervical femoral neck fracture in young adult

Tips to Avoid Injury: Lateral Femoral Cutaneous Nerve

The LFCN commonly is commonly found exiting the lesser pelvis underneath the inguinal ligament medial to the ASIS. The anterior approach to the hip places this nerve at risk, and previous authors, particularly in the context of total hip arthroplasty (THA), have reported it as a unique complication. Injury to the LFCN has been reported between 14% and 81% in the literature [27, 28], and a recent review of 1871 patients reported 16% of patients experiencing persistent neuropathic pain at a mean of 3.9 years from surgery [28]. A recent meta-analysis of 24 studies (n = 1720 subjects) reported the most common exit point from the pelvis to be medial to the sartorius muscle (86.8%) as a single branch (79.1%) on an average 1.9 (1.65–2.14) cm medial to the ASIS. When dividing the TFL fascia, this nerve must be identified and carefully protected to avoid injury.

Placement of the incision as lateral and distal as possible will help to protect the LFCN; however, it will not exactly correspond to the internervous plane and thus may limit exposure; 32% of patients have a fan-type pattern of the LFCN in the proximal thigh where multiple branches course across the tensor fascia lata and anterior border of sartorius. Risk of injury is highest in these patients, and some argue, it is inevitable [29]. The LFCN is also most at risk between 2.7 and 9.2 cm distal to the ASIS where it most commonly crosses the anterior border of the tensor fascia lata [30].

By staying within the fascial sheath of the TFL muscle, you will decrease the risk of injury to the LFCN. The TFL muscle fibers are sharply dissected from the anterior flap of the fascia. The iliac origin of the TFL is then released to further develop the internervous plane, and the TFL muscle belly is retracted laterally and the sartorius medially. The fascia overlying the rectus femoris muscle (femoral nerve) and gluteus medius muscle (superior gluteal nerve) is encountered, which represents the deep internervous plane. The rectus femoris muscle has two heads: the direct head which originates from the anterior inferior iliac spine (AIIS), and the reflected head which originates from the superior acetabulum and anterior capsule. To achieve appropriate surgical exposure, both heads of the rectus femoris are elevated, and the direct head may be released to improve visualization. Next, the gluteus medius attachment to the iliac crest is elevated and released, and with a periosteal elevator the muscle bellies of the gluteus medius and minimus are subperiosteally elevated from the lateral surface of the ilium. At this point, the hip capsule is exposed, and the arthrotomy can be made to access the femoral head and neck.

10.2 Management of Nerve Injuries

10.2.1 "Border Nerves": Ilioinguinal, Iliohypogastric, Genitofemoral

Somatic pain secondary to iliohypogastric, ilioinguinal, and genitofemoral nerve injury can be difficult to differentiate from visceral pain due to "viscerosomatic convergence" [31]. This occurs due to the convergence of both the peripheral somatic nerves and visceral nerve synapses onto the same dorsal horn cell [32]. The overlapping sensory distributions of these three nerves and their often terminally anastomosing branches further complicate diagnosis. Patients often suffer symptoms for many years without a conclusive diagnosis and are commonly referred to multiple sub-specialists. Oftentimes the lack of definitive abnormal investigations relegates the patient to being labelled as having psychogenic pain or accused of malingering.

Electromyography studies have low sensitivity and not frequently helpful to make the diagnosis [33]. There is dual innervation of the abdominal wall muscles from the intercostal nerves, and thus denervation is rarely seen on EMG. Use of MR neurography has been described to identify abnormalities within the nerve. Focal or diffuse enlargement of the nerve can be detected on T2-weighted images and perineural fibrosis can be seen on T1-weighted images as low intensity signals [34].

Diagnosis is made based on clinical symptoms with pain in the inguinal region, sensory disturbances (hypoesthesia, hyperalgesia, allodynia) in the expected cutaneous distribution, tenderness with palpation over expected compression sites, and relief of symptoms with a targeted nerve block. Targeted peripheral nerve blocks are extremely valuable both as a therapeutic and diagnostic modality. Only patients with significant pain relief following targeted nerve blocks should be considered for surgical intervention and neurectomy.

10.2.1.1 Ilioinguinal and Iliohypogastric Neuralgia

Iliohypogastric and ilioinguinal neuralgias are known complications of hernia repair, Pfannenstiel incisions, laparoscopic surgery, and uro-gynecological procedures resulting from entrapment from scar tissue, mesh, or suture ligature [35, 36]. Injury to the ilioinguinal nerve manifests as referred groin and lower abdominal pain [37]. Patients may experience discomfort with internal rotation and extension of the hip [37]. Abnormal gait patterns such as walking with the back in a forward flexed position, to avoid tightening of the lower abdominal muscles, is a non-specific sign. Radiographic findings of a "aspheric" femoral head, describing a deviation from a round appearance, may be suggestive of ilioinguinal injury [37]. Compression medial and anterior to the ASIS may elicit a positive Tinel's sign with pain or intensifying the symptoms. Patients may also have a positive modified Carnett's test with increased pain with tensing abdominal musculature [33].

Surgical Approaches

The iliohypogastric nerve is approached through an oblique incision overlying the ASIS. The external oblique is split in line with its fibers. A second oblique split may be necessary within the external oblique fascia, 2 cm more cephalad to identify the iliohypogastric nerve [36]. The iliohypogastric nerve is then traced proximally and a neurectomy is performed so that the nerve lies within the pelvis and not within the abdominal wall musculature.

The ilioinguinal nerve is approached through an oblique incision overlying the ASIS. The fascia of the external oblique is split in between its fibers and the ilioinguinal nerve identified coursing over the internal oblique toward the groin

[36]. The ilioinguinal nerve is then traced proximally and neurectomy is performed so that the nerve lies within the pelvis [36].

Clinical Outcomes

Kim describes 10 patients with combined ilioinguinal and iliohypogastric neuralgias, resulting either from iatrogenic injury or blunt abdominal trauma; 90% of patients had pain relief following combined ilioinguinal and iliohypogastric neurectomy. Lee also describes excellent outcomes following isolated iliohypogastric neurectomy with complete pain relief in 83% of patients following neurectomy [36].

Starling et al. described 19 patients with ilioinguinal neuralgia and 17 patients had complete relief of symptoms following neurectomy [38]. Lee reports similar outcomes with 78% of patients with complete resolution of pain following neurectomy and 11% no pain relief [39].

10.2.1.2 Genitofemoral Neuralgia

Magee first described seven cases of "genitofemoral causalgia" in 1942, most commonly resulting from nerve entrapment from adhesions of the terminal ileum and psoas muscles following appendectomy [40]. This was renamed "genitofemoral neuralgia" by Lyon, who further noted the neuropathic nature of the symptoms [41]. Gynecology or pelvic surgery, herniorrhaphy, appendectomy, Pfannenstiel incisions, and blunt abdominal trauma have been reported causes of genitofemoral neuralgias [42]. Symptoms include constant burning pain in the inguinal region and upper medial thigh exacerbated with walking, running, or hyperextension of the hip. Lying down and hip flexion may mitigate the pain. Patients do not typically have a discrete Tinel's sign, unlike the ilioinguinal nerve [42].

Targeted nerve blocks can distinguish between genitofemoral nerve–related dysesthesias from ilioinguinal neuralgia. Patients first undergo a direct ilioinguinal nerve block and if this provides substantial relief then a diagnosis of ilioinguinal neuralgia is made. If no relief is experienced, then a trans-psoas genitofemoral nerve block should be performed. If there is significant relief from this second block, then a diagnosis of genitofemoral neuralgia is suggested. If partial relief is achieved with both blocks, then symptoms may be a result of a combination of both ilioinguinal and genitofemoral neuralgia [42]. Furthermore, in genitofemoral neuralgia, maximal passive hip flexion will exacerbate symptoms of dysesthesias in the labial majora and scrotum, but not in the thigh [43]. The genitofemoral nerve also gives motor innervation for the cremasteric reflex, which can be used clinically to detect nerve dysfunction in male patients.

Surgical Approach

Genitofemoral nerve decompression is performed either through a pre-existing incision from abdominal or pelvic surgery or through a lateral extraperitoneal approach. A transverse incision is made superior and lateral to the umbilicus, extending to the anterior axillary line [44]. The retroperitoneum is then exposed by dividing the external oblique, internal oblique, and transversus abdominis muscles as necessary. The ureter is identified and protected prior to dissection of the genitofemoral nerve as it pierces through the psoas. Both the genital and femoral branches must be identified, and neurectomy is performed either proximal to the bifurcation if visualized or to both branches separately [44]. If only the genital branch of the genitofemoral nerve is compressed, resection of the nerve can be performed at the external inguinal ring to avoid entering the retroperitoneum.

Clinical Outcomes

Patients who undergo either genitofemoral or ilioinguinal neurectomy and fail to see any improvement may have involvement of a different nerve. Starling describes 17 cases of genitofemoral neuralgias, in which 12 patients had substantial or complete pain relief after neurectomy. In another series by Lee, 50% of patients with genitofemoral neuralgia had excellent pain relief following neurectomy, 25% with moderate relief, and 25% with no pain relief [36]. Murovic also reports considerable relief of symptoms in 10 patients who underwent neurectomy [42].

10.2.2 Femoral Nerve

Femoral nerve injury can result in motor weakness in hip flexion and knee extension, interfering with a patient's ability to stand from a sitting position and to walk, especially on an incline or upstairs. Patients may also experience sensory deficits in the anteromedial thigh, medial knee, lower leg, and foot. Compression of the femoral nerve at the inguinal ligament or more proximally between the iliacus and psoas muscles can present with pain in the inguinal region that worsens with hip extension and internal rotation.

Idiopathic compression neuropathy of the femoral nerve is rare. The most common cause of femoral neuropathy is iatrogenic injury during femoral artery cannulation, herniorrhaphy, pelvic surgery, or as part of oncologic resection [45]. The incidence of femoral nerve palsy after primary total hip arthroplasty is 0.21–2.27% [46, 47]. Patients undergoing a direct anterior or anterolateral approach have a 14.8-fold higher incidence of femoral nerve injury compared to a direct lateral or posterolateral approach [46]. Revisional procedures carry a higher incidence of nerve injury of 7.5% [48]. In its course between the iliacus and psoas muscles, the femoral nerve is susceptible to compression from hematomas following pelvic surgery, especially in anticoagulated patients [49]. Iatrogenic injury can also be caused by thermal injury, direct lacerations, implant extrusion, and retractor placement.

The femoral nerve is in close proximity to anterior acetabular rim and at risk of injury during total hip arthroplasty. The femoral nerve is in closest proximity to the acetabulum 90° to a reference line through the ASIS and center of the acetabulum, measuring only 1.6 cm away [50]. The tip of a retractor placed over the anterior acetabular wall can either directly compress the femoral nerve or cause compression through the iliopsoas muscle. During the posterior approach to THA, the anterior retractor must maintain contact with the anterior acetabular wall, deep to the iliopsoas to avoid nerve injury [51]. Measurement of intraoperative nerve pressures of the femoral nerve in 10 patients show a baseline pressure of 2–8 mmHg. Peak pressures of 25–220 mmHg were recorded during acetabular preparation and placement of a retractor over the anterior lip [52].

10.2.2.1 Treatment

Early identification of postoperative femoral nerve injury with a thorough clinical exam is crucial to minimizing the risk of falls and periprosthetic complications. Imaging should be obtained to rule out prosthetic or cement extrusion, pseudoaneurysm, and hematoma causing compression on the femoral nerve. If a reversible cause is identified, immediate surgical re-exploration should be performed to alleviate extrinsic sources of nerve compression and provide the best opportunity for nerve recovery. Similarly, if a sharp lacerating injury to the nerve is suspected, then prompt exploration will facilitate the best chance for primary nerve repair, without the need for nerve grafting. This requires microsurgical expertise, and if this is not immediately available, then the nerve ends should be marked with a brightly colored suture (e.g., a 4-0 polypropylene) so that they can later be easily identified.

10.2.2.2 Conservative Management

For patients with blunt or traction injuries, the initial management is conservative with education on fall prevention, engagement in physiotherapy, and the use of assistive walking devices. A locking knee brace can provide stability and prevent involuntary knee buckling when walking. Initial EMG studies should be performed 4–6 weeks after injury. Needle EMG and nerve conduction studies can help to differentiate femoral nerve palsy from lumbar radiculopathy or plexus lesions.

Based on a study of 36 femoral nerve palsies in a consecutive series of 17,350 patients undergoing primary total hip arthroplasty (THA), the majority of patients did not notice improvement until more than 6 months post surgery [46]. By 2.5 years, motor weakness had resolved spontaneously in 75% of patients, with those remaining experiencing minor deficits that did not require assistive walking devices or bracing [46]. In contrast, 80% of these patients had persistent sensory deficits [46]. In another study of 273 consecutive primary THA, the incidence of femoral nerve injury was 1.1% and in all three cases, the patients recovered full motor function within a year without surgical intervention [53].

10.2.2.3 Neurolysis and Nerve Grafting

Surgical intervention is recommended in cases without any EMG evidence of recovery by 3–6 months. The use of intra-operative nerve action potentials (NAPs) can aid in decision-making at the time of exploration. The presence of intact NAPs is associated with good return of nerve function with decompression and neurolysis alone [45]. If the nerve is in discontinuity, then either direct repair, if possible, or autologous interposition sural cable grafting should be performed. Prior to nerve grafting, the proximal and distal nerve ends should be resected until healthy fascicles are visualized. Multiple sural cable grafts are then used to match the cross-sectional area and span the defect.

Results from nerve grafting for femoral nerve lesions is mixed. Surgical intervention less than 3 months from the time of injury and younger patient correspond with better motor recovery [54, 55]. Tsuchihara reports on two cases of femoral nerve reconstruction using sural nerve grafts greater than 10 cm and both patients recovering MRC grade 4 [55]. Kim reports on 27 patients undergoing sural nerve grafting with lengths ranging from 2.5 to 14 cm with variable results in motor recovery ranging from MRC grade 2 to 4 by 2 years postoperatively [45]. In this study, functional outcomes were not correlated with nerve graft lengths and may be more influenced by the mechanism and time from initial injury [45].

10.2.2.4 Nerve Transfers

Nerve transfer techniques have been described in small case series to reinnervate the quadriceps using motor donors from the obturator nerve when a proximal nerve stump is not available [56–59]. The anterior branch of the obturator nerve to gracilis can be transferred to the rectus femoris and vastus medialis branches [57]. A variation of this technique involves transfer of the nerve to the tensor fascia lata to the vastus medialis in addition to transfer of anterior obturator branch to the rectus femoris [57]. Tung describes outcomes of one patient undergoing each procedure with MRC grade 4 hip flexion and knee extension using the first technique and MRC grade 4+ hip flexion and knee extension with the second technique [57]. Rastrelli describes one case with anterior obturator nerve transfer following a femoral defect from tumor resection with MRC grade 2 recovery after 1 year [58]. Dubois describes a single case with transfer of the motor branch to gracilis and adductor longus and MRC grade 4 recovery of knee extension at 34 months [59].

10.2.2.5 Surgical Approach

Exploration, decompression, or grafting of the femoral nerve can be performed through a preexisting incision if it will allow for adequate exposure or through a longitudinal incision starting proximal to the inguinal ligament and extending through the femoral triangle with a Z-incision across the inguinal crease. Dissection through the iliacus fascia will reveal the femoral nerve, and neurolysis can be performed after protecting the femoral artery and vein. If more proximal exposure is necessary, then a combined femoral triangle and retroperitoneal approach is required. The incision extends proximally across the inguinal ligament curving laterally toward the flank. The inguinal ligament is divided across the nerve and the external oblique, internal oblique and transversalis fascia is incised to enter the retroperitoneal space.

10.2.3 Lateral Femoral Cutaneous Nerve

The term "meralgia paresthetica" was coined by Roth in 1895, originating from the Greek words for "thigh" and "pain," and describes dysesthesias or anesthesia in the LFCN distribution [60]. Sigmund Freud, interestingly, published a description of bilateral meralgia paresthetica in himself in that same year [61].

LFCN neuropathy can result from compression from obesity, pregnancy, seat belt use, prolonged sitting or squatting, and trauma [62]. Sports-related causes of meralgia paresthetica include gymnasts from repetitive trauma from the uneven bar and scuba divers from compression from their weight belt [63]. The high degree of variability in LFCN branching patterns and exit point from the pelvis places it especially at risk for iatrogenic injury with reported rates ranging widely from 2% to 81% [27, 64]. This can include sharp injury or transection and traction or compression injury from retraction. The LFCN is especially at risk during the ilioinguinal approach for anterior column pelvic fractures or osteotomy, direct anterior approach for total hip arthroplasty, iliac crest bone graft harvest, inguinal herniorrhaphy, and appendectomy [65]. The LFCN may also be injured or compressed within its intrapelvic course from retroperitoneal or uterine masses, appendiceal abscesses, and laparoscopic surgery [60, 66].

Patients with meralgia paresthetica experience pain, dysesthesia, paresthesia, or anesthesia in the LFCN distribution over the anterolateral thigh. Symptoms may be exacerbated with walking or standing in some patients, and with sitting and squatting in others. Patients may also have a distinct Tinel's sign at a site of entrapment which most commonly occurs at the point where the LFNC exits the pelvis. Here, it is frequently found in a narrow space deep to the inextensible inguinal ligament and medial to the ASIS.

The diagnosis is made predominantly based on clinical exam and predictable response to nerve blocks. Lumbar radiculopathy, lumbar facet joint pain, and spondylolisthesis should be ruled out as possible differential diagnoses. As the LFCN is a purely sensory nerve, there should not be any accompanying motor deficits, lumbar pain, or tenderness over the sciatic notch. Nerve conduction studies are difficult to perform given the anatomic variation within the nerve, and only 26% of patients with meralgia paresthetica show slowed sensory conduction [67, 68]. EMG findings do not correlate highly with the severity of symptoms, and can also remain normal despite debilitating symptoms [69]. Directed LFCN nerve blocks are helpful in confirming the diagnosis and to rule out more proximal sources of pain originating from the lumbar roots or aberrant anatomy with genitofemoral or ilioinguinal contributions to LFCN.

Patients should initially be managed conservatively with oral or topical analgesics, nonsteroidal anti-inflammatory medications, activity modification such as avoidance of prolonged sitting, encouragement of weight loss, and local anesthetic or corticosteroid injections [70]. A vast majority of patients will have significant improvement in symptoms with time. Of patients with LFCN injury from a direct anterior approach for THA, Ozaki reports that 96% had spontaneous improvement of their symptoms at an average of 26 months follow-up, which also correlated with improved quality of life scores [71]. In another study, Patton shows 89% resolution of symptoms at 6–8 years following LFCN injury from THA [28].

Patients who fail conservative therapy and have a considerable response to targeted nerve blocks may be considered for surgery. Surgical treatment for idiopathic meralgia paresthetica includes neurolysis and decompression or neurectomy [70, 72–74]. Successful decompression necessitates careful division of all potential constriction points including the inguinal ligament, arcuate fibers of the iliac fascia, and fascia bands of the musculotendinous sartorius origin which lies *deep* to the nerve [70, 73–75]. Fascial bands superficial and overlying the LFCN are almost always released during decompression; however, exploration deep to the nerve is not always undertaken and these remaining fascial bands can result in failed decompression and recurrent symptoms [70, 72]. Neurectomy is most often performed after failed decompression, rather than as an index operation [70, 73]; however, some authors still advocate for primary neurectomy [76, 77].

For patients with LFCN neuropathy following prior hip or abdominal surgery, exploration can be performed through the previous incision if adequate exposure is possible. Depending on the intraoperative findings, neurolysis can be performed if the nerve is tethered by scar, mesh, or suture material. Neurectomy can also be performed if a neuroma is identified, provided the patient is aware and accepting of the resulting permanent anesthesia.

10.2.3.1 Surgical Approach

LFCN decompression is performed through a 5–7 cm incision parallel to and along the inferior margin of the inguinal ligament centered over the ASIS. If the patient has an incision from previous surgery that allows adequate access, this can alternatively be used. Due to the variable location of the LFCN, care should be taken when dissecting through subcutaneous tissues and deep fascia. The LFCN lies within a fascial tunnel which is more easily identified and dissected from a distal to proximal direction. Once identified, the fascial tunnel should be fully released on the superficial surface of the nerve including the tendinous arcuate fibers of the iliac fascia and deep to the nerve along the deep fascia of the thigh. At the level of the ASIS deep to the nerve, there is a tight fascia band formed by the musculotendinous origin of the sartorius which should be incised over sartorius. This fascial band is not commonly described and should be identified in each case [70]. Proximally, the inferior portion of the inguinal ligament is released. The thigh is then brought into full flexion, extension, and abduction to identify any further points of compression. Any remaining tight fascial bands are incised.

10.2.3.2 Clinical Outcomes

The results of LFCN neurolysis and decompression are generally favorable with 77–100% of patients experiencing significant relief [69, 70, 78, 79]. Siu reports 93% of patients with significant pain relief following decompression at 4.1-year follow-up, with no recurrences or re-operations [70]. In this cohort of 42 patients, multivariate analysis did not show any correlation of symptom duration with surgical outcome. This is in contrast to other studies reporting poorer outcomes with increased duration of symptoms. Benezis reports 85% recovery with surgery within 6 months, 65% within 6–12 months, and only 55% recovery if surgery is greater than 1 year after symptom onset [69]. Patients with idiopathic causes of LFCN neuropathy had a higher incidence of recovery following surgery (84%) compared to patients with iatrogenic injury from previous hip surgery (55–62.5%) [69]. Patients with a BMI greater than 30, however, have a six-time increased risk of incomplete relief following surgery [70]. Obese patients may have a combined traction and compression type injury [70, 80]. The weight of a large abdominal pannus places traction on Scarpa's fascia, the inguinal ligament, and the LFCN, in addition to exerting a compressive force. Thus, neurolysis and decompression alone may not completely alleviate the tractional source of nerve irritation.

Studies comparing results of decompression and neurectomy are conflicting and limited to small sample sizes. In de Ruiter's series of 22 consecutive patients, 93.3% (14 of 15 patients) experienced pain relief following neurectomy compared to 37.5% (3 of 8 patients) with decompression [76]. Benezis' series of 167 patients demonstrate the opposite with 78% (119 of 153 patients) improvement following decompression and 35% (5 of 14 patients) with neurectomy. These variable results may be influenced by differing surgical techniques for decompression and criteria for patient selection. Accurate diagnosis, aided by targeted nerve blocks, is important to rule out genitofemoral or ilioinguinal contributions to a patients' pain in order to ensure success following either decompression or neurectomy.

10.2.4 Obturator Nerve

Idiopathic obturator neuralgia is rare and described in case reports as resulting from compression within the obturator canal [81]. This has been described in pregnancy with increasing intra-abdominal pressures and in high-level athletes with groin pain and weakness following intense exercise [82, 83]. Within its intrapelvic course, the nerve is also susceptible to compression from pelvis fractures, pelvic hematomas, retroperitoneal masses, and obturator hernias [83]. Acetabular fractures with more than 24 mm of medial displacement of the quadrilateral plate and anterior wall and column comminution are associated with high incidence of obturator nerve injury. Iatrogenic injury of the obturator nerve has been reported in total hip arthroplasty, pelvic tumor exenteration and pelvic lymph node dissections, and trans-obturator sling procedures. Nerve injury in THA can result from improper retractor placement, intrapelvic penetration while drilling anchoring holes, and extrusion of bone cement [84, 85]. Patients with weak bony acetabular substance are especially at risk as bone cement can extrude during press-fitting of the polyethylene cup [85].

Patients with obturator neuropathy present predominantly with sensory symptoms without significant motor weakness, due to the common dual innervation of the pectineus and adductor magnus from the femoral and sciatic nerves, respectively. Patients may have a positive Howship-Romberg sign with pain in the medial thigh and knee, exacerbated by hip extension, abduction, external rotation, and weight-bearing on the affected side [86]. Patients may also describe a deep aching pain at the adductor origin at the public tubercle radiating to the medial thigh and knee. With severe injuries, loss of motor strength in adduction an internal rotation may present as abnormal gait pattern with outward movement of the leg during the swing phase.

The diagnosis is made based on clinical examination, EMG studies, and response to targeted nerve blocks. EMG studies may show selective denervation of the hip adductors and help to exclude a more proximal lesion. CT-guided targeted nerve blocks of the obturator canal are helpful to confirm the diagnosis. Due to its proximity and often overlapping sensory distribution, pudendal neuralgia should be ruled out with targeted nerve blocks in Alcock's pudendal nerve canal.

10.2.4.1 Treatment

The treatment of obturator neuropathy is guided by the nature of the injury. Urgent surgical exploration should be performed in the case of identifiable reversible causes of nerve compression such as postoperative hematoma or cement extrusion following THA. Iatrogenic sharp transection of the nerve should be immediately repaired to avoid the need for interposition grafting. If the nerve is in discontinuity with a gap, then multiple autologous sural nerve graft cables can be used [87]. Use of the ipsilateral genitofemoral nerve as an interposition graft has also been described in case reports for obturator nerve repair [88].

For patients with idiopathic obturator neuralgia, the initial management is conservative with physical therapy, to aid in adductor strengthening, and multi-modal pain management, including targeted nerve blocks. If the patient has good response to nerve blocks, then neurolysis or neurectomy can be performed through either a laparoscopic or open approach. Commonly, the nerve is compressed within the obturator canal. Tipton describes the thick fascia overlying the adductor brevis muscle as another point of compression that requires release [89].

In cases of delayed identification or traction injuries, conservative management can be initiated, and EMG studies performed at 4–6 weeks to determine the potential of spontaneous recovery. Surgical exploration should be performed if there is no improvement clinically or on EMG studies by 6 months. The use of intraoperative nerve action potentials (NAPs) can aid in decision-making. The presence of intact NAPs is predictive of good functional recovery with decompression and neurolysis alone. If the nerve is found to be in discontinuity, then either direct repair, if possible, or autologous interposition cable grafting should be performed. Nerve transfer techniques for obturator neuropathy have been described in one case study with transfer of the branch to vastus medialis to the obturator nerve at 7 months post-injury resulting in return of MRC grade 5 function at 1 year [90].

Due to the rarity of obturator neuropathy, treatment outcomes are limited to small case series. Generally, results are favorable with the majority of patients finding resolution of sensory symptoms and regaining at least MRC Grade 3 thigh adduction strength [91].

10.2.4.2 Surgical Approach

The obturator nerve can be accessed through a transabdominal, inguinal, extraperitoneal, or laparoscopic approach depending on surgeon expertise and the exposure required. The transabdominal approach allows for visualization of the nerve from the psoas to the obturator foramen. In the inguinal approach, an oblique incision is made at the inguinal crease and the nerve first identified within the obturator canal and then traced proximally. The extraperitoneal approach allows access to the intrapelvic portion of the obturator nerve after division of the external and internal oblique muscles.

10.2.5 Sciatic Nerve

Sciatic nerve injury proximal to the innervation of the hamstrings is severely debilitating, resulting in the loss of knee flexion and a flail foot. Injury distal to the hamstring innervation results in preserved knee flexion but still necessitates the use of an ankle foot orthoses. Patients also lose protective plantar sensation resulting in high risk of infection, chronic wounds, and significant morbidity.

The incidence of sciatic nerve injury after primary THA through a posterior approach is 0.17% [92]; however, this increases up to 7.6% in revision surgery. Iatrogenic injury during surgery can result from direct trauma, thermal damage, retractor placement, leg lengthening, cement extrusion, postoperative hematoma, femoral stem perforation, and use of trochanteric wires [93–95]. During the posterior approach, the sciatic nerve moves in closer proximity to the femoral neck with increasing hip flexion. The sciatic nerve lies 3.61 cm, 2.88 cm, and 1.91 cm to the femoral at 30°, 60°, and 90° of hip flexion, respectively [96]. Nerve injury has also been reported following both-column acetabular fractures, with the nerve entrapped within the posterior column, and after closed reduction of a dislocated total hip arthroplasty, with the nerve entrapped over the femoral neck stem [95, 97].

Sciatic nerve entrapment and compression under an intact "gluteal sling" during THA has also been implicated as a possible cause of postoperative neuropathy. The deep fibers of the inferior portion of the gluteus maximus inserts into the gluteal tuberosity of the femur forming a "sling." Hip flexion and internal rotation during the posterior approach for THA can result in tightening of the gluteal sling, compressing the sciatic nerve against the ischial tuberosity [98]. Hurd demonstrated MRI evidence of focal sciatic nerve compression between the distal tip of the ischial tuberosity and gluteus maximus femoral insertion in two cases of patients with postoperative sciatic nerve palsy following THA [99]. Biomechanical studies support this with pressures on the sciatic nerve reaching critical levels during acetabular exposure when the gluteal sling was left intact, but decreasing to below threshold levels after release [100]. This has led some to advocate for release of at least two-thirds of the gluteal sling during the posterior approach for THA [98–100].

10.2.5.1 Treatment

Treatment of sciatic nerve palsy is based on the mechanism and nature of the injury. Urgent surgical exploration should be undertaken in the case of an identifiable reversible cause, such as contact with implants, cement extrusion, or postoperative hematoma. Sciatic nerve palsy from a postoperative hematoma may present in a delayed fashion and has been reported to occur up to 18 days postoperatively [101]. Immediate decompression following diagnosis is ideal, as delayed decompression more than 12 h after symptom onset is associated with persistent sensory and motor deficits [101–103].

In cases of suspect sharp laceration, immediate primary repair should be performed when possible to avoid the necessity of cable grafting. If there is any concern for tension across the nerve coaptation, cabled nerve autograft reconstruction is utilized. For patients with a suspected traction injury, initial EMG studies are performed 4–6 weeks after injury. Early conservative management involves physiotherapy to maintain full passive range motion, the use of ankle-foot orthoses and assistive walking devices, and observation for spontaneous recovery. Surgical exploration should be performed if there is no improvement clinically or on EMG studies by 6 months.

Intraoperatively, the presence of intact NAPs is predictive of good functional recovery with decompression and neurolysis alone [104]. A review of 46 patients with sciatic nerve injury following THA shows significant reduction in pain by the visual analogue scale following exploration and neurolysis [105]. Following neurolysis, better recovery is seen in the tibial division compared to the peroneal division. Kim reports on eight patients undergoing neurolysis for sciatic nerve dysfunction following THA. All patients had intact NAPs intraoperatively and 75% regained MRC Grade 3 or better function in the tibial division, whereas only 25% recovered functional recovery in the peroneal division [104].

If the nerve is found to be in discontinuity or there is an absence of NAPs intraoperatively, then the zone of injury must be delineated with careful intrafascicular dissection until healthy fascicles. Either direct repair, if possible, or autologous interposition cable grafting should be performed. Following end-to end repair, 73% of patients with buttock-level lesions and 93% with thigh-level lesions achieved MRC Grade 3 or higher function in the tibial division, compared to 30% and 69% in the peroneal division, respectively [104]. Outcomes were slightly worse following graft repair ranging from 6 to 10 cm; 62% of patients with buttock-level and 80% of thigh-level lesions achieved MRC Grade 3 or better function in the tibial division and 24% and 45% in the peroneal division, respectively [104]. Recovery in the tibial division also occurred earlier starting at 12 months postoperatively, compared to 18 months in the peroneal division [104].

10.2.5.2 Surgical Approach

The proximal sciatic nerve can be approached with the patient positioned prone and through a curvilinear incision starting at the posterior inferior iliac spine, curving laterally, and then extending in the midline of the posterior thigh. If a limited approach is sufficient, then the incision may be placed within the gluteal crease for a more aesthetic scar.

Following the skin incision, the gluteus maximus muscle is detached laterally, leaving a 2–3 cm cuff of muscle for later repair. Alternatively, the gluteus maximus tendon can be reattached using suture anchors. The gluteus maximus is then retracted superomedially and blunt dissection performed to expose the sciatic nerve. From here neurolysis can proceed proximally toward the sciatic notch while protecting the hamstring, posterior femoral cutaneous branches, and superior and inferior gluteal nerves and arteries. Proceeding distally, neurolysis can be performed as the sciatic nerve divisions traverse under or through the piriformis. If distal exposure is required, then the incision can be extended toward the popliteal fossa. The hamstrings can then be split in the midline and the long head of the biceps femoris retracted to expose the sciatic nerve distally.

References

1. Judet R, Judet J, Letournel E. Fractures of the acetabulum: classification and surgical approaches for open reduction. Preliminary report. J Bone Joint Surg Am. 1964;46:1615–46.
2. Letournel E. The treatment of acetabular fractures through the ilioinguinal approach. In: Clinical orthopaedics and related research. Philadelphia: Lippincott; 1993. p. 62–76.
3. de Ridder VA, de Lange S, Popta JV. Anatomical variations of the lateral femoral cutaneous nerve and the consequences for surgery. J Orthop Trauma [Internet]. 1999;13(3):207–11. Available from: http://www.ncbi.nlm.nih.gov/pubmed/10206253.
4. Helfet DL, Schmeling GJ. Management of complex acetabular fractures through single nonextensile exposures. Clin Orthop Relat Res [Internet]. 1994;(305):58–68. Available from: http://www.ncbi.nlm.nih.gov/pubmed/8050248.
5. Mayo KA. Open reduction and internal fixation of fractures of the acetabulum: results in 163 fractures. In: Clinical orthopaedics and related research. Springer New York LLC; 1994. p. 31–7.
6. Høgh J, Macnicol MF. The Chiari pelvic osteotomy. A long-term review of clinical and radiographic results. J Bone Joint Surg Br [Internet]. 1987;69(3):365–73. Available from: http://www.ncbi.nlm.nih.gov/pubmed/3584186.
7. Aszmann OC, Dellon ES, Dellon AL. Anatomical course of the lateral femoral cutaneous nerve and its susceptibility to compression and injury. Plast Reconstr Surg [Internet]. 1997;100(3):600–4. Available from: http://www.ncbi.nlm.nih.gov/pubmed/9283556.
8. den Brave PS, Vas Nunes SE, Bronkhorst MWGA. Anatomical variations of the lateral femoral cutaneous nerve and iatrogenic injury after

autologous bone grafting from the iliac crest. J Orthop Trauma [Internet]. 2015;29(12):549–53. Available from: http://www.ncbi.nlm.nih.gov/pubmed/26595594.
9. Tomaszewski KA, Popieluszko P, Henry BM, Roy J, Sanna B, Kijek MR, et al. The surgical anatomy of the lateral femoral cutaneous nerve in the inguinal region: a meta-analysis. Hernia [Internet]. 2016;20(5):649–57. Available from: http://www.ncbi.nlm.nih.gov/pubmed/27115766.
10. Anloague PA, Huijbregts P. Anatomical variations of the lumbar plexus: a descriptive anatomy study with proposed clinical implications. J Man Manip Ther [Internet]. 2009;17(4):e107–14. Available from: http://www.ncbi.nlm.nih.gov/pubmed/20140146.
11. Sürücü HS, Tanyeli E, Sargon MF, Karahan ST. An anatomic study of the lateral femoral cutaneous nerve. Surg Radiol Anat [Internet]. 1997;19(5):307–10. Available from: http://www.ncbi.nlm.nih.gov/pubmed/9413078.
12. Astik RB, Dave UH. Anatomical variations in formation and branching pattern of the femoral nerve in iliac fossa: a study in 64 human lumbar plexuses. Peoples J Sci Res. 2011;4(2):14–9.
13. Anagnostopoulou S, Kostopanagiotou G, Paraskeuopoulos T, Chantzi C, Lolis E, Saranteas T. Anatomic variations of the obturator nerve in the inguinal region: implications in conventional and ultrasound regional anesthesia techniques. Reg Anesth Pain Med [Internet]. 2009;34(1):33–9. Available from: http://www.ncbi.nlm.nih.gov/pubmed/19258986.
14. Darmanis S, Lewis A, Mansoor A, Bircher M. Corona mortis: an anatomical study with clinical implications in approaches to the pelvis and acetabulum. Clin Anat [Internet]. 2007;20(4):433–9. Available from: http://www.ncbi.nlm.nih.gov/pubmed/16944498.
15. Rives J, Stoppa R, Fortesa L, Nicaise H. Dacron patches and their place in surgery of groin hernia. 65 cases collected from a complete series of 274 hernia operations. Ann Chir [Internet]. 1968;22(3):159–71. Available from: http://www.ncbi.nlm.nih.gov/pubmed/4247384.
16. Stoppa RE, Rives JL, Warlaumont CR, Palot JP, Verhaeghe PJ, Delattre JF. The use of Dacron in the repair of hernias of the groin. Surg Clin North Am [Internet]. 1984;64(2):269–85. Available from: http://www.ncbi.nlm.nih.gov/pubmed/6233733.
17. Hirvensalo E, Lindahl J, Kiljunen V. Modified and new approaches for pelvic and acetabular surgery. Injury [Internet]. 2007;38(4):431–41. Available from: http://www.ncbi.nlm.nih.gov/pubmed/17445529.
18. Cole JD, Bolhofner BR. Acetabular fracture fixation via a modified stoppa limited intrapelvic approach: description of operative technique and preliminary treatment results. In: Clinical orthopaedics and related research. Springer New York LLC; 1994. p. 112–23.
19. Karunakar MA, Le TT, Bosse MJ. The modified ilioinguinal approach. J Orthop Trauma [Internet]. 2004;18(6):379–83. Available from: http://www.ncbi.nlm.nih.gov/pubmed/15213504.
20. Güvençer M, Iyem C, Akyer P, Tetik S, Naderi S. Variations in the high division of the sciatic nerve and relationship between the sciatic nerve and the piriformis. Turk Neurosurg [Internet]. 2009;19(2):139–44. Available from: http://www.ncbi.nlm.nih.gov/pubmed/19431123.
21. Beaton LE, Anson BJ. The relation of the sciatic nerve and of its subdivisions to the piriformis muscle. Anat Rec. 1937;70(1):1–5.
22. Patel S, Shah M, Vora R, Zalawadia A, Rathod SP, Patel SM. A variation in the high division of the sciatic nerve and its relation with piriformis muscle. Natl J Med Res. 2011;1(2):27–30.
23. Smoll NR. Variations of the piriformis and sciatic nerve with clinical consequence: a review. Clin Anat [Internet]. 2010;23(1):8–17. Available from: http://www.ncbi.nlm.nih.gov/pubmed/19998490.
24. Rachbauer F, Kain MSH, Leunig M. The history of the anterior approach to the hip. Orthop Clin North Am [Internet]. 2009;40(3):311–20. Available from: http://www.ncbi.nlm.nih.gov/pubmed/19576398.
25. Smith-Petersen MN. A new supra-articular subperiosteal approach to the hip joint. J Bone Joint Surg Am. 1917;s2-15(8):592–5.
26. Smith-Petersen MN. Approach to and exposure of the hip joint for mold arthroplasty. J Bone Joint Surg Am. 1949;31A(1):40–6.
27. Goulding K, Beaule PE, Kim PRFA. Incidence of lateral femoral cutaneous nerve neuropraxia after anterior approach hip arthroplasty. Clin Orthop Relat Res. 2010;468(9):2397–404.
28. Patton RS, Runner RP, Lyons RJ, Bradbury TL. Clinical outcomes of patients with lateral femoral cutaneous nerve injury after direct anterior total hip arthroplasty. J Arthroplast. 2018;33(9):2919–2926.e1.
29. Rudin D, Manestar M, Ullrich O, Erhardt J, Grob K. The anatomical course of the lateral femoral cutaneous nerve with special attention to the anterior approach to the hip joint. J Bone Joint Surg Am [Internet]. 2016;98(7):561–7. Available from: http://www.ncbi.nlm.nih.gov/pubmed/27053584.
30. Ropars M, Morandi X, Huten D, Thomazeau H, Berton E, Darnault P. Anatomical study of the lateral femoral cutaneous nerve with special reference to minimally invasive anterior approach for total hip replacement. Surg Radiol Anat. 2009;31(3):199–204.
31. Perry CP. Peripheral neuropathies and pelvic pain: diagnosis and management. Clin Obstet Gynecol. 2003;46(4):789–96.
32. Viswanathan A, Kim DH, Reid N, Kline DG. Surgical management of the pelvic plexus and lower abdominal nerves. Neurosurgery. 2009;65(4):44–51.
33. Knockaert DC, Boonen AL, Bruyninckx FL, Bobbaers HJ. Electromyographic findings in ilioinguinal-iliohypogastric nerve entrapment syndrome. Acta Clin Belg. 1996;52(3):156–60.

34. Poh F, Xi Y, Rozen S, Scott K, et al. Role of MR neurography in groin and genital pain: ilioinguinal, iliohypogastric, and genitofemoral neuralgia. Am J Roentgenol. 2019;212(3):632–43.
35. Kim DH, Murovic JA, Tiel RL, Kline D. Surgical management of 33 ilioinguinal and iliohypogastric neuralgias. J Neurosurg. 2005;56(5):1013–20.
36. Lee CH, Dellon AL. Surgical management of groin pain of neural origin. J Am Coll Surg. 1997;7515:137–42.
37. Kopell HP, Thompson WA, Postel A. Entrapment neuropathy of the ilioinguinal nerve. N Engl J Med. 1962;266:16–9.
38. Harms BA, DeHaas DR, Starling JR. Diagnosis and Management of Genitofemoral Neuralgia. Arch Surg. 1984;119(3):339–341. https://doi.org/10.1001/archsurg.1984.01390150071017.
39. Kim JE, Lee SG, Kim EJ, Min BW, Ban JS, Lee JH. Ultrasound-guided lateral femoral cutaneous nerve block in meralgia paresthetica. Korean J Pain. 2011;24(2):115–8.
40. Magee RK. Genitofemoral causalgia: a new syndrome. Can Med Assoc J. 1942;46(4):326–9.
41. Lyon EK. Genitofemoral causalgia. Can Med Assoc J. 1945;53(3):213–6.
42. Murovic J, Kim D, Tiel R, Kline D. Surgical management of 10 genitofemoral neuralgias at the Louisiana State University Health Sciences Center. Neurosurgery. 2005;56(2):298–303.
43. Verstraelen H, De Zutter E, De Muynck M. Genitofemoral neuralgia: adding to the burden of chronic vulvar pain. J Pain Res. 2015;8:845–9.
44. Starling JR, Harms BA. Diagnosis and treatment of genitofemoral and ilioinguinal neuralgia. World J Surg. 1989;9:586–91.
45. Orleans N, Population P. Intrapelvic and thigh-level femoral nerve lesions: management and outcomes in 119 surgically treated cases. J Neurosurg. 2004;100:989–96.
46. Fleischman AN, Rothman RH, Parvizi J. Femoral nerve palsy following total hip arthroplasty: incidence and course of recovery. J Arthroplast. 2018;33(4):1194–9.
47. Simmons C Jr, Izant TH, Rothman RH, Booth RE Jr, Balderston R. Femoral neuropathy following total hip arthroplasty. Anatomic study, case reports, and literature review. J Arthroplast. 1991;6:S57–66.
48. Amstutz HC, Ma SM, Jumah RHML. Revision of aseptic loose total hip arthroplasties. Clin Orthop Relat Res. 1982;170:21–32.
49. Andreani L, Nucci AM, Giuntoli M, et al. Compressive femoral neuropathy associated with iliopsoas hematoma complicating hip hemiarthroplasty: a case report. J Orthop Case Rep. 2017;7(5):3–6.
50. Yoshino K, Nakamura J, Hagiwara S, Suzuki T, Kawasaki Y, Ohtori S. Anatomical implications regarding femoral nerve palsy during a direct anterior approach to total hip arthroplasty. J Bone Joint Surg Am. 2020;102(2):137–42.
51. Mcconaghie FA, Payne AP. The role of retraction in direct nerve injury in total hip replacement: an anatomical study. Bone Joint Res. 2014;3(6):212–6.
52. Slater N, Singh R, Senasinghe N, Gore R, Goroszeniuk T, James D. Pressure monitoring of the femoral nerve during total hip replacement: an explanation for iatropathic palsy. J R Coll Surg Edinb. 2000;45(4):231–3.
53. Hoshino C, Koga D, Koyano G, Yamauchi Y. Femoral nerve palsy following primary total hip arthroplasty with the direct anterior approach. PLoS One. 2019;14(5):1–12.
54. Kim D, Murovic JA, Tiel RL, Kline D. Intrapelvic and thigh-level femoral nerve lesions: management and outcomes in 119 surgically treated cases. J Neurosurg. 2004;100:989–96.
55. Tshuchihara T, Nemoto K, Arino H, Amako M, Murakami H, Yoshizumi Y. Sural nerve grafting for long defects of the femoral nerve after resection of a retroperitoneal tumour. J Bone Joint Surg Br. 2008;90B(8):1097–100.
56. Moore AM. Nerve transfers to restore upper extremity function: a paradigm shift. Front Neurol. 2015;5:40.
57. Tung T, Chao A, Moore A. Obturator nerve transfer for femoral nerve reconstruction: anatomic study and clinical application. Plast Reconstr Surg. 2012;130(5):1066–74.
58. Rastrelli M, Tocco-tussardi I, Tropea S, Riccardo C, Rizzato S, Vindigni V. CASE REPORT – OPEN ACCESS International Journal of Surgery Case Reports. Transfer of the anterior branch of the obturator nerve for femoral nerve reconstruction and preservation of motor function: a case report. Int J Surg Case Rep. 2018;51:58–61.
59. Dubois E, Popescu IA, Sturbois Nachef N, Teboul F, Goubier JN. Repair of the femoral nerve by two motor branches of the obturator nerve: a case report. Microsurgery. 2020;40(3):387–90.
60. Lee FC. Meralgia paresthetica. Int Clin. 1936;1:210.
61. Schiller F. Sigmund Freud's meralgia paresthetica. Neurology. 1985;35(4):557–8.
62. Williams PH, Trzil K. Management of meralgia paresthetica. Neurosurgery. 1991;74:76.
63. McCrory P, Bell S. Nerve entrapment syndromes as a cause of pain in the hip, groin, and buttock. Sports Med. 1992;27:261–74.
64. Restrepo C, Parvizi J, Pour AE, Hozack W. Prospective randomized study of two surgical approaches for total hip arthroplasty. J Arthroplast. 2010;25(5):671–9.
65. Sugano M, Nakamura J, Hagiwara S, Suzuki T, Nakajima T, Orita S, et al. Anatomical course of the lateral femoral cutaneous nerve with special reference to the direct anterior approach to total hip arthroplasty. Mod Rheumatol. 2020;30(4):752–7.

66. Pecina M, Kimpotic-Nemanic J, Markiewitz A. Tunnel syndromes. CRC Press; 1991. p. 105–11.
67. Sarala PK, Nishihara T, Oh S. Meralgia paresthetica: electrophysiologic study. Arch Phys Med Rehabil. 1979;60:30.
68. Tataroglu C, Coban A, Sair A, Kızilay Z. Inguinal segmental nerve conduction of the lateral femoral cutaneous nerve in healthy controls and in patients with meralgia paresthetica. J Clin Neurosci. 2019;67:40–5.
69. Benezis I, Boutaud B, Leclerc J, Fabre T, Durandeau A. Lateral femoral cutaneous neuropathy and its surgical treatment: a report of 167 cases. Muscle Nerve. 2007;36:659–63.
70. Siu TLT, Chandran KN, Ed F, Eng F. Neurolysis for meralgia paresthetica: an operative series of 45 cases. Surg Neurol. 2005;63:19–23.
71. Ozaki Y, Homma Y, Baba T, Sano K, Desroches A, Kaneko K. Spontaneous healing of lateral femoral cutaneous nerve injury and improved quality of life after total hip arthroplasty via a direct anterior approach. J Orthop Surg (Hong Kong). 2017;25(1):1–7.
72. Hanna A. Transposition of the lateral femoral cutaneous nerve. J Neurosurg. 2019;130:496–501.
73. Malessy MJA, Eekhof J, Pondaag W. Dynamic decompression of the lateral femoral cutaneous nerve to treat meralgia paresthetica: technique and results. J Neurosurg. 2018:1–9. https://doi.org/10.3171/2018.9.JNS182004.
74. Sugawara A, Isu T, Morita A. Deep decompression of the lateral femoral cutaneous nerve under local anesthesia. World Neurosurg. 2018;118:e659–65.
75. Mowlavi A, Schall J, Wilhelmi BJ. Extensor hallucis longus tenorrhaphy by using the Massachusetts General Hospital repair. J Foot Ankle Surg. 2004;43(6):412–8.
76. de Ruiter G, Kloet A. Comparison of effectiveness of different surgical treatments for meralgia paresthetica: results of a prospective observational study and protocol for a randomized controlled trial. Clin Neurol Neurosurg. 2015;134:7–11.
77. van Eerten PV, Polder TW, Broere C. Operative treatment of meralgia paresthetica: transection versus neurolysis. Neurosurgery. 1995;37:63–5.
78. Ducic I, Ph D, Dellon AL, Taylor NS. Decompression of the lateral femoral cutaneous nerve in the treatment of meralgia paresthetica. J Reconstr Microsurg. 2006;22(2):113–8.
79. Nahabedian MY, Dellon AL. Meralgia paresthetica: etiology, diagnosis, and outcome of surgical decompression. Ann Plast Surg. 1995;35:590–4.
80. de Ruiter GCW, et al. Histopathologic changes inside the lateral femoral cutaneous nerve obtained from patients with persistent symptoms of meralgia paresthetica. Acta Neurochir (Wien). 2019;161(2):263–9.
81. Rigaud J, Labat JJ, Riant T, Bouchot O, Robert R. Obturator nerve entrapment: diagnosis and laparoscopic treatment. Neurosurgery. 2007;61:E175.
82. Nogajski JH, Shnier RC, Zagami AS. Postpartum obturator neuropathy. Neurology. 2004;63(12):2451–2451.
83. Bradshaw C, McCrory P. Obturator nerve entrapment. Clin J Sport Med. 1997;7(3):217–9.
84. Pec M. Case report. Surgical treatment of obturator nerve palsy resulting from extrapelvic extrusion of cement during total hip arthroplasty. J Arthroplast. 2001;16(4):515–7.
85. Zwolak P, Eysel P, Michael JW. Femoral and obturator nerves palsy caused by pelvic cement extrusion after hip arthroplasty. Orthop Rev (Pavia). 2011;3:24–5.
86. Vasilev SA. Obturator nerve injury: a review of management options. Gynecol Oncol. 1994;53(2):152–5.
87. Dias AR Jr, Silva A, Carvalho JP, Baracat EC, Favero G. Correction of iatrogenic injury of the obturator nerve during pelvic laparoscopic lymphadenectomy by the use of sural nerve grafts. Gynecol Oncol Rep. 2014;10:16–8.
88. Scaletta G, Bizzarri N, Lauretti L, Scambia G, Fagotti A. Obturator nerve regeneration using a genito-femoral graft placed only by fi brin sealant (Tisseel®). Gynecol Oncol. 2019;153(3):703–4.
89. Tipton JS. Obturator neuropathy. Curr Rev Musculoskelet Med. 2008;1(3–4):234–7.
90. Spiliopoulos K, Williams Z. Femoral branch to obturator nerve transfer for restoration of thigh adduction following iatrogenic injury. J Neurosurg. 2011;114(6):1529–33.
91. Kitagawa R, Kim D, Reid N, Kline D. Surgical management of obturator nerve lesions. Neurosurgery. 2009;65(4):24–8.
92. Farrell CM, Springer BD, Haidukewych GJ, Morrey BF. Motor nerve palsy following primary total hip arthroplasty. J Bone Joint Surg Am. 2005;87:2619–25.
93. Colegate-Stone TJ, Hussain S. Iatrogenic sciatic nerve palsy following hemiarthroplasty of the hip. Eur J Trauma Emerg Surg. 2008;34(2):2007–8.
94. Yacoubian SV, Sah AP, Estok DM II. Incidence of sciatic nerve palsy after revision hip arthroplasty through a posterior approach. J Arthroplast. 2010;25(1):31–4.
95. Dunbar RP, Gardner MJ, Cunningham B, Routt MLC. Sciatic nerve entrapment in associated both-column acetabular fractures: a report of 2 cases and review of the literature. J Orthop Trauma. 2009;23:80–3.
96. Kanawati AJ, Facchetti G, Smith A, Stewart F. The change in position of the sciatic nerve during the posterior approach to the hip. Bone Joint J. 2015;97-B(8):1056–62.
97. Maeder B, Goetti P, Mahlouly J, et al. Entrapment of the sciatic nerve over the femoral neck stem after closed reduction of a dislocated total hip arthroplasty. J Am Acad Orthop Surg Glob Res Rev. 2019;3(2):e081.

98. Isik C, Apaydin N, Acar HI, Zahar A, Bozkurt M. The gluteal sling: an anatomical study. Surg Radiol Anat. 2014;36(6):595–9.
99. Hurd JL, Potter HG, Dua V, Ranawat C. Sciatic nerve palsy after primary total hip arthroplasty: a new perspective. J Arthroplast. 2006;21(6):796–802.
100. Gay DP, Desser DR, Parks BG, Boucher HR. Sciatic nerve injury in total hip resurfacing: a biomechanical analysis. J Arthroplast. 2010;25(8):1295–300.
101. Austin MS, Kelin GR, Sharkey PF, Hozack WJ, Rothman R. Late sciatic nerve palsy caused by hematoma after primary total hip arthroplasty. J Arthroplast. 2004;19(6):790–2.
102. Beksac BP, Della Valle AG, Salvati EA. Acute sciatic nerve palsy as a delayed complication of low-molecular-weight heparin prophylaxis after total hip arthroplasty. Am J Orthop (Belle Mead NJ). 2009;38(2):E28–30.
103. Sorenson JV, Christensen K. Wound hematoma induced sciatic nerve palsy after total hip arthroplasty. J Arthroplast. 1992;7(4):551.
104. Kim DH, Murovic JA, Tiel R, Kline DG. Management and outcomes in 353 surgically treated sciatic nerve lesions. J Neurosurg. 2004;101(1):8–17.
105. Kyriacou S, Pastides PS, Jeyaseelan L, Sinisi M, Fox M. Exploration and neurolysis for the treatment of neuropathic pain in patients with a sciatic nerve palsy after total hip replacement. Bone Joint J. 2013;95-B:20–2.

Nerve Injury After Total Hip Arthroplasty

11

Steve Key, John Skinner, and Tom Quick

11.1 Introduction

Whilst the mechanism(s) and associated cellular and tissue pathology of nerve injury following hip arthroplasty are well understood, this knowledge has failed to translate into any clear clinical protocol. Although the reported rate of nerve injury is relatively low (ranging 0.17–3.7% during primary hip arthroplasty [1, 2] for primary cases, rising to 7.5% in revision surgery [3]), there is a growing burden of disease given the increasing utilisation of total hip arthroplasty [4, 5]. The impact is always prolonged (1 year or more), and in 80% of cases, it creates permanent impairment and thus a growing prevalence [4, 6, 7].

Iatropathic injuries in the upper limb attract much interest, and in most experts' hands attract a high rate of intervention which is often associated with high rates of functional recovery. Outcomes from lower limb injuries are often poor, with very few cases seeming to produce satisfactory outcomes with or without surgery. We believe that the reasons driving this discrepancy are complex and multifactorial:

- In the lower limb, there is a need for strong muscular function is necessary to enable gait.
- In the setting of THA, the injuries are proximally located and severe in nature, leaving the difficult challenge of substantial lengths of neural regeneration at a location that is far from the end-target.
- Currently available imaging modalities do not consistently provide assessments with diagnostic clarity and prognostic information.
- The mechanism of injury is often clouded in the routine of frequent elective surgery: 'I don't know what I did different this time, I've done thousands of these and this is the first nerve injury I've noticed'. Consequently, assessment turns into repeated watchful waiting with an atavistic urge quite out of kilter with modern medicine, that 'things will just get better', and then a delayed referral, often after a point where intervention may have been helpful.

The common presentation in nerve injury is a loss of motor and sensory function in the nerve territory, with or without pain. Sensory reduction alone is not commonly reported as a major patient concern, but sympathetic dysfunction can often

Supplementary Information The online version of this chapter (https://doi.org/10.1007/978-3-030-84428-8_11) contains supplementary material, which is available to authorized users.

S. Key · J. Skinner
Joint Replacement Unit, Royal National Orthopaedic Hospital, Stanmore, UK
e-mail: john.skinner@ucl.ac.uk

T. Quick (✉)
Peripheral Nerve Injury Unit, Royal National Orthopaedic Hospital, Stanmore, UK

Centre for Nerve Engineering, University College London, London, UK
e-mail: tom.quick@nhs.net

C. J. Dy et al. (eds.), *Peripheral Nerve Issues after Orthopedic Surgery*,
https://doi.org/10.1007/978-3-030-84428-8_11

produce a concerning dryness, cracked skin, and propensity to infection. The presence of neuropathic pain in any nerve injury worsens outcome and is a major factor in the received history which would prompt a clear indication for intervention. Although the vast majority of the literature does not collectively consider all aspects of assessment of nerve injury (motor, sensory, autonomic, and pain), all are pertinent to function. A limb with good motor recovery but persisting severe pain will be as much of a limitation to the patient's engagement and participation as a completely insensate leg with functioning motor, or an entirely flail leg.

In addition to the purely neurologic aspects of the injury, individual patient personality characteristics contribute substantially to both subjective and objective outcomes after nerve injury [8]. These patient characteristics may play an even larger role within the context of sustaining of a nerve injury after elective THA. The relative ubiquity of THA has led to a perception of it being a 'low risk' operation with high rates of success in providing functional improvement and pain relief. Thus, the difference between the outcome that patients expect and the actual outcome received is substantial if a severe nerve injury occurs [9]. This must be addressed and the peripheral nerve surgeon must be aware of this burden, which can be a block to treatment and recovery. Trust must be re-established and this relies on timely assessment and a clear plan. Being realistic about the expected outcome and likely range of possibilities is important, and a team approach is necessary to establish realistic expectations and optimise chances of success.

This chapter reviews the background of the problem for nerve injuries following hip arthroplasty and discusses mechanisms of injury and their implications for treatment, the possible application of current imaging and neurophysiology to inform diagnosis, and the possibilities for the future. A systematic review carried out by De Fine et al. in 2017 [10] ascertained (1) the influence of leg length, (2) the risk factors, (3) prognosis, and (4) treatments. They state:

> The existing literature about this fundamental topic is contrasting and confusing, and many concerns remain about risk factors, treatment, and prognosis of post-arthroplasty sciatic nerve injuries.

This, sadly, is the state of the literature in this field; there is much expert opinion concerning this pathology from anecdotal experience and extrapolating from knowledge of assessment and treatment of nerve injuries in other anatomic areas and sustained through differing mechanisms. These aspects will be explored.

An overview of the literature is presented, not because there is a body of data which assists the clinician with their individual case but quite the opposite: the lack of such data highlights the challenges faced by us all in deciding on a diagnosis, appreciating the likely natural history, and deciding if intervention will improve upon this after weighing the implications of possible complications and likely outcome in each individual case. In the face of this uncertainty, we present our opinion on a method for management, admitting freely that we have not (yet) attempted to produce robust prospective data in this field to support these recommendations. Recognising that there is a range of opinion, we provide what we feel is a reasoned argument for this approach.

11.2 Background

The challenge in a nerve injury sustained at the hip is analogous to an injury to the ulnar nerve above the elbow; conduction block injuries have some potential for recovery but a degenerative lesion will be unable to regenerate the distance to its intended target muscles before becoming recalcitrant to reinnervation. The results of any major degenerative lesion (Sunderland II–V) are likely to be poor.

Injuries to the sciatic nerve account for the majority of clinically apparent nerve injuries sustained as a result of hip arthroplasty, possibly as many as 90% [4]. The femoral nerve has been reported to account for 2.3% of all hip arthroplasty-related nerve injuries [11]. The superior gluteal nerve has a high rate of electrophysiologically detected injury [12], but this does not correlate with the clinical findings as approximately 2/3 of such patients will have a negative Trendelenburg sign, while a positive Trendelenburg sign has multiple possible causes and may be seen in roughly 25% of patients without nerve injury [13]. Injury to the lateral femoral cutaneous nerve may be seen after direct anterior approaches, with a recent meta-analysis estimating this incidence as 2.8% [14], which is in line with reports of rates of other nerve injuries after posterior approaches. The incidence appears unrelated to the use of bikini or longitudinal incisions [15, 16] but is higher with smaller femoral offset [17] and does decrease with greater surgeon experience [18–20]. Moreover, as a purely sensory nerve, its impact is often limited [21], although painful neuromas can occur. Obturator nerve injury may be seen in any approach but is the rare subject of case reports, its true incidence being largely unknown.

Multiple risk factors for nerve injury after THA have been proposed. It is generally accepted that revision surgery and more complex reconstructions, such as dysplasia or post-trauma, are higher risk [1]. This may be due to scarring from previous injury/surgery, the need for more forceful retraction or the distorted underlying anatomy. While lengthening, such as may occur during arthroplasty for a dysplastic hip, certainly plays a role in nerve injury [22], it is far from the only cause in such cases. A correlation with the difficulty of the procedure, rather than lengthening, is well established [23]. A recent New York Statewide database analysis of 207,981 primary hip arthroplasties identified younger age, coexisting spinal stenosis, and females as higher risk, in line with existing literature [5]. Various reasons for these observations have been proposed, including an association with dysplasia in females and younger patients, generally shorter stature of females, and possibly the need for more forceful retraction in more muscular younger patients. An association with chronic anaemia and diabetes is thought to be related to an underlying predisposition to nerve injury at the cellular level. A correlation with post-operative anaemia and thromboembolic events may be related to the use of anticoagulation and the increased risk of haematoma formation.

Numerous mechanisms of nerve injury following hip arthroplasty have been described, although in many cases the exact cause remains uncertain [4, 24–26]. Recognised causes of direct intra-operative trauma to the nerve include the following:

- Laceration by scalpels, electrocautery, or drills (Fig. 11.1).
- Compression or laceration by retractors [27] or the implants themselves, including screws, wires, and cables [28–34] (Fig. 11.2).
- Compression or thermal injury due to cement extrusion [35–38] (Fig. 11.3).
- Transneural sutures [39].
- Intraneural injection [40].

Indirect injury, which probably accounts for the majority of the unidentified causes, may occur through compression or traction on the nerve during positioning of the limb [41–43] (Video 11.1), overzealous retraction [44–46], or lengthening [22], and may result from vascular insult to the nerve as well as the mechanical effect on the nerve itself.

In the early post-operative period, compression by haematoma is a well-established cause of nerve injury, and may be related to anticoagulation [47–49]. Haematomas can create an injurious environment around the nerve through

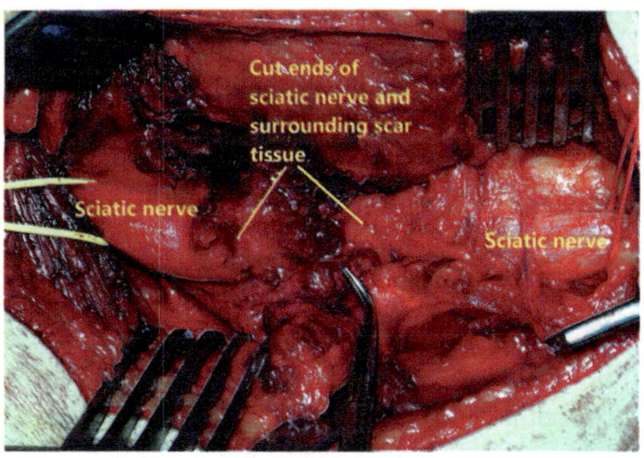

Fig. 11.1 Intra-operative photograph during sciatic nerve exploration showing complete transection of the nerve

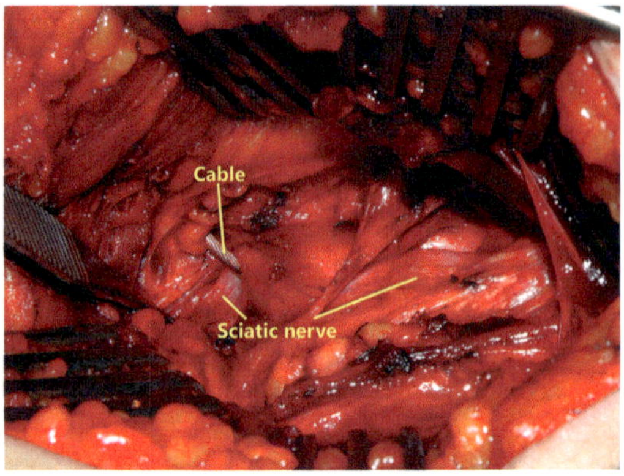

Fig. 11.2 Intra-operative photograph during sciatic nerve exploration showing nerve entrapped beneath cerclage cable

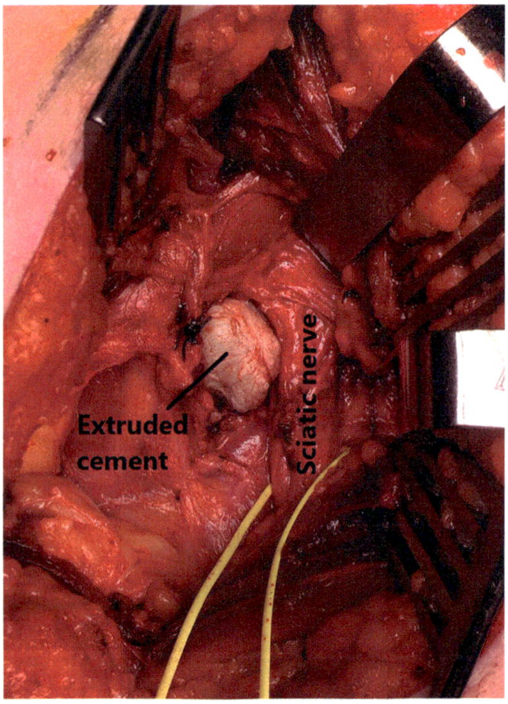

Fig. 11.3 Intra-operative photograph during sciatic nerve exploration showing compression of the nerve by extruded cement

pressure (causing hypoxia), chemical effects of blood breakdown and, over a delayed period, the development of adhesions and contractile scar which affect the nerve and its blood supply. Other documented causes of nerve injury include the effects of wear debris [50–55], bursitis [56], tethering in scar tissue [57], or even entrapment during closed reduction of a dislocated prosthetic hip [58–60].

Although not the primary focus of this chapter, it is worth noting that distant nerve injuries are also described following hip arthroplasty, resulting from patient positioning [61–66], complications of regional anaesthesia [67] or coexisting spinal stenosis [68]. Accordingly, careful positioning, protection and padding of pressure areas, and anaesthetic expertise are important in avoiding such injuries. Rarely, post-operative inflammatory neuropathies have been reported, and neurological advice may be necessary if no other explanation can be found [69–71]. Simply stated 'prevention is better than cure'.

11.3 Anatomy

11.3.1 Sciatic Nerve

The sciatic nerve is formed from the ventral rami of the L4–S3 nerve roots. The posterior divisions form the common peroneal component of the sciatic nerve, while the tibial component arises from the anterior divisions. In approximately 85% of cases, it exits the pelvis as a single nerve through the greater sciatic foramen, anterior to the gluteus maximus and piriformis muscles and courses posterior to the short external rotators of the hip (superior gemellus, obturator internus, and inferior gemelli). However, surgeons should be aware of the multiple variants of the sciatic nerve, both regarding its relationship to piriformis (possibly passing though the muscle or coursing posterior rather than anterior to the muscle) and whether it emerges as a single nerve or in its two components parts [72]. Such variants have been proposed as potential risk factors for traction or compression injuries following piriformis tenotomy during posterior approaches to the hip [73]. Distal to its course along the posterior aspect of the short external rotators, it descends into the posterior thigh between the greater trochanter and ischial tuberosity, remaining deep to gluteus maximus.

The tibial component supplies the hamstring muscles (except for the short head of biceps femoris, which is supplied from the common peroneal) and part of adductor magnus. The division into tibial and common peroneal branches proximal to the knee is highly variable [74]. The tibial nerve continues to supply the muscles of the posterior leg and foot, while the common peroneal, through its deep and superficial branches, supplies the anterior and lateral compartments of the leg, respectively. Cutaneous sensory supply is to the posterior leg and sole of the foot via the tibial nerve, and anterolateral leg and dorsum of the foot through the common peroneal.

The common peroneal component functions primarily to pre-position the foot during the swing phase of gait, enabling the toes and foot to clear the ground and producing eccentric muscle action to control the passive plantar flexion that occurs at initial contact. The tibial component actively plantar-flexes the ankle during terminal stance and toe-off, as well as playing a role in knee flexion and hip extension through the gastrocnemius and hamstrings. Protective sensation to the sole of the foot is also important. The interaction between the two branches balances inversion and eversion, through proprioception and balanced coordinated contraction.

During the posterior approach to the hip, the sciatic nerve is deep to gluteus maximus as it overlies the short external rotators (Fig. 11.4). The peroneal division of the nerve is more laterally positioned and therefore closer to the surgical field during a posterior approach. The peroneal division is more commonly injured during total hip arthroplasty, being involved in 94% of sciatic nerve injuries, while isolated tibial involvement was found in only 2%, in the series published by Schmalzried et al. [4]. In addition to its more lateral position, other proposed factors for the higher risk of peroneal injury rather than tibial include its relatively more tethered location at the fibular neck making it more vulnerable to stretch between the greater sciatic notch and the knee, its superficial location at the fibular neck making it vulnerable to compression injury, and its more tightly packed fascicles with relatively sparse connective tissue affording less protection against injury [75].

The relationship of the sciatic nerve to the hip changes with hip position (Video 11.1). It is closer to both the posterior acetabular wall and femoral neck with increasing flexion [76, 77] but has been shown to be further away following gluteus maximus release during extensile posterior exposures of the hip [76].

Although not directly encountered, the sciatic nerve remains at risk during (antero)lateral and direct anterior approaches to the hip through indirect injury as well as direct injury by, for example, retractors and acetabular screws [78, 79]. Its position within the greater sciatic foramen and adjacent to the posterior acetabulum must therefore be considered during such approaches. Distance from the posterior acetabular rim varies in the region of 1–3 cm and appears

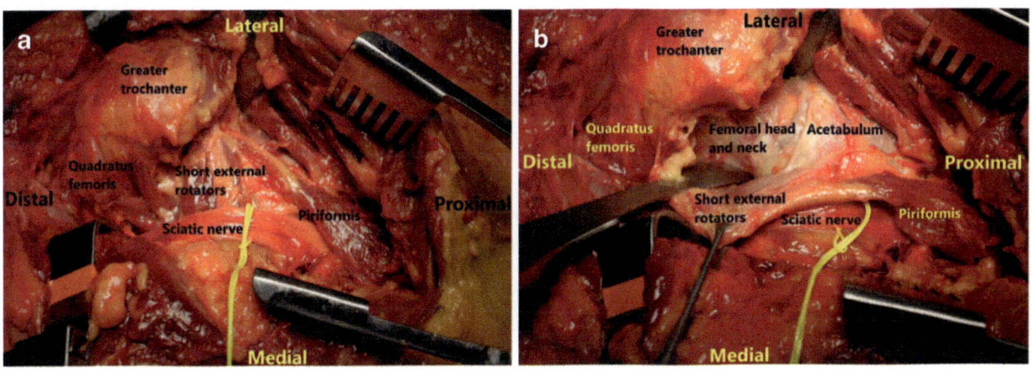

Fig. 11.4 Cadaveric dissection demonstrating posterior approach to the hip. (**a**) The sciatic nerve emerges beneath piriformis and overlies the short external rotators. (**b**) The piriformis, short external rotators, and posterior capsule are reflected medially to expose the hip, and used to provide some protection for the nerve against posteriorly placed retractors

to be related to patient's height. While it is generally closer in women, this seems to be a function of shorter stature rather than an independent predictor of the distance between the nerve and the acetabulum [80].

11.3.2 Superior Gluteal Nerve

The superior gluteal nerve arises from the posterior divisions of the ventral rami of L4, L5, and S1 in the lumbosacral plexus. It exits the pelvis through the greater sciatic foramen, accompanied by the superior gluteal vascular bundle, emerging between the inferior aspect of the gluteus minimus and superior aspect of the piriformis (Fig. 11.5a). It courses superiorly and anteriorly in the plane between gluteus minimus and gluteus medius where it divides into superior and inferior branches [81]. The superior branch supplies gluteus medius and occasionally minimus, the inferior branch supplies gluteus medius, gluteus minimus, and tensor fascia lata [82], although multiple variants of this are described [83]. These muscles are hip abductors, stabilising the pelvis during single leg stance and maintaining the centre of gravity over the base of support by preventing the pelvis from dropping on the contralateral side.

Injury to the superior gluteal nerve is typically considered to be a risk of the direct lateral approach to the hip [75, 84]. Within a 'safe zone' 5 cm proximal to the tip of the greater trochanter [85], it is proposed that gluteus medius and minimus can be safely incised without damage to branches of the superior gluteal nerve (Fig. 11.5b). However, abnormalities of the proximal femur may alter this relationship, and it is recognised that this distance may be affected by the height of the patient [81]. Additionally, the course of the inferior branch has been found to be oblique from posterosuperior to anteroinferior between medius and minimus, such that it is closer to the greater trochanter tip anteriorly than it is posteriorly [86]. Consequently, the safe zone may be considerably less than 5 cm, with branches as close as 2–3 cm being described in some reports [81, 87, 88].

In addition to direct injury during splitting of the medius and minimus, traction injury may occur with excessively forceful retraction of the anterior parts of these muscles [85], or during development of the plane between gluteus medius and tensor fascia lata during an anterolateral approach, resulting in damage to the termination in tensor fascia lata.

Superior gluteal nerve injury is not restricted to the lateral or anterolateral approaches. Electromyographic studies confirm a significant incidence of injury during the posterior approach [12] where the proximal extent of the exposure is limited by the emergence of the superior gluteal

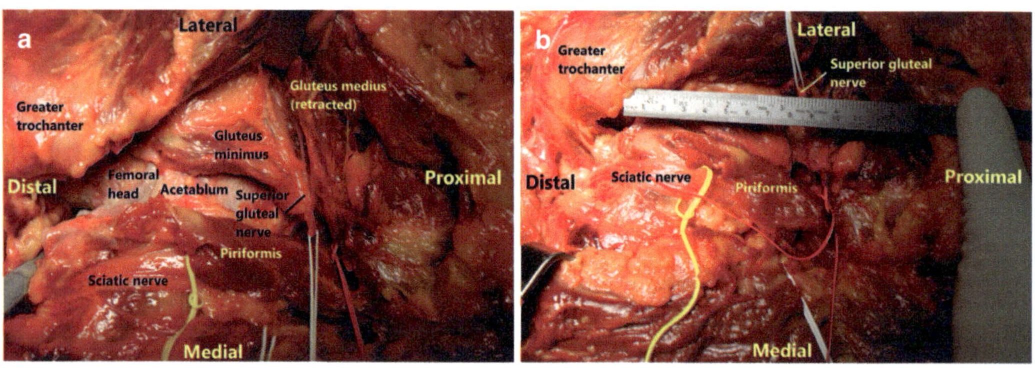

Fig. 11.5 Cadaveric dissection of superior gluteal nerve emerging from greater sciatic foramen between piriformis (released from femur as part of posterior approach to hip) and gluteus minimus to pass anteriorly between gluteus medius and minimus (**a**), and illustrating the safe zone proximal to the greater trochanter (**b**). The red sling is around the superior gluteal artery

nerve through the greater sciatic foramen and its passage between medius and minimus, although this posterior safe zone is greater than that anteriorly [86]. An extensile posterior approach for complex acetabular reconstruction can be performed by mobilising the superior gluteal neurovascular bundle as it emerges from the greater sciatic foramen and elevating both medius and minimus to expose the ilium [89]. In direct anterior exposures, the plane between tensor fascia lata and sartorius is used, so direct injury to the superior gluteal nerve should be prevented [90]. However, entry of branches into the muscle occurs close to the ascending branch of the lateral circumflex femoral artery, and it is proposed that injury may occur during ligation and cautery of that vessel or due to excessive traction on tensor fascia lata [91]; greater tensor fascia lata atrophy has been reported in the direct anterior approach when compared with an anterolateral approach [92].

11.3.3 Femoral Nerve

The femoral nerve is derived from the posterior divisions of the ventral rami of the second to fourth lumbar nerve roots within the lumbar plexus. It forms between the psoas and iliacus muscles, both of which it supplies, before emerging at the lateral border of psoas to descend into the anterior thigh deep to the midpoint of the inguinal ligament, lateral to the femoral artery (Fig. 11.6). It divides into multiple motor branches high within the femoral triangle to supply the quadriceps, sartorius, and pectineus. Cutaneous sensation is supplied to the anterior and medial thigh, and through the saphenous nerve to the medial leg, malleolus, and inner foot.

The direct anterior approach uses the internervous plane between the femoral and superior gluteal nerves [93]. When the appropriate plane is developed, the femoral nerve should not normally be encountered directly. As with other nerves, however, misplaced instruments, implants, or other causes of indirect injury have the potential to produce femoral nerve damage [94], although the actual cause is often unidentified [4]. Due to the proximity of the femoral nerve to the anterior acetabulum as it passes under the inguinal ligament, anterior acetabular retractors have been implicated, regardless of the approach [11, 78, 45, 95] (Fig. 11.7). The femoral nerve is in the region of 1.5–2.5 cm from the anterior acetabular wall [80, 96]; the separation is reduced in shorter individuals [80]. Sullivan et al. [97] demonstrated that the tip of a retractor placed against the superior aspect of the anterior

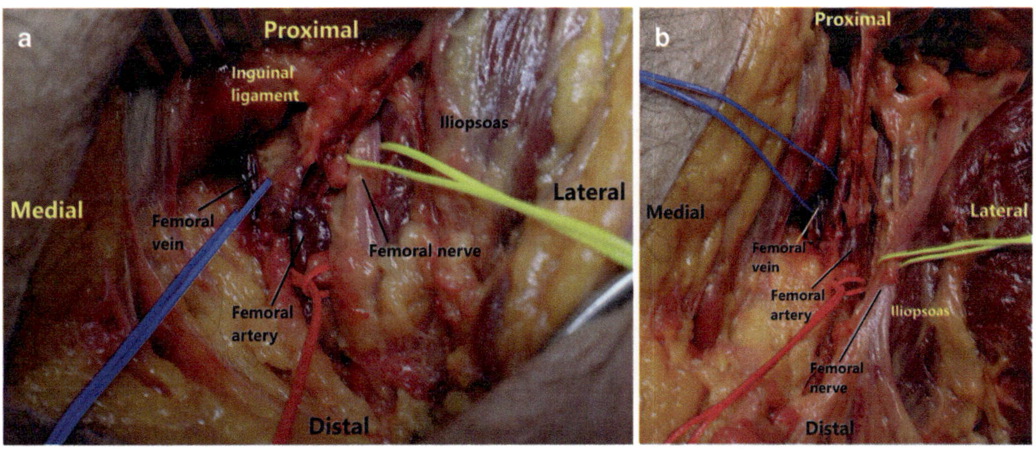

Fig. 11.6 Cadaveric dissection of the femoral triangle. The femoral nerve enters the thigh deep to the inguinal ligament and lateral to the femoral artery (**a**). In (**b**) the inguinal ligament has been released off the anterior superior iliac spine and retracted to illustrate the femoral nerve's passage through the pelvis, while distal extension reveals its terminal branches within the femoral triangle

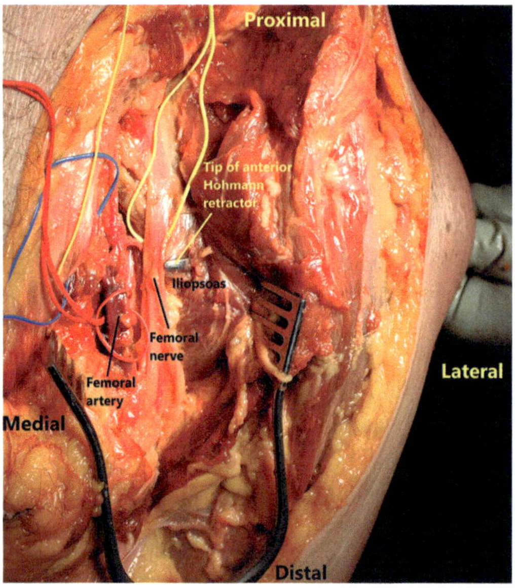

Fig. 11.7 Cadaveric dissection of the femoral triangle (inguinal ligament released and retracted). The tip of an anterior Hohmann retractor, placed inappropriately through the iliopsoas rather than directly against bone, risks compression of the femoral nerve

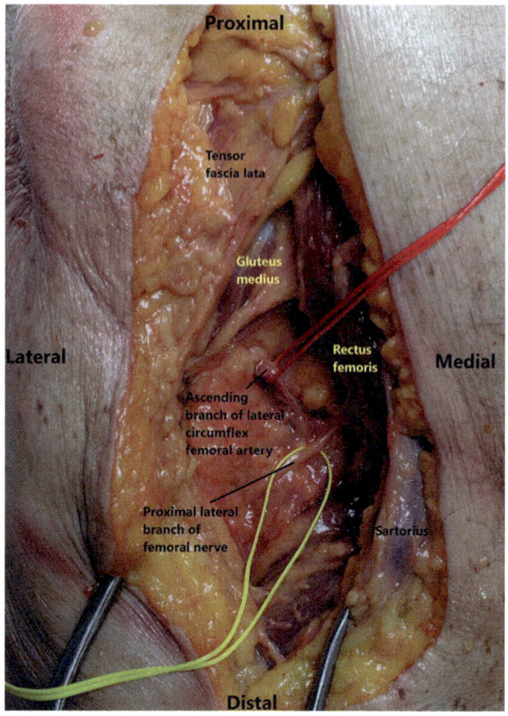

Fig. 11.8 Cadaveric anterior approach to the hip. The proximal of two lateral branches of the femoral nerve, supplying vastus intermedius and lateralis, can be seen emerging from deep to rectus femoris to cross the surgical field, limiting distal extension of the approach

acetabular wall moves from a mean position 2.8 mm lateral to the femoral nerve, to a mean of 4.8 mm medial to it as the retractor is positioned more inferiorly, increasing the potential for the nerve to be compressed by the retractor tip if placed more inferiorly [79, 97]. The iliopsoas is interposed between the acetabulum and femoral nerve and affords some protection, provided retractors are placed directly against the bone. However, loss of contact between the retractor tip and anterior acetabulum again risks entrapment of the nerve [27].

One criticism of the direct anterior approach has been the difficulty of distal extension when greater access to the femur is required. This is due to the threat to anterolateral quadriceps innervation, as branches cross the surgical field deep to rectus femoris to supply the vastus lateralis and vastus intermedius [98] (Fig. 11.8). In cadaveric specimens, two predictable bundles have been demonstrated: a proximal bundle which is a mean of 1.6 cm distal to upper margin of the lesser trochanter with the transverse branch of the lateral femoral circumflex artery (LFCA), and a distal bundle in the region of 3.3 cm distal to the proximal bundle with the descending branch of the LFCA [99]. Attempting to identify and work around these bundles has been proposed as one route to access the femur through a direct anterior approach, but femoral nerve injury and subsequent quadriceps denervation may occur [100].

11.3.4 Lateral Femoral Cutaneous Nerve

Lateral femoral cutaneous nerve injury is well recognised following direct anterior approaches to the hip. It arises from the ventral rami of the second and third lumbar nerve roots, emerging from the lateral border of psoas major proximal to the femoral nerve, before passing over iliacus, and entering the thigh beneath the inguinal liga-

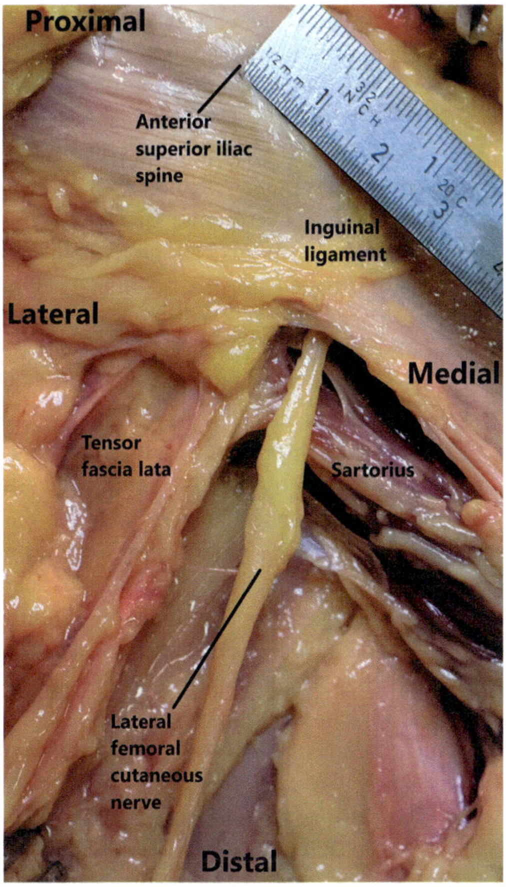

Fig. 11.9 Cadaveric dissection of the lateral femoral cutaneous nerve. It enters the thigh deep to the inguinal ligament and adjacent to the anterior superior iliac spine

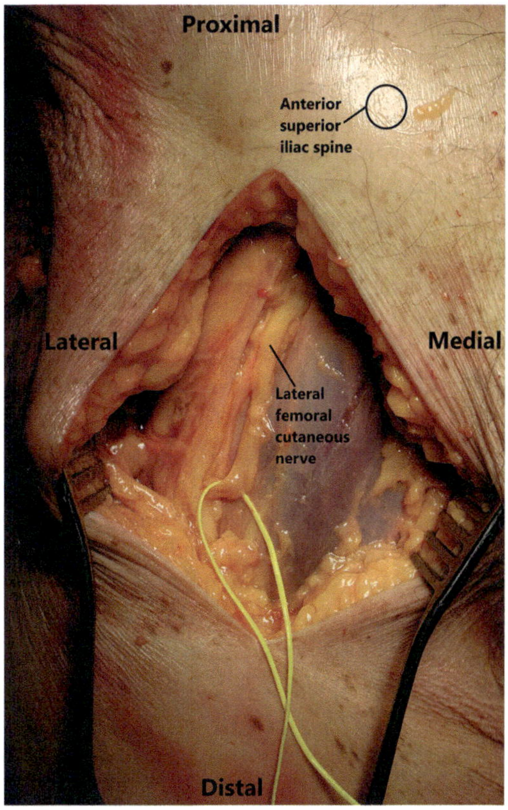

Fig. 11.10 Cadaveric dissection of the lateral femoral cutaneous nerve. Its path in relation to sartorius and tensor fascia lata, and the point at which it pierces the deep fascia, are highly variable

ment adjacent to the anterior superior iliac spine (ASIS) (Fig. 11.9). Two main branches, anterior and posterior, are described, but the precise path, branching pattern, and point at which the deep fascia is pierced are highly variable [101, 102]. It supplies cutaneous sensation to the anterolateral thigh.

The nerve, or its branches, may lie within or cross the plane between tensor fascia lata and sartorius between approximately 3 to 9 cm below the ASIS (Fig. 11.10), and are at risk during development of this plane during the anterior approach [101]. Incision of the deep fascia over the tensor fascia lata, and development of the intermuscular plane from within the fascia, has been described in an effort to reduce the risk to the nerve which classically pierces the deep fascia in a more medial position, through or over sartorius, and can then be retracted medially [103]. Due to the highly variable path of this nerve, however, it may nonetheless be at risk of direct injury despite such measures, or due to indirect injury through excessive traction [101, 104].

11.3.5 Obturator Nerve

The anterior divisions of the second to fourth lumbar ventral rami form the obturator nerve. It descends through the inner fibres of psoas major to emerge from its medial border before passing over the pelvic brim and entering the thigh through the obturator foramen. It has anterior and posterior branches on either side of adductor brevis, respectively. The anterior branch, therefore, lies between adductor brevis posteriorly, and adductor longus and pectineus anteriorly; it supplies brevis, longus, gracilis, and an occasional branch to pectineus, as well as cutaneous innervation to the medial thigh. The posterior branch pierces obturator externus, which it supplies, and lies between adductor brevis anteriorly, and adductor magnus, which it also supplies, posteriorly.

Obturator nerve injuries are rare, but they can occur following medial penetration of the acetabulum [105, 106]. In common with other nerves, retractor placement about the acetabulum is a threat to the obturator nerve. The tip of an inferiorly placed retractor has been found to pierce the obturator externus, internus and obturator membrane, making contact with the intra-pelvic obturator nerve in many cases, though the extra-pelvic anterior and posterior branches were seen not to be in close proximity [27].

11.4 Prevention

As with all nerve injuries, but especially considering the difficulty in managing nerve injuries about the hip, and their limited outcomes, prevention is of paramount importance. The following strategies are proposed:

- Planning – With the aforementioned risk factors in mind, surgeons should recognise cases with a higher risk of nerve injury and discuss with patients during the informed consent process. Intra-operative monitoring may decrease incidence of injury [107, 108], but its use is not widespread. The surgeon should be cognizant of bone defects that may allow cement extrusion, whether occurring pre- or intra-operatively.
- Careful and gentle positioning – Taking care to avoid excessive pressure or tension on nerves throughout the lower limb, including the distal continuations of the peroneal and femoral nerves.
- Sound anatomical knowledge – Although the sciatic nerve is not routinely visualised or palpated during total hip arthroplasty from a posterior approach, the surgeon should be able to expose the nerve if there is a question regarding its safety. Routinely visualising the lateral femoral cutaneous nerve through a direct anterior approach is prudent. In cases where there is a specific concern intra-operatively, for example when using cables or if there is a chance of cement extrusion, additional nerves may also need to be explored. The use of intra-operative nerve stimulation to confirm motor function will also highlight any cases where there has been a change in neurologic status.
- Retractor placement – Careful and accurate placement, directly against bone, coupled with sound anatomical knowledge of the surrounding nerve anatomy and avoiding excessively forceful retraction. If using a Charnley retractor, the posterior blade must be carefully placed onto muscle under direct vision, without applying tension until it is certain the sciatic nerve is not interposed (Fig. 11.11).
- Screw placement – The quadrant system for acetabular screw placement is well established, with the safest zones being postero-superior and postero-inferior [109] (Fig. 11.12). In more complex reconstructions, additional planning may be required given the available bone stock, and this should take account of the surrounding nerve anatomy. 3-D imaging, and possibly custom

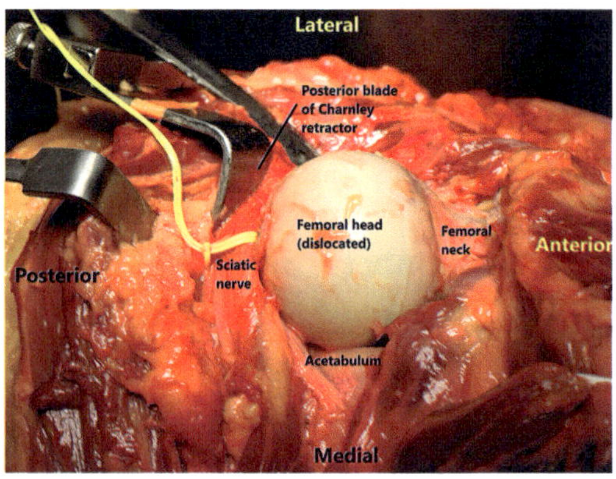

Fig. 11.11 Cadaveric dissection of a posterior approach to the hip. The hip has been dislocated posteriorly. Note the proximity of the sciatic nerve to the posterior blade of the Charnley bow retractor and the femoral head

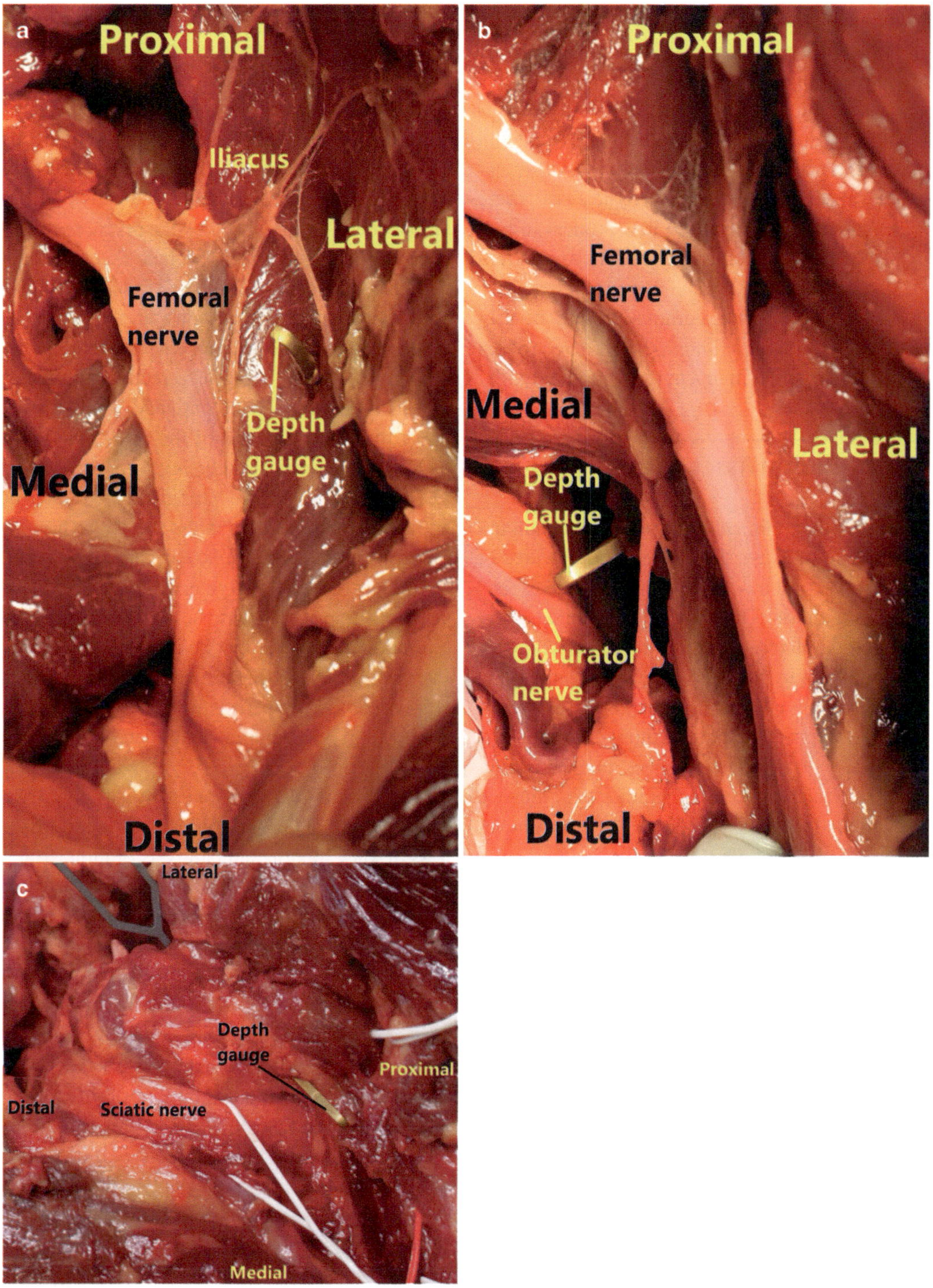

Fig. 11.12 Cadaveric dissection demonstrating risks of misplaced acetabular screws. A depth gauge has been placed in holes drilled in the anterosuperior (**a**) and anteroinferior (**b**) quadrants to illustrate the proximity to the femoral and obturator nerves, as well as the iliac vessels. A posteroinferior screw longer than 20 mm threatens the sciatic nerve (**c**)

implants planned accordingly, may be useful in such cases.

- Lengthening – While it is not possible to give an absolute value for safe lengthening, as it is likely instead to be related to strain, and therefore starting length of the nerve, rather than absolute change [43, 110], in cases where lengthening has occurred it is prudent to palpate the sciatic nerve to check for excess tension. If concern exists then intra-operative monitoring or nerve stimulation may be useful, and the surgeon should be prepared to perform shortening manoeuvres if necessary.

11.5 Clinical Assessment

In assessing the clinical history, it is of paramount importance to *listen*. There are many features of the history which will present themselves and inform diagnosis. The current condition and presenting complaint should be explored with specific attention to pain, movement, sensation, and also sweating and hair growth. Current treatments in terms of therapy, orthoses, medications and other pain therapies (patches, creams, stimulators, alternative medical therapies etc.) must be documented and asked if the patient believes these to be efficacious and in what way.

In the past history, understanding the circumstances leading to THA is important: whether this was considered a standard operation or a difficult procedure, or a revision and if there was any predisposing DDH, known intra-operative complication, problems with anticoagulation, or associated pain, swelling, or infection. Lumbar spine pathology must be noted (with any sciatica, back, or buttock pain documented) and the presence of diabetes and/or smoking confirmed.

Often the most informative period of the history is the patient's first recollections on waking from general anaesthesia or sedation. Many have persistent anaesthesia from regional blockade, but the presence of motor function, paraesthesia, and pain (noting character and distribution) is very informative. Furthermore, the evolution of these signs over the first post-operative day and beyond is also important to note.

Although presence of neuropathic pain in the distribution of that nerve is not accounted for in most of the published literature, we believe it is the most important part of the history and examination. Patients will be very clear on spontaneous and evoked elements of their pain. Evoked pain (allodynia) is pain brought on by touch or stimulation, and is often noticed by the severe pain created by the light touch of bed sheets and is pathognomonic of an ongoing irritation or injury to the nerve. Allodynia demonstrates there is neuronal continuity (some nerves are sensing the touch even if it is being incorrectly interpreted) but also that there is a continued insult to that nerve that is the genesis of the pain. Thus, *in a painful post-operative palsy, exploration must be undertaken*, the nerve explored for any tether or entrapment, and any compressive lesion (haematoma, cement, suture) removed. This exploration can be performed by a general orthopaedic surgeon and does not require the skillset of a peripheral nerve specialist. We believe this is the one intervention that is most likely to provide long-term benefit to the patient as it will arrest further damage to the nerve and deterioration of function.

The aspect of function that is universally assessed in sciatic nerve injury is motor weakness of knee flexion and paralysis of motor function distal to the knee. Sensation can be absent or altered, the skin unity can be affected, and pain can be present and may be severe.

The high steppage slapping gait of a foot drop is easily recognisable, but one should assess the position of the foot in swing, initial contact, and stance. It is useful to evaluate whether the foot is inverted by unopposed tibialis posterior action, whether the peroneus longus and brevus muscles are functioning, or whether there is a concomitant tibial nerve injury paralysing inversion, plantar flexion, or toe gripping.

With the support of a talented orthotist, foot drop can be addressed to lead to little functional loss. The impairment of active dorsiflexion and eversion can be mitigated by a passive or sprung ankle foot orthosis (AFO). A patient who demonstrated an inability to function well with a suitable and well-fitting AFO would raise concerns that the nerve injury extends beyond the peroneal nerve and predicts the likelihood of a poor outcome regardless of intervention.

We prefer to evaluate motor and sensory function using the Louisiana State University system (Tables 11.1 and 11.2), acknowledging that there is no mention of neuropathic pain. We assess muscle wasting in the thigh and calf. Hamstring wasting is consistent with sciatic injury, but quadriceps bulk must also be assessed, being aware that a more proximal or associated lesion may be present in other nerve territories.

Assessment of each muscle group in the lower limb then follows. Motor paralysis is very different from 'weakness': any function, even MRC1/5, is an important finding, as it demonstrates continuity of the nerve to the muscle. A complaint of MRC4/5 is *not* a significant finding in relation to the assessment of a peripheral nerve lesion.

One important competing diagnosis to consider for a common peroneal nerve (CPN) injury is an L5 nerve root lesion. In such a condition, often seen due to para-central L4/5 or far lateral L5/S1 disk herniation, there is loss of tibialis anterior and tibialis posterior with maintained peronei function (S1). The sensory loss for CPN and L5 root dysfunction can easily be confused but often involves the plantar surface of the great toe in an L5 lesion where the loss is restricted to the dorsum of the foot and shin in a CPN. Sciatic stretch tests will be positive in a lumbar spinal pathology as well as peripheral nerve injury.

Physical examination must include assessment of passive range of movement, with particular attention to tightness in the calf muscles and the presence of an equinus/plantar-flexion contracture of the Achilles tendon. If such a flexion contracture has developed, it will make recovery of function substantially more challenging.

It is important to document if the common loss of sensation over the dorsum of the foot is present, requesting that the patient rate it out of 10 (0/10 being no sensation and 10/10 being normal), and recording any descriptors of altered sensation such as 'sharp', 'bright', 'fluffy',

Table 11.1 Louisiana State University Health Sciences Center motor grading system for the buttock and thigh-level tibial divisions [8]

Grade	Evaluation	Description
0	Absent	No gastrocnemius-soleus function; no inversion; no too flexion; little or no sensation on the plantar surface of the foot
1	Poor	Trace gastrocnemius, but no other tibial muscle; trace to poor plantar sensation
2	Fair	Gastrocnemius contracts against gravity only; plantar surface sensation usually grade 2 or better
3	Moderate	Gastrocnemius-soleus contracts against gravity and some force; trace or better inversion; plantar sensation is grade 3 or better
4	Good	Gastrocnemius contracts against moderate resistance; inversion grade 3 or better, either a trace or no toe flexion; sensation grade 4 or better
5	Excellent	Gastrocnemius has full function; inversion grade 4 or better; toe flexion present; plantar sensation grade 4 or better

Table 11.2 Louisiana State University Health Sciences Center motor grading system for the buttock and thigh-level peroneal divisions [8]

Grade	Evaluation	Description
0	Absent	No or little function in the short head of biceps, no peroneal function, no AT, no EHL or ED function
1	Poor	Short head of biceps contracts; no distal peroneal-innervated muscle function
2	Fair	Short head of biceps contracts, peroneus muscles contract against gravity or better, no trace of AT; no other distal motor function
3	Moderate	Short head of biceps contracts, peroneus muscles are grade 3 or better, AT contracts against gravity, but the function of EHL and ED for toes is usually absent
4	Good	Short head of biceps and peroneus muscles contract, as does AT, which is grade 3 or better; EHL and ED may have trace function
5	Excellent	Short head of biceps and peroneus muscles contract, AT grade 4 or better; EHL and ED contract at least against gravity

AT anterior tibialis, *EHL* extensor hallucis longus, *ED* extensor digitorum 'numb', etc. Also, it is important to record any paraesthesiae (strange sensations, tingling, sparkling, etc.) as monitoring changes in the function of these fibres can demonstrate important improvements prior to motor recovery. Sympathetic dysfunction, leading to dry, cracked skin, must be recognised and treated with emollients as cellulitis can easily develop, be missed due to anaesthesia of the skin, and lead to local complications or delay surgery intended to improve outcome.

Non-sciatic lesions may also present with pain. The LFCN is well known and recognised as the clinical entity often called meralgia paraesthetica. Operative neurolysis can provide very good outcomes [111]. However, in an intractably damaged nerve, often neurectomy proximal to the area of injury is the only intervention which may be able to provide relief [112]. Injury to other cutaneous branches of the lumbar plexus (iliohypogastric, ilioinguinal, genitofemoral nerves) can create similar sensory presentations.

Femoral nerve injury leads to a severe limitation of gait function. Hip flexion and knee extension are essential functions to ambulate (along with hip extension via the gluteal nerves). Patients can develop the ability to lock the leg with hyper-extension of the knee through stretching of the posterior capsule. If the knee will not allow the centre of gravity to fall ventral to the centre of rotation of the knee, then gait is very difficult. The sensory pain and sympathetic symptoms affect the anterior thigh and medial lower leg.

Superior gluteal nerve injury presents with hip abductor weakness, leading to the characteristic Trendelenburg gait and positive Trendelenburg test. During single-leg stance, the pelvis is not stabilised and drops down on the contralateral side, with compensatory body sway to the ipsilateral side to maintain the centre of gravity over the base of support. Diagnosis is difficult, however, as there are many causes of abductor insufficiency following hip arthroplasty, there is no sensory loss, and neurophysiological evidence of nerve injury does not correlate with clinical features in many cases, as detailed above [13].

Obturator nerve injury can produce difficulty with gait and the development of an unstable leg in stance. Pain is often described as a deep ache in the region of the adductor origin and may radiate into the medial aspect of the thigh. Numbness over this area is frequently reported. Many patients, however, can mobilise well with no obturator nerve function; the tibial innervated part of adductor magnus, and some adduction also possible through the pectineus form the femoral territory, often compensate.

11.6 Diagnostic Investigations

A plain pelvic radiograph can demonstrate any gross lengthening or misplacement of implants, extruded cement, etc. Ultrasound can demonstrate a deep collection or post-operative haematoma, and can track the sciatic nerve along its length and may identify any nerve entrapment. MRI or CT can demonstrate threatening placement of acetabular screws in the pelvis or any mass lesion around the nerve. Occasionally a nerve tumour may be identified as the underlying cause of ongoing symptoms, brought on by operative intervention stretching the tethered nerve or creating oedema. MRI is also used to assess the lumbar disks for any herniation that may contribute to symptoms.

Electrodiagnostic studies are a tool that, when properly utilised, can provide useful information to differentiate between a conduction block (neurapraxic, Sunderland 1) injury and a degenerative lesion; monitor recovery in the form of re-innervation of sequential muscle groups with serial studies; and assess the presence of concomitant compressive neuropathy. It is important to recognise that neuropathic pain can exist in the face of entirely normal nerve conduction tests and EMGs. This is because signals from the small fibres, whose dysfunction can create the symptoms, are not easily assessed through the strong signals from the large and myelinated fibres.

Intra-operative neurophysiology is a very useful tool to exclude proximal injury (through assessing somatosensory evoked potentials), to aid careful dissection (using stimulation of functioning fibres), and to assess the conduction of the injured segment. Also, assessing a segment of nerve distal to the injury will allow the degree of degeneration from the more proximal lesion to be evaluated.

11.7 Treatment

Following diagnosis, it is essential first to offer any necessary anti-neuropathic analgesia and institute early conservative treatment. Protection against contractures is most effectively undertaken at point of diagnosis: a resting night splint (well-moulded and padded, especially over the anaesthetic areas), physical therapy, and orthoses to improve gait will assist in rehabilitation and maintaining the best environment for any subsequent recovery. Analgesia for any persistent pain will allow elective rehabilitation.

The importance of the interventions of nerve exploration and decompression in a painful palsy cannot be emphasised enough. There are few cases without pain where there is a clear indication for acute treatment. Most pathologies that have an unequivocal indication for intervention create pain, but often this is masked by post-operative epidural/analgesia. Therefore, if there is any suspicion that there is a direct insult to the nerve (e.g. injury from a suture or cable, from herniated cement, from a misplaced bone fragment, acetabular screw, or the rim of an implant), we believe there is a clear indication to re-explore and confirm if the nerve is in continuity and any damage is not ongoing.

11.7.1 Nerve Surgical Techniques

It is known that neurolysis of the sciatic nerve provides a significant possibility for a meaningful reduction in pain [113] even after significant delay since onset (Fig. 11.13). A recent study [114] has shown improvements in motor, sensation, and pain outcomes in 92% of patients who underwent sciatic nerve decompression, as well

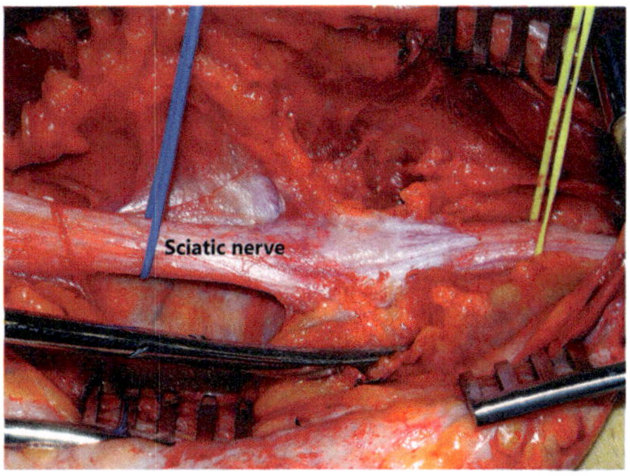

Fig. 11.13 Intra-operative photograph of sciatic neurolysis. The sciatic nerve is in continuity but tethered by adhesions at the injured segment

as improvements in Harris Hip Score, Short Form-36, and UCLA activity scores. It is likely this effect is most efficacious if undertaken early in the presentation. The ability for a nerve injury with a degenerative lesion at the level of the hip to recover function to below the knee is limited, making the aim of intervention to reduce or remove pain by resolving any element of conduction block.

Exposure of the sciatic nerve: We believe that exploration of the sciatic nerve at the site of the injury is foundational to establish diagnosis and prognosis, and also provides an opportunity for definitive intervention. In our practice, the approach to the sciatic nerve is undertaken with the patient comfortably placed prone, with attention to pressure areas, especially those of other peripheral nerves. The patient is prepped and draped with particular caution when extending the hip, so as not to cause a prosthetic dislocation. The bony landmarks of the sacrum, ischium, and posterior aspect of the greater trochanter are marked. The course of the sciatic nerve is then marked and, centred on this line, a trans-gluteal approach incision is marked (Fig. 11.14). This oblique incision is placed across the buttock from supero-medially to infero-laterally. The skin is infiltrated with adrenalised local anaesthetic, and the incision is taken down to fascia over the gluteus maximus without undermining. On incising this fascia, muscle splitting dissection proceeds

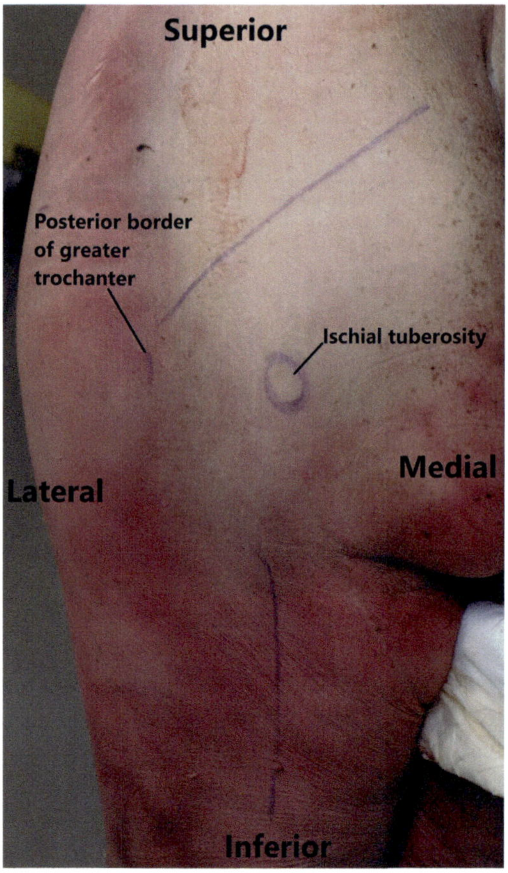

Fig. 11.14 Surface landmarks for sciatic nerve exploration

(not using monopolar cautery due to the strong muscular contractions seen on stimulation), dissecting any neuro-vascular pedicle encountered. A deep self-retaining retractor is inserted, and often a Deaver or other deep angled retractor used at the medial superior aspect of the wound. At this point in the approach, many deep veins are encountered and dissection can be a considerable challenge. It must be noted that significant bleeding can be encountered if dissection is not meticulous, and that, if divided, some of these local vessels can retract into the pelvis through the sciatic notch, and this presents a serious risk of dangerous bleeding. The sciatic nerve can be identified from its exit from the sciatic notch, usually under piriformis, right down to the inferior border of gluteus maximus. Often a second incision in the midline of the thigh is undertaken, running distally from the inferior gluteal crease to expose the nerve more distally or to facilitate delivery of graft (Fig. 11.14). Other approaches described divide the insertion of the gluteus maximus. We would not advocate this approach as it further risks the function of the hip.

Once the sciatic nerve is exposed, the determination is made as to whether the nerve is structurally intact (and scarred at the site of injury) or whether it has been divided. In cases where the nerve is intact, removal of external adhesions is performed to alleviate any potential conduction block pathology. If the nerve is more severely injured with varying degrees of axonopathy (e.g. when the nerve is entrapped at the implant-bone interface, crushed against the bone by cables, or burned by cement to a level of severe scarring) or with complete nerve division, there is nearly no chance of natural recovery, leaving graft reconstruction as the only option. In such cases, depending on cause, the pain is often severe and treated by dissecting the nerve free and excising the damaged segment.

Technical aspects of nerve grafting: Neurolysis of the segment of nerve above and below the point of injury will allow mobilisation of the nerve and a thorough assessment of the zone of injury. A local anaesthetic blockade is then undertaken by bathing the nerve, proximal to the level it will be transected, with plain levobupivacaine. The temptation to use adrenalised solutions to control intraneural vessel bleeding must be resisted (and, instead, addressed through a haemostatic material, application of pressure, or very judicious low voltage bipolar cautery), as we consider direct neural adrenalin is likely to exacerbate or trigger neuropathic pain states. The proximal and distal ends must be transected back to a fascicular structure that looks amenable to grafting.

The nerve gap is then measured in both knee flexion and extension. In paediatric cases and some very select adult patients, one might consider a primary repair if the nerve ends can be approximated under no tension, facilitated by knee flexion. The advantages of this technique are often offset by the problems of rehabilitation in a knee flexion brace and the subsequent stiffness. Nerve grafting can be achieved with cabled autograft (most commonly sural nerve) or allograft of a suitable diameter (commercially available as Avance graft: Axogen Alachua, FL, USA). When using cabled autograft, given the large diameter of the sciatic nerve, bilateral sural nerve harvest is often needed. This brings about the concern that harvested the ipsilateral sural nerve will (A) widen the area of existing sensory loss and (B) lead to the potential development of neuropathic pain in the sural distribution. If nerve allograft is being considered, it should be noted that the current literature does not universally support its use for mixed and motor nerves. Repair with epineural microsuture is undertaken with the leg in neutral hip flexion/extension and full knee extension and ankle dorsiflexion to allow easy rehabilitation.

11.7.2 Treatment of Persistent Foot Drop

The first and most important aspect of treatment is maintaining passive range of movement. Any degree of secondary equinus or equinovarus contracture will contribute significantly to a poor outcome. Thus early recognition of the foot drop, and assessment of the muscle imbalance and any sensory impact of the nerve injury, will allow a regimen of passive stretch, provision of a well-padded orthosis (with regular checks for skin damage if there is sensory disturbance under the splint), and mobilisation in the orthosis (many are available and patients may require one for night resting splintage, and one or two for differing activities when mobilising).

The injury itself must be diagnosed and treated. Neuronal reconstruction at the level of the injury at the hip to restore function is, as has been stated, infrequently successful, and then only in those cases of a majority non-degenerative (majority conduction block) injury. There are, though, often un-recognised injuries from intra-operative compression at more distal levels (commonly the level of the knee or fibular neck) which can be well treated by neurolysis and can demonstrate good results after grafting in the case of an unfavourable degenerative lesion (Sunderland III and IV).

In the case of a degenerative lesion in the upper thigh or at hip level, if there has been little recovery following neurolysis, then nerve transfer can offer a further treatment option. There have been numerous reports of transferring fascicles from the tibial nerve to the CPN to reinnervate the anterior compartment. Often the nerve to tibialis anterior is targeted for a specific nerve transfer [115].

The concerns regarding the outcomes from nerve transfer for this indication are many. The enthusiasm of success from upper limb transfers has not been seen in this application; results are often unimpressive, with reinnervation being documented on electrodiagnostic studies, but often a mismatch with clinical outcome. Furthermore, the nerve transfer is non-synergistic, and much of gait is not cerebral but a spinal level process; therefore, relearning is more challenging than in the upper limb following nerve transfer. Patient selection, pre-habilitation, and rehabilitation are likely highly influential factors when undertaking these procedures.

11.7.3 Salvage Techniques – Tendon Transfer for Foot Drop

While the outcome from tendon transfer surgery depends on a number of factors, a reliable functional result can be obtained in a majority of patients [116, 117].

There are a number or techniques, but most use the tibialis posterior tendon alone and transfer it to the anterior aspect of the foot. In our experience, the following tips have been learned: using tibialis posterior only (provided it has not itself undergone a nerve injury), dissecting a long segment of the muscle belly free to allow increased excursion, and ensuring no kinking or tenting of the tendon in its course. An anterior subcutaneous course avoids the risk of fibrosis and scarring seen in the interosseous route, and has poorer cosmesis as its only disadvantage. Insertion of the transferred tendon not just to the tibialis anterior tendon but also to the tendon of EHL (and perhaps, if enough length is available, to EDL and peroneus tertius too) allows the balance of inversion-eversion to be recreated and also avoids the drawback seen, if the toes are not reanimated, of ankle dorsiflexion creating tenodesis toe flexion, leading to the toes being trodden under the foot when walking without shoes. The Stanmore assessment questionnaire is a useful tool in subjectively and objectively assessing outcome from tendon transfer (Table 11.3) [118, 119].

In a patient placed supine on the operating table, with the ability to rotate the hip freely, incisions are marked over the tibialis posterior (TP) tendon from its insertion onto the navicular up to the level of the inferior border of the gastrocnemius bulk. The heel should be at the end of the bed and a full passive excursion of ankle dorsiflexion is confirmed. A second incision is made transversely at the level of the ankle joint. The TP tendon is dissected from the navicular and freed up to be delivered through the tendon tunnel behind the medial malleolus. Placing a strong monofilament suture through the end of the tendon facilitates its manipulation and passage. When the tendon has been passed proximally, it can be grasped to put tension on the muscle so it may be dissected free from its attachment to bone and septum to allow a significant excursion. One or two motor branches and vessels may be sacrificed at this lower and mid end in order to gain sufficient excursion without adversely affecting the perfusion or innervation significantly. In grasping and manipulating the musculotendinous unit, ensure it is handled cleanly, kept warm and moist, and is not allowed to contact the skin. The senior author favours a subcutaneous passage of the tendon superior to the medial malleolus. This course is dissected and the suture-bearing distal tendon end is then delivered into the anterior wound. The TP tendon is then again protected. It is best to wash and close the medial wound at this stage. The cutaneous nerves and anterior neurovascular bundle are dissected and protected. The TP tendon is then passed through the tibialis anterior (TA) tendon whilst maintaining the ankle in full passive dorsiflexion (a robust and well-fed paunch is an asset in this stage of the operation as the foot can be rested on the surgeon's abdomen). When the tendon has been passed and three sutures placed in mattress orientation across the TA recipient and TP tendon donor with a strong

Table 11.3 Stanmore assessment questionnaire

Pain	(15 points)
Never	15
Occasionally	10
Sometimes	5
Serious pain	0
Need for orthosis	(15 points)
No need	15
Rarely (once a week)	10
Sometimes (twice a week)	5
Frequent (more than twice a week)	0
Ability to wear normal shoes	(5 points)
Yes	5
Only special model	3
No	0
Functions	(10 points)
Normal daily activity and normal recreation	10
Normal daily activity and limited recreation	6
Limited daily activity and limited recreation	3
Seriously limited daily activity and recreation	0
Degree of active dorsiflexion	(25 points)
Grade 4–5	25
Grade 4	20
Grade 3	10
Grade 2 and lower	0
Degree of active dorsiflexion	(25 points)
More than 6°	25
0–5°	20
−5/−1°	10
−10/−6°	0
Less than −11°	25
Foot posture (5 points)	(5 points)
Plantigrade, balanced, no deformity	5
Plantigrade; mild deformity	3
Obvious deformity, misalignment	0
Grading	
100–85 points	Very good
84–70 points	Good
69–55 points	Fair
<55 points	Poor

braided suture (1-0 Ticron Ethilon), the foot can be released and assessed briefly. Balance is then attained by tensioning the extensor hallucis longus tendon with the TP tendon passing through this at a tension that allows the toe to extend passively as the ankle flexes, but not so tight that the toe is 'cocked-up', and sutures again placed. The long lesser toe extensors are next to be traversed by the TP tendon and sutured. Finally, if there is a peroneus tertius, then this may again be used to balance the foot. Often there is then a short length of TP tendon left and this can be folded over the tenorrhaphies and sutured back on to itself. The anterior wound can now be lavaged and haemostasis ensured before closure. A plaster is placed from beyond the knee to beyond the toes with the ankle in neutral or slight dorsiflexion, and the toes in extension. This requires a dorsal slab, stirrups, and toe reinforcement. This can be reinforced with lightweight fibreglass after 48 hours to allow partial weightbearing.

The advantages of tendon transfer are many: it is reliable, creates a balanced active movement of the foot and toes, and can be undertaken at any point following surgery; there is no clinical urgency to complete the surgery, such that full passive range of movement and rehabilitation of other injuries can be undertaken in an AFO prior to committing to the surgery, therefore presenting a patient who is fully pre-treated and 'prehabilitated' for the procedure, ensuring optimal outcomes. It provides function within 6 weeks of the procedure. It does not restore sensation, but nor does motor nerve transfer. Like all surgeries it will be dependent on patient selection and engagement with rehabilitation. Timing of surgery, in our view, should depend on the assessment of the primary injury and the likelihood for recovery along with discussion with the patient. Some have recommended early tendon transfer [119] for the reason that it reduces rates of equinus contracture. We would be reticent to undertake surgery to avoid a complication that is readily avoidable through appropriate nonoperative management in cases where there may be spontaneous recovery. Surgery is not without negative implications: the loss of the donor function can lead to acquired flat foot deformity and the scars around the foot and ankle can be problematic. The risks of infection, deep vein thrombosis, and the chance of failure of tendon transfer can produce a much worse condition than if surgery had not been undertaken.

In femoral palsy, many patients can and do end up developing the compensatory backkneeing which is necessary to mobilise with quadriceps paralysis. For those who cannot mobilise without a brace following rehabilitation for their nerve injury, hamstring transfer [120], which has a long history in poliomyelitis treatment [121], is an effective but disfiguring operation, necessitating long scars, widespread dissection, and significant risks. For this reason, obturator nerve transfer, if indicated, can offer a useful option [122].

11.8 Outcomes

Pritchett et al. [9] reported on public perception on nerve injury following hip arthroplasty and noted that direct and indirect nerve injuries were deemed by patients to violate the expected standard of care according to 17% and 9% of participants, respectively. Importantly, this publication emphasised the necessity of preserving communication in the context of a nerve injury.

Sciatic injuries: Without active management, the outcome from sciatic nerve injury following THA is poor with only 35% [1] to 50% [123] of patients demonstrating recovery without surgical intervention. In those patients who have neuropathic pain following THA with over-lengthening, the intervention of revising the implant can offer improvement both in symptoms of pain and motor dysfunction [22].

Neurolysis of the sciatic nerve following a painful palsy can offer reduction in the patient's pain [113], with enduring improvement at 24 months following surgery [124]. Regev reports that the impact of delay to treatment was a significant negative factor for motor when assessing those treated before and after 12 months [124]. Chughtai et al. [114], in a retrospective assessment of 19 patients who sustained a partial sciatic nerve injury following THA, of whom 12 accepted the offer of surgery to decompress the nerve at a point 12–16 weeks post injury while seven declined surgery, there were significant differences in outcomes for pain, sensation, and motor function. All patients following decompression had demonstrable recovery and only four out of seven of those managed non-operatively demonstrated improvement.

There are no series of outcomes of THA-related damage of the sciatic nerve necessitating primary repair or graft, as this is rarely indicated and reported. However, results from repair or graft following traumatic laceration of the sciatic in the thigh have historically been seen to produce acceptable results, with around a third of cases gaining useful motor recovery and two-thirds good sensory recovery in the CPN division. Much better outcomes are seen in the tibial distribution with up to 80% functional results. It is stated that the trend in this small series was that the more proximal the repair the less satisfactory the result [125]. More recent reports suggest that these historic figures may be improved upon with modern techniques [126]. It must be recognised that these reports relate mainly to lacerations of the nerve and not stretch injuries over the length of the nerve as are seen in the majority of nerve injuries related to THA; any translation of these outcomes must be done with an understanding of the mechanisms involved.

Non-sciatic nerve injuries: The low rate of non-sciatic nerve injuries means that meaningful descriptions of any cohorts are limited. Fleischman et al. [127] reported on a 0.21% incidence of femoral nerve palsy in 17,350 primary total hip replacements, more so in anterior and anterolateral approaches. They found little recovery before 6 months, but by 33 months 75% complete motor recovery and only mild residual weakness in the remaining 25%. Sensory improvement occurred in nearly all, but was complete in less than 20%. In a report of 54 patients treated surgically for persistent complete intra- and extra-pelvic femoral nerve lesions (various causes), 13 were found to have recordable nerve action potentials intra-operatively and recovered to at least grade 3 power following neurolysis alone, while 27 patients had sural graft repairs performed, with graft lengths varying from 2.5 to 14 cm, and most patients had some nerve regeneration and regained function to grade 3–4 levels by 2 years. Four of five patients with suture repairs recovered to grade 3 or better within 2 years [128].

The most common complaint following lateral femoral cutaneous nerve injury is numbness and was found by Patton et al. [129] to improve significantly with time. This is supported by Ozaki et al. [130] who found spontaneous improvement in 96% at 2 years, which was also seen to correlate with improved quality of life. Both decompression (88%) and neurectomy (94%) have been shown to produce good outcomes in the treatment of painful meralgia paraesthetica [131], although neither has shown a definite benefit over the other [132]. Laparoscopic LFCN neurectomy has been performed successfully for meralgia paraesthetica, including following direct anterior hip arthroplasty [133].

11.9 Pearls and Pitfalls

1. Prevention is better than cure.
2. Assess all functions of nerve – motor, touch, sympathetics, and pain.
3. Do not miss the ‘painful palsy’. Urgent surgical exploration should be performed in cases of nerve palsies associated with severe pain.
4. Actively maintain passive range of ankle joint motion with physical therapy and splintage.
5. Consider using electrodiagnostic studies, including distal to the injury, to informed decision-making.
6. Examine and document neurologic function before and after any surgical procedure, and be honest to yourself and your patient if this has changed.
7. Seek expert support, advice, and guidance in the event of a nerve injury, and do so at the earliest opportunity.

Suggested Protocol for Sciatic Nerve Injury (CPN/Total Sciatic)
From the a priori and literature-based discussion, we suggest the following adaptation of our colleagues' recommendations:

Initial clinical review:

- Palsy with neuropathic pain in distribution of the sciatic nerve – operate.
- Neuropathic pain in distribution of the sciatic nerve resistant to anti-neuropathic medication – operate.
- Painless palsy – assess for Tinel along full length of tibial and peroneal divisions, from distal up to level of hip, and accurately document location if present. Obtain MRI of hip (with metal artifact reduction) and lumbar spine; reassess in 6 weeks.
- All of the above cases – arrange for resting splint, give advice about ankle stretches and skin care.

6-week clinical review:

- Ensure no onset of contracture or skin damage in anaesthetic or hypo-aesthetic areas.
- Pain commenced or no longer controlled by anti-neuropathic analgesia – operate.
- No change – order electrodiagnostic studies (with an assessment of distal conduction in SNAP and CMAP distal to the lesion) – if significant conduction block, then operate.

3–6-month review

- Ensure no onset of contracture or skin damage in anaesthetic or hypo-aesthetic areas of skin.
- Pain commenced or no longer controlled by anti-neuropathic analgesia – operate.
- If degenerative lesion and no advancing Tinel – consider nerve transfer. While some surgeons would advocate for a nerve transfer, we do not utilise this procedure due to the concerns described above.

12 months (now little chance of any novel recovery of function)

- Ensure good understanding – functions that are now returned will strengthen and become less fatigable but unlikely any novel function will now accrue.
- If no motor recovery – ensure no onset of contracture or skin damage in anaesthetic or hypo-aesthetic areas of skin.
- Ensure best orthotic support is available and plan to meet in 6/12.
- Ensure understanding around equinus contracture.
- If tibial palsy with recovering CPN, be aware of claw toes – strapping and stretching required to avoid claw deformity.

18–24 months (now no chance of any further recovery in motor, but perhaps in discomfort and sensation)

- If happy with orthosis – discharge.
- If not happy offer tendon transfer:
  - If full CPN palsy with intact tibial – tib post to tib ant and EHL – EDL.
  - If deep peroneal palsy and recovering superficial peroneal – then peroneus longus to tib ant and EHL – EDL.
- If tibial palsy with recovering CPN be aware of claw toes – strapping and stretching required to avoid claw deformity.

References

1. Farrell CM, Springer BD, Haidukewych GJ, Morrey BF. Motor nerve palsy following primary total hip arthroplasty. J Bone Joint Surg Am. 2005;87(12):2619–25.
2. Wilson JN, Scales JT. The Stanmore metal on metal total hip prosthesis using a three pin type cup. A follow-up of 100 arthroplasties over nine years. Clin Orthop Relat Res. 1973;(95):239–49.
3. Amstutz HC, Ma SM, Jumah RH, Mai L. Revision of aseptic loose total hip arthroplasties. Clin Orthop Relat Res. 1982;170:21–32.

4. Schmalzried TP, Amstutz HC, Dorey FJ. Nerve palsy associated with total hip replacement. Risk factors and prognosis. J Bone Joint Surg Am. 1991;73(7):1074–780.
5. Christ AB, Chiu YF, Joseph A, Westrich GH, Lyman S. Risk factors for peripheral nerve injury after 207,000 total hip arthroplasties using a New York state database (Statewide Planning and Research Cooperative System). J Arthroplasty. 2019;34(8):1787–92.
6. Johanson NA, Pellicci PM, Tsairis P, Salvati EA. Nerve injury in total hip arthroplasty. Clin Orthop Relat Res. 1983;(179):214–22.
7. Oldenburg M, Müller RT. The frequency, prognosis and significance of nerve injuries in total hip arthroplasty. Int Orthop. 1997;21(1):1–3.
8. Wilson TJ, Chang KW, Yang LJ. Depression and anxiety in traumatic brachial plexus injury patients are associated with reduced motor outcome after surgical intervention for restoration of elbow flexion. Neurosurgery. 2016;78(6):844–50.
9. Pritchett JW. Public perceptions about nerve injury from hip replacement surgery. J Arthroplasty. 2018;33(4):1200–1204.e1.
10. De Fine M, Romagnoli M, Zaffagnini S, Pignatti G. Sciatic nerve palsy following total hip replacement: are patients personal characteristics more important than limb lengthening? A systematic review. Biomed Res Int. 2017;2017:8361071.
11. Simmons C Jr, Izant TH, Rothman RH, Booth RE Jr, Balderston RA. Femoral neuropathy following total hip arthroplasty. Anatomic study, case reports, and literature review. J Arthroplasty. 1991;6 Suppl:S57–66.
12. Abitbol JJ, Gendron D, Laurin CA, Beaulieu MA. Gluteal nerve damage following total hip arthroplasty. A prospective analysis. J Arthroplasty. 1990;5(4):319–22.
13. Kenny P, O'Brien CP, Synnott K, Walsh MG. Damage to the superior gluteal nerve after two different approaches to the hip. J Bone Joint Surg Br. 1999;81(6):979–81.
14. Lee GC, Marconi D. Complications following direct anterior hip procedures: costs to both patients and surgeons. J Arthroplasty. 2015;30(9 Suppl): 98–101.
15. Lanting BA, Hartley KC, Raffoul AJ, Burkhart TA, Sommerville L, Martin GR, Howard JL, Johnson M. Bikini versus traditional incision direct anterior approach: is there any difference in soft tissue damage? Hip Int. 2017;27(4):397–400.
16. Leunig M, Faas M, von Knoch F, Naal FD. Skin crease 'bikini' incision for anterior approach total hip arthroplasty: surgical technique and preliminary results. Clin Orthop Relat Res. 2013;471(7):2245–52.
17. Ozaki Y, Homma Y, Sano K, Baba T, Ochi H, Desroches A, Matsumoto M, Yuasa T, Kaneko K. Small femoral offset is a risk factor for lateral femoral cutaneous nerve injury during total hip arthroplasty using a direct anterior approach. Orthop Traumatol Surg Res. 2016;102(8):1043–7.
18. York PJ, Logterman SL, Hak DJ, Mavrogenis A, Mauffrey C. Orthopaedic trauma surgeons and direct anterior total hip arthroplasty: evaluation of learning curve at a level I academic institution. Eur J Orthop Surg Traumatol. 2017;27(3):421–4.
19. den Hartog YM, Mathijssen NM, Peters SJ, Vehmeijer SB. The anterior supine intermuscular approach for total hip arthroplasty: reducing the complication rate by improving the procedure. Hip Int. 2015;25(1):28–33.
20. Post ZD, Orozco F, Diaz-Ledezma C, Hozack WJ, Ong A. Direct anterior approach for total hip arthroplasty: indications, technique, and results. J Am Acad Orthop Surg. 2014;22(9):595–603.
21. Homma Y, Baba T, Sano K, Ochi H, Matsumoto M, Kobayashi H, Yuasa T, Maruyama Y, Kaneko K. Lateral femoral cutaneous nerve injury with the direct anterior approach for total hip arthroplasty. Int Orthop. 2016;40(8):1587–93.
22. Pritchett JW. Nerve injury and limb lengthening after hip replacement: treatment by shortening. Clin Orthop Relat Res. 2004;(418):168–71.
23. Eggli S, Hankemayer S, Müller ME. Nerve palsy after leg lengthening in total replacement arthroplasty for developmental dysplasia of the hip. J Bone Joint Surg Br. 1999;81(5):843–5.
24. Birch R, Giddins G. Peripheral nerve injuries. In: Foy F, editor. Medicolegal reporting in orthopaedic trauma. Edinburgh: Churchill Livingstone; 1995.
25. Navarro RA, Schmalzried TP, Amstutz HC, Dorey FJ. Surgical approach and nerve palsy in total hip arthroplasty. J Arthroplasty. 1995;10(1):1–5.
26. Yang IH. Neurovascular injury in hip arthroplasty. Hip Pelvis. 2014;26(2):74–8.
27. McConaghie FA, Payne AP, Kinninmonth AW. The role of retraction in direct nerve injury in total hip replacement: an anatomical study. Bone Joint Res. 2014;3(6):212–6.
28. Nozawa M, Matsuda K, Maezawa K, Kim S, Maeda K, Kaneko K. Delayed sciatic nerve injury by posterior flange of reinforcement ring after acetabular revision surgery. J Arthroplasty. 2013;28(1):197. e5–7.
29. Darmanis S, Pavlakis D, Papanikolaou A, Apergis E. Neurovascular injury during primary total hip arthroplasty caused by a threaded acetabulum cup. J Arthroplasty. 2004;19(4):520–4.
30. Bose WJ, Petty W. Femoral artery and nerve compression by bulk allograft used for acetabular reconstruction. An unreported complication. J Arthroplasty. 1996;11(3):348–50.
31. McLean M. Total hip replacement and sciatic nerve trauma. Orthopedics. 1986;9(8):1121–7.
32. Yoon SJ, Park MS, Matsuda DK, Choi YH. Endoscopic resection of acetabular screw tip to decompress sciatic nerve following total hip arthroplasty. BMC Musculoskelet Disord. 2018;19(1):184.

33. Asnis SE, Hanley S, Shelton PD. Sciatic neuropathy secondary to migration of trochanteric wire following total hip arthroplasty. Clin Orthop Relat Res. 1985;(196):226–8.
34. Mallory TH. Sciatic nerve entrapment secondary to trochanteric wiring following total hip arthroplasty. A case report. Clin Orthop Relat Res. 1983;(180):198–200.
35. Zwolak P, Eysel P, William-Patrick Michael J. Femoral and obturator nerves palsy caused by pelvic cement extrusion after hip arthroplasty. Orthop Rev (Pavia). 2011;3(1):e6.
36. O'Brien S, Bennett D, Blair PH, Beverland DE. Femoral nerve compression after migration of bone cement to the groin after hip arthroplasty. J Arthroplasty. 2011;26(8):1571.e11–3.
37. Jerosch J. Femoral nerve palsy in hip replacement due to pelvic cement extrusion. Arch Orthop Trauma Surg. 2000;120(9):499–501.
38. Birch R, Wilkinson MC, Vijayan KP, Gschmeissner S. Cement burn of the sciatic nerve. J Bone Joint Surg Br. 1992;74(5):731–3.
39. Marchese M, Sinisi M, Anand P, Di Mascio L, Humphrey J. Neuropathic pain following hip resurfacing due to a transneural suture. J Bone Joint Surg Br. 2011;93(4):555–7.
40. Uppal HS, Gwilym SE, Crawfurd EJ, Birch R. Sciatic nerve injury caused by pre-operative intraneural injection of local anaesthetic during total hip replacement. J Bone Joint Surg Br. 2007;89(2):242–3.
41. Hurd JL, Potter HG, Dua V, Ranawat CS. Sciatic nerve palsy after primary total hip arthroplasty: a new perspective. J Arthroplasty. 2006;21(6):796–802.
42. Stone RG, Weeks LE, Hajdu M, Stinchfield FE. Evaluation of sciatic nerve compromise during total hip arthroplasty. Clin Orthop Relat Res. 1985;(201):26–31.
43. Fleming P, Lenehan B, O'Rourke S, McHugh P, Kaar K, McCabe JP. Strain on the human sciatic nerve in vivo during movement of the hip and knee. J Bone Joint Surg Br. 2003;85(3):363–5.
44. Pereles TR, Stuchin SA, Kastenbaum DM, Beric A, Lacagnino G, Kabir H. Surgical maneuvers placing the sciatic nerve at risk during total hip arthroplasty as assessed by somatosensory evoked potential monitoring. J Arthroplasty. 1996;11(4):438–44.
45. Ishimatsu T, Kinoshita K, Nishio J, Tanaka J, Ishii S, Yamamoto T. Motor-evoked potential analysis of femoral nerve status during the direct anterior approach for total hip arthroplasty. J Bone Joint Surg Am. 2018;100(7):572–7.
46. Slater N, Singh R, Senasinghe N, Gore R, Goroszeniuk T, James D. Pressure monitoring of the femoral nerve during total hip replacement: an explanation for iatropathic palsy. J R Coll Surg Edinb. 2000;45(4):231–3.
47. Lachmann M. Lower limb paresis after total hip arthroplasty. A rare differential diagnosis. Orthopade. 2013;42(10):874–8.
48. Fritzsche H, Kirschner S, Hartmann A, Hamann C. Femoral nerve palsy as delayed complication after total hip replacement: delayed hematoma formation in unexpected screw malpositioning. Orthopade. 2013;42(8):651–3.
49. Butt AJ, McCarthy T, Kelly IP, Glynn T, McCoy G. Sciatic nerve palsy secondary to postoperative haematoma in primary total hip replacement. J Bone Joint Surg Br. 2005;87(11):1465–7.
50. Wodowski AJ, Rider CM, Mihalko WM. Local tissue reaction and necrosis-induced femoral nerve palsy in a patient with a metal-on-metal total hip arthroplasty: a case report. J Long-Term Eff Med Implants. 2014;24(1):7–12.
51. Kayani B, Rahman J, Hanna SA, Cannon SR, Aston WJ, Miles J. Delayed sciatic nerve palsy following resurfacing hip arthroplasty caused by metal debris. BMJ Case Rep. 2012;2012:bcr2012006856.
52. Mann BS, Whittingham-Jones PM, Shaerf DA, Nawaz ZS, Harvie P, Hart AJ, Skinner JA. Metal-on-metal bearings, inflammatory pseudotumours and their neurological manifestations. Hip Int. 2012;22(2):129–36.
53. Beaver WB Jr, Fehring TK. Abductor dysfunction and related sciatic nerve palsy, a new complication of metal-on-metal arthroplasty. J Arthroplasty. 2012;27(7):1414.e13–5.
54. Fokter SK, Repse-Fokter A, Takac I. Case report: femoral neuropathy secondary to total hip arthroplasty wear debris. Clin Orthop Relat Res. 2009;467(11):3032–5.
55. Schuh A, Werber S, Zeiler G, Craiovan B. Femoral nerve palsy due to excessive granuloma in aseptic cup loosening in cementless total hip arthroplasty. Zentralbl Chir. 2004;129(5):421–3.
56. Liman J, von Gottberg P, Bähr M, Kermer P. Femoral nerve palsy caused by ileopectineal bursitis after total hip replacement: a case report. J Med Case Rep. 2011;5:190.
57. Wettstein M, Garofalo R, Mouhsine E. Painful total hip replacement due to sciatic nerve entrapment in scar tissue and lipoma. Musculoskelet Surg. 2010;94(2):77–80.
58. Maeder B, Goetti P, Mahlouly J, Mustaki L, Buchegger T, Guyen O. Entrapment of the sciatic nerve over the femoral neck stem after closed reduction of a dislocated total hip arthroplasty. J Am Acad Orthop Surg Glob Res Rev. 2019;3(2):e081.
59. Haque S, Sundararajan S. Entwinement of sciatic nerve around a total hip prosthesis following closed reduction of dislocated total hip replacement. Pol Orthop Traumatol. 2013;78:273–5.
60. Chan JH, Ballal MS, Dheerendra S, Sanchez-Ballester J, Pydisetty RV. Entrapment of the sciatic nerve following closed reduction of a dislocated revision total hip replacement. J Bone Joint Surg Br. 2011;93(2):274–6.
61. Nercessian OA, Macaulay W, Stinchfield FE. Peripheral neuropathies following total hip arthroplasty. J Arthroplasty. 1994;9(6):645–51.

62. Schwarzman G, Schwarzman L, MacGillis K, Chmell S. A case report of a radial nerve palsy following uncomplicated total hip arthroplasty. J Orthop Case Rep. 2018;8(2):107–9.
63. Logroscino G, Del Tedesco F, Cambise C, Coraci D, Donati F, Santilli V, Padua L. Fibular nerve palsy after hip replacement: not only surgeon responsibility. Hereditary neuropathy with liability to pressure palsies (HNPP) a rare cause of nerve liability. Orthop Traumatol Surg Res. 2016;102(4):529–31.
64. Verhagen CV, Verhagen WI, Van Norel GJ. Left recurrent laryngeal palsy after left total hip arthroplasty; stretch injury due to inappropriate positioning in the lateral approach? Acta Neurol Belg. 2007;107(4):115–7.
65. Lee CT, Espley AJ. Perioperative ulnar neuropathy in orthopaedics: association with tilting the patient. Clin Orthop Relat Res. 2002;(396):106–11.
66. Posta AG Jr, Allen AA, Nercessian OA. Neurologic injury in the upper extremity after total hip arthroplasty. Clin Orthop Relat Res. 1997;(345):181–6.
67. Shields LBE, Iyer VG, Zhang YP, Shields CB. Acute cauda equina syndrome following orthopedic procedures as a result of epidural anesthesia. Surg Neurol Int. 2018;9:81.
68. Pritchett JW. Lumbar decompression to treat foot drop after hip arthroplasty. Clin Orthop Relat Res. 1994;303:173–7.
69. Ahn KS, Kopp SL, Watson JC, Scott KP, Trousdale RT, Hebl JR. Postsurgical inflammatory neuropathy. Reg Anesth Pain Med. 2011;36(4):403–5.
70. Heyworth BE, Fabricant PD, Pizzurro MM, Beksac B, Salvati EA. Guillain-barré syndrome mimicking nerve injury after total hip arthroplasty. HSS J. 2011;7(3):286–9.
71. Laughlin RS, Dyck PJ, Watson JC, Spinner RJ, Amrami KK, Sierra RJ, Trousdale RT, Staff NP. Ipsilateral inflammatory neuropathy after hip surgery. Mayo Clin Proc. 2014;89(4):454–61.
72. Tomaszewski KA, Graves MJ, Henry BM, Popieluszko P, Roy J, Pękala PA, Hsieh WC, Vikse J, Walocha JA. Surgical anatomy of the sciatic nerve: a meta-analysis. J Orthop Res. 2016;34(10):1820–7.
73. Pokorný D, Jahoda D, Veigl D, Pinskerová V, Sosna A. Topographic variations of the relationship of the sciatic nerve and the piriformis muscle and its relevance to palsy after total hip arthroplasty. Surg Radiol Anat. 2006;28(1):88–91.
74. Kanawati AJ. Variations of the sciatic nerve anatomy and blood supply in the gluteal region: a review of the literature. ANZ J Surg. 2014;84(11):816–9.
75. DeHart MM, Riley LH Jr. Nerve injuries in total hip arthroplasty. J Am Acad Orthop Surg. 1999;7(2):101–11.
76. Kanawati AJ, Narulla R, Lorentzos P, Graham E. Position of the sciatic nerve and effect of gluteus maximus release during hip arthroplasty. J Orthop. 2017;14(2):281–6.
77. Dikici F, Kale A, Ugras AA, Gayretli O, Gurses IA, Kaya I. Sciatic nerve localization relative to the position of the hip, an anatomical study. Hip Int. 2011;21(2):187–91.
78. Weale AE, Newman P, Ferguson IT, Bannister GC. Nerve injury after posterior and direct lateral approaches for hip replacement. A clinical and electrophysiological study. J Bone Joint Surg Br. 1996;78(6):899–902.
79. Shubert D, Madoff S, Milillo R, Nandi S. Neurovascular structure proximity to acetabular retractors in total hip arthroplasty. J Arthroplasty. 2015;30(1):145–8.
80. Wang TI, Chen HY, Tsai CH, Hsu HC, Lin TL. Distances between bony landmarks and adjacent nerves: anatomical factors that may influence retractor placement in total hip replacement surgery. J Orthop Surg Res. 2016;11:31.
81. Eksioglu F, Uslu M, Gudemez E, Atik OS, Tekdemir I. Reliability of the safe area for the superior gluteal nerve. Clin Orthop Relat Res. 2003;(412):111–6.
82. Miguel-Pérez M, Ortiz-Sagristà JC, López I, Pérez-Bellmunt A, Llusá M, Alex L, Combalia A. How to avoid injuries of the superior gluteal nerve. Hip Int. 2010;20(Suppl 7):S26–31.
83. Lavigne P, Loriot de Rouvray TH. The superior gluteal nerve. Anatomical study of its extrapelvic portion and surgical resolution by trans-gluteal approach. Rev Chir Orthop Reparatrice Appar Mot. 1994;80(3):188–95.
84. Hasija R, Kelly JJ, Shah NV, Newman JM, Chan JJ, Robinson J, Maheshwari AV. Nerve injuries associated with total hip arthroplasty. J Clin Orthop Trauma. 2018;9(1):81–6.
85. Jacobs LG, Buxton RA. The course of the superior gluteal nerve in the lateral approach to the hip. J Bone Joint Surg Am. 1989;71(8):1239–43.
86. Baker AS, Bitounis VC. Abductor function after total hip replacement. An electromyographic and clinical review. J Bone Joint Surg Br. 1989;71(1):47–50.
87. Ince A, Kemper M, Waschke J, Hendrich C. Minimally invasive anterolateral approach to the hip: risk to the superior gluteal nerve. Acta Orthop. 2007;78(1):86–9.
88. Pérez MM, Llusá M, Ortiz JC, Lorente M, Lopez I, Lazaro A, Pérez A, Götzens V. Superior gluteal nerve: safe area in hip surgery. Surg Radiol Anat. 2004;26(3):225–9.
89. Solomon LB, Hofstaetter JG, Bolt MJ, Howie DW. An extended posterior approach to the hip and pelvis for complex acetabular reconstruction that preserves the gluteal muscles and their neurovascular supply. Bone Joint J. 2014;96-B(1):48–53.
90. Putzer D, Haselbacher M, Hörmann R, Thaler M, Nogler M. The distance of the gluteal nerve in relation to anatomical landmarks: an anatomic study. Arch Orthop Trauma Surg. 2018;138(3):419–25.
91. Grob K, Manestar M, Ackland T, Filgueira L, Kuster MS. Potential risk to the superior gluteal nerve during the anterior approach to the hip joint: an anatomical study. J Bone Joint Surg Am. 2015;97(17):1426–31.

92. Takada R, Jinno T, Miyatake K, Hirao M, Kimura A, Koga D, Yagishita K, Okawa A. Direct anterior versus anterolateral approach in one-stage supine total hip arthroplasty. Focused on nerve injury: a prospective, randomized, controlled trial. J Orthop Sci. 2018;23(5):783–7.
93. Onyemaechi N, Anyanwu E, Obikili E, Ekezie J. Anatomical basis for surgical approaches to the hip. Ann Med Health Sci Res. 2014;4(4):487–94.
94. Heller KD, Prescher A, Birnbaum K, Forst R. Femoral nerve lesion in total hip replacement: an experimental study. Arch Orthop Trauma Surg. 1998;117(3):153–5.
95. Fox AJ, Bedi A, Wanivenhaus F, Sculco TP, Fox JS. Femoral neuropathy following total hip arthroplasty: review and management guidelines. Acta Orthop Belg. 2012;78(2):145–51.
96. Mehta CR, Constantinidis A, Farhat M, Suthersan M, Graham E, Kanawati A. The distance of the femoral neurovascular bundle from the hip joint: an intraoperative guide to reduce iatrogenic injury. J Orthop Surg Res. 2018;13(1):135.
97. Sullivan CW, Banerjee S, Desai K, Smith M, Roberts JT. Safe zones for anterior acetabular retractor placement in direct anterior total hip arthroplasty: a cadaveric study. J Am Acad Orthop Surg. 2019;27(21):e969–76.
98. Grob K, Monahan R, Gilbey H, Yap F, Filgueira L, Kuster M. Distal extension of the direct anterior approach to the hip poses risk to neurovascular structures: an anatomical study. J Bone Joint Surg Am. 2015;97(2):126–32.
99. Ghijselings SGM, Driesen R, Simon JP, Corten K. Distal extension of the direct anterior approach to the hip: a cadaveric feasibility study. J Arthroplasty. 2017;32(1):300–3.
100. Ghijselings SGM, Driesen R, Simon JP, Corten K. Distal extension of the anterior approach to the hip using the femoral interbundle technique: surgical technique and case series. J Arthroplasty. 2017;32(7):2186–90.
101. Ropars M, Morandi X, Huten D, Thomazeau H, Berton E, Darnault P. Anatomical study of the lateral femoral cutaneous nerve with special reference to minimally invasive anterior approach for total hip replacement. Surg Radiol Anat. 2009;31(3):199–204.
102. Sugano M, Nakamura J, Hagiwara S, Suzuki T, Nakajima T, Orita S, Akazawa T, Eguchi Y, Kawasaki Y, Ohtori S. Anatomical course of the lateral femoral cutaneous nerve with special reference to the direct anterior approach to total hip arthroplasty. Mod Rheumatol. 2019;22:1–6.
103. Oinuma K, Eingartner C, Saito Y, Shiratsuchi H. Total hip arthroplasty by a minimally invasive, direct anterior approach. Oper Orthop Traumatol. 2007;19(3):310–26.
104. Ozaki Y, Baba T, Homma Y, Tanabe H, Ochi H, Bannno S, Watari T, Kaneko K. Preoperative ultrasound to identify distribution of the lateral femoral cutaneous nerve in total hip arthroplasty using the direct anterior approach. SICOT J. 2018;4:42.
105. Siliski JM, Scott RD. Obturator-nerve palsy resulting from intrapelvic extrusion of cement during total hip replacement. Report of four cases. J Bone Joint Surg Am. 1985;67(8):1225–8.
106. Fricker RM, Troeger H, Pfeiffer KM. Obturator nerve palsy due to fixation of an acetabular reinforcement ring with transacetabular screws. A case report. J Bone Joint Surg Am. 1997;79(3): 444–6.
107. Sutter M, Hersche O, Leunig M, Guggi T, Dvorak J, Eggspuehler A. Use of multimodal intra-operative monitoring in averting nerve injury during complex hip surgery. J Bone Joint Surg Br. 2012;94(2):179–84.
108. Kong X, Chai W, Chen J, Yan C, Shi L, Wang Y. Intraoperative monitoring of the femoral and sciatic nerves in total hip arthroplasty with high-riding developmental dysplasia. Bone Joint J. 2019;101-B(11):1438–46.
109. Wasielewski RC, Cooperstein LA, Kruger MP, Rubash HE. Acetabular anatomy and the transacetabular fixation of screws in total hip arthroplasty. J Bone Joint Surg Am. 1990;72(4):501–8.
110. Kerns J, Piponov H, Helder C, Amirouche F, Solitro G, Gonzalez M. Mechanical properties of the human tibial and peroneal nerves following stretch with histological correlations. Anat Rec (Hoboken). 2019;302(11):2030–9.
111. Malessy MJA, Eekhof J, Pondaag W. Dynamic decompression of the lateral femoral cutaneous nerve to treat meralgia paresthetica: technique and results. J Neurosurg. 2019;131:1552–60.
112. Birch R, Bonney G, Wynn Parry CB. Surgical disorders of the peripheral nerves. Edinburgh: Churchill Livingstone; 1998.
113. Kyriacou S, Pastides PS, Singh VK, Jeyaseelan L, Sinisi M, Fox M. Exploration and neurolysis for the treatment of neuropathic pain in patients with a sciatic nerve palsy after total hip replacement. Bone Joint J. 2013;95-B(1):20–2.
114. Chughtai M, Khlopas A, Gwam CU, Elmallah RK, Thomas M, Nace J, Mont MA. Nerve decompression surgery after total hip arthroplasty: what are the outcomes? J Arthroplasty. 2017;32(4):1335–9.
115. Giuffre JL, Bishop AT, Spinner RJ, Levy BA, Shin AY. Partial tibial nerve transfer to the tibialis anterior motor branch to treat peroneal nerve injury after knee trauma. Clin Orthop Relat Res. 2012;470(3):779–90.
116. Yeap JS, Birch R, Singh D. Long-term results of tibialis posterior tendon transfer for drop-foot. Int Orthop. 2001;25(2):114–8.
117. Hove LM, Nilsen PT. Posterior tibial tendon transfer for drop-foot: 20 cases followed for 1–5 years. Acta Orthop Scand. 1998;69(6):608–10.
118. Yeap JS, Singh D, Birch R. A method for evaluating the results of tendon transfers for foot drop. Clin Orthop Relat Res. 2001;383:208–13.

119. Lingaiah P, Jaykumar K, Sural S, Dhal A. Functional evaluation of early tendon transfer for foot drop. J Orthop Surg. 2018;26(3):1–7.
120. Fansa H, Meric C. Reconstruction of quadriceps femoris muscle function with muscle transfer. Handchir Mikrochir Plast Chir. 2010;42(4):233–8.
121. Shahcheraghi GH, Javid M, Zeighami B. Hamstring tendon transfer for quadriceps femoris paralysis. J Pediatr Orthop. 1996;16(6):765–8.
122. Tung TH, Chao A, Moore AM. Obturator nerve transfer for femoral nerve reconstruction: anatomic study and clinical application. Plast Reconstr Surg. 2012;130(5):1066–74.
123. Park JH, Hozack B, Kim P, Norton R, Mandel S, Restrepo C, Parvizi J. Common peroneal nerve palsy following total hip arthroplasty: prognostic factors for recovery. J Bone Joint Surg Am. 2013;95(9):e55.
124. Regev GJ, Drexler M, Sever R, Dwyer T, Khashan M, Lidar Z, Salame K, Rochkind S. Neurolysis for the treatment of sciatic nerve palsy associated with total hip arthroplasty. Bone Joint J. 2015;97-B(10):1345–9.
125. Clawson DK, Seddon HJ. The results of repair of the sciatic nerve. J Bone Joint Surg Br. 1960;42-B(2):205–12.
126. Aydin A, Ozkan T, Aydin HU, Topalan M, Erer M, Ozkan S, Yildirim ZH. The results of surgical repair of sciatic nerve injuries. Acta Orthop Traumatol Turc. 2010;44(1):48–53.
127. Fleischman AN, Rothman RH, Parvizi J. Femoral nerve palsy following total hip arthroplasty: incidence and course of recovery. J Arthroplasty. 2018;33(4):1194–9.
128. Kim DH, Kline DG. Surgical outcome for intra- and extrapelvic femoral nerve lesions. J Neurosurg. 1995;83(5):783–90.
129. Patton RS, Runner RP, Lyons RJ, Bradbury TL. Clinical outcomes of patients with lateral femoral cutaneous nerve injury after direct anterior total hip arthroplasty. J Arthroplasty. 2018;33(9):2919–2926.e1.
130. Ozaki Y, Homma Y, Baba T, Sano K, Desroches A, Kaneko K. Spontaneous healing of lateral femoral cutaneous nerve injury and improved quality of life after total hip arthroplasty via a direct anterior approach. J Orthop Surg (Hong Kong). 2017;25(1):2309499016684750.
131. Khalil N, Nicotra A, Rakowicz W. Treatment for meralgia paraesthetica. Cochrane Database Syst Rev. 2008;3:CD004159.
132. Payne R, Seaman S, Sieg E, Langan S, Harbaugh K, Rizk E. Evaluating the evidence: is neurolysis or neurectomy a better treatment for meralgia paresthetica? Acta Neurochir. 2017;159:931–6.
133. Hong J, Trus TL, Ball PA. Laparoscopic-assisted intra-abdominal section of the lateral femoral cutaneous nerve for meralgia paresthetica following anterior hip arthroplasty. World Neurosurg. 2019;126:415–7.

Nerve Injury After Hip Arthroscopy, Hip Preservation Surgery, and Proximal Hamstring Repair

12

John M. Apostolakos, Kenneth M. Lin, Daniel A. Osei, and Anil S. Ranawat

12.1 Introduction

Surgical intervention to address pathologies within the hip is common in the field of orthopedics. As with any procedure, the potential for iatrogenic complication exists. For the purposes of this chapter, the focus will be directed on neurologic structures, their function, anatomic course, and level of risk during specific interventions. The detailed text below provides the surgeon with a precise description of normal anatomy of the hip and its surrounding nerves, surgical anatomy with commonly utilized arthroscopic portal placements and open approaches, technical pearls for avoiding iatrogenic nerve injury, and an overview of specific physical examination findings and electrodiagnostic tests/imaging studies to evaluate peripheral nerve injuries.

12.2 Detailed Neural Anatomy of the Hip/Thigh

A detailed understanding of the neurological anatomy of the hip and thigh begins with the lumbar plexus which is formed by the first four lumbar nerves (L1-4) with contributions from the subcostal nerve (T12). The anterior division of the lumbar plexus gives off the genitofemoral (L1-2) and obturator (L2-4) nerves [1]. The genitofemoral nerve pierces through the psoas and divides into its two sensory branches, the femoral branch which provides sensation to the proximal anterior thigh and the genital branch which provides sensation to the scrotum/labia [1]. The obturator nerve exits the pelvis through the obturator canal to provide cutaneous sensation to the inferomedial thigh via the cutaneous branch of the obturator nerve and motor innervation to the gracilis, adductor longus, adductor brevis, and the adductor magnus [1, 2].

The posterior division of the lumbar plexus gives off the lateral femoral cutaneous nerve (LFCN, L2-3) and the femoral nerve (L2-4). The LFCN is a purely sensory nerve providing innervation to the lateral thigh. The femoral nerve (L2-4) is the largest branch of the lumbar plexus and provides innervation to the anterior thigh via the anterior/intermediate cutaneous nerves [1, 2]. After originating in the psoas muscle, it courses posterolaterally within the pelvis before passing deep to the inguinal ligament and through the femoral triangle, just lateral to the femoral vessels [2]. Once distal to the femoral triangle, the nerve gives off several branches to the anterior thigh while also providing articular branches to the hip and knee as well as cutaneous branches to the medial thigh [2]. The femoral nerve provides

J. M. Apostolakos (✉) · K. M. Lin · D. A. Osei
A. S. Ranawat
Department of Orthopaedic Surgery, Hospital for Special Surgery, New York, NY, USA
e-mail: apostolakosj@hss.edu; oseid@HSS.EDU; RanawatAnil@HSS.EDU

C. J. Dy et al. (eds.), *Peripheral Nerve Issues after Orthopedic Surgery*,
https://doi.org/10.1007/978-3-030-84428-8_12

motor innervation to the psoas, pectineus, sartorius, and the quadriceps (rectus femoris, vastus lateralis, vastus intermedialis, vastus medialis) [1].

The sacral plexus (L4-S4) provides several nerves supplying the gluteal region via the superior and inferior gluteal nerves, the perineum via the pudendal nerve, and the sciatic nerve in the posterior thigh, which divides into the tibial and common peroneal nerves in the distal thigh [1, 2]. More specifically, the superior gluteal nerve (posterior divisions of anterior rami of L4-S1 spinal nerves) enters the gluteal region via the greater sciatic foramen, superior to the piriformis [2]. It then courses laterally between the gluteus minimus and gluteus medius with a branch of the superior gluteal artery [2]. Along its course, it divides into superior and inferior branches which provide motor innervation to the gluteus medius and the gluteus medius, gluteus minimus, and tensor fascia lata, respectively [2]. The inferior gluteal nerve (posterior divisions of anterior rami of L5-S2 spinal nerves) also enters the gluteal region via the grater sciatic foramen [2]. Relative to the superior gluteal nerve, the inferior gluteal nerve courses inferior to the piriformis along with branches of the inferior gluteal artery to provide motor sensation to the gluteus maximus [2].

Continuing with the deep gluteal nerves, the nerve to quadratus femoris (anterior divisions of anterior rami of L4-S1 spinal nerves) exits the pelvis through the greater sciatic foramen inferior to the piriformis and anterior to the sciatic nerve and obturator internus [2]. It then continues to course posterior to the hip joint and provides motor innervation to the inferior gemellus and quadratus femoris [2]. The posterior cutaneous nerve of thigh (anterior and posterior divisions of anterior rami of S1-3 spinal nerves) also enters the gluteal region via the greater sciatic foramen. It travels inferior to the piriformis while remaining deep to the gluteus maximus before descending distally in the posterior thigh deep to the fascia lata [2]. The nerve provides a great deal of cutaneous innervation via the anterior divisions of S2 and S3 which supply the skin of the perineum while some fibers from the posterior divisions of the anterior rami of S1 and S2 supply the inferior part of the buttocks [2]. More distally, the nerves continue to give off branches to supply the skin of the posterior thigh and proximal leg [2]. Although this nerve is described as a "cutaneous" nerve, a majority of the structure remains deep to the fascia lata. Continuing with the nerves of the gluteal region, the pudendal nerve (anterior divisions of anterior rami of S2-S4 spinal nerves) also exits the pelvis via the greater sciatic foramen. More specifically, it is the most medial nerve to exit the greater sciatic foramen and continues inferior to the piriformis, posterolateral to the sacrospinous ligament, before entering the perineum via the lesser sciatic foramen [2]. It does not innervate any structures in the gluteal region but is instead a major innervator to the perineum. The nerve to obturator internus (posterior divisions of anterior rami of L5-S2 spinal nerves) courses in parallel to the pudendal nerve [2]. It enters the gluteal region through the greater sciatic foramen inferior to the piriformis, posterior to the sacrospinous ligament, and enters the perineum through the lesser sciatic notch [2]. It supplies motor innervation to the superior gemellus and obturator internus.

The major nerve continuing from the sacral plexus, and the largest nerve in the body, is the sciatic nerve (anterior and posterior divisions of anterior rami of L4-S3 spinal nerves). The sciatic nerve enters the gluteal region via the greater sciatic foramen inferior to piriformis and deep to gluteus maximus [2]. The sciatic nerve becomes a thick, flattened nerve approximately 2 cm wide and is the most lateral structure which courses through the greater sciatic foramen [2]. It then courses distally in an inferomedial direction beneath the gluteus maximus, in between the greater trochanter of the femur and the ischial tuberosity [2]. In regard to motor supply, the sciatic nerve does not provide any innervation to gluteal muscles. It does supply motor innervation to all posterior thigh muscles as well as all leg and foot muscles via tibia and peroneal divisions [2]. The sciatic nerve demonstrates substantial anatomic variation. In approximately 12% of people, the tibial and peroneal nerves separate as they leave the pelvis with the tibial nerve coursing inferior to the piriformis and the peroneal nerve piercing through and coursing superior to the piriformis [2].

12.3 Surgical Anatomy

When describing the anatomy, the human "hip" should be subdivided into the following three categories: the superficial/surface anatomy, the deep femoroacetabular joint and capsule, and the "associated" structures including muscles, nerves, and vasculature [3].

12.3.1 Superficial/Surface Anatomy

The hip has several palpable bony landmarks to assist the clinician/surgeon. To begin, the anterosuperior iliac spine (ASIS) and the anteroinferior iliac spine (AIIS) and anteriorly located structures serve as the muscular origin for the sartorius and rectus femoris, respectively. Posteriorly, additional structures can be palpated. The greater trochanter can be palpated posterolaterally and serves as the insertion of the gluteus medius, the gluteus minimus, the obturator externus, the obturator internus, the femelli, and the piriformis [1–3]. An additional structure palpable posteriorly is the posterosuperior iliac spine which is the attachment point for the oblique portion of the posterior sacroiliac ligaments and multifidus [3]. All of these structures are utilized when planning portal sites, open procedures, and conducting a physical examination.

12.3.2 Deep Femoroacetabular Joint and Capsule

The femoroacetabular ("hip") joint can be described as a synovial, diarthrodial, ball-and-socket joint [3]. It is an articulation of the femoral head (proximal femur) and the acetabulum. The acetabulum is a cartilaginous convergence of the ilium, ischium, and pubis. In general, the acetabular is included roughly 55 degrees and anteverted roughly 20 degrees [3]. The femoral head articulates with the acetabulum while there is a tapered femoral neck creating a 130 degree neck-shaft angle [3].

In addition, capsular ligaments of the hip play a significant role in functional mobility and stability [4]. More specifically, the iliofemoral ligament is composed of lateral (superior) and medial (inferior) branches that insert onto the anterior inferior iliac spine (AIIS) and extend out to attach on the femoral intertrochanteric line forming an inverted Y-shaped ligament of Bigelow [4]. The functional importance of the iliofemoral ligament is to provide support during external rotation and extension. Next, the ischiofemoral ligament inserts in the ischium and attaches to the posterior intertrochanteric line providing stability during internal rotation in neutral positions and during flexion, adduction, and internal rotation (FADIR) [4]. Finally, the pubofemoral ligament inserts onto the superior ramus converging with the medial iliofemoral and inferior ischiofemoral ligaments before attaching onto the femur to provide stability within the inferior capsule for abduction and external rotation during hip extension [4].

12.3.3 "Associated" Structures

The term "associated" structures encompasses muscles, nerves, and vasculatures pertaining to the hip joint [3]. There are 27 muscles that cross the hip, making the joint a complex interaction between flexors, extensors, adductors, abductors, internal rotators, and external rotators [3]. The purpose of this text is specifically related to peripheral nerve anatomy as it relates to surgical procedures and approaches which will be discussed more thoroughly in the following section.

12.3.3.1 Arthroscopic Approaches

During hip arthroscopy, palpable structures are utilized to create portals. A 2008 investigation by Robertson and Kelly [6] evaluated 11 portals (4 central, 4 peripheral, and 3 peritrochanteric) in cadavers to determine location as they relate to neurovascular structures. Historically, three arthroscopic portals were created (anterior, anterolateral, and posterolateral) [7] with newer techniques utilized to access the peripheral and peritrochanteric compartments [6, 8, 9]. Although numerous arthroscopic hip portals have been described, we will describe the most commonly utilized below. To begin, the surgeon marks out the tip of the greater trochanter and ASIS with a line drawn down the anterior thigh in line with the ASIS. To clarify, hip arthroscopic portal can be described as "central" providing access to the hip joint proper, "peripheral" providing access to the femoral neck and acetabular rim, and "peritrochanteric" providing access to the space between the iliotibial band and the proximal femur [6].

12.3.4 Anteroposterior (AP)

This portal is placed 1 cm lateral to the ASIS in line with the AL portal [6]. Based on cadaveric dissections, this portal penetrates the tensor fascia latae (TFL) muscle belly, through the interval between the gluteus minimus and rectus femoris, then enters the joint through the anterior capsule (Figs. 12.1, 12.3, 12.4) [6]. The structure most at risk during AP portal placement is the LFCN, with an average distance from the portal to the LFCN of 15.4 mm [6]. In some cases, the LFCN may divide into two branches proximal to the AP portal placement; in these variants (3/10 cases per a cadaveric dissection by Robertson and Kelly [6]), the portal was found to be even closer to the lateral branch of the LFCN (1, 6, and 10 mm, respectively, in the specimens of the investigation). Additionally, when using the AP portal to access the central compartment, it is 54 mm from the femoral nerve at the sartorius, 45 mm from the femoral nerve at the rectus femoris, and 35 mm from the femoral nerve at the capsule [3, 6].

12.3.5 Anterolateral (AL)

This portal is placed 1 cm superior and 1 cm anterior to the tip of the greater trochanter (Figs. 12.1, 12.2, 12.3, and 12.4) [6, 10]. In many young and active patients, the posterior border of the TFL and the anterior border of the gluteus maximus fascia merge together at the anterior

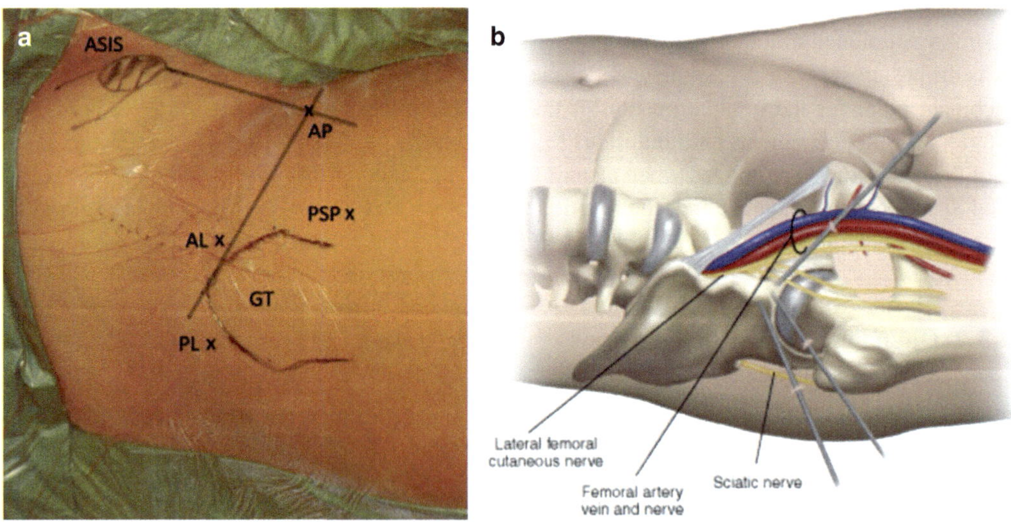

Fig. 12.1 Surface anatomy of the anterior, anterolateral, and posterolateral portals. (**a**) Superficial landmarks for the anterior portal (AP) at the intersections of a vertical line from the ASIS and a horizontal line drawn from the superior aspect of the GT. The anterolateral (AL) and the posterolateral (PL) portals are made anterior and posterior to the superolateral aspect of the GT. Peritrochanteric space portal (PSP). (**b**) Neuromuscular structures that are in close proximity to the three arthroscopic portals. (*As published in the Gerhadt et al. [5])

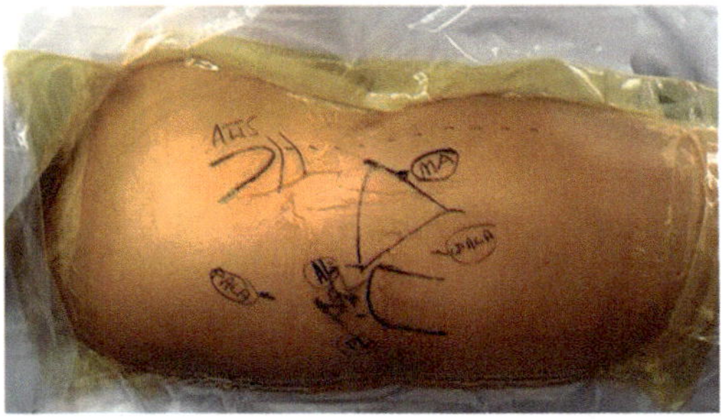

Fig. 12.2 Right hip (proximal on the left, distal on the right), illustrating 5 outlined incisions for 11 possible portal entry sites. The greater trochanter, AIIS, anterolateral (AL) portal, posterolateral (PL) portal, mid-anterior (MA) portal, proximal anterolateral accessory (PALA) portal, and distal anterolateral accessory (DALA) portal are outlined

aspect of the greater trochanter and provide a palpable ridge along the anterolateral thigh when traction is applied to the leg [6]. Placing the portal through this ridge allows the surgeon to access the intermuscular interval between the abductors and the TFL [6]. When utilizing the AL portal to access the central compartment, it has been found to be 64 mm from the superior gluteal nerve and 40 mm from the sciatic nerve [3, 6]. When this portal is used to access the peripheral compartment, it has been found to be 69 mm to the superior gluteal nerve and 58 mm from the sciatic nerve [3, 6].

12.3.6 Posterolateral (PL)

This portal is placed 1 cm superior and 1 cm posterior to the tip of the greater trochanter (Figs. 12.1, 12.2, 12.3, and 12.4) [6, 10]. During placement of this portal, the sciatic nerve is at the greatest risk. The nerve is most at risk when accessing the central compartment where it has been reported to be a mean distance of 22 mm away from the portal, whereas when accessing the peripheral compartment it is a mean of 34 mm from the portal [3, 6].

12.3.7 Mid-Anterior Portal (MAP) and Proximal Mid-Anterior Portal (PMAP)

As described by Robertson and Kelly [6], after establishing the AP and AL portals, the measured distance between these two portals is used to create an equilateral triangle with the third point making the MAP (Figs. 12.2, 12.3, and 12.4). The MAP can be used to access both the central and peripheral compartments. In both cases, the portal penetrated the TFL then extending through the gluteus minimus and rectus femoris interval [6]. At this level, the LFCN has been divided into two or more branches. With the MAP placed in the central compartment, it has been found to be 25 mm from the LFCN, 64 mm from the femoral nerve at the sartorius, 53 mm from the femoral nerve at the rectus femoris, and 40 mm from the femoral nerve at the capsule [3, 6]. When utilizing the MAP to access the peripheral compartment, it has been found to be 30 mm from the LFCN, 70 mm from the femoral nerve at the sartorius, 57 mm from the femoral nerve at the rectus femoris, and 39 mm from the femoral nerve at the capsule [3, 6].

Similarly, the PMAP (Figs. 12.3 and 12.4) is created more proximally utilizing the same measure distance to create an equilateral triangle. This portal is used to access the peripheral compartment and has been found to be 50 mm from the superior gluteal nerve and 58 mm from the sciatic nerve [3, 6].

12.3.8 Peritrochanteric Portals

Three portals are commonly used to access the peritochanteric space. These portals are established laterally in line with the anterior border of the femur [6]. The proximal anterolateral accessory (PALA) portal (Figs. 12.2, 12.3, and 12.4) is created directly posterior to the PMAP. Next, the peritrochanteric space portal (PSP) is at the level

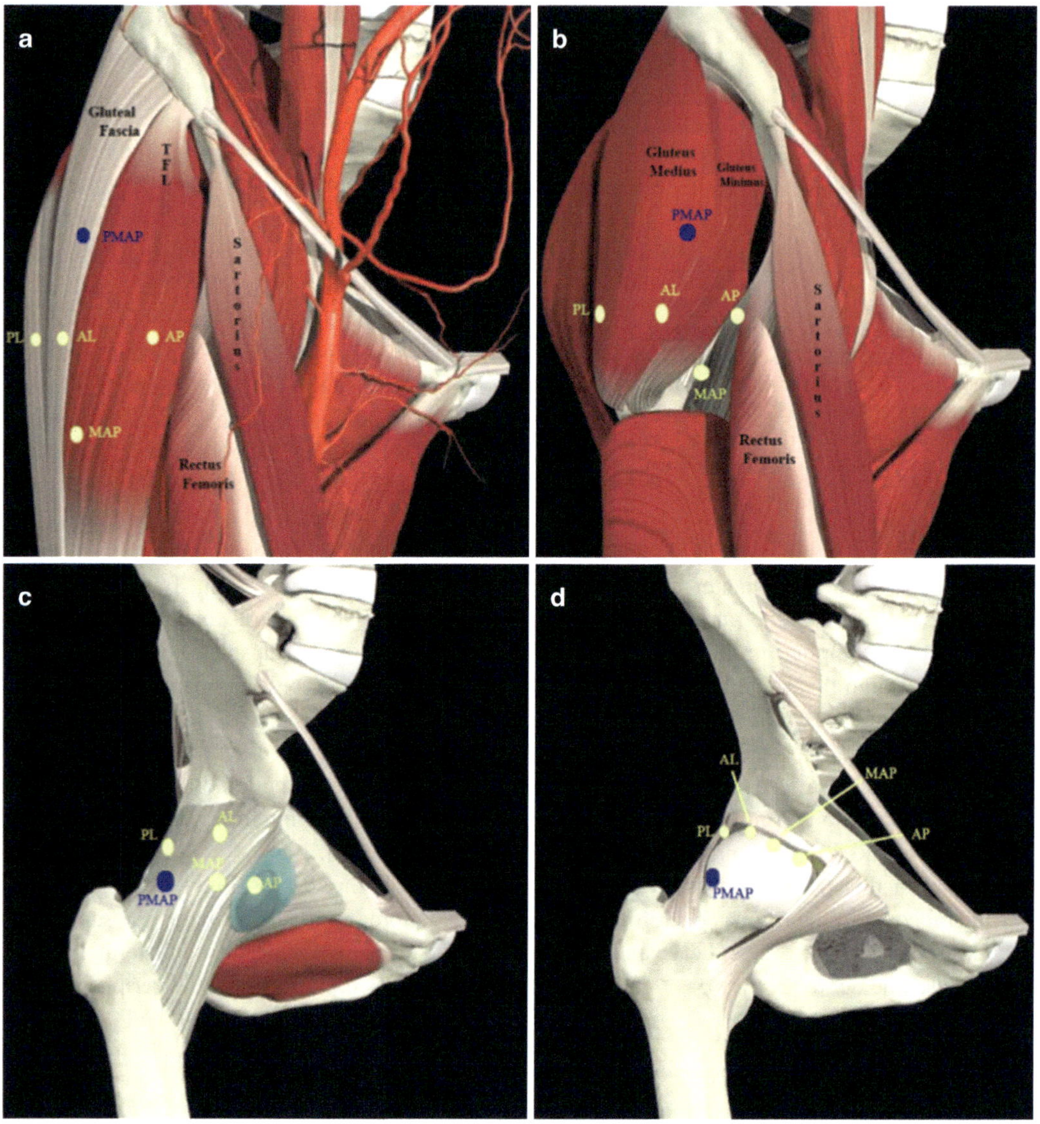

Fig. 12.3 "Central and peripheral compartment portal locations as they traverse soft tissues surrounding hip from superficial to deep. (**a**) The AL portal enters the junction of the posterior TFL fibers and the anterior gluteal fascial fibers. The AP portal and MAP pierce the TFL. (**b**) The AP portal and MAP pass between the gluteus minimus and the rectus femoris via a deep intermuscular plane. The AL portal passes anterior to the hip abductors and should meet little resistance before reaching the hip capsule. (**c**, **d**) Portal entry through capsule to access hip joint and head-neck junction." (As published by Robertson and Kelly [6])

of the MAP. Finally, distal anterolateral accessory (DALA) portal (Figs. 12.2, 12.3, and 12.4) is established distally from the PSP at a measured distance equivalent to the PMAP and MAP [6].

The PALA portal courses through the dermis and subcutaneous fat into the peritrochanteric space, while the PSP enters through the anterior fibers of the iliotibial band toward the lateral aspect of the greater trochanter [6]. The DALA portal courses though the overlying fascial layer anterior to the iliotibial band before entering the peritrochanteric space [6]. None of the peritro-

Compartment	Portal	Anatomic Structure	Mean Distance
Central	Anterior	Lateral femoral cutaneous nerve	15 mm
		Femoral nerve at sartorius	54 mm
		Femoral nerve rectus femoris	45 mm
		Femoral nerve at capsule	35 mm
		Ascending lateral femoral cutaneous artery	31 mm
		Terminal branch of ascending lateral femoral cutaneous artery	15 mm
	Anterolateral	Superior gluteal nerve	64 mm
		Sciatic nerve	40 mm
	Mid-anterior	Lateral femoral cutaneous nerve	25 mm
		Femoral nerve at sartorius	64 mm
		Femoral nerve at rectus femoris	53 mm
		Femoral nerve at capsule	40 mm
		Ascending lateral femoral cutaneous artery	19 mm
		Terminal branch of ascending lateral femoral cutaneous artery	10 mm
	Posterolateral	Sciatic nerve	22 mm
Peripheral	Anterolateral	Superior gluteal nerve	69 mm
		Sciatic nerve	59 mm
	Mid-anterior	Lateral femoral cutaneous nerve	30 mm
		Femoral nerve at sartorius	70 mm
		Femoral nerve at rectus femoris	57 mm
		Femoral nerve at capsule	39 mm
		Ascending lateral femoral cutaneous artery	21 mm
		Terminal branch of ascending lateral femoral cutaneous artery	15 mm
		Sciatic nerve	58 mm
	Posterolateral	Sciatic nerve	34 mm

Fig. 12.4 "Proximity of Arthroscopic Portals to Neurovascular Structures." (*As published in the Gerhadt et al. [5]. Original data adapted from Robertson and Kelly [6])

chanteric portals pose a significant risk for neurologic injury, with the DALA portal the only one of the three which poses a potential threat to a transverse branch of the lateral circumflex femoral artery (LFCA) [6].

12.3.8.1 Open Surgical Approaches

Anterior Approach to the Hip

This approach is also referred to as the Smith-Peterson approach and provides the surgeon access to the hip joint and ilium [11]. This approach can be utilized for open reduction of congenital dislocations of the hip, biopsy, intra-articular fusions, arthroplasty, or pelvis osteotomies (when utilizing the proximal aspect of the approach) [11]. An incision is made along the anterior half of the iliac crest toward the ASIS. It is then carried down distally and laterally 8–10 cm in the direction of the lateral aspect of the patella [11]. This approach actually utilizes two internervous planes: the first (more superficial) is developed between the sartorius (femoral nerve) and TFL (superior gluteal nerve), while a second (deeper plane) is established between the rectus femoris (femoral nerve) and the gluteus medius (superior gluteal nerve) [11]. During the superficial portion of the dissection, the surgeon should be aware of the LFCN, which pierces the deep fascia of the thigh close to the intermuscular interval between the sartorius and TFL [11]. By remaining on the medial side of the deep fascia of the TFL, the sheath will protect to surgeon from damaging the LFCN as the nerve courses over the fascia of the sartorius. Next, retraction of the sartorius proximally and medially while retracting the TFL downward and laterally will expose the deeper portion of the approach. The rectus femoris has two origination points: the direct head from the AIIS and the reflected head which is intimate with the joint capsule entering the superior acetabulum [11]. Once identified, the two heads of the rectus femoris can be retracted medially while simultaneously retracting the gluteus medius laterally exposing the underlying joint capsule [11].

Anterolateral Approach to the Hip

This approach is also known as the Watson-Jones approach and is most commonly used for total hip arthroplasty and open reduction and internal fixation of the femoral neck by utilizing the intermuscular plane between the TFL and gluteus medius [11]. An 8–15-cm longitudinal incision is made centered over the tip of the greater trochanter down the shaft of the femur. The superficial dissection is carried through the deep fascia of the thigh at the posterior margin of the greater trochanter in line with the skin incision. Dividing the fascia at this point, the surgeon now enters the underlying bursa and the fascial incision can then be extended proximally/anteriorly toward the ASIS and distally/anteriorly exposing the underlying vastus lateralis [11]. Blunt dissection is then carried down between the TFL and gluteus medius. A retractor is then placed under the gluteus medius and minimus to mobilize them proximally and laterally exposing the superior joint capsule above the femoral neck [11]. Deep dissection can then be performed to partially or fully detach the abductor mechanism utilizing either a trochanteric osteotomy or soft tissue dissection for full exposure.

Lateral Approach to the Hip

This direct approach is transgluteal allowing for exposure of the hip joint during arthroplasty without the need for osteotomy and preserving a bulk of the gluteus medius permitting early mobilization postoperatively [11]. An incision is made roughly 5 cm superior to the tip of the greater trochanter extending distally across the tip of the greater trochanter and in line with the femoral shaft. As is the case with the anterolateral approach, this approach also does not have a true internervous plane as the dissection is carried down through the fibers of the gluteus medius. The underlying fascia is incised in line with the skin incision, and the TFL is retracted anteriorly with the gluteus maximus retracted posteriorly. The gluteus medius fibers are then dissected in the direction of its muscular fibers beginning in the middle of the greater trochanter. The surgeon must be aware that this intermuscular dissection places the superior gluteal nerve at risk which courses proximally near the muscular insertion into the iliac crest. Next, the fibers of the vastus lateralis are split and a retractor is placed to create an anterior flap consisting of the anterior gluteus medius, gluteus minimus, and the anterior aspect of the vastus lateralis [11]. The surgeon will continue developing the plane beneath the anterior flap until the anterior hip joint capsule is exposed.

Posterior Approach to the Hip

The posterior approach to the hip is most commonly used for arthroplasty, open reduction and internal fixation of posterior acetabular fractures, incision and drainage of infected joint, and open reduction of posterior hip dislocations [11]. Beginning proximal and posterior to the tip of a greater trochanter, a 10–15-cm incision continues over the posterior aspect of the greater trochanter before continuing down the shaft of the femur. After dissecting through fascia, the gluteus maximus muscle belly is then split in line with its fibers revealing the posterolateral aspect of the hip joint [11]. At this point, the surgeon must recall that the sciatic nerve exits the greater sciatic foramen to the posterior thigh over the short external rotators before crossing the obturator internus, inferior and superior gemelli, and quadratus femoris [11]. Keeping in mind the close proximity of the sciatic nerve, the short external rotators are carefully released from the posterolateral aspect of the greater trochanter and laid back over the posteriorly located sciatic nerve for protection. The posterior aspect of the hip capsule is now fully exposed.

Medial Approach to the Hip

The medial approach was initially described by Ludloff and designed to approach the hip in flexed, abducted, and externally rotated hips such as those found in congenital hip dislocations [11]. It can be utilized for open reduction of the hip, psoas release, and obturator neurectomy. A longitudinal skin incision is made beginning 3 cm below the pubic tubercle and continuing distally over the adductor longus [11]. The superficial plane of dissection is bluntly carried through the plane between the adductor longus and gracilis which are both innervated by the anterior division of the obturator nerve [11]. Deep dissection is then carried down between the adductor brevis (anterior division of the obturator nerve) and the adductor magnus (the adductor portion is innervated by the posterior division of the obturator nerve while its ischial division is supplied by the tibial aspect of the sciatic nerve) down to the lesser trochanter [11].

Exposing the Ischium for Proximal Hamstring Repair

With the patient in a prone position, the chest and all bony prominences are well padded. The gluteal crease is identified and an 8-cm incision is drawn out, centered over the ischium (Fig. 12.5) [12]. Superficial dissection is then carried down through the subcutaneous tissue to expose the inferior aspect of the gluteus maximus. The gluteus maximus is then mobilized proximally with the underlying ischium now exposed. The gluteal fascia is released to allow for proximal mobilization of the gluteus maximus and to allow for visualization of the ischial tuberosity. The posterior cutaneous nerve of the thigh is typically encountered first superficially in the lateral aspect of the incision and can be carefully dissected proximally until the sciatic nerve is encountered (Figs. 12.6 and 12.7). The pudendal nerve is further medial than the typical

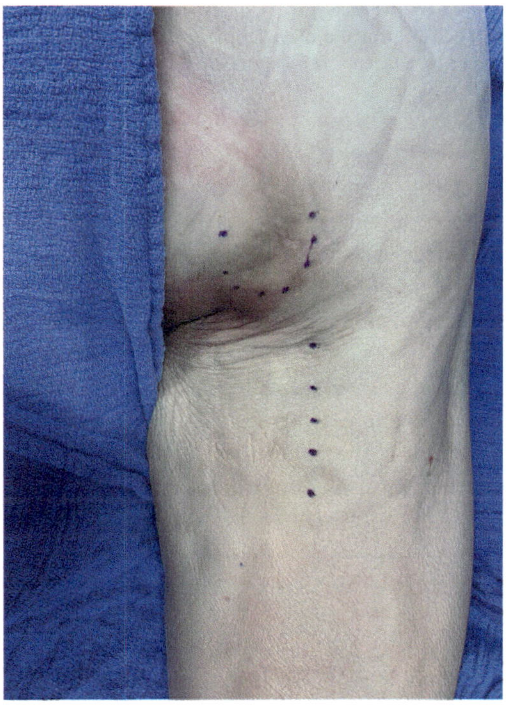

Fig. 12.5 Surgical approach to the right ischium with the patient in a prone position. Semi-circular marking at the top of the image marks out the ischium, while the vertical makings distally represent the proposed surgical approach

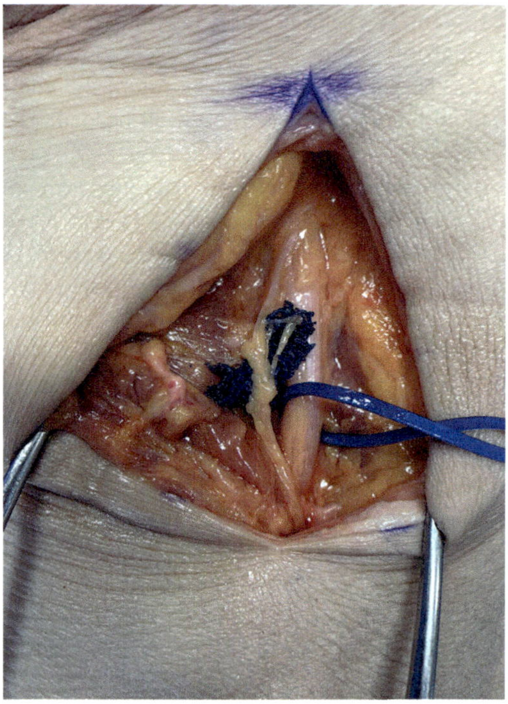

Fig. 12.6 The blue vessel loop is surrounding the sciatic nerve. The structure over the piece of blue towel is the posterior cutaneous nerve of the thigh

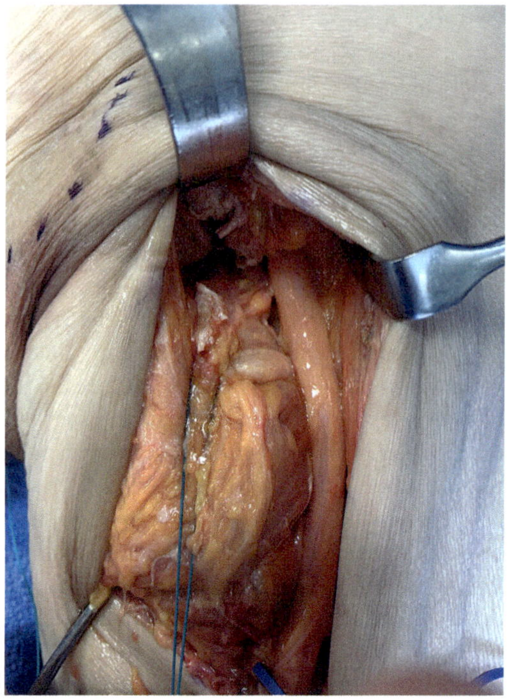

Fig. 12.7 For demonstration purposes, the origin of the hamstring tendons from the ischium is tagged with a blue suture. The sciatic nerve can be seen in the lateral aspect of the wound

surgical exposure for proximal hamstring repair, emerging along the inferior/medial border of the piriformis at a location 6.3 ± 1.4 cm from the superior aspect of the proximal hamstring origin before it courses deep to the sacrotuberous ligament (Fig. 12.8). However, the shortest distance between the pudendal nerve and the superior original of the hamstring origin was 2.6 ± 0.5 cm, placing it at risk with medial and superomedial retractor placement when exposing the hamstring origin site (Fig. 12.9).

12.4 Prevention Strategies

12.4.1 Hip Arthroscopy

In addition to a thorough understanding of surgical anatomy, careful consideration of position techniques is an additional component to preventing neurological injury. Hip arthroscopy can be performed in both supine and lateral positions. In regard to supine positioning, it is common for the surgeon to request full paralysis of the patient in order to optimize the use of traction to allow for distraction of the hip [3]. The patient can be positioned onto a traction table with both legs placed into secure traction boots with a well-padded peroneal post placed firmly against the perineum slightly lateralized toward the operative hip [3]. It is critical to remain aware of potential injury to the pudendal nerve with the peroneal post. In addition to padding, risk of pudendal nerve injury can also be mitigated by placing gentle traction to the leg in roughly 10 degrees of abduction which slightly lateralizes the pelvis leading to the post resting on the inner upper thigh and therefore decreasing the amount of pressure on the perineum and consequently the pudendal nerve [3].

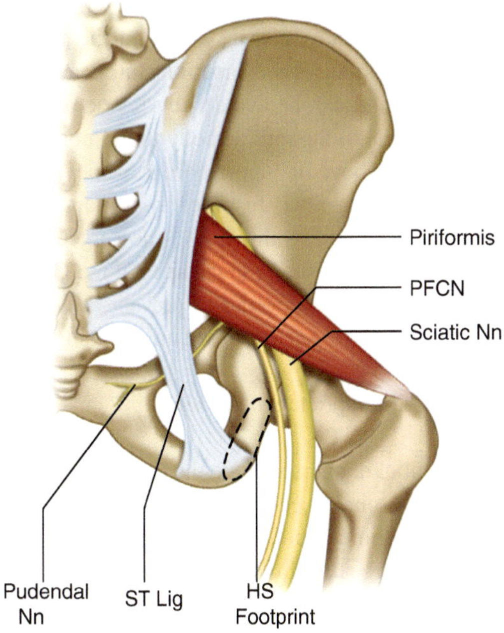

Fig. 12.8 Course of the pudendal nerve, posterior femoral cutaneous nerve (PFCN), and sciatic nerve relative to the hamstring (HS) footprint and the sacrotuberous (ST) ligament. (Redrawn from: Cvetanovich et al. [24])

- Positioning during supine hip arthroscopy with care to protect the pudendal nerve from pressure between the pelvis and peroneal post of the operative traction table [3].
- Historically, the AP portal placement is in line with the ASIS; however, by placing this portal 1 cm lateral to the ASIS, the surgeon is able to decrease risk to the LFCN [6].
- In addition, reports of the LFCN branching proximal to the AP portal site necessitate the need for stab incisions through the skin with careful blunt dissection superficially through the subcutaneous tissue [6].
- During placement of the posterolateral portal, consider the orientation of the lower extremity. When the leg is externally rotated, the posteriorly positioned greater trochanter results in a sharp angle for placing a spinal needle, thereby increasing a potential injury to the sciatic nerve [3]. Similarly, hip flexion also moves the sciatic nerve closer to the joint [3].

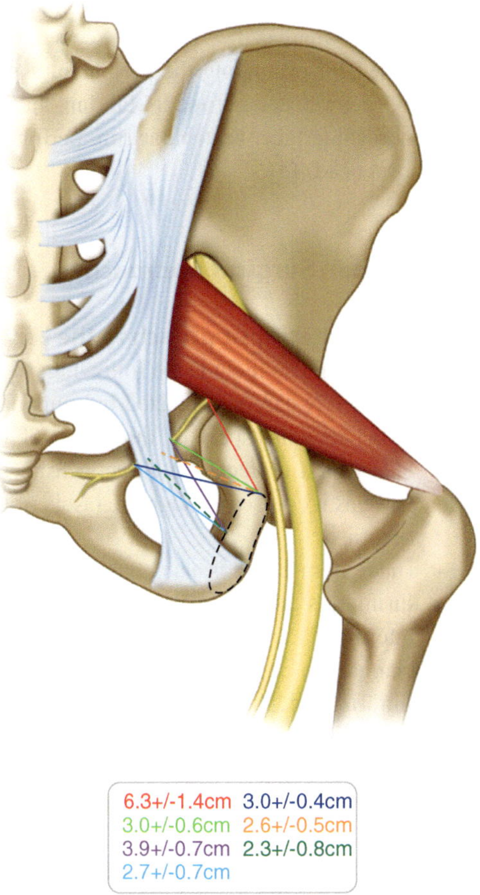

Fig. 12.9 Distances from proximal hamstring footprint/origin to the pudendal nerve at the various points of the latter's course. The blue, green, and purple lines demonstrate the distance between the pudendal nerve at the medial edge of the proximal hamstring footprint, while the red, green, and orange lines demonstrate the distance to the superior edge of the footprint. (Redrawn from: Cvetanovich et al. [24])

- In general, fluoroscopy can be utilized when directing spinal needles into the joint for possible portal placement.
- Portals should be placed under direct visualization, when possible.
- Utilizing both a 30 and 70 degree lens may improve arthroscopic visualization while minimizing the number of portals that need to be established. In general, a 30 degree scope will provide improved access to the center femoral

head, deep acetabular fossa, and the ligamentum teres, whereas the 70 degree scope is ideally used for evaluating the peripheral aspect of the central compartment (labrum, labral-chondral interface, acetabular rim, peripheral femoral head) [3].

12.4.2 Open Surgical Approaches

12.4.2.1 Anterior Approach to the Hip

- Potential dangers include the following:
  - The LFCN can be protected by remaining in the medial aspect of the fascia of the TFL which protects the surgeon from the nerve as it courses through the fascia of the sartorius.
  - The femoral nerve is also potentially at risk during this procedure as it courses directly anterior to the hip joint within the femoral triangle. It courses medial to the rectus femoris and should be protected during deep dissection as long as the surgeon remains in the correct place during dissection.

Anterolateral approach *to the hip:*

- Potential dangers include the following:
  - As this is an intermuscular plane, the superior gluteal nerve needs to be protected as it crosses the TFL close to its origin into the iliac crest. The superior gluteal nerve should be protected by refraining from dissection toward the muscular origins of the TFL and gluteus medius onto the iliac crest.
  - The femoral nerve is also a potential danger during this approach as it is the most lateral neurovascular structure in the femoral triangle and therefore the closest to the operative field during this approach. Commonly, neurapraxia can be encountered due to compression due to medial retraction [11].

Lateral approach *to the hip:*

- Potential dangers include the following:
  - The intermuscular dissection of the gluteus medius places the superior gluteal nerve at risk and can be avoided by restricting dissection of the muscle belly to no more than 3 cm above the upper border of the greater trochanter [11]. In order to prevent iatrogenic injury to this nerve, the surgeon can place a stay suture in the apex of the gluteus medius split in order to prevent accidental proximal extension of the muscle belly [11].

Posterior approach *to the hip:*

- Potential dangers include the following:
  - The sciatic nerve can be protected before detachment of the short external rotators by placing the limb into internal rotation which places the short external rotators on stretch and bringing the operative field away from the sciatic nerve.
  - The nerve also must be considered during retraction of the posterior aspect of the gluteus maximus to avoid compression.
  - As discussed previously in this text, the sciatic nerve does occasionally split into the tibial and common peroneal nerves within the pelvis. If the surgeon encounters a nerve that appears too small to be considered the sciatic, they should further explore for a possible second branch [11].

Medial approach *to the hip:*

- Potential dangers include the following:
  - The anterior division of the obturator nerve resides at the superior aspect of the obturator externus before extending distally between the adductor longus and adductor brevis [11].
  - The posterior division of the obturator nerve resides within the obturator externus before extending distally on the adductor magnus, beneath the adductor brevis [11].

Exposing the Ischium for Proximal Hamstring Repair

- Potential dangers include the following:
  - Sciatic nerve

    When the proximal hamstring is retracted posteriorly and scarred, the anatomy is altered and the nerve can be displaced. Beginning the nerve dissection distally where the anatomy is more normal and the nerve is less scarred can be helpful.

    Neurolysis throughout the entire affected region will untether the sciatic nerve from the hamstring. When the hamstring is repaired and pulled proximally into its normal anatomic position, adhesions between the nerve and the muscle can lead to traction of the nerve and potential neurologic compromise. Neurolysis prior to repair can mitigate this risk.

    The nerve does not need to be skeletonized with all scar tissue removed. It only needs to be separated from the muscle so that differential gliding can occur between nerve and muscle. Removing all scar tissues circumferentially from the nerve increases the risk of neurologic compromise.
  - Pudendal nerve

    Retractors positioned medially and superomedially to the hamstring origin site may place the pudendal nerve at risk, as it lies 2–3 cm superior and medial to the proximal hamstring origin
  - Posterior cutaneous nerve of the thigh

    The nerve, while relatively large for a cutaneous nerve, can easily be missed if the surgeon is not looking for it. Once the dissection proceeds deep to the fascia lata, care must be taken to identify and protect the PCN.

12.5 Initial Evaluation and Physical Exam:

The initial clinical evaluation allows the physician to determine the level and severity of any injury and provides a baseline for serial assessment. Sensory evaluation includes several instruments and measurements; however, there remains little consensus regarding a gold standard for assessment [13]. In general, clinical assessment of sensory receptors may include evaluation of sensory threshold meaning the minimal stimulus required to elicit a response, and innervation density meaning the number of innervated sensory receptors [13]. Light moving touch can provide a simple assessment and can be completed with the Ten Test method as initially described by Strauch et al. [14] and allows the patient to subjectively compare sensation between the distribution of the affected side and the normal contralateral side with normal sensation described as a 10/10. The sensory threshold may also be evaluated using vibration and can be assessed either qualitatively or quantitatively or with the use of cutaneous pressure thresholds which are commonly tested utilizing Semmes-Weinstein monofilaments [14]. Evaluation of innervation density can be assessed with two-point discrimination which has been hypothesized to indicate the quantity of innervated sensory receptors [14].

Motor evaluation can also be assessed qualitatively and quantitatively. The physician can evaluate for muscular atrophy (more relevant in subacute versus chronic presentations) and strength. In cases of suspected compressive neuropathy, patients may initially present with insignificant muscular complaints with concerns more related to sensation such as paresthesias and numbness [14]. In comparison, patients presenting after a traumatic or iatrogenic nerve injury may present with a more abrupt and severe loss of muscular function. The most commonly utilized description of muscular testing on physical examination was described in 1943 by the British Medical Research Council with grades of 0–5: (0) indicating no muscle contraction, (1) indicating a flicker of contraction, (2) indicating movement with gravity eliminated, (3) indicating full motion against gravity, (4) indicating full motion against resistance, and (5) indicating normal strength [14, 15].

A detailed neurological examination of the lower extremity would include evaluation of motor strength, sensation, and reflexes. In general, motor innervation of the lower extremity can be broken down into hip flexion (L2-3), hip extension (L5-S1), knee flexion (L5-S1), knee extension (L3-4), ankle dorsiflexion (L4-L5), ankle plantarflexion (S1-S2), foot inversion (L4-L5), and foot eversion (L5-S1) [16]. Zones of autonomous sensation display a spiral dermatomal pattern within the lower limb as a result of its embryonic medial rotation [16]. While there is considerable overlap and variability in dermatomal patterns, in general the inguinal region is supplied by L1, the anterior knee by L4, the second toe by L5, and the posterior leg/thigh by S1-S2 [16]. A more specific evaluation of the lower extremity requires a detailed examination of the following nerves:

Femoral Nerve *(L2-4):* Innervates the anterior compartment of the thigh and motor strength is evaluated via extension of thigh. The cutaneous branches of the nerve include the lateral cutaneous nerve of the thigh, anterior cutaneous nerve of the thigh, and the saphenous nerve to the medial knee, leg, and ankle. The patellar tendon reflex (L3-4) also evaluates the integrity of the femoral nerve via knee extension [16].

Obturator Nerve *(L2-4)*: As the major innervator of the medial thigh compartment, motor strength from this nerve is evaluated through the adductor muscles. When evaluating the sensory supply, it innervates a small field on the medial thigh. There is no reflex to be evaluated for this nerve distribution [16].

Sciatic Nerve *(L4-S3)*: The nerve innervates the muscles of the posterior compartment of the thigh, and motor strength is tested by evaluating hip extension and knee flexion. There is no sensory supply derived from the sciatic nerve directly as sensation to the posterior thigh is supplied by the *posterior cutaneous nerve of the* thigh which derives directly from the rami of S1-3 nerve roots. As the sciatic nerve courses below the knee, the sciatic nerve divides into tibial and common peroneal (fibular) nerves which should be evaluated separately [16].

Tibial Nerve *(L4-S3)*: The tibial nerve supplies motor innervation to the posterior compartment of the leg and the plantar aspect of the foot. The motor strength provided by this nerve is evaluated with plantarflexion and/or inversion of the foot. Sensory innervation is tested by evaluating the plantar foot and the calcaneal (Achilles) tendon reflex (S1-2) can also be examined within this nerve distribution [16].

Common Peroneal (Fibular) Nerve (L4-S2): The fibular nerve supplies motor innervation to the lateral compartment of the leg via its superficial branch, and the anterior compartment of the leg/dorsum of the foot via the deep branch. As dorsiflexors of the foot, footdrop and steppage gait are physical exam findings that present in patients with a common peroneal or deep peroneal injury. Sensory innervation is testing by evaluating the anterolateral leg and dorsum of the foot (superficial fibular nerve) and the first dorsal web space of the foot (deep fibular nerve) [16].

12.6 Diagnostic Tests and Imaging

The electrodiagnostic examination of peripheral nerve injuries may assist the clinician with determining lesion localization, quantitative severity, and prognostic information [13]. The most common nerve fiber pathology encountered is axon loss where the affected nerve fibers are incapable of conducting action potentials [13]. Motor nerve fiber involvement presents with muscular weakness and atrophy, while sensory nerve involvement causes impairment of both large diameter (vibration, proprioception, and light touch) and small diameter (pain and temperature) deficits [13]. Overall, the examination for peripheral nerves can be categorized into nerve conduction studies (NCSs) and electromyography (EMG) [13]. Motor NCSs and EMG studies are utilized to assess motor axons from the cell bodies of origin such as the lower motor neurons of the brain stem or the spinal cord to the respective muscular fibers they are innervating, while sensory NCSs evaluate sensory axons from their cell body of origin to their respective site of action [13]. A standard EMG evaluates the distal, middle, and proximal limb muscles innervated by motor nerve fibers traversing nerve roots, plexus elements, and nerve trunks [13]. During examination, the electrical activity of each muscle is recorded during insertion, rest, and activation phases. It is the most sensitive examination for detecting motor axon injury. NCSs can be classified as sensory, motor, or mixed. For sensory and mixed studies, the electrodes are placed over the nerve being studied, while motor testing is conducted with the electrode over the motor point and tendon of the muscle group of the nerve being tested [13]. Sensory and mixed responses represent nerve fiber action potentials traversing large diameter myelinated nerve fibers and are recorded as sensory nerve action potentials (SNAPs) while motor responses represent muscle fiber action potentials and are termed compound muscle fiber action potentials (CMAPs) [13].

Historically, peripheral nerve injury severity has been based on the Seddon and Sunderland classifications [17–19]. The Seddon classification defines nerve injuries as neurapraxia, axonotmesis, and neurotmesis. Neurapraxis and axonotmesis are milder forms of nerve injury, whereas neurotmesis is the most severe injury with an end-result similar to transection [18]. A more extensive classification was described by Sunderland who categorized peripheral nerve injuries into five histological grades based on successive involvement of the functional axonal conduction or myelin sheath (grade I), axonal continuity (grade II), endoneurial tube (grade III), perineurium (grade IV), and epineurium/entire nerve trunk (grade V) [19]. The Sunderland classification can also be used to anticipate recovery: grades I and II undergo spontaneous recovery, grade III undergoes partial recovery at a rate of 1 inch/month, and grades IV and V do not undergo spontaneous recovery and require surgical intervention [13].

MRI evaluation of peripheral nerve injuries is also an evolving field. It allows for noninvasive evaluation of injury which can include gap distance between lacerated segments, adjacent structures such as fracture fragments or hematomas, and denervation edema-like signal within days on injury [17, 20–22]. A 2018 investigation evaluated diagnostic accuracy of MRI for characterization of sciatic nerve injury as high grade (Sunderland grade IV and V) versus low grade (Sunderland I-III) and found no significant difference in signal intensity but did note features of high-grade injuries included bulbous enlargement, perineural fibrosis, muscle denervation changes, and nerve discontinuity [17]. The investigation serves as another example that imaging modalities for the characterization of peripheral nerve injuries remains challenging.

12.7 Management of Peripheral Nerve Injuries

When considering evaluation strategies for peripheral nerve injuries, neurapraxia (Sunderland grade I) and axonotmesis (Sunderland II) are managed nonoperatively, as full spontaneous recovery is expected. The challenge lies in differentiating Sunderland II injuries (with a good prognosis, typically treated with observation) from Sunderland III injuries (with a more guarded prognosis, with a potential role of surgical intervention), as the classification is predicated on recovery. For these cases, serial examinations and electrodiagnostic studies can help make this distinction. With higher grade lesions (Sunderland grade IV and V), surgical intervention is often performed given the poor prognosis for spontaneous recovery.

During hip arthroscopy, traction injuries to the pudendal nerve are most commonly caused due to pulling the operative leg against the perineal post. This typically results in a low-grade nerve injury which resolves spontaneously without surgical intervention. In support of this management, a 2018 systematic review of 24 studies which included 3405 patients reported a 1.8% rate (62 patients) of pudendal nerve traction injuries following hip arthroscopy [23]. By 6 weeks to 3 months postoperatively, all 62 patients experienced a full spontaneous recovery.

In regard to sciatic nerve injuries during operative fixation of proximal hamstring repair, the most likely scenario is the possibility of nerve entrapment by suture material or excessive tension along the sciatic nerve if remains adhered to the proximal hamstring tendon as it is reattached. To minimize the risk of these issues, it is important to visualize the sciatic nerve and perform an appropriate amount of neurolysis to free it from the hamstring tendon and to directly visualize and protect it during the placement of suture anchors and attachment of the proximal tendon. During the immediate postoperative recovery period, if the patient has signs of neurologic compromise on motor or sensory testing, or distinct neuropathic pain in a distribution supplied by the sciatic nerve or one of its branches, imaging and/or re-exploration to evaluate for nerve injury or compressive hematoma should be considered. During proximal hamstring repair, neurotmesis is extremely rare and represents a potentially devastating complication. If intraoperative nerve transection occurs and is recognized, immediate reconstruction should be considered, incorporating standard nerve reconstruction techniques.

12.8 Conclusion

Arthroscopic and open surgical management of hip conditions are common procedures in the field of orthopedic surgery. With a precise understanding of anatomic structures surrounding the hip, the surgeon is able to minimize neurological injuries during management. Fortunately, hip arthroscopic traction–related nerve injuries are low grade and have been shown to spontaneously recover fully without intervention. Direct iatrogenic injuries to the sciatic nerve are also extremely rare but would cause significant and devastating consequences. The anatomic descriptions and technical pearls provided in this chapter should allow for safe surgical management of patients presenting with pathology of the hip. In the event of intraoperative iatrogenic injury, the clinician should utilize the information obtained during a thorough physical examination, electrodiagnostic studies, and MRI to determine the exact location of the peripheral nerve injury and predict potential recovery.

References

1. Thompson J. Netter's concise orthopaedic anatomy. 2nd ed. Philadelphia: Saunders Elsevier; 2010.
2. Moore K, Dalley A, Agur A. Clinically oriented anatomy. Philadelphia: Lippincott Williams & Wilkins; 2014.
3. Sekiya J, Safran M, Ranawat A, Leunig M. Techniques in hip arthroscopy and joint preservation surgery. Philadelphia: Elsevier Saunders; 2011.
4. Ng KCG, Jeffers JRT, Beaule PE. Hip joint capsular anatomy, mechanics, and surgical management. J Bone Joint Surg Am. 2019;101(23):2141–51.
5. Gerhadt M, Logishetty K, Meftah M, Ranawat A. Techniques in hip arthroscopy and joint preservation surgery. Philadelphia: Elsevier Publishing; 2011. p. 9–22.
6. Robertson WJ, Kelly BT. The safe zone for hip arthroscopy: a cadaveric assessment of central, peripheral, and lateral compartment portal placement. Arthroscopy. 2008;24(9):1019–26.
7. Byrd JW, Pappas JN, Pedley MJ. Hip arthroscopy: an anatomic study of portal placement and relationship to the extra-articular structures. Arthroscopy. 1995;11(4):418–23.
8. Dienst M, Godde S, Seil R, Hammer D, Kohn D. Hip arthroscopy without traction: in vivo anatomy of the peripheral hip joint cavity. Arthroscopy. 2001;17(9):924–31.
9. Voos JE, Rudzki JR, Shindle MK, Martin H, Kelly BT. Arthroscopic anatomy and surgical techniques for peritrochanteric space disorders in the hip. Arthroscopy. 2007;23(11):1246, e1241-1245.
10. Philippon MJ, Stubbs AJ, Schenker ML, Maxwell RB, Ganz R, Leunig M. Arthroscopic management of femoroacetabular impingement: osteoplasty technique and literature review. Am J Sports Med. 2007;35(9):1571–80.
11. Hoppenfeld S, deBoer P, Buckley R. Surgical exposures in orthopaedics: the anatomic approach. Philadelphia: Lippincott Williams & Wilkins; 2009.
12. Moatshe G, Chahla J, Vap AR, et al. Repair of proximal hamstring tears: a surgical technique. Arthrosc Tech. 2017;6(2):e311–7.
13. Mackinnon S, Yee A. Nerve surgery. New York: Thieme; 2015.
14. Strauch B, Lang A, Ferder M, Keyes-Ford M, Freeman K, Newstein D. The ten test. Plast Reconstr Surg. 1997;99(4):1074–8.
15. Medical research council of the U.K. Aids to the investigation of peripheral nerve injuries (War Memorandum No. 7). 1943.
16. Hansen J. Lower limb. In: Netter's clinical anatomy. 4th ed. Philadelphia: Elsevier; 2019.
17. Ahlawat S, Belzberg AJ, Fayad LM. Utility of magnetic resonance imaging for predicting severity of sciatic nerve injury. J Comput Assist Tomogr. 2018;42(4):580–7.

18. Seddon HJ, Medawar PB, Smith H. Rate of regeneration of peripheral nerves in man. J Physiol. 1943;102(2):191–215.
19. Sunderland S. A classification of peripheral nerve injuries producing loss of function. Brain. 1951;74(4):491–516.
20. Grant GA, Britz GW, Goodkin R, Jarvik JG, Maravilla K, Kliot M. The utility of magnetic resonance imaging in evaluating peripheral nerve disorders. Muscle Nerve. 2002;25(3):314–31.
21. Mitchell CH, Brushart TM, Ahlawat S, Belzberg AJ, Carrino JA, Fayad LM. MRI of sports-related peripheral nerve injuries. AJR Am J Roentgenol. 2014;203(5):1075–84.
22. Ahlawat S, Belzberg AJ, Montgomery EA, Fayad LM. MRI features of peripheral traumatic neuromas. Eur Radiol. 2016;26(4):1204–12.
23. Habib A, Haldane CE, Ekhtiari S, et al. Pudendal nerve injury is a relatively common but transient complication of hip arthroscopy. Knee Surg Sports Traumatol Arthrosc. 2018;26(3):969–75.
24. Cvetanovich GL, Saltzman BM, Ukwuani G, Frank RM, Verma NN, Bush-Joseph CA, Nho SJ. Anatomy of the pudendal nerve and other neural structures around the proximal hamstring origin in males. Arthroscopy. 2018;34(7):2105–10. https://doi.org/10.1016/j.arthro.2018. PMID: 29606539

Distal Femur, Tibial Plateau, and Tibial Shaft Fractures

13

Kitty Wu, Mitchel R. Obey, Christopher J. Dy, and Marschall B. Berkes

13.1 Introduction

Peripheral nerve injury (PNI) in the lower extremity accounts for only 20% of all peripheral nerve lesions; however, it is associated with a much worse prognosis compared to the upper extremity [1–3]. The majority of lower extremity PNI results from high-energy trauma and motor vehicle collisions, resulting in fractures about the knee including those of the distal femur and tibial plateau, as well as fractures of the tibial shaft. In these patients, the common peroneal nerve (CPN) tends to be the most frequently injured [4], with an incidence ranging from 3% in tibial plateau fractures to up to 50% in posterolateral knee dislocations with multi-ligamentous injury [5, 6]. Even in cases where these nerves remain largely unharmed by the initial trauma, they can be injured by a variety of other mechanisms throughout the course of fracture treatment. These include preoperative or intraoperative intraneural local anesthetic injection, improper patient positioning, prolonged tourniquet time, excessive traction during surgery, impingement or penetration by surgical implants, and inadvertent nerve transection either during the surgical approach or during fracture fixation [7, 8].

The incidence of iatrogenic CPN injury is underestimated and reported to be as high as 7% of all lower extremity PNI [7]. Iatrogenic CPN injuries have been reported with high tibial osteotomies, arthroscopic and open repair of lateral meniscus tears, total knee arthroplasties, and external fixator placement [7, 9–12]. Distal branches of the CPN, such as the deep peroneal nerve (DPN) and superficial peroneal nerve (SPN), may also be injured in isolation during fasciotomies, external fixation pin placement, plate fixation of tibial plateau and shaft fractures, and percutaneous placement of proximal locking screw during placement of intramedullary fixation. Injuries to these nerve branches may present with motor, sensory, or mixed deficits postoperatively. The saphenous nerve may also be injured during plating of tibial plateau and shaft fractures. Injuries to this nerve can result in sensory deficits, paresthesias, or painful neuromas.

Lower extremity PNI results in significant morbidity, causing severe gait abnormalities, absence of protective foot sensation, and neuropathic pain [13]. Patients experience loss of phys-

K. Wu
Department of Plastic and Reconstructive Surgery, Western University, London, ON, Canada
e-mail: kwu92@uwo.ca

M. R. Obey · M. B. Berkes (✉)
Department of Orthopedic Surgery, Washington University School of Medicine, St. Louis, MO, USA
e-mail: obeym@wustl.edu; mberkes@wustl.edu

C. J. Dy
Department of Orthopedic Surgery, Washington University, St. Louis, MO, USA
e-mail: dyc@wustl.edu

C. J. Dy et al. (eds.), *Peripheral Nerve Issues after Orthopedic Surgery*,
https://doi.org/10.1007/978-3-030-84428-8_13

ical independence, decreased productivity, and psychosocial distress. This emphasizes the importance of a thorough understanding of not only the normal anatomy but also its variations to prevent iatrogenic injury and to maintain a high index of suspicion in trauma evaluation. In this chapter, we focus on peripheral nerve injuries associated with surgical treatment of fractures of the distal femur, tibial plateau, and tibial shaft.

13.2 Surgical Anatomy

13.2.1 Common Peroneal Nerve

The superficial nature and tethered course of the common peroneal nerve around the knee renders it especially vulnerable to trauma, traction, compression, and iatrogenic injuries. Thirty percent of lower extremity nerve injuries are to the CPN, and the results following exploration and repair are the worst of all peripheral nerves [14–16].

The peroneal division of the sciatic nerve is composed of the posterior L4–S2 lumbosacral roots and descends in the upper leg between the adductor magnus and hamstring muscles. Within the sciatic nerve, the peroneal fascicles are smaller and more superficially located compared to the tibial contribution [17, 18].

The sciatic nerve bifurcates into the common peroneal and tibial nerves 8–10 cm proximal to the knee joint [19, 20]. High pelvic origins of the CPN have been described, where early branching from the sciatic nerve occurs, and the CPN passes above or through the piriformis [21, 22]. From its usual bifurcation from the sciatic nerve, the CPN descends in an oblique inferolateral direction at an angle of 20.2° from a line perpendicular to the medial and lateral malleolus [20]. The mean diameter of the CPN is 3.75 mm and its fascicular pattern very consistent along the length of the nerve with the DPN fascicles located lateral to the SPN [19]. The number of fascicles of the CPN more than doubles, from an average of 7.5 fascicles within the popliteal region to 18.2 fascicles at the proximal fibular head [23]. At the level of the femoral inter-epicondylar line, the CPN is only 3.4 cm from the common tibial nerve and thus concurrent nerve injuries must be considered [20]. Iatrogenic injury to the CPN varies from 0.3% to 1.3% in primary total knee arthroplasty [24, 25]. Imaging studies show that the CPN is 15 mm (range 8.5–22.3 mm) from the closest edge of the inner surface of the joint capsule at the joint line and 14 mm (range 8–23.2 mm) from the posterolateral corner of the proximal tibia [26].

The CPN innervates the short head of the biceps femoris and travels along the lateral gastrocnemius before curving around the fibular neck. Within this course, the CPN lies in an exposed subcutaneous position for 8 cm (range 4.75–12.4 cm) before entering the fibular tunnel [21]. The fibular tunnel is defined by the peroneus longus aponeurosis, dorsomedial fibers from the soleus fascia, and the fibula [27–29]. Being tethered at both the sciatic notch and within the fibular tunnel, the CPN is exceptionally susceptible to traction injuries [30].

Within the fibular tunnel, the CPN most commonly trifurcates 3.3 cm distal to the fibular head into the anterior tibial recurrent nerve (ATRN), deep peroneal nerve (DPN), and superficial peroneal nerve (SPN) [27] (Fig. 13.1). Three locations of CPN branching have been described, with 82% dividing distal to the fibular neck, 10% branching proximal to the joint line of the knee, and 8% branching distal to the joint line but proximal to the fibular neck [22]. The ATRN and DPN pierce the anterior crural fascia. The ATRN recurs toward the knee joint before terminating in the tibialis anterior muscle, and the DPN continues distally to innervate the muscles in the anterior compartment. Various branching patterns are described with the ATRN and DPN further branching either before or after piercing the anterior crural septum [27].

13.2.2 Superficial Peroneal Nerve

The SPN trifurcates from the CPN and provides innervation to the peroneus longus (PL) and peroneus brevis (PB) muscles for ankle eversion. Classically, the SPN descends within the lateral compartment of the lower leg, deep to PL, and between the PB and extensor digitorum longus (EDL) muscles [31, 32]. Variable courses of the

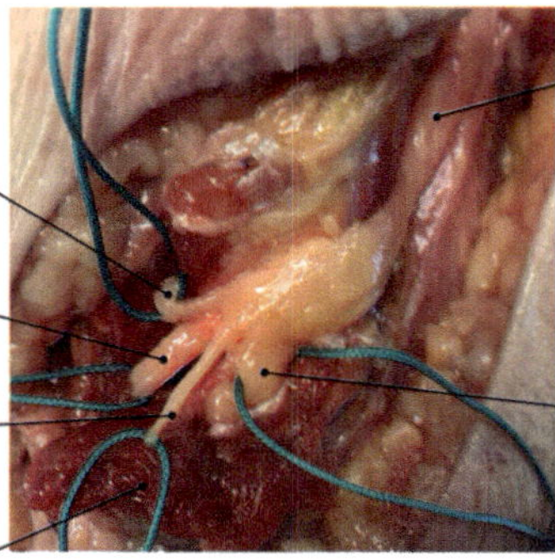

Fig. 13.1 Trifurcation and branches of common peroneal nerve. The common peroneal nerve trifurcates into the anterior tibial recurrent nerve, superficial peroneal nerve, and deep peroneal nerve. The motor branch to the peroneus longus. (Image copyright the authors, used with permission)

SPN have been described with 73% descending entirely within the lateral compartment, 14% traversing the anterior crural septum and descending within the anterior compartment, 12% with branches in both lateral and anterior compartments, and 1% descending in the lateral compartment but superficial to the PL, just deep to fascia (Fig. 13.2) [33].

The SPN gives three motor branches to the PL between 6.7 and 13.4 cm from the apex of the fibular head [34, 35]. The PB contributes to only 28% of the eversion capacity of the foot but is a more effector evertor than the peroneus longus [36]. Most often the SPN gives two motor branches to the PB between 13.4 and 20 cm from the fibular head; however, in 10% of cases, the PB is innervated with only one motor branch [34, 37]. Within the SPN, fascicles to the PL and PB are not easily distinguishable due to the interfascicular connections [4].

After giving branches to PL and PB, the SPN then pierces the crural fascia 13 cm (range 3–18 cm) proximal to the lateral malleolus, either directly on or anterior to a straight line from the fibular head to the lateral malleolus [34, 35, 38]. The SPN then continues distally in a subcutaneous course

before dividing into its terminal sensory branches, the medial dorsal cutaneous (MDC) and intermediate dorsal (IDC) cutaneous nerves, providing sensation to the majority of the dorsum of the foot [31, 32]. Three distinct terminal sensory branching patterns are described [39]. In Type A (72%), the SPN pierces the crural fascia and then divides into the MDC and IDC 4.4 cm proximal to the ankle. In Type B (16%), the MDC and IDC branch independently from the SPN, and the IDC pierces the crural fascia *posterior* to the fibula and courses anteromedially across the lateral fibula 4.5 cm proximal to the ankle joint. In Type C (12%), the MDC and IDC also branch independently from the SPN but the IDC pierces the crural fascia *anterior* to the fibula 4.9 cm proximal to the ankle joint [39]. Type B and C branching patterns may represent cases where the SPN descends as separate branches within the anterior and lateral compartments, with the anterior branch continuing as the MDC and the lateral branch continuing as the IDC nerve [33] (Fig. 13.3). Recognition of the anatomic variations of the SPN and its terminal branches is especially important when performing lower leg fasciotomies. Dangerous branching patterns include a superficial course of SPN just deep to fascia instead of deep to PL and Type B MDC/IDC branching where the IDC courses anteromedially across the fibula.

The accessory deep peroneal nerve (ADPN) arises from the SPN and is an anatomical variant present in 18.8% of patients [40]. When present, the ADPN innervates the EDB, which is normally supplied by the deep peroneal nerve. After branching from the SPN, the ADPN courses within the lateral compartment posterior to the PB before descending posteriorly to the lateral malleolus and provides sensation to the periosteum of the tarsal bones, metatarsals, and fibula [41]. Isolated traumatic injury to the ADPN

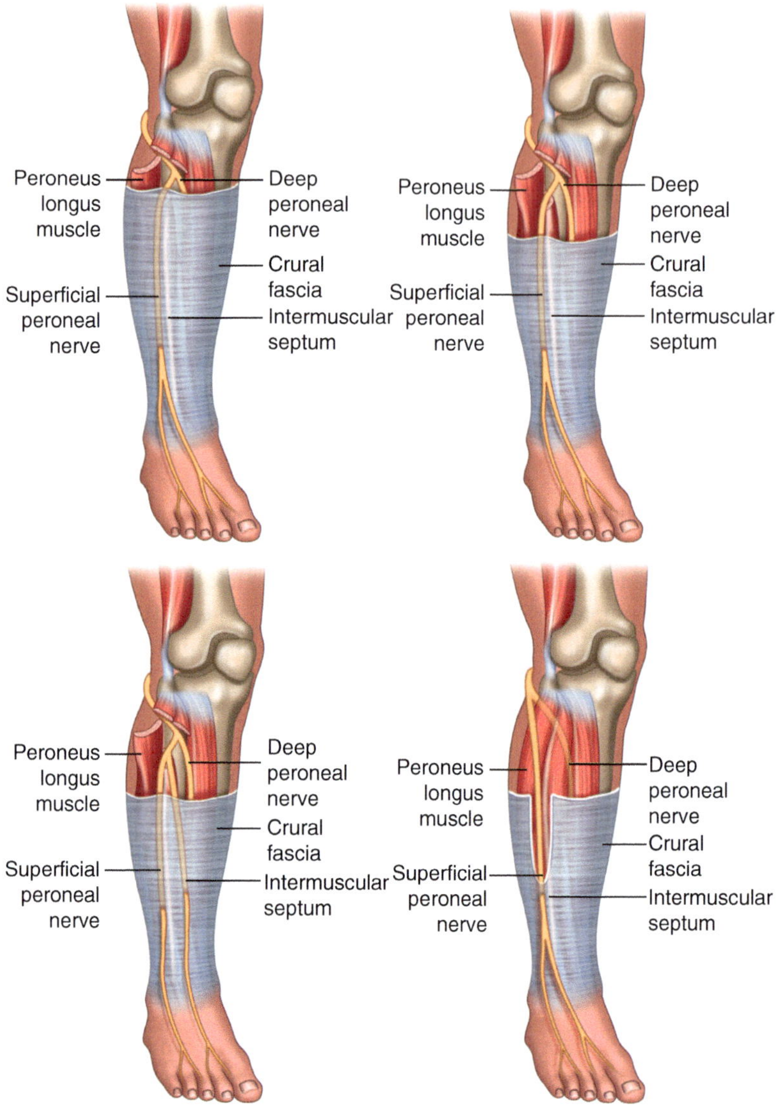

Fig. 13.2 Variations in the course of the superficial peroneal nerve. Classically, the SPN descends within the lateral compartment of the leg between the peroneus brevis and extensor digitorum longus muscles (Type A). Variations have been described with the SPN traversing the anterior crural septum and descending within the anterior compartment (Type B), or bifurcating and descending in both the lateral and anterior compartments (Type C), or descending in the lateral compartment, superficial to peroneus longus and just deep to fascia (Type D)

should be considered as part of the differential for isolated EDB atrophy or chronic lateral ankle pain [42] and care should be taken to protect the ADPN during lateral approaches to the ankle and sural nerve harvest.

13.2.3 Deep Peroneal Nerve

The DPN trifurcates from the CPN at an angle of 28.1° to the axis of the fibula and then remains in the lateral compartment for 3.3 cm before piercing the anterior crural septum [43]. In the anterior compartment, the DPN innervates the tibialis anterior (TA), extensor hallucis longus (EHL), and extensor digitorum longus (EDL) for ankle dorsiflexion and toe extension [21, 43]. The DPN divides into an average of three branches that pierce the anterior crural septum 7 cm below the apex of the fibula [21]. The most proximal branch directly pierces the anterior crural septum and passes deep to the EDL to innervate the tibialis anterior, while the remaining branches pass through an osteofibrous hiatus formed by the anterior crural septum and the fibula [44]. In 80% of cases, three motor branches innervate the tibi-

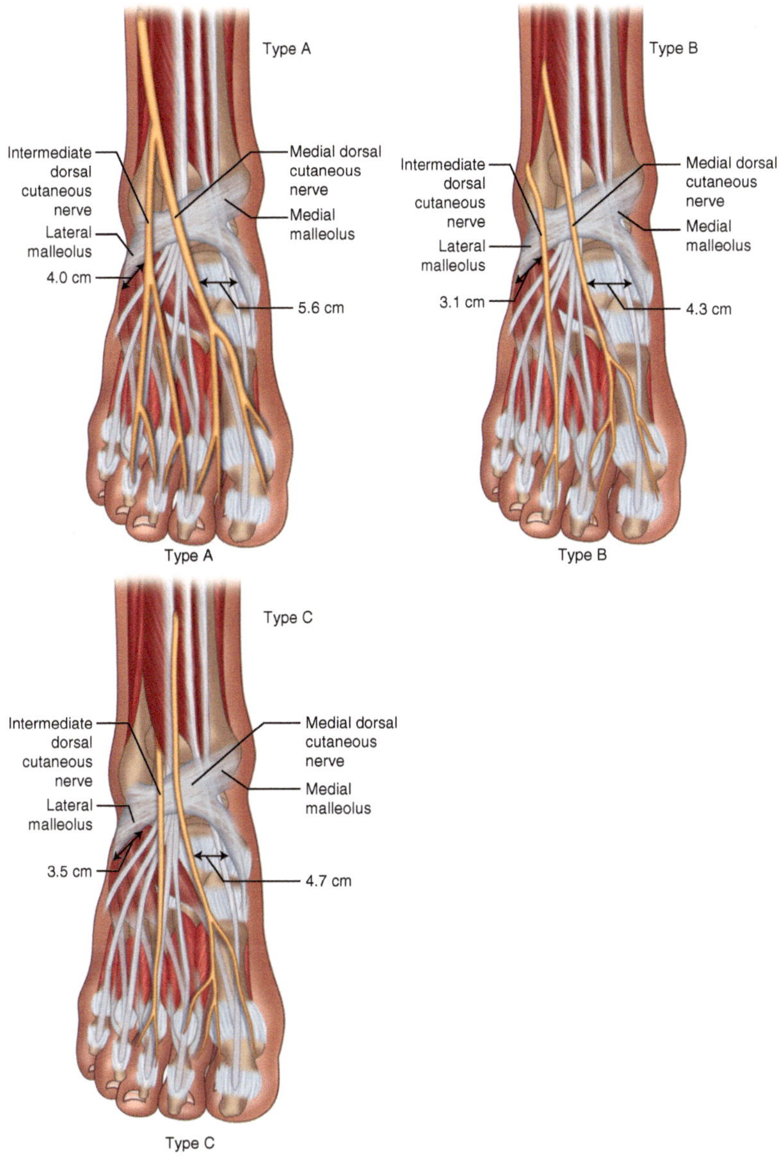

Fig. 13.3 Variable branching patterns of the terminal sensory branches of the superficial peroneal nerve. Most commonly, the SPN pierces the crural fascia and divides into the medial dorsal cutaneous (MDC) and intermediate dorsal cutaneous (IDC) branches (Type A). Variations have been described with the MDC and IDC branching independently from the SPN, with the IDC either piercing the crural fascia posterior (Type B) or anterior (Type C) to the fibula

alis anterior and the remaining 20% containing two motor branches [37]. The tibialis anterior and EHL have a mean of 3363 and 2062 axons, respectively [45].

Within the anterior compartment, the DPN travels along the anterior border of the fibula and interosseous membrane and gives branches to EDL and EHL 8.8 cm and 10.5 cm from the fibular head, respectively [35, 37]. The EDL and EHL are most commonly innervated by three motor branches each; however, the EHL is reported in cases to have only a single motor branch [37, 46]. Due to these branches passing medially toward the anterior crural septum, the zone of highest risk of iatrogenic injury is between 6.8 and 15.3 cm distal to the fibular head [47]. A described "safe zone" for distal external fixation Steinmann pin placement is between 4 and 6 cm distal to the fibular tubercle, which should remain proximal to even the most proximal DPN branch to tibialis anterior [21].

The DPN passes deep to EHL 1.25 cm proximal to the ankle and travels between EHL and EDL before bifurcating into medial and lateral terminal branches [48]. The DPN may bifurcate distal (76.5%), at the same level (11.8%), or proximal (2.9%) to the talocrural joint or remain as a single branch to the first webspace (8.8%) [49]. The lateral branch innervates the EDB muscle and the medial branch courses toward the forefoot providing sensation to the first dorsal webspace.

13.2.4 Tibial Nerve

The tibial division of the sciatic nerve is composed of the anterior L4–S3 lumbosacral roots. Within the sciatic nerve, the tibial fascicles are located in a more protected position, deeper and surrounded by thicker extra-fascicular adipose and collagen tissue compared to the peroneal division [4, 19, 50, 51]. Furthermore, the tibial nerve has twice as many fascicles and only one tether point at the sciatic notch compared to the CPN [51]. All of these factors contribute to the tibial nerve being less vulnerable to injury; however, isolated tibial nerve injuries have been described with distal femur and tibia fractures, high tibial osteotomies, total knee arthroplasties, and knee arthroscopic surgery [50, 52, 53].

The sciatic nerve divides into its peroneal and tibial divisions 8–10 cm proximal to the knee joint, and then the tibial nerve crosses the popliteal fossa lateral to the posterior tibial artery and vein to enter the posterior compartment. The tibial nerve innervates the medial and lateral gastrocnemius, soleus, plantaris, and tibialis posterior for plantarflexion and eversion at the ankle; flexor hallucis longus (FHL) and flexor digitorum longus (FDL) for toe flexion; and intrinsic musculature of the foot. The tibial nerve sends its most proximal branches to the medial and lateral gastrocnemius and soleus at 3.6 cm, 4.5 cm, and 7.6 cm distal to the femoral intercondylar line, respectively [54]. Most commonly, each muscle has at least two motor entry points with the most distal points ranging from 14 to 17 cm distal to the femoral intercondylar line. The branching pattern is highly variable in this region and common trunks between each of the three muscles described; however, in 46% of cases, there are no common trunks and each muscle receives innervation separately from the tibial nerve proper [55].

The tibial nerve then descends within the deep posterior compartment of the leg and demonstrates variable branching patterns to the popliteus, tibialis posterior, FDL, and FHL [56] (Fig. 13.4). The tibial nerve innervates the FHL, with either one (39%) or two (61%) motor branches. The most proximal branch to FHL is 6.7 cm distal to the fibular head and the second branch, if present, is 19.7 cm distal [56]. Innervation to the tibialis posterior originates from the fibular side of the nerve with an average of two motor branches 7.6 cm distal to the fibular head. The FDL is innervated, most commonly, with only one distal branch 19.8 cm distal to the fibular head. Thus, care must be taken when considering using the FDL and FHL for

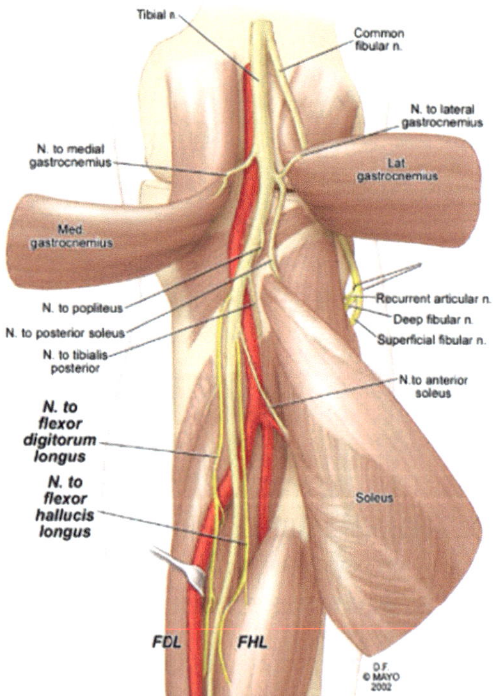

Fig. 13.4 Course of the tibial nerve and its branches in the posterior knee and lower leg. Medial and lateral gastrocnemius and soleus muscles reflected. (Image from Bodily et al. [57]. Permission for reprint from the Mayo Foundation for Medical Education and Research)

nerve transfers as each may have only a single motor terminal branch [56].

Distally, the tibial nerve courses subcutaneously and bifurcates into the medial and lateral plantar nerves, providing sensation to the sole of the foot [58]. In 95% of patients, the bifurcation occurs within 1 cm of the medial malleolar–calcaneal axis and within the fibro-osseous tarsal tunnel [58]. The tarsal tunnel, located posteriorly and inferiorly to the medial malleolus, is a common compression point formed by the medial wall of the talus, calcaneus, distal tibia, and flexor retinaculum [59]. Both distal and proximal divisions of the plantar nerves, in relation to the tarsal tunnel, are also described [60, 61].

13.2.5 Saphenous Nerve

The saphenous nerve is the largest and longest cutaneous sensory branch of the femoral nerve, supplying sensation to the anteromedial aspect of the leg. In the proximal thigh, the saphenous nerve originates from the femoral nerve 7.9 cm distal to the inguinal crease and is lateral to the femoral artery [62]. Within Hunter's adductor canal, the saphenous nerve crosses medially over the femoral artery and exits the canal 6.5–9 cm proximal to the upper border of the patella [62].

The saphenous nerve divides into the anterior sartorial branch and one to three infrapatellar branches. The infrapatellar branches bifurcate 2.3 cm proximal to the joint line of the knee and 6 cm posterior to the midpoint of the medial patellar margin [63, 64]. The upper infrapatellar branch courses anteroinferiorly at a 55.5° angle to the joint line, providing sensation to the anteromedial knee and proprioception to the anteromedial ligaments of the knee [64]. At the joint line, the sartorial branch is deep to sartorius fascia in the majority of cases (66%) and then becomes subcutaneous between the sartorius and gracilis tendons [65]. The saphenous nerve pierces the fascia between 3.7 cm proximal and 3 cm distal to the joint line of the knee [65]. Distally the saphenous nerve travels vertically in a subcutaneous plane along with the saphenous vein and provides sensation to the medial foot, terminating either at the ankle (72%) or at the first metatarsal head (28%) [66].

13.2.6 Sural Nerve

The sural nerve is commonly used as nerve grafts or site of nerve biopsy due to its superficial location and long length [67]. Injury to the sural nerve is reported in up to 13% of Achilles tendon repairs and can also occur with lesser saphenous vein harvest, peroneal tendon procedures, and posterolateral ankle surgery [68].

The sural nerve provides sensation to the posterolateral lower limb and lateral foot, with various branching patterns are described [65]. In 52% of cases, the sural nerve is formed by the union of the medial sural cutaneous nerve (MSCN) arising from the tibial nerve and the peroneal communicating nerve (PCN) either arising from the lateral sural cutaneous (LSCN) or the common peroneal nerve directly [69]. Other branching patterns occur with the sural nerve forming as a continuation of the MSCN with absent PCN and LSCN (32%) or forming from the union of the MSCN and LSCN (14%). Less common branching patterns, collectively comprising 1.8% of cases, include the sural nerve arising from the PCN alone, LSCN alone, or directly from the sciatic nerve [69]. The sural nerve then crosses the lateral border of the Achilles tendon 8–10 cm proximal to the calcaneal tuberosity and is consistently 1–2 cm posterior to the posterior border of the lateral malleolus [70, 71]. Although usually considered a pure sensory nerve, motor fibers to the intrinsic musculature of the foot are present in 6.2% of patients, leading some to advocate for EMG/NCS prior to its use as a nerve graft [72].

13.3 Neuroanatomy and the Surgical Approach

13.3.1 External Fixation

The application of external fixation constructs is commonly used for fractures of the distal femur, proximal tibia, and tibial shaft. They are often utilized in patients with open fractures who will require multiple debridements in the operating room, fractures with extensive soft tissue devitalization, and in cases where temporary stabilization is required in accordance with the guidelines of damage control orthopedics (DCO). It is commonly favored in fractures of the metaphyseal junction and, in some instances, can serve as definitive treatment. Configurations consist of the traditional monolateral constructs of Steinmann pins connected longitudinally by bars or circular external fixators which include a series of wires and/or pins connected to rings. Regardless of the construct configuration or location, the general principles remain the same: restore length, alignment, and rotation of the injured limb. Pin insertion technique is the same in the femur and tibia. It includes sharp incision of the overlying skin directly at the site of pin insertion, and then with a blunt instrument, the dissection is taken down to bone. This avoids inadvertent injury to any neurovascular structures in the area and particularly important to keep in mind when drilling the pin sites. A soft tissue protector should be used to avoid entanglement of neurovascular structures and soft tissues within the drill bit and pin during application.

13.3.1.1 Safe Zones in the Femur

When placing knee spanning external fixator constructs for distal femur fractures, the safest anatomical zones for pin insertion are the anterolateral and direct lateral aspects of the femur. Pins may also be placed directly anterior; however, the major neurovascular structures are located medially, and incidental drilling medially places those structures are risk. In the midshaft to distal shaft of the femur, pins may be placed anterolaterally through the interval between the rectus femoris and vastus lateralis muscle bellies (Fig. 13.5a). When approaching the femur direct laterally, pins are placed trans-muscularly through the vastus lateralis muscle belly (Fig. 13.5b). Direct anterior pin placement will be trans-muscularly through the muscle belly of the rectus femoris. In the femur, the neurovascular structures are located posteriorly and medially, and when placing pins from a lateral aspect, care must be taken not to plunge through the medial or posterior cortices to avoid injury to these structures.

13.3.1.2 Safe Zone in the Tibia

When placing knee spanning external fixator constructs for proximal tibia fractures, the safest anatomical zone for pin insertion are the anteromedial aspect of the tibia. Pins should be inserted

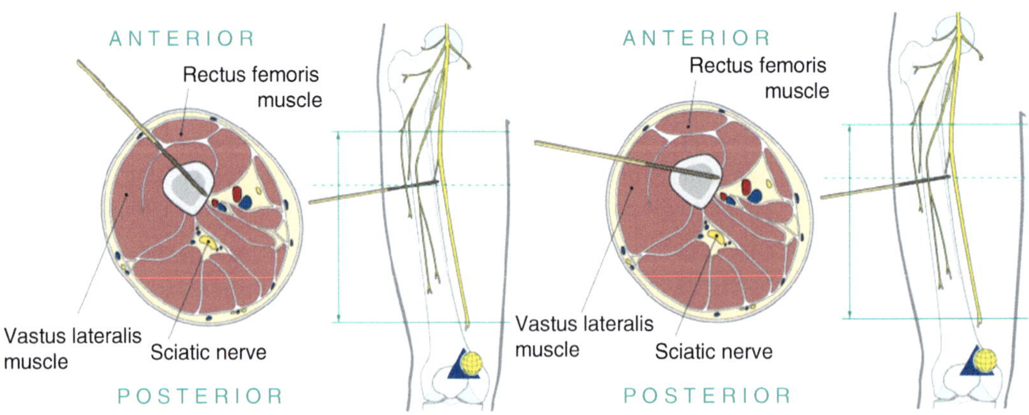

Fig. 13.5 Anterolateral and direct anterior pin placement with external fixation. (**a**) Anterolateral pin placement through the interval between the rectus femoris and vastus lateralis. (**b**) Direct anterior pin placement is trans-muscular through the vastus lateralis muscle belly. (Copyright by AO Foundation, Switzerland. Source: AO Surgery Reference, www.aosurgery.org. Reprinted with permission)

approximately 1 cm medial to the tibial crest and perpendicular with the anteromedial aspect of the tibia (Fig. 13.6). In the tibia, the neurovascular structures at risk (anterior tibial artery/vein and deep peroneal nerve) are located posterolateral to the posterior cortex of the tibia just anterior to the anterior intermuscular septum. Care must be taken not to direct pins toward the neurovascular bundle and not to plunge through when drilling or inserting pins.

13.3.2 Fractures of the Distal Femur

Fractures of the distal femur are difficult and complex injuries that represent less than 1% of all fractures in adults and approximately 3–6% of all femoral fractures [73–75]. Their incidence is largely bimodal, occurring after high-energy trauma in young males and low-energy trauma in elderly women [74, 76]. They may also occur above or around the femoral component of a total knee arthroplasty (TKA), with an incidence of 0.3–2.5% [77]. The tibial nerve is at risk in these injures due to its proximity to the femur. With the leg in extension, it is located 10.29 ± 4.41 mm posterior to distal femoral condyle at 1 cm proximal to the joint line and 13.1 ± 4.15 mm posterior to the proximal tibia cortex at the level of the joint line [78]. Alternatively, with knee flexed to 90 degrees, it is located 26.24 ± 7.70 mm posterior to distal femoral condyle at 1 cm proximal to the joint line and 21.52 ± 10.67 mm posterior to the proximal tibia cortex at the level of the joint line [78]. In patients where surgical fixation is indicated, a variety of treatment options and surgical approaches exist, and the appropriate choice is often dictated by fracture pattern and surgeon experience.

13.3.2.1 Direct Lateral/Anterolateral Approach to the Distal Femur

This approach allows for visualization, reduction, and fixation of many fractures of the distal femur, including extra- and intra-articular patterns (Fig. 13.7). In essence, this approach is an extension of the lateral approach to the femur, and visualization of the femur relies on elevation of the vastus lateralis off from the lateral intermuscular septum to expose the femur and lateral joint capsule. The skin incision is centered over the mid-lateral aspect of the femoral shaft and is often extended distally in a curvilinear fashion anteriorly over the lateral femoral condyle toward the tibial tubercle. Alternatively, it may be extended to Gerdy's tubercle rather than curving the incision anteriorly. In this approach, there is no internervous plane, and no major nerves are located in or near the area. The 8- to 10-cm skin incision is drawn out, and sharp dissection is taken down through the skin to the level of the iliotibial band. The iliotibial band is then split in line with the fibers, which distally slope anteriorly toward the tibial tubercle. The surgeon can now visualize the overlying fascia of the vastus

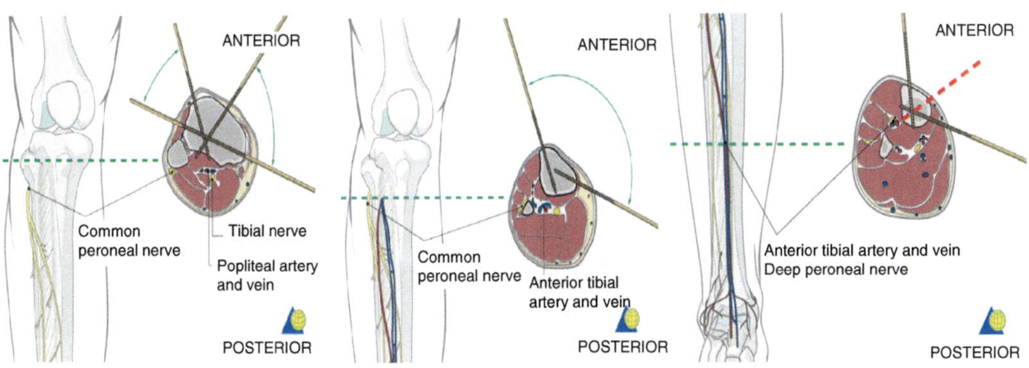

Fig. 13.6 Pin placement in knee spanning external fixation application. (Copyright by AO Foundation, Switzerland. Source: AO Surgery Reference, www.aosurgery.org. Reprinted with permission)

lateralis. Incise the fascia just anterior to the lateral intermuscular septum, and retract the muscle belly anteromedially to visualize the distal femur. Several perforating vessels from the profunda femoris artery and vein will be encountered as the muscle is elevated, but there will be no major nerves.

Tips to Avoid Injury: Sciatic Nerve

The sciatic nerve bifurcates into the common peroneal and tibial nerves 8–10 cm proximal to the knee joint [19, 20]. The tibial nerve then crosses the popliteal fossa lateral to the posterior tibial artery and vein to enter the posterior compartment, and the common peroneal nerve branches to innervate the short head of the biceps femoris and then travels along the lateral gastrocnemius before curving around the fibular neck. Within this course, the CPN lies in an exposed subcutaneous position for 8 cm (range 4.75–12.4 cm) before entering the fibular tunnel [21]. Care must be taken during the dissection to not veer posteriorly to the lateral intermuscular septum and also to avoid overretraction of posterior structures and prevent inadvertent neurovascular injury.

13.3.2.2 Direct Medial Approach to the Distal Femur

This approach allows for visualization, reduction, and fixation of mainly fractures of the medial distal femur, including Hoffa-type fractures, extra- and intra-articular patterns (Fig. 13.8). It relies on proper identification of the interval between the sartorius and vastus medialis to expose the femur and medial joint

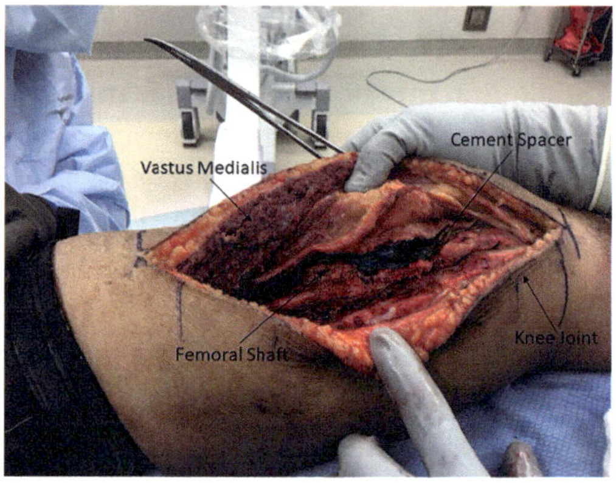

Fig. 13.8 Intraoperative image while performing the Masquelet technique in the distal femur for significant bone loss via direct medial approach. Image copyright the authors, used with permission

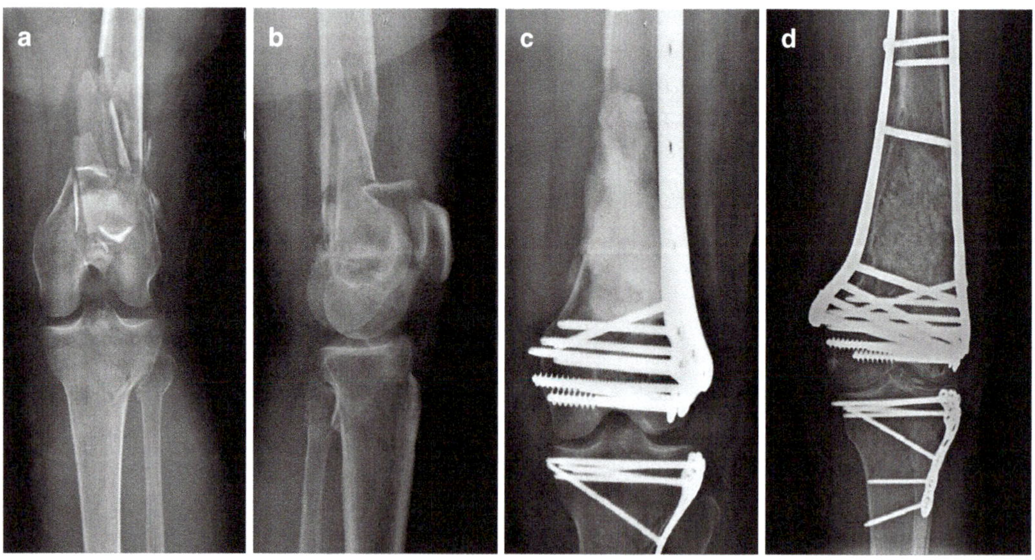

Fig. 13.7 Comminuted intra-articular left distal femur fracture radiographs (**a**–**b**), open reduction internal fixation via direct lateral approach and masquelet technique via direct medial approach (**c**), interval open reduction internal fixation via direct medial approach to the distal femur (**d**)

capsule. The incision is centered over the mid-medial aspect of the femoral shaft in line with the tendon of the adductor magnus muscle. An 8- to 10-cm skin incision is utilized and is often extended several centimeters distal to the joint line. The skin is sharply incised, and the dissection is taken down to the fascia overlying the sartorius and vastus medialis muscles. The anterior leading edge of the sartorius is identified and the fascia is incised in line with the edge. To expose the femur, sartorius is retracted posteriorly and the vastus medialis anteriorly to expose the adductor magnus tendon, which can now be retracted posteriorly with the sartorius. The popliteal neurovascular bundle lies posteriorly to the femur and can be identified through blunt dissection behind the adductor magnus.

Tips to Avoid Injury: Saphenous Nerve

In the medial approach to the distal femur, the surgeon must be mindful of the medially based neurovascular structures as they exit the adductor canal 6.5–9 cm proximal to the upper border of the patella [62] or approximately 8.5–9 cm proximal to the adductor tubercle [79, 80]. The saphenous nerve can be found emerging between the sartorius and gracilis muscles 11.7 cm proximal to the adductor tubercle and traveling distally along the posterior edge of the sartorius with the long saphenous vein. The infrapatellar branches bifurcate 2.3 cm proximal to the joint line of the knee 6 cm posterior to the midpoint of the medial patellar margin [63, 64]. Injury to this nerve can be avoided by careful retraction away from the surgical field.

13.3.3 Fractures of the Tibial Plateau

Fractures of the tibial plateau are intra-articular injuries of the knee that represent approximately 1–2% of all adult fractures [73]. They have a bimodal distribution of incidence with high-energy fractures occurring in younger patients and lower-energy mechanisms occurring in the elderly [81]. They carry a high association with neurovascular injuries, compartment syndrome, and other concurrent fractures. They are most commonly classified in accordance with the Schatzker classification first described in 1979 [82], which includes Types I through VI and can offer guidance on treatment.

13.3.3.1 Anterolateral Approach to the Proximal Tibia

This approach allows for visualization, reduction, and fixation of fractures of the lateral proximal tibia, including tibial plateau patterns (Fig. 13.9). This approach to the proximal tibia relies on proper identification of the insertion of the iliotibial band at Gerdy's tubercle, and careful elevation of the tibialis anterior muscle from its proximal attachment to expose the lateral tibial plateau and lateral joint capsule. The skin incision begins 1–2 cm lateral to the tibial crest, crosses the center of Gerdy's tubercle, and extends proximally to 8 cm proximal to the joint line just lateral to the patella. The incision is often a straight line, hockey stick, or "lazy S" in shape, depending on surgeon preference. The anterior compartment fascia is incised 5–10 mm lateral to the tibial crest and anterior to the iliotibial band, and the tibialis anterior is elevated subperiosteally to expose the proximal tibia. If needed, the dissection can be taken proximally by incising the iliotibial band in line with its fibers and then elevating it both anteriorly and posteriorly. The dissection is then taken posterolaterally until the anterior capsule of the proximal tibiofibular joint is encountered. The common peroneal nerve here runs posterior to the biceps femoris tendon at its attachment to the fibular head.

Tips to Avoid Injury: Common Peroneal Nerve

The common peroneal nerve is most at risk in surgical treatment of these injuries as it courses along the lateral aspect of the fibular neck to enter the anterior and lateral compartments of the leg (Fig. 13.10). Within the fibular tunnel, the CPN most commonly trifurcates 3.3 cm distal to the fibular head into the anterior tibial recurrent nerve (ATRN), deep peroneal nerve (DPN), and superficial peroneal nerve (SPN) [27]. Three locations of CPN branching have been described with 82% dividing distal to the fibular neck, 10%

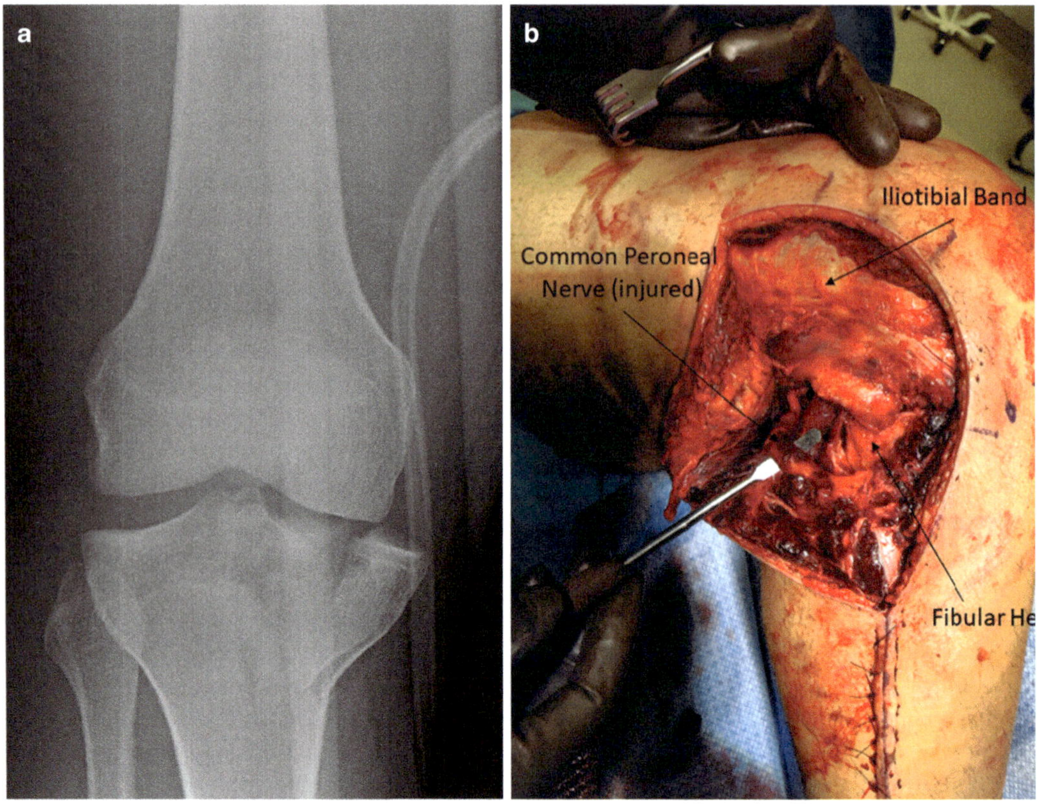

Fig. 13.9 Right tibial plateau fracture dislocation (**a**) with intraoperative image (**b**), while performing an anterolateral approach to the tibial plateau for posterolateral corner and common peroneal nerve injuries. (Image copyright the authors, used with permission)

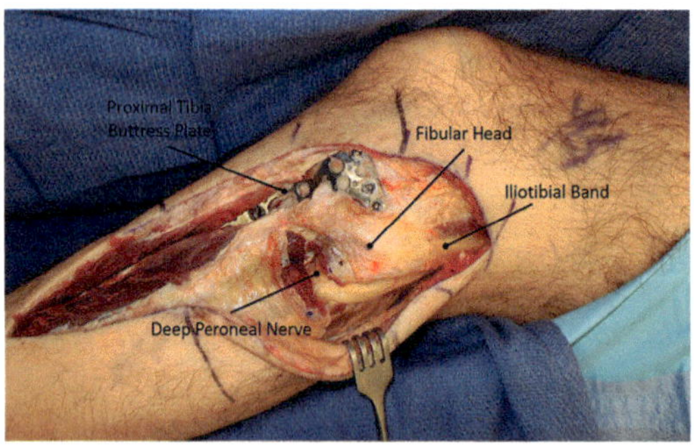

Fig. 13.10 Intraoperative images of anterolateral proximal tibia buttress plate in relation to the common and deep peroneal nerves. (Image copyright Dr. Christopher Dy, used with permission)

branching proximal to the joint line of the knee, and 8% branching distal to the joint line but proximal to the fibular neck [22]. After it branches from the CPN, within the anterior compartment the deep peroneal nerve travels along the anterior border of the fibula and interosseous membrane and gives branches to EDL and EHL 8.8 and 10.5 cm from the fibular head, respectively [35, 37].

13.3.3.2 Direct Posterior Approach to the Proximal Tibia

This approach was first described in the German literature by Galla and Lobenhoffer in the context of tibial plateau fracture dislocations with a posteromedial split [135]. In contrast to alternative posterior approaches of the knee, this approach minimizes soft tissue dissection and does not involve a dissection of the neurovascular bundle. With the patient in the prone position, a 6- to 8-cm skin incision is made longitudinally along the border of the medial head of the gastrocnemius muscle ending proximally at the medial joint line. Sharp dissection is taken down through the subcutaneous tissues to the level of the popliteal fascia. In the traditional exposure, the popliteal fossa is not crossed; however, in cases where further exposure is required, the incision can be continued is a "lazy S" pattern across the fossa to the posterolateral thigh. The popliteal fascia is incised, and the small saphenous vein can then be identified in the sulcus between the two heads of the gastrocnemius musculature. There is no internervous plane during this level of the dissection. Located lateral to the saphenous vein will be the medial sural cutaneous nerve, a cutaneous branch of the tibial nerve. It should be identified and protected, but the dissection will remain medial and away from the nerve. Blunted dissect around the medial and lateral aspects of the medial head of the gastrocnemius to free up any surrounding adhesions. The muscle is carefully retracted laterally to expose the underlying semimembranosus tendon, which is retracted medially with blunt dissection. The popliteus muscle belly is now identified, and bluntly dissected and subperiosteally elevated to expose the underlying posterior surface of the proximal tibia. If this does not provide adequate exposure, the semimembranosus can be subperiosteally elevated from its medial insertion on the proximal tibia, and the soleus can be elevated from its insertions distally on the posterior fibula and tibia. This will now give the surgeon access to the posteromedial proximal tibia.

Tips to Avoid Injury: Tibial and Common Peroneal Nerve

The sciatic nerve divides into its peroneal and tibial divisions 8–10 cm proximal to the knee joint, and then the tibial nerve crosses the popliteal fossa lateral to the posterior tibial artery and vein to enter the posterior compartment. By staying medial to the saphenous vein during the superficial dissection of the approach, injury to the sural nerve and cutaneous branches of the tibial nerve can be avoided. The tibial nerve lies lateral to the popliteal vessels and sends its most proximal branches to the medial and lateral gastrocnemius and soleus at 3.6 cm, 4.5 cm, and 7.6 cm distal to the femoral intercondylar line, respectively [54], and injury to these nerves can be avoided by staying medial to the popliteal artery and vein during the deep dissection.

13.3.3.3 Posteromedial Approach to the Proximal Tibia

This approach allows for visualization, reduction, and fixation of bicondylar or medial unicondylar fractures of the tibial plateau. The skin incision is made 1–2 cm posterior to the posteromedial tibial border and can be extended proximally along medial femoral epicondyle and distally along the tibial crest. Dissection is taken down to the fascia overlying the pes anserinus tendons. Incise the overlying fascia and retract the pes tendons anteriorly and the medial head of the gastrocnemius posteriorly to expose the medial tibial plateau and joint capsule. The saphenous nerve and its infrapatellar branches are at risk during this approach, and care should be taken to avoid injury.

Tips to Avoid Injury: Saphenous Nerve

The saphenous nerve can be found traveling distally along the posterior edge of the sartorius with the long saphenous vein. The infrapatellar branches bifurcate 2.3 cm proximal to the joint line of the knee 6 cm posterior to the midpoint of the medial patellar margin [63, 64]. The saphenous nerve pierces the fascia between 3.7 cm proximal to 3 cm distal to the joint line of the knee [65] and travels vertically in a subcutaneous plane along with the saphenous vein in the lower leg (Fig. 13.11).

13.3.4 Fractures of the Tibial Shaft

Fractures of the tibial shaft occur with an incidence of 16.9/100,000 per year with the highest incidence seen in males between the ages of 10 and 20 [83]; however, there is a second peak seen around the age of 50 [84]. High-energy trauma accounts for those seen in younger patients, whereas standing level falls tend to account for those in the elderly [84]. In nearly 60% of cases, they are accompanied by an associated injury, and roughly 39% are open fractures [84]. The

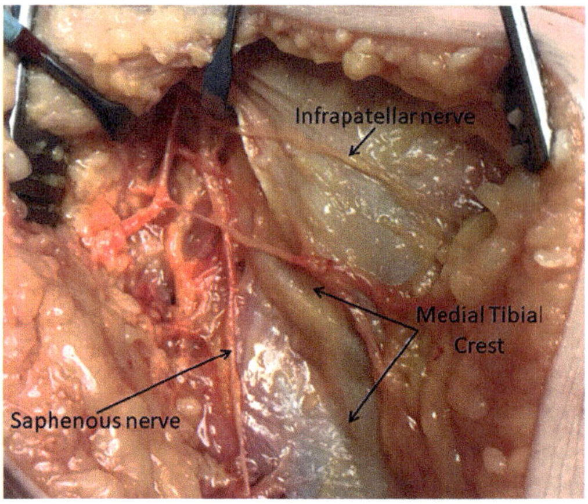

Fig. 13.11 Posteromedial proximal tibia cadaveric dissection displaying at-risk saphenous nerve and its branches to the patella. (Image copyright the authors, used with permission)

majority of proximal third and midshaft tibia fractures are treated via intramedullary nailing techniques, which limits soft tissue dissection (Fig. 13.12). However, the common peroneal nerve, as well as the sural and saphenous nerves, remains at risk during the procedure. It is during placement of the proximal [85, 86] and distal interlocking screws [87] when these nerves can be injured, and thus, care must be taken not to plunge when drilling and also to use the "nick and spread" technique.

13.3.4.1 Intramedullary Nailing of the Tibia

- *Suprapatellar Approach*: 3- to 5-cm skin incision made beginning at the superomedial edge of the patella and extended proximally. Full-thickness soft-tissue flaps are elevated, and an arthrotomy is made through the extensor mechanism.
- *Infra- or Transpatellar Approach*: 3- to 5-cm skin incision made beginning at the inferior pole of the patella and extended distally. Full-thickness soft-tissue flaps are elevated, the paratenon of the patellar tendon at its midpoint is incised, and medial/lateral flaps are elevated. An incision is made in the midline of the patellar tendon taking care not to incise the capsule of the knee joint.
- *Medial Parapatellar Approach*: 3- to 5-cm skin incision made beginning at the inferomedial edge of the patella and extended distally along the medial border of the patellar tendon. Full-thickness soft-tissue flaps are elevated down to the level of retinaculum which is incised to retract the patellar tendon laterally. The capsule of the knee joint is not incised.
- *Lateral Parapatellar Approach*: 3- to 5-cm skin incision made beginning at the inferolateral edge of the patella and extended distally along the lateral border of the patellar tendon. Full-thickness soft-tissue flaps are elevated down to the level of retinaculum which is incised to retract the patellar tendon medially. The capsule of the knee joint is not incised.

Tips to Avoid Injury: Peroneal and Saphenous Nerve

Aside from the suprapatellar approach, the incision in each of these approaches places the infrapatellar branch of the saphenous nerve at risk of injury. Care can be taken during the superficial and deep dissection to avoid severing these branches; however, in many cases, it is often unavoidable. When placing proximal and distal interlocking screws, it is key to only incise the skin and utilize a "nick and spread technique" to dissect down to bone with a blunt instrument to avoid injury to branches of the common peroneal nerve proximally [85, 86]. Previous authors have reported on incidental injury to the peroneal nerve during placement of proximal interlocking screws, and injury rates have been as high as 19% with approximately 5.3% experiencing weakness of the extensor halluces longus [85]. An anatomical study reported the common peroneal nerve was on average 2.6 mm (1.0–10.7 mm) from the proximal oblique interlock screws [86]. Distally, branches of the saphenous or superficial peroneal nerves are also at risk of injury when placing the distal interlock screws (Fig. 13.13). In general, screws are placed from medial to lateral to minimize risk of injury to the superficial peroneal nerve. Medially, branches of the saphenous can be found running just proximal and directly

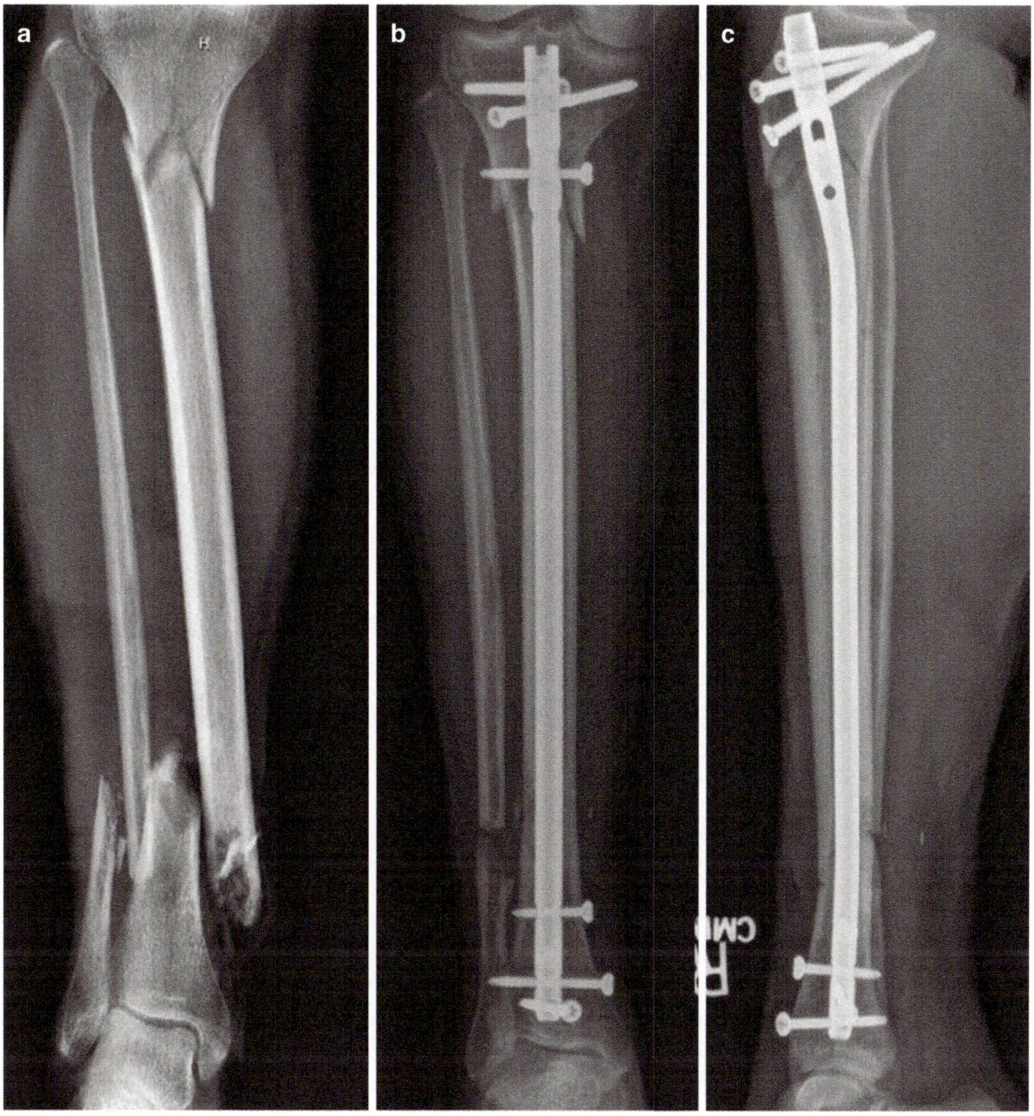

Fig. 13.12 Right proximal tibial and distal tibia and fibula fractures (**a**) and status post intramedullary nailing (**b**, **c**)

superficial to the medial malleolus. Laterally, branches of the superficial peroneal nerve are found superficial to the fascia running just anterior to the fibula as they cross the anterolateral aspect of the ankle joint. Care must be taken to perform a clean, complete dissection down to bone and to use a soft tissue protector when drilling tunnels for the interlock screws.

13.3.4.2 Tibial Plating

- *Anterolateral Approach:* this approach allows for visualization, reduction, and fixation of the middle two-thirds of the tibia shaft (Fig. 13.14). The skin incision is made longitudinally overlying the shaft of the fibula. The incision is commonly centered over the fracture site and can be extended proximally and distally as needed for exposure. Dissection is taken down to the fascia overlying the lateral compartment and then incised to identify the interval between the anterior aspect of the peroneus brevis muscle and the extensor digitorum muscle of the anterior compartment. As the dissection is taken down to the anterolat-

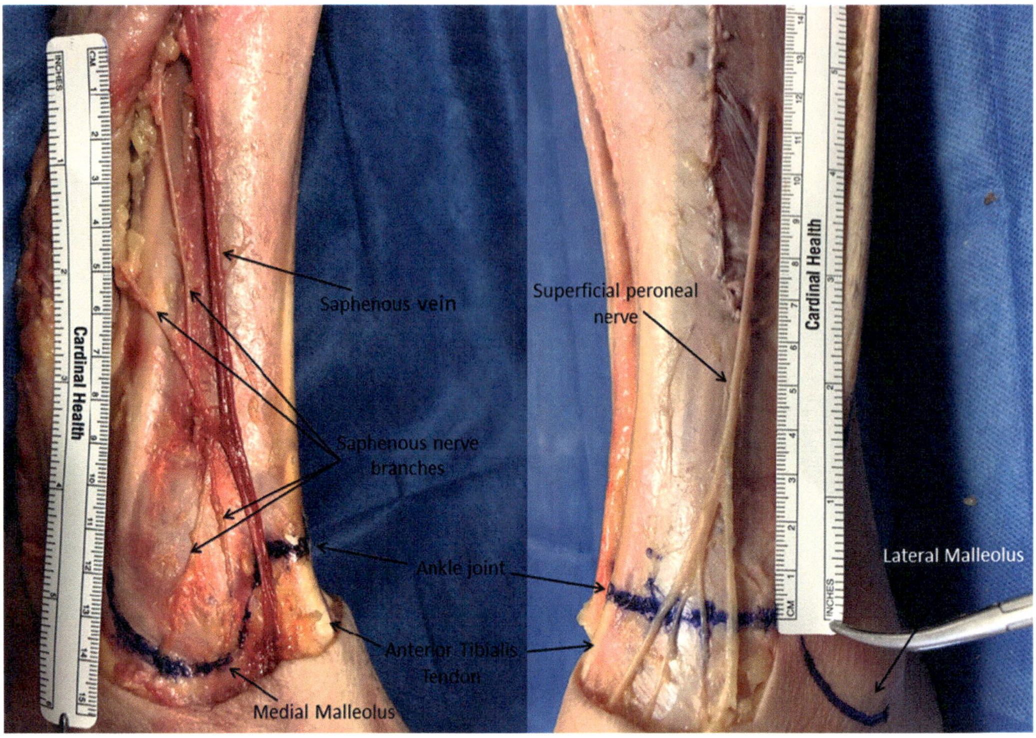

Fig. 13.13 Cadaveric dissection of saphenous nerve and vein (left) and superficial peroneal nerve and its branches just proximal to the ankle joint to demonstrate their potential injury during placement of medial-to-lateral distal interlock screws. (Image copyright the authors, used with permission)

eral aspect of the fibular, the superficial peroneal nerve can be seen lying on the peroneus brevis muscle. This must be protected. Next the extensor muscles of the anterior compartment are gently elevated off the interosseous membrane with the anterior tibial artery/vein and deep peroneal nerve to expose the lateral border of the tibia.

- *Anteromedial Approach*: this approach allows for visualization, reduction, and fixation of fractures along the distal two-thirds of the tibia. The skin incision is made 1–2 cm lateral to the tibia crest and is extended distally along the medial edge of the tibialis anterior in a gentle curve in the direction of the medial malleolus. Full-thickness subcutaneous flaps are elevated to expose the fracture, and dissection is kept superficial to the fascia layer of the anterior compartment. Distally, the saphenous vein and nerve are at risk during the approach and must be identified and protected. Minimally invasive fixation can also be done through a medial approach and utilized two incisions, one proximal and one distal, both 5 cm in length along the medial tibia. The plate can then be passed subcutaneously and fixed percutaneously. Again, care must be taken distally to protect branches of the saphenous vein and nerve.

13.3.4.3 Tips to Avoid Injury

During the anterolateral approach to the tibia, the superficial peroneal nerve is at risk during the superficial dissection and must be identified on the anterior surface of the peroneus brevis and protected throughout the procedure. Motor branches to the lateral compartment leave the superficial peroneal nerve proper in the proximal third of the tibia, and at the level of the midshaft primarily sensory branches remain. In the anteromedial approach, the saphenous vein and nerve cross the surgical field distally, and should be identified and protected.

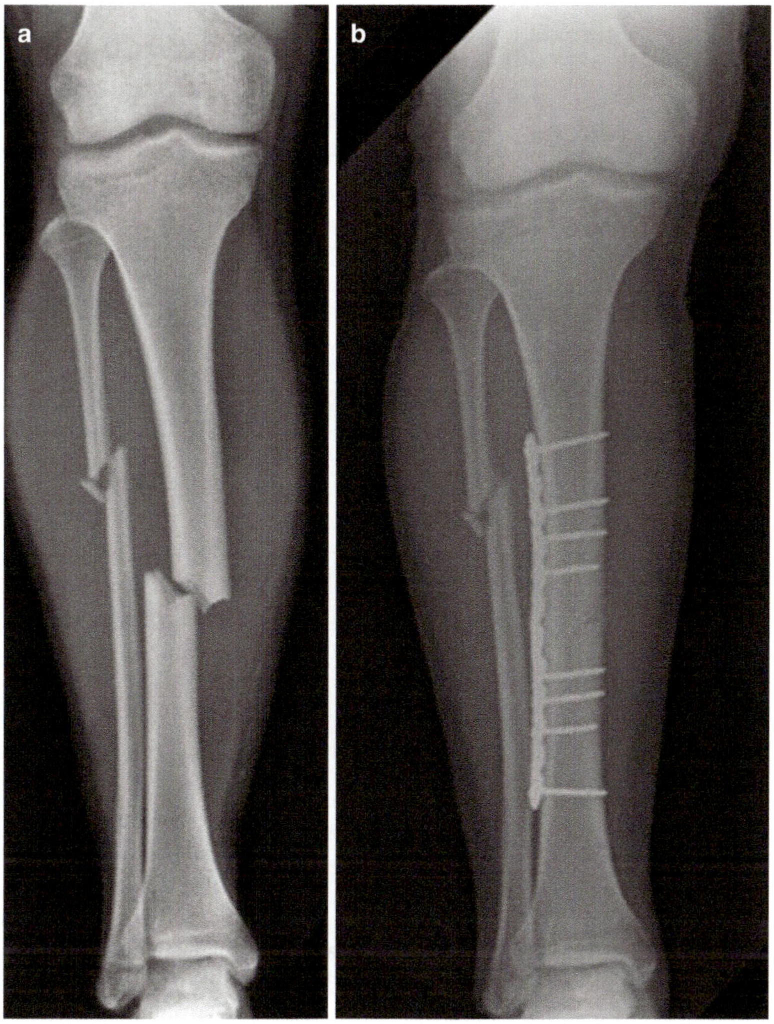

Fig. 13.14 Right mid-shaft tibia and fibula fractures (**a**), status open reduction internal fixation via lateral approach (**b**)

13.3.5 Compartment Releases of the Lower Leg

Acute compartment syndrome (ACS) is among the most devastating of orthopedic conditions, and if misdiagnosed can lead to significant morbidity, and in some cases mortality, for patients (Fig. 13.15). ACS is considered an orthopedic emergency that requires prompt diagnosis, and immediate treatment. It has numerous causes, but tibial fractures are among the most common. Following fracture, pressures within the impermeable fascial compartments of the lower leg rise to levels greater than arteriolar perfusion pressures within muscle units leading to decreased blood flow, decreased oxygen delivery, and eventual cell death. Hargens et al. [88] reported muscle undergoes irreversible change after 8 hours of ischemia, whereas nerves can undergo irreversible damage after as early as 6 hours of ischemia. The lower leg has four muscular compartments: anterior, lateral, superior posterior, and deep posterior. Fasciotomy is considered the standard of care for ACS, and two techniques have been described: double-incision technique and single-incision technique. Regardless of approach, it is critical to achieve a complete release of the involved or all compartments and avoid unnecessary damage to local neurovascular structures during the procedure.

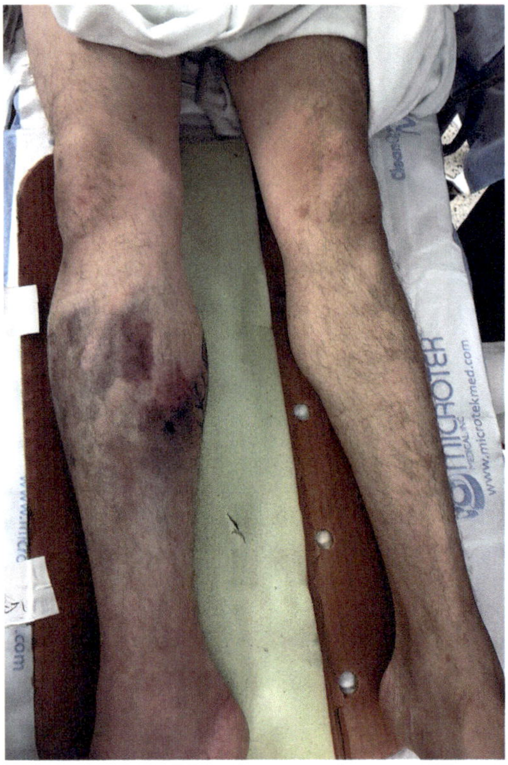

Fig. 13.15 Right lower extremity compartment syndrome after a crush injury. (Image copyright the authors, used with permission)

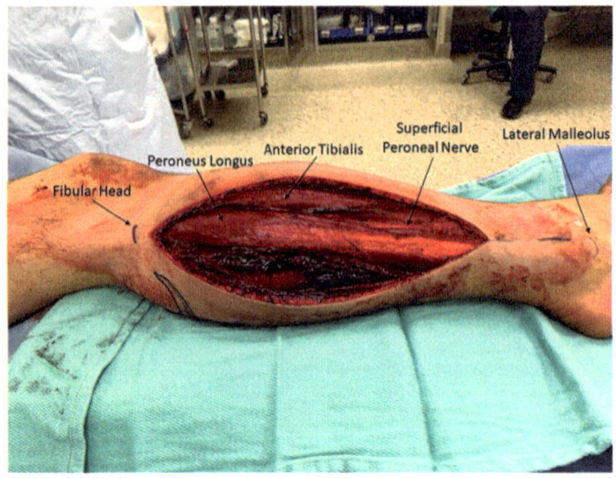

Fig. 13.16 Anterolateral incision of lower leg fasciotomy. (Image copyright the authors, used with permission)

13.3.5.1 Double-Incision Technique

The anterolateral incision is 10–15 cm in length and is made approximately midway between the fibula and tibial cortex, overlying the intermuscular septum between the anterior and lateral compartments (Fig. 13.16). A small incision is then made perpendicular to the septum to open the compartments, and the fascia of each compartment is then split longitudinally. During this step, care must be taken to avoid injuring the superficial peroneal nerve running along an anterior groove between the lateral compartment muscles.

Tips to Avoid Injury: Superficial Peroneal Nerve

The superficial peroneal nerve (SPN) pierces the crural fascia on the lateral aspect of the lower leg approximately 13 cm proximal to the lateral malleolus. It travels distally in a subcutaneous position and divides into the terminal sensory branches (medial dorsal cutaneous [MDC] and intermediate dorsal cutaneous [IDC] nerves) that provide sensation to the foot. Three distinct branch patterns have been described (Types A–C) that one must be aware of when performing fasciotomies in order to avoid iatrogenic injury. In Type A (72%), the SPN pierces the crural fascia and then divides into the MDC and IDC 4.4 cm proximal to the ankle. In Type B, (16%) the MDC and IDC branch independently from the SPN and the IDC pierces the crural fascia posterior to the fibula and courses anteromedially across the lateral fibula 4.5 cm proximal to the ankle joint. In Type C (12%), the MDC and IDC also branch independently from the SPN but the IDC pierces the crural fascia anterior to the fibula 4.9 cm proximal to the ankle joint [38]. Type B and C branching patterns may represent cases where the SPN descends as separate branches within the anterior and lateral compartments, with the anterior branch continuing as the medial dorsal cutaneous nerve and the lateral branch continuing as the intermediate dorsal cutaneous nerve [32]. Recognition of the anatomic variations of the SPN and its terminal branches is especially important when performing lower leg fasciotomies. Dangerous branching patterns include a superficial course of SPN just deep to fascia instead of deep to peroneus longus and Type B MDC/IDC branching where the IDC courses anteromedially across the fibula.

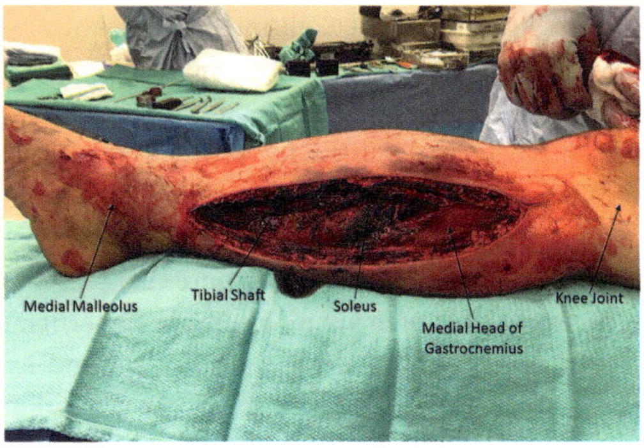

Fig. 13.17 Medial incision of lower leg fasciotomy

The posteromedial incision is made 2 cm posterior to the posterior tibial margin to visualize the intermuscular septum between the deep and superficial posterior compartments (Fig. 13.17). Care must be taken to avoid injury to the saphenous vein and nerve running subcutaneously along the medial lower leg, which should be retracted anteriorly and protected.

13.3.5.2 Single-Incision Technique

A single extensile longitudinal incision is made slightly posterior and parallel to the fibula at the level of the fibular head and ended distally just proximal to the tip of the lateral malleolus. The posterior compartments are accessed and released posterior to the fibula, and care must be taken to avoid injury to the posterior tibial artery/vein and tibial nerve. The anterior and lateral compartments are then released through dissection anterior to the fibula, and again care must be taken to avoid injury to the superficial peroneal nerve in the lateral compartment.

13.4 Initial Evaluation/Exam

The clinical evaluation of the peripheral nerve injuries after surgical procedures for distal femur, tibial plateau, and tibial shaft fractures should follow a standardized algorithm [12]. Patients will often give a history of neuropathic pain beginning after surgery. It is important to elicit exactly when the pain began (immediately after surgery vs. weeks to months later), because it can give insight into the etiology of injury. Symptoms immediately after surgery often represent acute injury either from nerve transection during the surgical approach or entrapment by implants. Motor strength tests and grading of the lower extremity, especially in the CPN distribution, monitor recovery or progression weakness after the index orthopedic surgery. Serial examination of muscle function by the same examiner is helpful to assess recovery. Sensory testing in the superficial peroneal, saphenous, and sural nerve distributions must be assessed via light tough, pin prick, and vibratory sense tests. Finally, the presence of a Tinel sign at the site of injury indicates axonal disruption. Advancement of the Tinel sign distally often represents axonal regeneration, whereas, a Tinel sign that is persistently located at the site of suspected injury likely represents neuroma formation [12].

13.5 Diagnostic Tests/Imaging

Imaging and electrodiagnostic testing are helpful components of the evaluation of potential peripheral nerve injuries following orthopedic surgery. Workup should begin with plain radiographs to determine the proximity of peripheral nerves to adjacent hardware. Less frequently, fracture or implant gapping may be indicative of possible nerve entrapment. Magnetic resonance imaging (MRI) may be utilized; however, even with specific metal subtraction sequences, the degree of metal artifact can make detailed evaluation of neurovascular structures difficult. Thus, ultrasonography can visualize nerves longitudinally and has the ability to display nerves in continuity, sites of enlargement, nerve transection, and neuroma formation. However, it is technique- and operator-dependent – it is important that the peripheral nerve surgeon communicate with the ultrasonographer to provide clinical context. Finally, electromyography (EMG) and nerve conduction studies are helpful in localizing nerve injury, predicting prognosis of nerve recovery, and identifying potential donor nerves for transfer. These studies may show denervation changes as soon as 10 days after surgery [12, 89]. An absence of motor unit recruitment by 3 months after injury coupled with absence of an advancing Tinel sign suggests a non-recovering axonometic injury and potential surgical intervention. In this setting, it is advisable to consider surgical intervention. If there is progressive recovery on serial EMG studies, there is a greater likelihood that spontaneous reinnervation will occur and observation is recommended.

13.6 Management of Nerve Injuries

13.6.1 Peroneal Nerve Injuries

In the lower extremity, common peroneal nerve injury is among the most commonly encountered mononeuropathy after orthopedic surgery [90, 91]. This results in sensory deficits to the dorsum of the foot; functional limitations in ankle dorsiflexion and eversion, due to paralysis of the tibialis anterior and peroneal muscles; and potentially debilitating neuropathic pain. Patients experience gait disturbances with a "foot drop" and can develop supinated equinovarus contractures from the unopposed action of the tibialis posterior, and shortening of the FHL, and FDL muscles [92]. Ankle–foot–orthoses (AFO) provide static ankle dorsiflexion to help with mobility and prevent contracture formation but are uncomfortable, cumbersome, and not well tolerated as a long-term option. Surgical options include neurolysis and repair or grafting, nerve transfers, tendon transfers, and combined procedures.

13.6.1.1 Direct Inspection and Neurolysis

The majority of peroneal nerve injuries result from traction with a broad zone of injury. In addition to those that occur during the original mechanism of injury, peroneal nerve damage can occur with intraoperative retractor placement, nerve entanglement within drills, or nerve entrapment by hardware such as osteosynthesis plates. When sharp transection of the nerve is suspected, such as SPN injury during fasciotomy, immediate exploration and direct inspection are recommended to allow for the possibility of primary repair and avoid the necessity of nerve grafts. Microsurgical expertise is necessary to perform immediate primary repair. If immediate microsurgical consultation is not available, it is often advisable to tag the nerve ends with a brightly colored suture (such as 4-0 polypropylene) and suture them to superficial tissue, where they can be readily identified by the microsurgery team.

For patients with known blunt injuries to the nerve (based on prior intraoperative assessment), surgical treatment is delayed for 3–4 weeks to allow the zone of injury to declare itself. For patients with suspected nerve injuries from closed mechanisms, initial EMG studies are performed 4–6 weeks after injury. Early treatment involves the use of an AFO, physiotherapy to maintain full passive range of motion, and observation for signs of spontaneous recovery. Eighty-seven percent of patients with incomplete CPN palsy will regain full motor recovery [93]. Surgical intervention is recommended in cases of complete palsies with no clinical or electromyographic evidence of recovery by 3–6 months [94–96].

The use of intraoperative nerve action potentials (NAPs) can aid in decision-making at the time of surgical exploration. Because intraoperative NAPs are highly sensitive to technical variation, establishing a regular working relationship with the intraoperative electrophysiology team is advised. The presence of intact NAPs, despite absent clinical motor function, is predictive of good functional motor recovery and either decompression alone or external neurolysis is performed if epineural scarring is visible [97]. Internal neurolysis using microsurgical technique may be necessary if there is extensive perineural scarring. Large case series and systematic reviews of neurolysis for CPN injuries demonstrate 80–89% recovery of MRC 3 or greater ankle dorsiflexion [95, 97, 98]. After neurolysis, muscle contraction in the peroneus muscles was detected at 5 months and the anterior tibialis at 12 months, with an average recovery ranging from 12 to 30 months [97].

Surgical Technique: Common Peroneal Nerve Decompression and Neurolysis

Decompression and neurolysis of the common peroneal nerve are typically performed with the patient under a general anesthesia and with the use of a thigh tourniquet. Preoperative markings should include the location of any detectable Tinel's sign. The patient is positioned supine with padding under the ipsilateral hip, the knee placed in flexion, and a sandbag under the foot to help with immobilization. The incision is oriented just distal to the fibular head coursing obliquely from proximal posterior to distal anterior direction, following the expected course of the peroneal nerve. The skin incision can also be placed along preexisting incisions.

Dissection is taken down through skin and subcutaneous tissue to the level of the superficial fascia, taking care to protect any lateral cutaneous contributions from the peroneal nerve to the sural nerve (Fig. 13.23). The CPN is palpable just posterior to the peroneus longus and the superficial fascia can be incised over the nerve (Fig. 13.18). There are three points of decompression required for complete release of the CPN: the posterior crural septum, anterior crural septum, and innominate septum. Decompression starts laterally with first releasing the posterior crural septum (posterior fascia of the peroneus longus) which often contains a tendinous leading edge (Figs. 13.19 and 13.20). Tenotomy scissors can be used on either side of the fascia to separate it from the peroneus longus and soleus muscle bellies before careful release of the fascia from superficial to deep. Following decompression, the CPN then lies on the surface of soleus muscle, which can also be released if suspected to create a secondary point of compression. Next

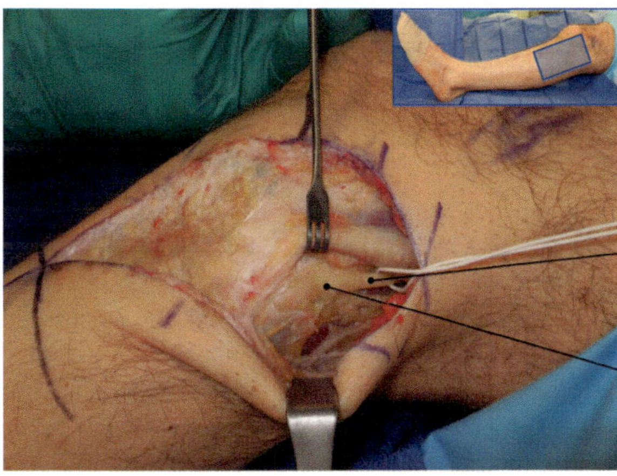

Fig. 13.18 Patient with previous open reduction and internal fixation of tibial plateau fracture with a plate undergoing hardware removal and neurolysis and decompression of the common peroneal nerve. Identification of the CPN passing under the posterior crural septum. (Image copyright Dr. Christopher Dy, used with permission)

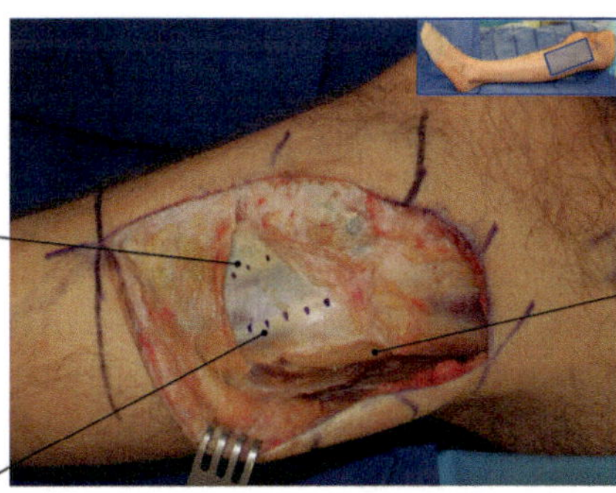

Fig. 13.19 Following decompression of the posterior crural septum, the anterior and innominate crural septae can be visualized through the fascia. The posterior crural septum has been released. (Image copyright Dr. Christopher Dy, used with permission)

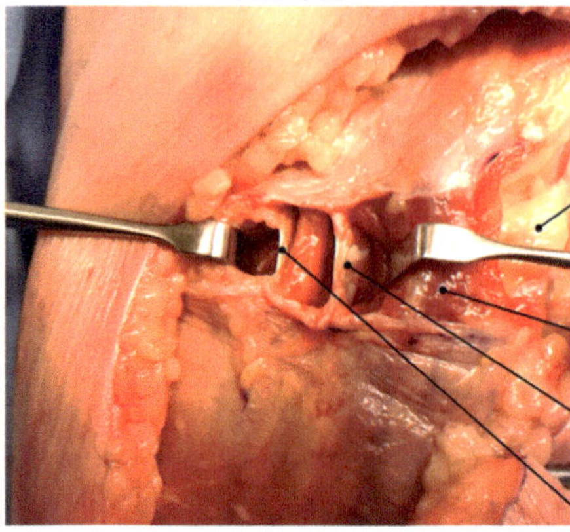

Fig. 13.20 Visualization of the anterior and innominate crural septae. (Image copyright the authors, used with permission)

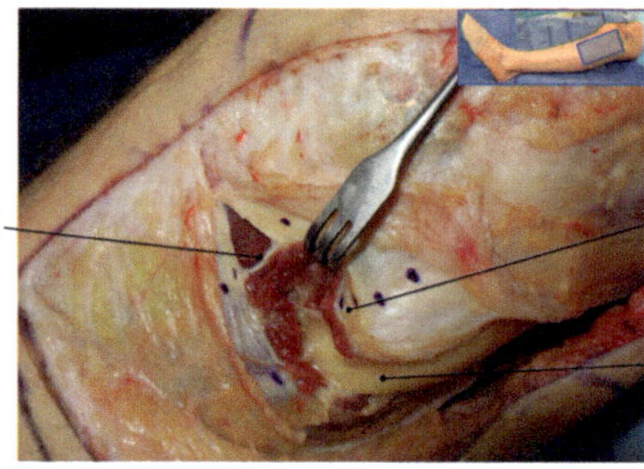

Fig. 13.21 Tendinous edges of the anterior and innominate crural septae. (Image copyright Dr. Christopher Dy, used with permission)

the anterior crural septum between the peroneus longus and EDL is divided in a similar fashion (Fig. 13.20). Lastly, the innominate septum between the EDL and tibialis anterior is visualized and divided (Fig. 13.21). Dissection can be carried further to visualize the CPN trifurcating into the anterior tibial recurrent, CPN, and DPN branches (Figs. 13.22 and 13.23).

13.6.1.2 Nerve Grafting

If the nerve is found to be discontinuous at the time of exploration, then either direct repair or autologous interposition cable grafting should be undertaken. Commonly, end-to-end repair is not possible in a tension-free manner due to the traction nature of the injury, extensive scarring, and internal neural fibrosis [97]. Following careful neurolysis and resection back to healthy fascicles, multiple sural cable grafts are used to match the cross-sectional area and bridge the defect. Difficult decisions arise when the nerve appears contiguous but is nonconducting and has palpable thickening or a visible neuroma in continuity. Initial external neurolysis is recommended followed by repeat intraoperative stimulation. Expeditious dissection is needed if a tourniquet is used, as tourniquet-related ischemia may create false-negative results from intraoperative stimulation as early as 20–30 minutes after tourniquet inflation. If there is persistence absence of recordable NAPs, then the zone of injury must be localized with careful intrafascicular dissection. Resection must be undertaken until healthy fascicles are visualized before grafting [99].

In cases of complete peroneal nerve injury, better outcomes are associated with shorter graft lengths and earlier time to surgical intervention [94, 97, 99]. In total, 64–75% of patients with grafts less than 6 cm in length achieved MRC 3 or greater ankle dorsiflexion, compared to 29–38% of patients with grafts between 6 and 12 cm and only 11% of patients with grafts

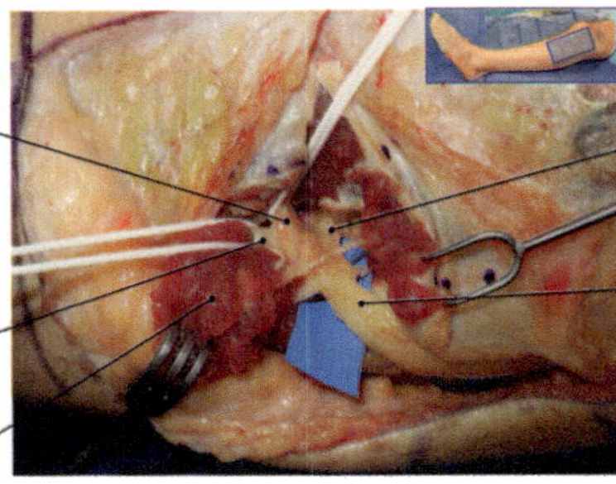

Fig. 13.22 Following decompression of the posterior, anterior, and innominate crural septae, the trifurcation of the common peroneal nerve is visualized. (Image copyright Dr. Christopher Dy, used with permission)

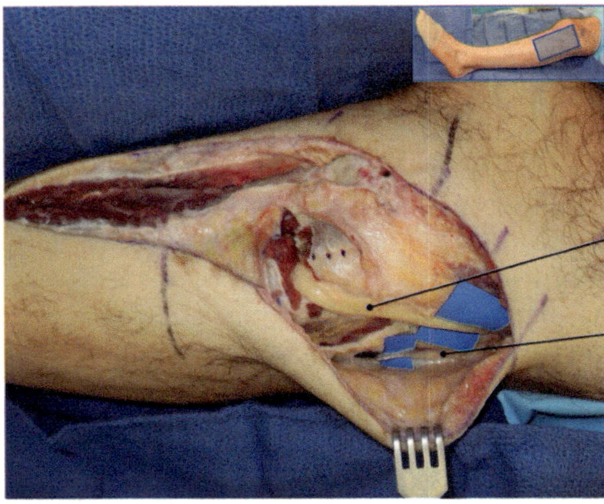

Fig. 13.23 Proximal dissection and release of common peroneal nerve. Lateral sural cutaneous nerve visualized showing its close proximity to the common peroneal nerve. Distal incision lengthened to allow for hardware removal. (Image copyright Dr. Christopher Dy, used with permission)

greater than 12 cm [95–97]. The necessity for longer grafts is also indicative of greater injury severity with higher energy mechanisms producing traction over a long segment. Similarly, outcomes also worsened with increased time to surgery. Forty-four percent of patients with surgical exploration within 6 months achieved MRC 3 or greater ankle dorsiflexion, compared to 28% of patients with surgery between 7 and 12 months, and only 12% in those with surgery more than 12 months from time of injury [95]. Although age was correlated with improved outcomes, this was not found to be statistically significant in a systematic review of 368 CPN nerve repairs [95].

13.6.1.3 Nerve Transfers

Nerve transfers have been successfully used in functional reconstruction of the upper extremity with predictable outcomes [100]. Advantages of nerve transfers include bypassing the zone of injury, avoiding use of long nerve grafts, and decreasing the time to reinnervation. While there have been some early promising results in the literature, the initial enthusiasm for use of nerve transfers has waned as more series have been published with mixed and poor outcomes. The specific challenge for nerve transfers, particularly those that use tibial nerve-based donors, are that motor reeducation can be challenging given the nonsynergistic pairing of donor and recipient. Use of these transfers by the senior author (CJD) is relatively limited for this reason.

The indications for nerve transfer in CPN injury include no clinical or electromyographic evidence of ankle dorsiflexion by 3 months, the absence of an advancing Tinel's at 3 months, the expectation of requiring greater than 6 cm of cabled nerve graft, and the presence of a healthy donor neuromuscular unit (preferably a synergistic donor) [94]. Contraindications include preexisting peripheral neuropathy, abnormal EMG testing in the tibial nerve, or greater than 12 months from the time of injury [94]. Surgical intervention must occur before 12 months, and preferably sooner, to allow time for nerve regeneration before irreversible muscle fibrosis and motor end-plate degeneration.

SPN Donor

In cases of isolated DPN injury with spared SPN function, partial transfer of the SPN to the tibialis anterior can be considered [101]. The SPN has an almost three times larger cross-sectional area compared to the tibialis anterior motor branch. Case reports of partial transfer of one-third of the SPN demonstrated that it was feasible without downgrading of foot eversion [101]. In another case series of SPN to tibialis anterior transfer, four of five patients regained MRC 4 strength in ankle dorsiflexion and patient achieved MRC 3 strength [101]. The use of SPN donors has the distinct advantage of synergism between donor and recipient. Unfortunately, its utilization is limited due to the relatively infrequent clinical presentation of a DPN palsy with intact SPN donors.

Proximal Tibial Motor Donors: Soleus, Gastrocnemius

Although many variations exist, the majority of nerve transfers involve using donors from the tibial nerve (gastrocnemius, soleus, FHL, FDL), which are often spared in CPN injuries. Tibial nerve donors can be transferred to either the CPN, DPN, or directly into the tibialis anterior [57, 102]. Motor transfer to the DPN allows for reinnervation of the EHL and EDL in addition to the anterior tibialis, and transfers to the CPN further reinnervates the peroneus longus and brevis for foot eversion. Donor motor nerve selection is dependent on the level of injury, patient-specific anatomy, and the ability to perform a direct transfer without using interposition nerve grafts. As stated above, the challenge of postoperative cortical reeducation has limited the widespread use of these nerve transfers in the senior author's practice.

For injuries of the CPN proximal to its trifurcation, the soleus, medial, and lateral head of gastrocnemius can be considered as possible donors. Anatomic studies show that the motor branch to the soleus had a mean length of 65 mm, lateral gastrocnemius 43 mm, and medial gastrocnemius 35 mm [102]. With intramuscular dissection, the soleus and lateral head of gastrocnemius motor branches can reach the CPN up to an average of 39.5 mm and 28.9 mm below the tibial plateau, respectively; however, this was not consistently sufficient to reach the tibialis anterior branch directly for primary repair [57]. Based on cross-section area of the tibialis anterior (0.255 mm), the lateral gastrocnemius was the best match (0.256 mm), and based on total number of axons of the tibialis anterior (3363 axons), the popliteus (3317 axons) or soleus (4941 axons) were the best matches [45]. Overall, the branch to the soleus was most similar to the tibialis anterior when considering both axonal count and cross-sectional area and distance from the site of coaptation to the muscle [45]. Furthermore, muscles with duel innervations (gastrocnemius) and similar actions (gastrocnemius and soleus) are preferentially used to minimize donor site morbidity and functional loss.

Outcomes from a case series by Flores et al. with 10 patients undergoing soleus to DPN nerve transfers, only 2 achieved MRC 3 or greater ankle dorsiflexion and the remaining 8 patients had MRC 0 or 1 function. They suspected either partial undetected preexisting injury to the tibial nerve or mismatch of axonal counts between the soleus and DPN to account for these poor outcomes. While the soleus is a good match to the tibialis anterior, it contains less than half the number of axons as the DPN [103]. Either use of two motor branch donors for the DPN or direct coaptation to the anterior tibialis may avoid axonal dispersion and produce more consistent results. Outcomes from several case series of lateral gastrocnemius transfer to tibialis anterior were more promising with most patients regaining MRC 4 or greater dorsiflexion strength by one year; however, in Nath et al. series of nine patients, two failed to gain any function with MRC 0 after 14–18 months [101, 104]. Donor morbidity included 5–10% reduction in calf circumference from lateral gastrocnemius denervation [101]. The modest and variable results reported by Flores [103] and Nath [104] suggest that additional work is needed to define the role of tibial-to-peroneal nerve transfers.

Distal Tibial Motor Donors: FHL, FDL

For direct neurotization to the tibialis anterior motor branch or for more distal coaptations to the DPN, the motor fascicles to the long toe-flexors FHL and FDL are possible donors that provide more length (Fig. 13.24). We do not recommend use of nerves to the posterior tibialis as donor nerves, given the high reliability of using the posterior tibialis for tendon transfer. The FHL and FDL together account for 45% of the cross-sectional area of the DPN [57]. Depending on the size of the donors and patient anatomy, various combinations of FDL, FHL, and more proximal donors can be combined. These branches can also be used as motor donors to reinnervate EHL directly for foot eversion. The cross-sectional area of the EHL (0.197 mm) was best matched with the FHL (0.234 mm). Proximal intraneural dissection of the DPN division of the CPN can also be performed to gain additional length [102]. To reach the tibialis anterior motor target, the donor nerve can be placed coursing superficially around the fibular head or passed directly through the interosseous membrane by developing a plane just deep to the fibula in order to gain more length [94, 103].

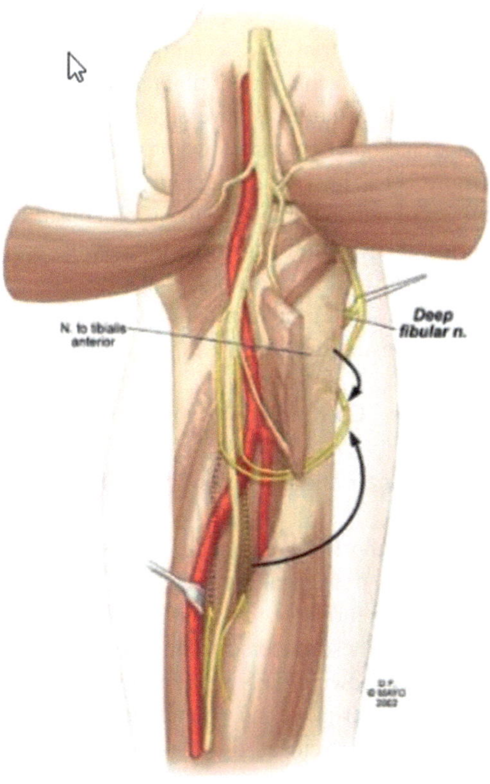

Fig. 13.24 Nerve transfer of flexor hallucis longus and flexor digitorum longus motor branches to the deep peroneal nerve distal to its bifurcation from the common peroneal nerve. (Image from Bodily et al. [57]. Permission for reprint from the Mayo Foundation for Medical Education and Research)

Outcomes with using distal tibial motor donors have been favorable, but skepticism remains regarding reproducibility of these outcomes. Ferris et al. report on nine patients undergoing transfer of either one, two, or three FDL branches alone, one or two FHL branches alone, or the two in combination to the tibialis anterior with good results [105]. Seven patients achieved MRC 3 or greater ankle dorsiflexion and two patients (one with three FDL branches, and one with one FDL and one soleus branch) did not recovery anti-gravity strength [105]. Giuffre et al. describe nine patients undergoing either FHL alone, FDL alone, or posterior tibial fascicle transfer to the tibialis anterior with mixed results. Three patients achieved MRC 3 or greater ankle dorsiflexion. Additional case series demonstrating reproducible and reliable results are needed to support widespread usage of tibial-to-peroneal nerve transfers.

13.6.1.4 Tendon Transfers

In patients where nerve-based reconstruction has either failed or is not an option, tendon transfer is the standard for restoration of functional dorsiflexion [106]. Any consideration for nerve transfer should preserve the posterior tibialis for use in tendon transfer as a salvage option. Many tendon transfer techniques have been previously described and choice often depends on surgeon preference and that functionality of proposed tendons for transfer. Ober first described use of the posterior tibial tendon for the surgical correction of peroneal nerve palsy to transfer the tendon medially across the tibial [107]. Since then further improvements have been suggested by Watkins with transfer of the tibial posterior tendon through the interosseous membrane and by Anderson and Srinivasan who split the tendon into two portions for insertion into the EHL and

EDL tendons [108–110]. The most well-known is the Riordan "Bridle procedure", which involves a transfer of the posterior tibialis tendon through the interosseous membrane to the dorsum of the foot with insertion into the tibialis anterior and peroneus longus tendons [91, 111]. Furthermore, in patients who are not candidates for tendon transfer procedures (such as those without a suitable donor tendon), alternative surgical procedures such as tibiotalar or tibiotalocalcaneal arthrodesis can be considered.

- Posterior Tibialis Tendon Transfer (i.e. Bridle Procedure [112, 113])
  - There should be a low threshold for lengthening of the gastric–soleus complex, as transferring of the posterior tibial tendon will decrease its strength by one grade (i.e. 5/5 to 4/5), thus preventing any antagonism of the transfer by an Achilles contracture is prudent.
  - In some patients, transfer of the posterior tibialis tendon through the interosseous membrane may lead to stenosis, and thus ensuring an adequate size pathway through the membrane to the anterior tibia is essential.
  - Balance of the foot with equal balancing of the tibialis and peroneus longus components of the construct to avoid varus or valgus deformity.
  - Surgeons should err toward over-tensioning rather than under-tensioning of the tendons at the time of procedure, as there is a degree of subsidence of the tendons with time.
- Tibiotalar or Tibiotalocalcaneal Arthrodesis
  - Identification of the neurovascular bundle (anterior tibial/dorsalis pedis artery and deep peroneal nerve) during the dissection and careful retraction out of the surgical field are critical.
  - As with all arthrodesis, joint surface preparation with meticulous removal of remaining cartilage is essential for fusion to occur. During this step, one must also take care to preserve subchondral bone architecture.
  - Proper positioning of the arthrodesis is key, and the optimal position is neutral dorsiflexion–plantarflexion, slight hindfoot valgus, and the second metatarsal aligned with the anterior tibial crest.

The outcomes of salvage procedures, specifically those for the treatment of common peroneal nerve injury leading to foot drop, have been described across the literature [91, 112, 113]. Regarding tendon transfers, specifically the Bridle procedure, outcomes are good to excellent in nearly all studies. In one study, the surgery has proven consistent ability to restore ankle dorsiflexion and strength with a high satisfaction rate demonstrated to 100% of patients reported good or excellent results and 100% reporting becoming brace free for normal daily activities [91]. Similar outcomes have been reported across the literature for the same procedure [113], or a similar tendon transfer technique [114–116]. Similarly, the techniques of tibiotalar and tibiotalocalcaneal arthrodesis have demonstrated good functional outcomes and low rates of revision or failure [117, 118]. The reliability and reproducibility of tendon transfers must be considered during decision-making for patients with peroneal nerve palsies. Peripheral nerve surgeons should preserve a salvage option when planning their reconstructive surgeries.

13.6.1.5 Combined Procedures

Nerve Repair and Posterior Tibialis Tendon Transfer

Several authors advocate for early posterior tibialis tendon transfer at the same time as decompression, neurolysis, or nerve grafting [15, 119–121]. These authors attribute the poor recovery seen following CPN repair to the imbalance from the over-powering plantar flexors against the passively stretched tibialis anterior and toe-extensors. This was thought to hinder full active range of motion upon reinnervation [122]. Ferraresi et al. hypothesized that the ability to return to ambulation earlier acts as "continuous rehabilitation" and helps to rebalance the flexion and extension forces [15]. They describe 39 patients undergoing posterior tibialis tendon transfer through the interosseous membrane anchored to the third cuneiform with simultaneous exploration and nerve grafting [15]. They report two patients obtaining MRC 3 or greater recovery with delayed surgical intervention at 13 and 18 months post-injury and also achievement of MRC 4 grade ankle dorsiflexion with graft lengths up to 20 cm [15]. Garozzo et al. describe 23 patients also undergoing early tendon transfers with 17 achieving at MRC grade 3 dorsiflexion [123]. However, in both studies, the length of graft used, time to surgery, and MRC grade were not provided for each specific patient, and thus, direct comparisons to neurolysis and grafting alone are difficult to make. Similar to concomitant tendon and nerve transfer for radial nerve palsy, combination strategies make it difficult to discern which "part" of the surgery was successful. Regardless, combination strategies provide optimal chance of recovery for patients after peroneal nerve palsy.

Gastrocnemius Neuromuscular Tendinous Transfer

The gastrocnemius neuromuscular tendinous transfer, first described by Ninkovic in 1994, involves transferring the medial gastrocnemius muscle and superficial portion of the Achilles tendon into the tibialis anterior, EHL, and EDL tendons with simultaneous transfer of the motor nerve to the gastrocnemius to the DPN [120, 121]. The transfer can also be performed using both heads of the gastrocnemius. The medial head is used for anterior compartment reconstruction as above, and the lateral head to restore lateral compartment function. The concept of "orthotopic reinnervation" with the lateral gastrocnemius being transferred and powered by the proximal intact CPN circumvents the need for muscle reeducation as is the case with traditional tendon transfers. However, this method crucially depends on a healthy proximal CPN stump with more than 70% normal fascicles [120]. CPN injury proximal to the gastrocnemius motor branch point would preclude a patient from undergo this procedure and traditional tendon transfers would be performed. Of 18 patients, all were able to ambulate without an AFO and none experienced any donor site morbidity. Fourteen patients regained good to excellent results with active dorsiflexion and range of motion greater than 30° [120].

13.6.2 Tibial Nerve Injuries

Isolated tibial nerve injury is rare due to its more protected position within the sciatic nerve and thicker surrounding extra-fascicular adipose tissue [4, 19, 50, 51]; however, they have been described with distal femur and tibia fractures, high tibial osteotomies, total knee arthroplasties, and knee arthroscopic surgery [50, 52, 53]. Patients experience loss of protective plantar foot sensation and decreased strength in pushing-off during the stance-to-swing phase of walking [122]. Results from neurolysis and grafting have been disappointing due to the often more proximal levels of injury and long distance to reinnervation to the foot [124]. Tibial nerve injury often occurs in combination with CPN injuries, leading to poor overall functional recovery.

In the case of concomitant tibial and peroneal injury, transfers from the obturator and femoral nerves have been described. Restoration of knee flexion and plantarflexion can be achieved with transfer of the anterior branch of the obturator nerve to the medial head of the gastrocnemius. This required, on average, a 21-cm interposition graft [125]. In a case series of five patients, three achieved MRC grade 3 or greater knee flexion and ankle plantarflexion at 12–15 months postoperatively [125].

Transfers using femoral nerve donors to restore tibial nerve function involve transfer of the vastus lateralis branch to the lateral gastrocnemius with an interpositional graft and concurrent vastus medialis transfer to the medial gastrocnemius with direct coaptation [126]. The first stage of sensory transfers to restore plantar sensation can be performed at the same time with direct coaptation of the saphenous nerve to the sural nerve. A second stage transfer is then later performed with transfer of the distal sural nerve to the tibial nerve at the ankle [126].

Results from a case report of two patients show recovery of MRC 3 and 3+ gastrocnemius motor function without any downgrading of quadricep strength [126].

If the DPN is intact, then sensory nerve transfers can also be performed with transferring the first webspace sensory branch of the DPN to the medial tibial nerve in the medial foot [124]. This transfer provides a one-stage procedure with relatively fast recovery given the proximity of the coaptation to the foot; however, it does not restore sensation to the heel.

13.6.3 Saphenous Nerve Injuries

Injuries to the saphenous nerve can occur after tibial fractures either due to the original injury or during intramedullary tibial nail fixation [127]. The infrapatellar branch of the saphenous nerve can be injured during arthroscopic meniscal surgery, total knee arthroplasty, and hamstring harvest resulting in painful neuromas and reflex sympathetic dystrophy of the knee [128, 129]. Patients experience dysesthesias in the upper medial thigh and lower leg. Sixty-nine percent of patients report significantly bothersome sensory changes following infrapatellar nerve injury with medial parapatellar incisions, and 7% experience debilitating pain preventing kneeling [63]. Anterior knee pain following tibial nailing may also be attributed to infrapatellar nerve injury during the surgical approach or irritation from a prominent nail [127, 130]. A randomized control trial of infrapatellar blocks with lidocaine compared to placebo in patients with chronic anterior knee pain following tibial nailing confirmed this diagnosis with effective pain relief [130].

The initial assessment for a saphenous neuroma should include a full history and physical exam to elicit symptoms of neuropathic pain and identify a Tinel sign if present. In addition, a full sensory and motor examination of the lower extremity should be performed to rule out other associated nerve injuries. Ultrasound-guided nerve blocks with local anesthetic can be both therapeutic and diagnostic of painful neuromas. Nerve blocks can also help to delineate saphenous neuromas from those arising from the femoral nerve proximally and the posterior tibial nerve distally given. Nonsurgical managements include pain medications, desensitization, and radiofrequency ablation. Surgical management includes neurolysis alone, neurectomy with muscle implantation, neuroma excision and nerve allograft repair, end to side neurorrhaphy, targeted muscle reinnervation, or regenerative peripheral nerve interfaces [131–134].

13.6.3.1 Surgical Technique: Saphenous Decompression in Hunter's Canal

Decompression and exploration of the saphenous nerve are performed under general anesthesia with a sterile upper thigh tourniquet. The patient is placed supine with the hip abducted and knee flexed into a "figure-4" position. A sandbag can be placed below the foot to help with immobilization. Preoperative markings should include the location of any detectable Tinel's sign An 8- to 10-cm incision is designed in the medial upper thigh just anterior to the sartorius (Fig. 13.25). Dissection is carried through skin and subcutaneous tissues until the fascia of the sartorius is visualized. The "fat stripe" in between the sartorius and adductor longus serves as a guide for identification of the saphenous nerve (Fig. 13.26). Once the nerve is identified, dissection proximally along the nerve will lead to the tight compressive fascia of Hunter's adductor canal. This is then carefully released to decompress the nerve (Figs. 13.27 and 13.28).

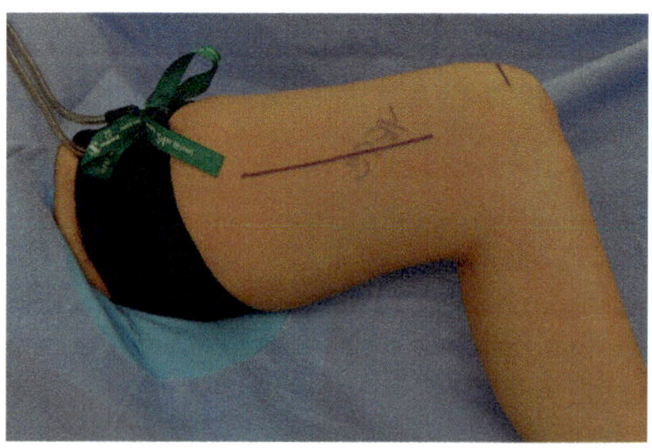

Fig. 13.25 Incision marked in medial upper thigh just anterior to sartorius. (Image copyright Dr. Christopher Dy, used with permission)

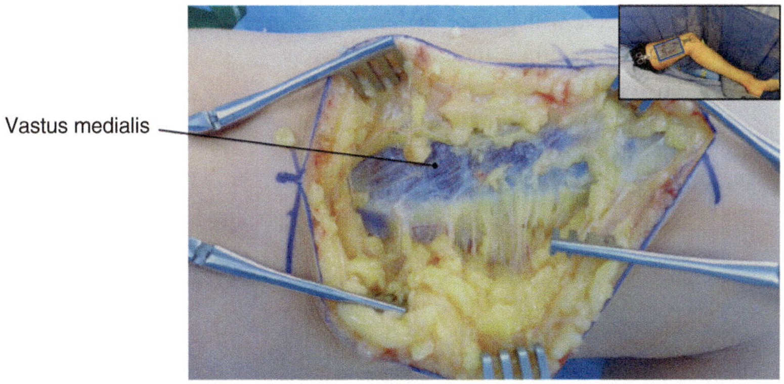

Fig. 13.26 Fat stripe visualized between vastus medialis and adductor muscles. (Image copyright Dr. Christopher Dy, used with permission)

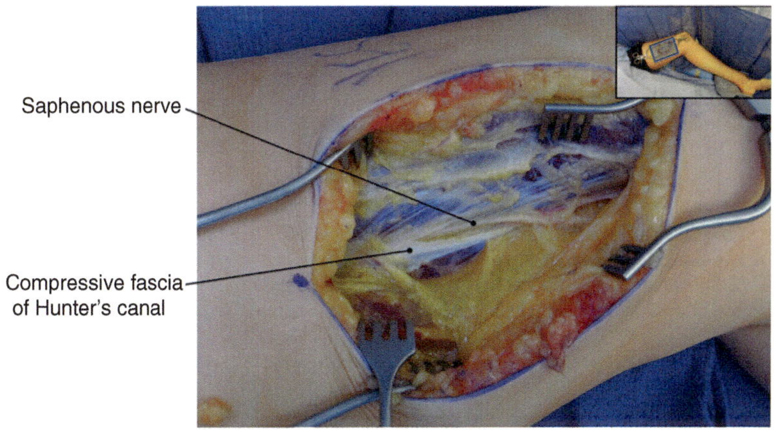

Fig. 13.27 Saphenous nerve coursing underneath tight compression fascia of Hunter's canal. (Image copyright Dr. Christopher Dy, used with permission)

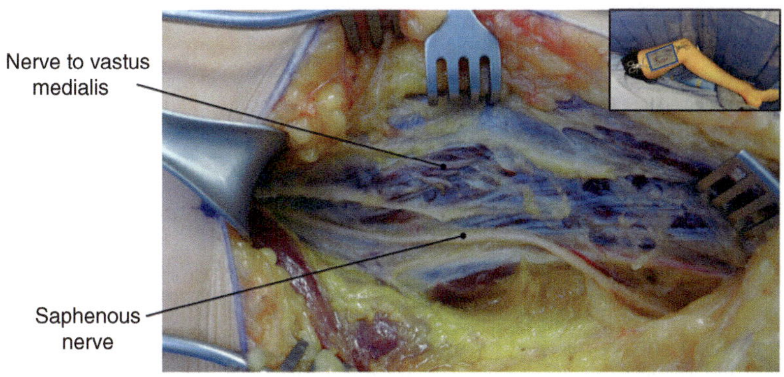

Fig. 13.28 Fascia of Hunter's canal released over saphenous nerve. Anteriorly, nerve to vastus medialis visualized. (Image copyright Dr. Christopher Dy, used with permission)

Exploration and neurolysis can also proceed distally to identify the presence of a neuroma use preoperative markings as guide. If desired after preoperative discussion with the patient, neurectomy is performed with a proximal crush injury to the nerve and distal transection. The nerve ending is then buried within the vastus medialis muscle belly after creating a small myotomy. The myotomy is loosely closed to prevent the nerve ending from dislodging, but care is taken to avoid creating a new site of compression. After taking the knee through passive motion to ensure that the nerve ending does not dislodge, fibrin glue is used to seal the myotomy site. These steps (multilevel injury to the saphenous nerve with a crush and intramuscular transposition) minimize the chances of recurrence of painful neuroma symptoms.

References

1. Matejčík V. Peripheral nerve reconstruction by autograft. Injury. 2002;33(7):627–31. https://doi.org/10.1016/S0020-1383(02)00073-6.
2. Kouyoumdjian JA, Graça CR, Ferreira VFM. Peripheral nerve injuries: a retrospective survey of 1124 cases. Neurol India. 2017;65(3):551–5. https://doi.org/10.4103/neuroindia.NI_987_16.
3. Gosk J, Rutowski R, Rabczyński J. The lower extremity nerve injuries - own experience in surgical treatment. Folia Neuropathol. 2005;43(3):148–52. http://www.ncbi.nlm.nih.gov/pubmed/16245209. Accessed October 12, 2019.
4. Immerman I, Price AE, Alfonso I, Grossman JAI. Lower extremity nerve trauma. Bull Hosp Joint Dis. 2014;72(1):43–52.
5. Cush G, Irgit K. Drop foot after knee dislocation. Sports Med Arthrosc. 2011;19(2):139–46. https://doi.org/10.1097/JSA.0b013e3182191897.
6. Shrestha BK, Bijukachhe B, Rajbhandary T, Uprety S, Banskota AK. Tibial plateau fractures: four years review at B & B Hospital. Kathmandu Univ Med J (KUMJ). 2(4):315–23. http://www.ncbi.nlm.nih.gov/pubmed/16388243. Accessed October 13, 2019.
7. Kretschmer T, Antoniadis G, Braun V, Rath SA, Richter HP. Evaluation of iatrogenic lesions in 722 surgically treated cases of peripheral nerve trauma. J Neurosurg. 2001;94(6):905–12. https://doi.org/10.3171/jns.2001.94.6.0905.
8. Antoniadis G, Kretschmer T, Pedro MT, König RW, Heinen C, Richter H-P. Iatrogenic nerve injuries. Dtsch Aerzteblatt Online. 2014;111(16):273–9. https://doi.org/10.3238/arztebl.2014.0273.
9. Rasulić L, Savić A, Vitošević F, et al. Iatrogenic peripheral nerve injuries—surgical treatment and outcome: 10 years' experience. World Neurosurg. 2017;103:841–51.e6. https://doi.org/10.1016/j.wneu.2017.04.099
10. Wootton JR, Ashworth MJ, MacLaren CAN. Neurological complications of high tibial osteotomy – the fibular osteotomy as a causative factor: a clinical and anatomical study. Ann R Coll Surg Engl. 1995;77(1):31–4.
11. Georgoulis AD, Makris CA, Papageorgiou CD, Moebius UG, Xenakis T, Soucacos PN. Nerve and vessel injuries during high tibial osteotomy combined with distal fibular osteotomy: a clinically relevant anatomic study. Knee Surgery, Sport Traumatol Arthrosc. 1999;7(2):15–9.
12. Pulos N, Shin EH, Spinner RJ, Shin AY. Management of Iatrogenic Nerve Injuries. J Am Acad Orthop Surg. 2019:1. https://doi.org/10.5435/jaaos-d-18-00510.
13. Decrouy-Duruz V, Christen T, Raffoul W. Evaluation of surgical treatment for neuropathic pain from neuroma in patients with injured peripheral nerves. J Neurosurg. 2018;128(4):1235–40. https://doi.org/10.3171/2017.1.JNS161778.
14. Khan R, Birch R. Latropathic injuries of peripheral nerves. J Bone Joint Surg Br. 2001;83(8):1145–8. https://doi.org/10.1302/0301-620x.83b8.12251.
15. Ferraresi S, Garozzo D, Buffatti P. Common peroneal nerve injuries: results with one-stage nerve repair and tendon transfer. Neurosurg Rev. 2003;26(3):175–9. https://doi.org/10.1007/s10143-002-0247-4.
16. Kline DG. Operative management of major nerve lesions of the lower extremity. Surg Clin North Am. 1972;52(5):1247–65. https://doi.org/10.1016/s0039-6109(16)39839-5.
17. Perineurium AL, Reina MA, Peyrano EC. Ch 39 ultrastructure of nerve root cuffs. Atlas Funct Anat Reg Anesth Pain Med. 2015:721–47. https://doi.org/10.1007/978-3-319-09522-6
18. Ribak S, Fonseca JR, Tietzmann A, Gama SAM, Hirata HH. The anatomy and morphology of the superficial peroneal nerve. J Reconstr Microsurg. 2016;32(4):271–5. https://doi.org/10.1055/s-0035-1568881.
19. Gustafson KJ, Grinberg Y, Joseph S, Triolo RJ. Human distal sciatic nerve fascicular anatomy: implications for ankle control using nerve-cuff electrodes. J Rehabil Res Dev. 2012;49(2):309–22. https://doi.org/10.1682/JRRD.2010.10.0201.
20. Hwang K, Jin S, Hwang JH, Han SH. Proximity of the common peroneal nerve to the tibial nerve entering the gastrocnemius muscle: the implications for calf reduction. Aesthet Plast Surg. 2008;32(1):116–9. https://doi.org/10.1007/s00266-007-9034-5.
21. Ryan W, Mahony N, Delaney M, O'Brien M, Murray P. Relationship of the common peroneal nerve and its branches to the head and neck of the fibula. Clin Anat. 2003;16(6):501–5. https://doi.org/10.1002/ca.10155.
22. Deutsch A, Wyzykowski RJ, Victoroff BN. Evaluation of the anatomy of the common peroneal nerve: defining nerve- at-risk in arthroscopically assisted lateral meniscus repair. Am J Sports Med. 1999;27(1):10–5. https://doi.org/10.1177/03635465990270010201.
23. Sunderland SBK. Stress-strain phenomena in human peripheral nerve trunks. Brain. 1961;84:102–19.
24. Nercessian OA, Ugwonali OFC, Park S. Peroneal nerve palsy after Total knee arthroplasty. J Arthroplast. 2005;20(8):1068–73. https://doi.org/10.1016/j.arth.2005.02.010.
25. Idusuyi OB, Morrey BF. Peroneal nerve palsy after total knee arthroplasty. Assessment of predisposing and prognostic factors. J Bone Joint Surg Am. 1996;78(2):177–84. https://doi.org/10.2106/00004623-199602000-00003.
26. Jia Y, Gou W, Geng L, Wang Y, Chen J. Anatomic proximity of the peroneal nerve to the posterolateral corner of the knee determined by MR imaging.

Knee. 2012;19(6):766–8. https://doi.org/10.1016/j.knee.2012.01.007.
27. Watt T, Hariharan AR, Brzezinski DW, Caird MS, Zeller JL. Branching patterns and localization of the common fibular (peroneal) nerve: an anatomical basis for planning safe surgical approaches. Surg Radiol Anat. 2014;36(8):821–8. https://doi.org/10.1007/s00276-013-1242-x.
28. Fabre T, Piton C, Andre D, Lasseur E, Durandeau A. Peroneal nerve entrapment*. J Bone Jt Surg. 1998;80(1):47–53. https://doi.org/10.2106/00004623-199801000-00009.
29. Gloobe H, Chain D. Fibular fibrous arch. Anatomical considerations in fibular tunnel syndrome. Acta Anat (Basel). 1973;85(1):84–7. https://doi.org/10.1159/000143983.
30. Nogueira MP, Paley D, Bhave A, Herbert A, Nocente C, Herzenberg JE. Nerve lesions associated with limb-lengthening. J Bone Jt Surgery-American Vol. 2003;85(8):1502–10. https://doi.org/10.2106/00004623-200308000-00011.
31. Canella C, Demondion X, Guillin R, Boutry N, Peltier J, Cotten A. Anatomic study of the superficial peroneal nerve using sonography. Am J Roentgenol. 2009;193(1):174–9. https://doi.org/10.2214/AJR.08.1898.
32. Darland AM, Kadakia AR, Zeller JL. Branching patterns of the superficial peroneal nerve: implications for ankle arthroscopy and for anterolateral surgical approaches to the ankle. J Foot Ankle Surg. 2015;54(3):332–7. https://doi.org/10.1053/j.jfas.2014.07.002.
33. Adkison DP, Bosse MJ, Gaccione DR, Gabriel KR. Anatomical variations in the course of the superficial peroneal nerve. J Bone Joint Surg Am. 1991;73(1):112–4. PMID: 1985980
34. Lee J-H, Lee B-N, An X, Chung R-H, Kwon S-O, Han S-H. Anatomic localization of motor entry point of superficial peroneal nerve to peroneus longus and brevis muscles. Clin Anat. 2011;24(2):232–6. https://doi.org/10.1002/ca.21076.
35. Rupp RE, Podeszwa D, Ebraheim NA. Danger zones associated with fibular osteotomy. J Orthop Trauma. 1994;8(1):54–8. https://doi.org/10.1097/00005131-199402000-00012. PMID: 8169696.
36. Otis JC, Deland JT, Lee S, Gordon J. Peroneus brevis is a more effective evertor than peroneus longus. Foot Ankle Int. 2004;25(4):242–6. https://doi.org/10.1177/107110070402500408.
37. Reebye O. Anatomical and clinical study of the common fibular nerve. Part 1: anatomical study. Surg Radiol Anat. 2004;26(5):365–70. https://doi.org/10.1007/s00276-004-0238-y.
38. Bowness J, Turnbull K, Taylor A, et al. Identifying the emergence of the superficial peroneal nerve through deep fascia on ultrasound and by dissection: implications for regional anesthesia in foot and ankle surgery. Clin Anat. 2019;32(3):390–5. https://doi.org/10.1002/ca.23323.
39. Blair JM, Botte MJ. Surgical anatomy of the superficial peroneal nerve in the ankle and foot. Clin Orthop Relat Res. 1994;(305):229–38. PMID: 8050234.
40. Tomaszewski KA, Roy J, Vikse J, Pękala PA, Kopacz P, Henry BM. Prevalence of the accessory deep peroneal nerve: a cadaveric study and meta-analysis. Clin Neurol Neurosurg. 2016;144:105–11. https://doi.org/10.1016/j.clineuro.2016.03.026.
41. Tzika M, Paraskevas GK, Kitsoulis P. The accessory deep peroneal nerve: a review of the literature. Foot. 2012;22(3):232–4. https://doi.org/10.1016/j.foot.2012.05.003.
42. Mathis S, Ciron J, du Boisguéheneuc F, et al. Study of accessory deep peroneal nerve motor conduction in a population of healthy subjects. Neurophysiol Clin. 2011;41(1):29–33. https://doi.org/10.1016/j.neucli.2010.12.002.
43. Chompoopong S, Apinhasmit W, Sangiampong A, et al. Anatomical considerations of the deep peroneal nerve for biopsy of the proximal fibula in thais. Clin Anat. 2009;22(2):256–60. https://doi.org/10.1002/ca.20752.
44. Schaffler GJ, Groell R, Schoellnast H, et al. Digital image fusion of CT and PET data sets–clinical value in abdominal/pelvic malignancies. J Comput Assist Tomogr. 2000;24(4):644–7. http://ovidsp.ovid.com/ovidweb.cgi?T=JS&PAGE=reference&D=med4&NEWS=N&AN=10966202
45. White CP, Cooper MJ, Bain JR, Levis CM. Axon counts of potential nerve transfer donors for peroneal nerve reconstruction. Can J Plast Surg. 2012;20(1):24–7. https://doi.org/10.1177/229255031202000104.
46. Stitgen SH, Cairns ER, Ebraheim NA, Niemann JM, Jackson WT. Anatomic considerations of pin placement in the proximal tibia and its relationship to the peroneal nerve. Clin Orthop Relat Res. 1992;(278):134–7. PMID: 1563143.
47. Kirgis A, Albrecht S. Palsy of the deep peroneal nerve after proximal tibial osteotomy. An anatomical study. J Bone Joint Surg Am. 1992;74(8):1180–5. http://www.ncbi.nlm.nih.gov/pubmed/1400546. Accessed October 14, 2019.
48. Lawrence SJ, Botte MJ. The deep peroneal nerve in the foot and ankle: an anatomic study. Foot Ankle Int. 1995;16(11):724–8. https://doi.org/10.1177/107110079501601110.
49. Ucerler H, Ikiz ZAA, Uygur M. A cadaver study on preserving peroneal nerves during ankle arthroscopy. Foot Ankle Int. 2007;28(11):1172–8. https://doi.org/10.3113/FAI.2007.1172.
50. Murovic JA. Lower-extremity peripheral nerve injuries: a Louisiana State University Health Sciences Center literature review with comparison of the operative outcomes of 806 Louisiana State University Health Sciences Center sciatic, common peroneal, and tibial nerve. Neurosurgery. 2009;65(SUPPL. 4):18–23. https://doi.org/10.1227/01.NEU.0000339123.74649.BE.
51. Schraut NB, Walton S, Monsef JADBOU, et al. What protects certain nerves from stretch injury? Anat Rec (Hoboken). 2016;299(1):111–7. https://doi.org/10.1002/ar.23286.

52. Freedman DM, Barron OA. Iatrogenic posterior tibial nerve division during ankle arthroscopy. Arthroscopy. 1998;14(7):769–72. https://doi.org/10.1016/s0749-8063(98)70109-4.
53. Taylor CA, Braza D, Rice JB, Dillingham T. The incidence of peripheral nerve injury in extremity trauma. Am J Phys Med Rehabil. 2008;87(5):381–5. https://doi.org/10.1097/PHM.0b013e31815e6370.
54. Kim MW, Kim JH, Yang YJ, Ko YJ. Anatomic localization of motor points in gastrocnemius and soleus muscles. Am J Phys Med Rehabil. 2005;84(9): 680–3. https://doi.org/10.1097/01.phm.0000176341.85398.a9.
55. Zhong S, Li G, Yang L, et al. Anatomic and ultrasonic study based on selective Tibial Neurotomy. World Neurosurg. 2017;99:214–25. https://doi.org/10.1016/j.wneu.2016.11.023.
56. Apaydin N, Loukas M, Kendir S, et al. The precise localization of distal motor branches of the tibial nerve in the deep posterior compartment of the leg. Surg Radiol Anat. 2008;30(4):291–5. https://doi.org/10.1007/s00276-008-0321-x.
57. Bodily KD, Spinner RJ, Bishop AT. Restoration of motor function of the deep fibular (peroneal) nerve by direct nerve transfer of branches from the Tibial nerve: an anatomical study. Clin Anat. 2004;17:201–5.
58. Dellon AL, Mackinnon SE. Tibial nerve branching in the tarsal tunnel. Arch Neurol. 1984;41(6):645–6.
59. Ahmad M, Tsang K, Mackenney PJ, Adedapo AO. Tarsal tunnel syndrome: a literature review. Foot Ankle Surg. 2012;18(3):149–52. https://doi.org/10.1016/j.fas.2011.10.007.
60. Lenchik L, Brigido MK, Shahabpour M, Marcelis S. Normal anatomy and compression areas of nerves of the foot and ankle: US and MR imaging with anatomic correlation. RadioGraphics. 2015;35(5):1469–82.
61. Norzana AG, Farihah HS, Fairus A, et al. Original article Higher division of the tibial nerve in the leg: gross anatomical study with clinical implications. Clin Ter. 2013;164(1):1–3. https://doi.org/10.7417/CT.2013.1501.
62. Ghosh A, Chaudhury S. Morphology of saphenous nerve in cadavers: a guide to saphenous block and surgical interventions. Anat Cell Biol. 2019;52(3):262–8.
63. Louis DS, Ricciardi JR, Connor GAO, Arbor A, Arbor A. The saphenous nerve: its course and importance in medial arthrotomy. Am J Sports Med. 1979;7(4):227–30.
64. Koch G, Kling A, Ramamurthy N, Edalat F. Anatomical risk evaluation of iatrogenic injury to the infrapatellar branch of the saphenous nerve during medial meniscus arthroscopic surgery. Surg Radiol Anat. 2017;39(6):611–8. https://doi.org/10.1007/s00276-016-1781-z.
65. Dunaway DJ, Steensen RN, Wiand W, Dopirak RM. The sartorial branch of the saphenous nerve: its anatomy at the joint line of the knee. Arthroscopy. 2005;21(5):547–51. https://doi.org/10.1016/j.arthro.2005.02.019.
66. Marsland D, Fracs AD, Tr NJLF, Tr MCSF. Foot and ankle surgery the saphenous nerve in foot and ankle surgery: its variable anatomy and relevance. Foot Ankle Surg. 2013;19(2):76–9. https://doi.org/10.1016/j.fas.2012.10.007.
67. Poppler LH, Davidge K, Lu JCY, Armstrong J, Fox IK, Mackinnon SE. Alternatives to sural nerve grafts in the upper extremity. Hand. 2015;10(1):68–75. https://doi.org/10.1007/s11552-014-9699-6.
68. Klein W, Lang DM, Saleh M. The use of the Ma-Griffith technique for percutaneous repair of fresh ruptured tendo Achillis. Chir Organi Mov. 1991;76(3):2230228.
69. Ramakrishnan PK, Henry BM, Vikse J, et al. Annals of anatomy anatomical variations of the formation and course of the sural nerve: a systematic review and meta-analysis. Ann Anat. 2015;202:36–44. https://doi.org/10.1016/j.aanat.2015.08.002.
70. Kavyashree AN, Prabha Subhash L, Asha KR, Bindu Rani MK. Anatomical variations in formation of sural nerve in adult Indian cadavers. J Clin Diagnostic Res. 2013;7(9):1838–41. https://doi.org/10.7860/JCDR/2013/6633.3328.
71. Blackmon JA, Atsas S, Clarkson MJ, et al. Locating the sural nerve during calcaneal (Achilles) tendon repair with confidence: a cadaveric study with clinical applications. J Foot Ankle Surg. 2013;52(1):42–7. https://doi.org/10.1053/j.jfas.2012.09.010.
72. Amoiridis G, Schöls L, Ameridis N, Przuntek H. Motor fibers in the sural nerve of humans. Neurology. 1997;49(6):1725–8. https://doi.org/10.1212/WNL.49.6.1725.
73. Court-Brown CM, Caesar B. Epidemiology of adult fractures: a review. Injury. 2006;37(8):691–7. https://doi.org/10.1016/j.injury.2006.04.130.
74. Martinet O, Cordey J, Harder Y, Maier A, Bühler M, Barraud GE. The epidemiology of fractures of the distal femur. Injury. 2000;31(Suppl. 3). https://doi.org/10.1016/s0020-1383(00)80034-0.
75. Gwathmey FW, Jones-Quaidoo SM, Kahler D, Hurwitz S, Cui Q. Distal femoral fractures: current concepts. J Am Acad Orthop Surg. 2010;18(10):597–607. https://doi.org/10.5435/00124635-201010000-00003.
76. Arneson TJ, Melton LJ, Lewallen DG, O'Fallon WM. Epidemiology of diaphyseal and distal femoral fractures in Rochester, Minnesota, 1965-1984. Clin Orthop Relat Res. 1988;234:188–94. https://doi.org/10.1097/00003086-198809000-00033.
77. Healy WL, Siliski JM, Incavo SJ. Operative treatment of distal femoral fractures proximal to total knee replacements. J Bone Joint Surg Am. 1993;75(1):27–34. https://doi.org/10.2106/00004623-199301000-00005.
78. Keyurapan E, Phoemphunkunarak W, Lektrakool N. Location of the neurovascular bundle of the knee

during flexed and extended position: an MRI study. J Med Assoc Thail. 2016;99(10):1102–9.
79. Checroun AJ, Mekhail AO, Ebraheim NA, Jackson WT, Yeasting RA. Extensile medial approach to the femur. J Orthop Trauma. 1996;10(7):481–6. https://doi.org/10.1097/00005131-199610000-00006.
80. Thiayagarajan M, Kumar S, Venkatesh S. An exact localization of adductor canal and its clinical significance: a cadaveric study. Anesth Essays Res. 2019;13(2):284. https://doi.org/10.4103/aer.aer_35_19.
81. Jeelani A, Arastu MH. Tibial plateau fractures – review of current concepts in management. Orthop Trauma. 2017;31(2):102–15. https://doi.org/10.1016/j.mporth.2016.10.005.
82. Schatzker J, McBroom R. The tibial plateau fracture. The Toronto experience 1968–1975. Clin Orthop Relat Res. 1979;138:94–104.
83. Larsen P, Elsoe R, Hansen SH, Graven-Nielsen T, Laessoe U, Rasmussen S. Incidence and epidemiology of tibial shaft fractures. Injury. 2015;46(4):746–50. https://doi.org/10.1016/j.injury.2014.12.027.
84. Anandasivam NS, Russo GS, Swallow MS, et al. Tibial shaft fracture: a large-scale study defining the injured population and associated injuries. J Clin Orthop Trauma. 2017;8(3):225–31. https://doi.org/10.1016/j.jcot.2017.07.012.
85. Hems TEJ, Jones BG. Peroneal nerve damage associated with the proximal locking screws of the AIM tibial nail. Injury. 2005;36(5):651–4.; discussion 655. https://doi.org/10.1016/j.injury.2004.10.005.
86. Jones BG, Mehin R, Young D. Anatomical study of the placement of proximal oblique locking screws in intramedullary tibial nailing. J Bone Joint Surg Br. 2007;89(11):1495–7. https://doi.org/10.1302/0301-620X.89B11.19018.
87. Bono CM, Sirkin M, Sabatino CT, Reilly MC, Tarkin I, Behrens FF. Neurovascular and tendinous damage with placement of anteroposterior distal locking bolts in the tibia. J Orthop Trauma. 2003;17(10):677–82. https://doi.org/10.1097/00005131-200311000-00003.
88. Hargens AR, Romine JS, Sipe JC, Evans KL, Mubarak SJ, Akeson WH. Peripheral nerve-conduction block by high muscle-compartment pressure. J Bone Joint Surg Am. 1979;61(2):192–200.
89. Lee DH, Claussen GC, Oh S. Clinical nerve conduction and needle electromyography studies. J Am Acad Orthop Surg. 2004;12(4):276–87. https://doi.org/10.5435/00124635-200407000-00008.
90. Mont MA, Dellon AL, Chen F, Hungerford MW, Krackow KA, Hungerford DS. The operative treatment of peroneal nerve palsy. J Bone Joint Surg Am. 1996;78(6):863–9.
91. Johnson JE, Paxton ES, Lippe J, et al. Outcomes of the bridle procedure for the treatment of foot drop. Foot Ankle Int. 2015;36(11):1287–96. https://doi.org/10.1177/1071100715593146.
92. Wiesseman GJ. Tendon transfers for peripheral nerve injuries of the lower extremity. Orthop Clin North Am. 1981;12:459–67.
93. Woodmass JM, Romatowski NPJ, Esposito JG, Mohtadi NGH, Longino PD. A systematic review of peroneal nerve palsy and recovery following traumatic knee dislocation. Knee Surg Sport Traumatol Arthrosc. 2015;23(10):2992–3002. https://doi.org/10.1007/s00167-015-3676-7.
94. Giuffre JL, Bishop AT, Spinner RJ, Shin AY. Surgical technique of a partial tibial nerve transfer to the tibialis anterior motor branch for the treatment of peroneal nerve injury. Ann Plast Surg. 2012;69(1):48–53. https://doi.org/10.1097/SAP.0b013e31824c94e5.
95. George SC, Boyce DE. An evidence-based structured review to assess the results of common peroneal nerve repair. Plast Reconstr Surg. 2014;134(2):302e–11e.
96. Wood MB. Peroneal nerve repair: surgical results. Clin Orthop Relat Res. 1991;267:206–10. https://doi.org/10.1097/00003086-199106000-00033.
97. Kim DH, Murovic JA, Tiel RL, et al. Management and outcomes in 318 operative common peroneal nerve lesions at the Louisiana State University Health Sciences Center. Neurosurgery. 2004;54(6):1421–9. https://doi.org/10.1227/01.NEU.0000124752.40412.03.
98. Tiel RL, Happel LTKD. Nerve action potential recording method and equipment. Neurosurgery. 1996;39(1):103–9.
99. O'Malley MP, Pareek A, Reardon P, Krych A, Stuart MJ, Levy BA. Treatment of peroneal nerve injuries in the multiligament injured/dislocated knee. J Knee Surg. 2016;29:287–92.
100. Moore AM. Nerve transfers to restore upper extremity function: a paradigm shift. Front Neurol. 2015;5:40.
101. Nath RK, Lyons AB, Paizi M. Successful management of foot drop by nerve transfers to the deep peroneal nerve. J Reconstr Microsurg. 2008;24(6):419–27. https://doi.org/10.1055/s-0028-1082894.
102. Flores LP. Proximal motor branches from the tibial nerve as direct donors to restore function of the deep fibular nerve for treatment of high sciatic nerve injuries: a cadaveric feasibility study. Neurosurgery. 2009;65(6 Suppl. 1):218–25. https://doi.org/10.1227/01.NEU.0000346329.90517.79.
103. Pirela-Cruz MA, Hansen U, Terreros DA, Rossum AWP. Interosseous nerve transfers for tibialis anterior muscle paralysis (foot drop): a human cadaver-based feasibility study. J Reconstr Microsurg. 2009;25(3):218–25.
104. Strazar R, White CP, Bain J. Foot reanimation via nerve transfer to the peroneal nerve using the nerve branch to the lateral gastrocnemius: case report. J Plast Reconstr Aesthetic Surg. 2011;64(10):1380–2. https://doi.org/10.1016/j.bjps.2011.02.025.
105. Ferris S, Maciburko SJ. Partial tibial nerve transfer to tibialis anterior for traumatic peroneal nerve palsy. Microsurgery. 2017;37(6):596–602. https://doi.org/10.1002/micr.30174.
106. Giuffre JL, Bishop AT, Spinner RJ, Levy BA, Shin AY. Partial tibial nerve transfer to the tibialis anterior motor branch to treat peroneal nerve injury after knee

trauma. Clin Orthop Relat Res. 2012;470(3):779–90. https://doi.org/10.1007/s11999-011-1924-9.
107. Ober FR. Tendon transposition in the lower extremity. N Engl J Med. 1933;209:52–9.
108. Watkins MB, Jones JB, Ryder CT Jr, Brown TJ. Transplantation of the posterior tibial tendon. J Bone Jt Surg Am. 1954;36:1181–9.
109. Andersen JG. Foot drop in leprosy and its surgical correction. Acta Orthop Scand. 1963;32:151–71.
110. Srinivasan H, Mukherjee SMSR. Two-tailed transfer of tibialis posterior for correction of drop-foot in leprosy. J Bone Jt Surg Br. 1968;50:623–8.
111. Schweitzer KM, Jones CP. Tendon transfers for the drop foot. Foot Ankle Clin. 2014;19(1):65–71. https://doi.org/10.1016/j.fcl.2013.12.002.
112. McCall RE, Frederick HA, McCluskey GM, Riordan DC. The Bridle procedure: a new treatment for equinus and equinovarus deformities in children. J Pediatr Orthop. 1991;11(1):83–9.
113. Rodriguez RP. The bridle procedure in the treatment of paralysis of the foot. Foot Ankle Int. 1992;13(2):63–9. https://doi.org/10.1177/107110079201300203.
114. Prahinski JR, McHale KA, Temple HT, Jackson JP. Bridle transfer for paresis of the anterior and lateral compartment musculature. Foot Ankle Int. 1996;17(10):615–9. https://doi.org/10.1177/107110079601701005.
115. Vigasio A, Marcoccio I, Patelli A, Mattiuzzo V, Prestini G. New tendon transfer for correction of drop-foot in common peroneal nerve palsy. Clin Orthop Relat Res. 2008;466(6):1454–66. https://doi.org/10.1007/s11999-008-0249-9.
116. Carayon A, Bourrel P, Bourges M, Touzé M. Dual transfer of the posterior tibial and flexor digitorum longus tendons for drop foot. Report of thirty-one cases. J Bone Joint Surg Am. 1967;49(1):144–8.
117. Haddad SL, Coetzee JC, Estok R, Fahrbach K, Banel D, Nalysnyk L. Intermediate and long-term outcomes of total ankle arthroplasty and ankle arthrodesis: a systematic review of the literature. J Bone Jt Surg – Ser A. 2007;89(9):1899–905. https://doi.org/10.2106/JBJS.F.01149.
118. Hendrickx RPM, Stufkens SAS, De Bruijn EE, Sierevelt IN, Van Dijk CN, Kerkhoffs GMMJ. Medium- to long-term outcome of ankle arthrodesis. Foot Ankle Int. 2011;32(10):940–7. https://doi.org/10.3113/FAI.2011.0940.
119. Gatskiy AA, Tretyak IB, Tretiakova AI, Tsymbaliuk YV. Choosing the target wisely: partial tibial nerve transfer to extensor digitorum motor branches with simultaneous posterior tibial tendon transfer. Could this be a way to improve functional outcome and gait biomechanics? J Neurosurg. 2019:1–9. https://doi.org/10.3171/2019.3.jns182866.
120. Ninkovic M, Ninković M. Neuromusculotendinous transfer: an original surgical concept for the treatment of drop foot with long-term follow-up. Plast Reconstr Surg. 2013;132(3):438e-45e.
121. Ninkovic N, Sucur DJ, Starovic B, Marković S. A new approach to persistent traumatic peroneal nerve palsy. Br J Plast Surg. 1994;47:185–9.
122. Millesi H. Lower extremity nerve lesions. In: Terzis J, editor. Microreconstruction of nerve injuries. Philadelphia: Saunders; 1987. p. 243–9.
123. Garozzo D, Ferraresi SBP. Common peroneal nerve injuries in knee dislocations: results with one-stage nerve repair and tibialis posterior tendon transfer. J Orthopaed Traumatol. 2002;2:135–7.
124. Koshima I, Nanba Y, Tsutsui T, Takahashi Y. Deep peroneal nerve transfer for established plantar sensory loss. J Reconstr Microsurg. 2003;19(7):451–4. https://doi.org/10.1055/s-2003-44632.
125. Yin G, Chen H, Hou C, Xiao J, Lin H. Obturator nerve transfer to the branch of the Tibial nerve innervating the gastrocnemius muscle for the treatment of sacral plexus nerve injury. Neurosurgery. 2015;78(4):546–51.
126. Moore AM, Krauss EM, Parikh RP, Franco MJ, Tung TH. Femoral nerve transfers for restoring tibial nerve function: an anatomical study and clinical correlation: a report of 2 cases. J Neurosurg. 2018;129(4):1024–33. https://doi.org/10.3171/2017.5.JNS163076.
127. Heare A, Mitchell JJ, Bravman JT. Posttraumatic saphenous neuroma after open tibial fracture. Am J Orthop (Belle Mead NJ). 2015;44(11):E461–4.
128. Sherman OH, Fox JM, Snyder SJ, et al. Arthroscopy–"no-problem surgery". An analysis of complications in two thousand six hundred and forty cases. J Bone Joint Surg Am. 1986;68(2):256–65. http://www.ncbi.nlm.nih.gov/pubmed/3753706. Accessed October 16, 2019.
129. Walshaw T, Karuppiah SV, Stewart I. The knee the course and distribution of the infra patellar nerve in relation to ACL reconstruction. Knee. 2015;22(5):384–8. https://doi.org/10.1016/j.knee.2014.11.003.
130. Leliveld MS, den Hartog D, Kleinrensink GJ. The surgical anatomy of the infrapatellar branch for anteromedial knee surgery. J Bone Joint Surg Am. 2013;95:2119–25.
131. Eberlin KR, Ducic I. Surgical algorithm for neuroma management: a changing treatment paradigm. Plast Reconstr Surg Glob Open. 2018;6(10):e1952.
132. Bi A, Park E, Dumanian GA. Treatment of painful nerves in the abdominal wall using processed nerve allografts. Plast Reconstr Surg Glob Open. 2018;6(3):e1670.
133. Souza JM, Cheesborough JE, Ko JH, Cho MS, Kuiken TADG. Targeted muscle Reinnervation: a novel approach to Postamputation neuroma pain. Clin Orthop Relat Res. 2014;472(10):2984–90.
134. Woo SL, Kung TA, Brown DL, Leonard JA, Kelly BM, Cederna PS. Regenerative peripheral nerve interfaces for the treatment of postamputation neuroma pain: a pilot study. Plast Reconstr Surg Glob Open. 2016;4(12):e1038.

14 Peripheral Nerve Injury in Total Knee Arthroplasty

Benjamin A. McArthur, Steven L. Henry, Alexander Rothy, and Laura E. Bashour

14.1 Epidemiology

Peripheral nerve injury after total knee arthroplasty (TKA) is a rare but potentially devastating cause of postoperative disability. Aside from sensory changes associated with disruption of the infrapatellar branch of the saphenous nerve as part of the anterior skin incision, the reported incidence of peripheral nerve injury after TKA ranges from approximately 0.3–1.3% in most series [66, 80, 89] and as high as 9% in rheumatoid patients [42]. Given that nerve injury exists on a spectrum ranging from subclinical to complete palsy, it is likely that mild cases may frequently be overlooked [89] and the true incidence may be under reported.

While sensory changes related to disruption of the infrapatellar branch of the saphenous nerve (IPBSN) appear to be nearly universal, fortunately the impact on patient satisfaction seems to be limited [56]. However, there are occasions in which the sensory disturbance may negatively affect patients, as Mistry et al. reported a 10% incidence of sensory changes resulting in decreased patient satisfaction [57], and there are case reports of painful neuromas and bothersome dysesthesias [60].

Injury to the peroneal nerve resulting in postoperative foot drop is by far the most common and the most dreaded functional deficit. Sciatic and tibial nerve mononeuropathies, lumbosacral plexopathies, and even sural neuropathies have also been reported, though the incidence is significantly lower [89].

14.2 Risk Factors

A number of risk factors have been identified in the literature, though significant discrepancies exist between studies as to which risk factors are most pertinent. While not all studies are in agreement, risk factors identified include valgus deformity, especially when combined with flexion contracture [2, 9, 28, 33, 35, 78], increased tourniquet time [28], younger age [12, 66], female gender [12, 84], rheumatoid arthritis (RA) [43, 80], higher body mass index (BMI) [66], epidural anesthesia [33], and history of previous spine disease or neuropathy [12, 33, 84]. Although causa-

B. A. McArthur (✉) · L. E. Bashour
Dell Medical School at the University of Texas at Austin, Austin, TX, USA
e-mail: bmcarthur@txortho.com; laura.bashour@utexas.edu

S. L. Henry
Institute of Reconstructive Plastic Surgery, Dell Medical School at the University of Texas at Austin, Austin, TX, USA
e-mail: steven.henry@austin.utexas.edu

A. Rothy
Joseph M. Abell Arthroplasty and Value-Based Health Care Delivery Fellow, Dell Medical School at the University of Texas at Austin, Austin, TX, USA
e-mail: alexander.rothy@austin.utexas.edu

C. J. Dy et al. (eds.), *Peripheral Nerve Issues after Orthopedic Surgery*,
https://doi.org/10.1007/978-3-030-84428-8_14

tion cannot be established, there are theoretical mechanisms tying each of these factors to the risk of nerve injury.

Preoperative valgus deformity and flexion contracture reduce the tension on the peroneal nerve. Consequently, the correction of these deformities results in an acute increase in tension that is thought to be the primary mechanism of peroneal nerve injury [34, 79]. This hypothesis is supported by a higher incidence of palsy in patients with higher degrees of deformity and is consistent with what is known about the tolerance of neurologic structures to traction injury. Lundborg et al. noted histologic changes after increases in strain as low as 4%, with impaired microcirculation after 8% strain and full ischemia after 15% [50]. Watanabe et al. noted that small but repetitive strain can result in subsequent dysfunction, particularly in patients with subclinical pathology [103]. As such, the combined effects of deformity correction and vigorous retraction in severely contracted patients may result in a higher frequency of cumulative and clinically apparent injury. It has been suggested that the increased incidence of nerve injury in patients with RA may be due in part to the increased incidence of severe deformity and combined valgus and flexion contractures in this particular patient population [33, 43], though some authors have noted RA to be an independent risk factor [81].

The mechanism underlying an increased risk in younger patients has been postulated to be multifactorial. Increased initial deformity and increased incidence of post-traumatic contractures in younger patient populations undergoing TKA could potentially be responsible for this finding. Furthermore, Christ et al. hypothesized that decreased tissue pliability and increased muscle mass might be associated with more vigorous retraction in this patient cohort [12]. Similarly, the association with increased BMI and neurologic injury has been proposed to be related to the need for more vigorous and forceful retraction in these patients [66].

Women have been noted to have a higher risk of nerve injury after TKA. This has been attributed to reduced muscle bulk, differential vascular anatomy, and reduced limb length [84]. The findings regarding increased nerve injury risk with both higher body mass index (in younger patients) and reduced muscle bulk (in women) seem to be at odds, demonstrating the lack of true understanding within the literature.

The role of tourniquet use in the causation of postoperative nerve dysfunction remains controversial. While Horlocker et al. identified tourniquet time >120 minutes to be a risk factor for postoperative peroneal nerve injury [28], other studies have failed to identify similar associations [33, 43, 78, 80]. Given that the vast majority of TKA cases are <120 minutes, the relationship between increased tourniquet time and postoperative nerve dysfunction may be confounded by complexity of the case. The impact of tourniquet use on peripheral nerves in extremity surgery has been evaluated in both animal models [64, 68] and clinical studies [65, 105]. While clinically relevant deficits after TKA are rarely attributed to tourniquet-induced injury, there is evidence that tourniquet pressures less than 350 mm Hg and tourniquet times less than 2 hours are likely to be well tolerated [29].

The potential role of epidural anesthesia as a causative factor has similarly been a source of controversy. The initial association was identified in a case report of a patient who had undergone an exploratory laparotomy [14]. The authors attributed the deficit to the prolonged compression of the leg against the bed rail, potentially resulting in compression of the peroneal nerve at the fibular neck. Subsequently, epidural anesthesia was identified as a significant risk factor among TKA patients by Idusuyi and Morrey [33]. The proposed mechanism was felt to be related to increased tolerance of excessive pressure either from postoperative positioning or tight postoperative dressings. Others have failed to identify an increased risk in this patient population [28], though it was noted that, when nerve injury was present, epidural anesthesia was associated with a delay in the diagnosis, which could potentially have an impact on early intervention and final prognosis [29].

Previous spine disease and baseline neuropathy, while not identified in all studies, are nearly universally recognized as relevant risk factors for postoperative nerve deficit [13, 29, 34, 63, 85]. This association is widely accepted to be a manifestation of the "double crush" phenomenon, where multiple points of neural compression along the anatomic course of a nerve result in a cumulative effect on downstream neural function [100]. Patients with pre-existing subclinical compressive neuropathy have reduced capacity to tolerate acute increases in neural strain, potentially increasing the risk of clinically evident postoperative nerve palsy.

14.3 Mechanisms of Injury

The potential mechanisms of injury vary by nerve. With regard to injury to the IPBSN, this is most commonly the result of direct surgical transection of this nerve as it crosses the surgical field for a midline anterior incision. The vulnerability of the peroneal nerve to injury is a result of both its proximity to the posterolateral corner of the knee and its physiologic tethers proximal and distal to the surgical field. Peroneal nerve injury can be caused by direct trauma due to aberrant and overly aggressive lateral retractor placement or during posterolateral capsular release. Furthermore, as described above, correction of significant valgus and/or flexion deformities may result in stretch injury to the peroneal nerve. Pressure-induced injury to the peroneal or tibial nerves may also be seen as a result of significant pseudoaneurysm (Fig. 14.1) [87] or hematoma within the popliteal fossa [48] or at the level of the fibular neck [22]. Injuries to the sciatic, tibial, or sural nerves and the lumbosacral plexus are generally the result of an indirect injury as the course of these nerves is somewhat further from the surgical field. Tourniquet-related compression injuries, traction neuropathies, or peripheral nerve block–related injuries to these structures are rare, but possible.

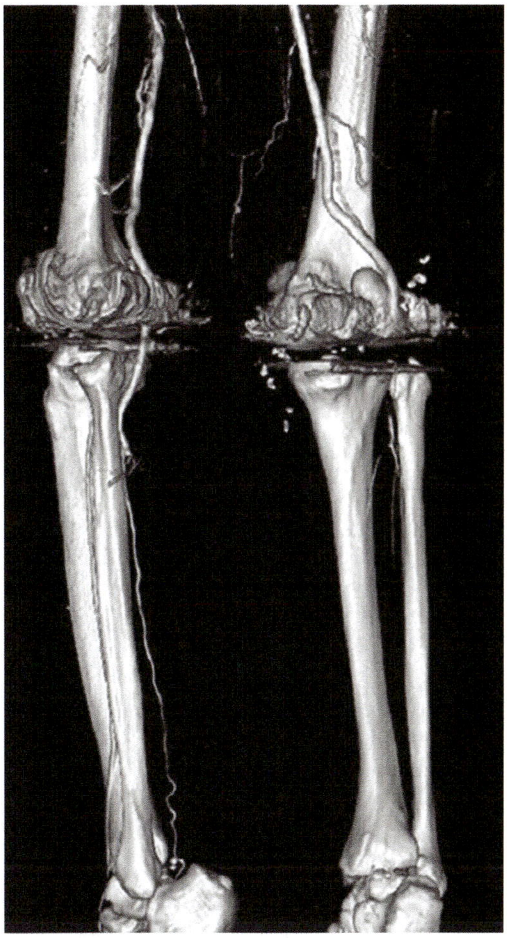

Fig. 14.1 Computed tomographic angiography of the right lower limb with three-dimensional reconstruction demonstrates a large pseudoaneurysm of the right popliteal artery. (Reproduced with permission from Shin et al. 'Popliteal artery pseudoaneurysm following primary total knee arthroplasty')

14.4 Pertinent Surgical Anatomy

14.4.1 Infrapatellar Branch of the Saphenous Nerve

Arising as a division of the femoral nerve, the saphenous nerve exits the adductor canal between the semitendinosus and gracilis tendons. Distally, the nerve bifurcates into the main saphenous branch, which courses down to the ankle, and the infrapatellar branch, which runs transversely across the anterior aspect of the knee from medial to lateral, trifurcating into three branches (Fig. 14.2). These branches, in combination with the anterior branch of the lateral cutaneous nerve, the intermediate cutaneous nerves of the thigh, and the anterior branch of the medial cutaneous nerve of the thigh, form the prepatellar plexus [7, 94]. The anatomic location of the IPBSN is such that a vertical midline incision extending from the inferior pole of the patella to the tibial tubercle will almost universally transect one or more of the branches (Fig. 14.3). Kartus et al. noted in their cadaveric study of 60 knees that in only 1 specimen did one of the branches of the IPBSN fail to cross in the interval between the inferior pole of the patella and the superior edge of the tibial tubercle [41]. As the IPBSN provides sensation over the inferolateral quadrant of the anterior aspect of the knee, its transection has traditionally been felt to be of little clinical import. However, case reports of complex regional pain syndrome, painful neuromas

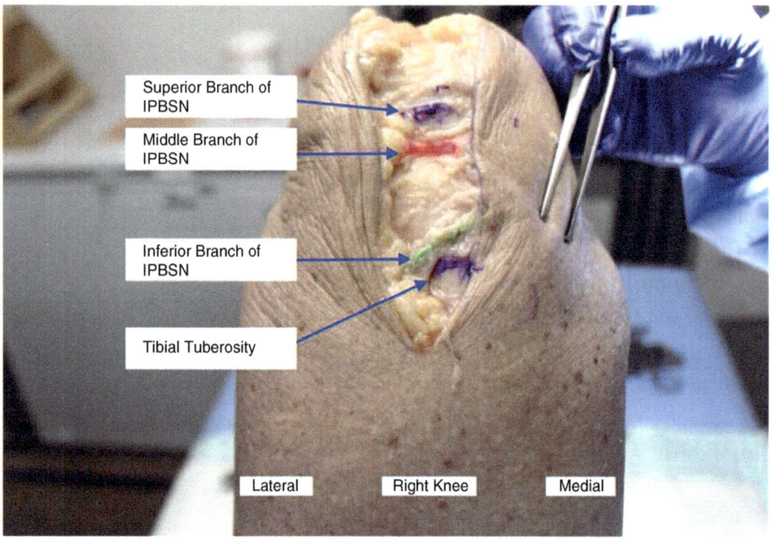

Fig. 14.2 Three branches of the IPBSN are identified running transversely between the inferior pole of the patella and the superior edge of the tibial tubercle. (Reproduced with permission from Leea et al. 'Cadaveric study of the infrapatellar branch of the saphenous nerve: Can damage be prevented in total knee arthroplasty?')

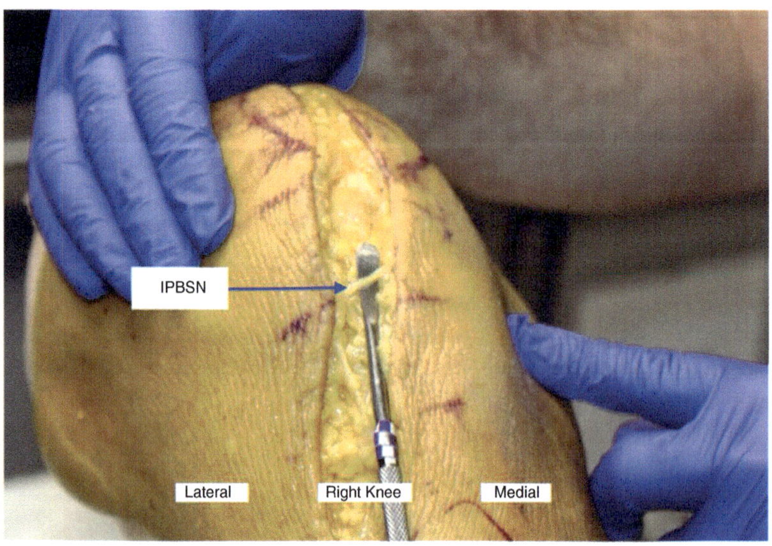

Fig. 14.3 A vertical anterior midline knee incision will almost universally transect one or more of the branches of the IPBSN. (Reproduced with permission from Leea et al. 'Cadaveric study of the infrapatellar branch of the saphenous nerve: Can damage be prevented in total knee arthroplasty?')

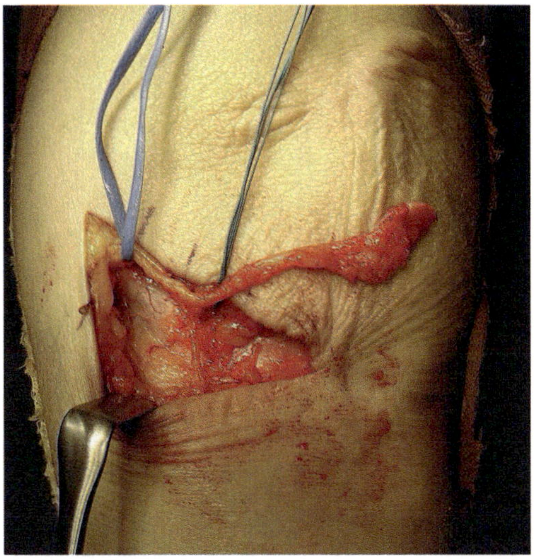

Fig. 14.4 Transection of the IPBSN, can on rare occasion, cause the formation of a painful neuroma. (Reproduced with permission from Nagai et al. 'Early-onset severe neuromatous pain of the infrapatellar branch of the saphenous nerve after total knee arthroplasty')

(Fig. 14.4), and patient dissatisfaction related to the associated sensory changes illustrate the point that its clinical impact may be underestimated [1, 32, 58, 61, 94, 95, 99, 110].

14.4.2 Sciatic Nerve

The sciatic nerve is the largest peripheral nerve of the body and arises from the roots of spinal nerves L4-S3. It exits the pelvis through the greater sciatic notch, and in the majority of patients runs deep to the piriformis muscle and over the conjoint tendon of the superior and inferior gemili and the obturator internus. Variant relationship to the piriformis muscle exists in 10–15% of cases and may predispose to increased risk of injury in these patients [6, 96, 101] (Fig. 14.5). In the posterior thigh, the nerve runs in the interval between the lateral biceps femoris and semitendinosus muscles (Fig. 14.6). The peroneal and tibial divisions, while often identifiable proximally at the level of the buttock, separate at approximately the junction of the middle and distal thirds of the posterior thigh bounded by the gluteal crease proximally and the popliteal crease distally [111] (Fig. 14.7).

14.4.3 Tibial Nerve

The posterior tibial nerve arises as the medial division of the sciatic nerve and remains in the posterior midline of the distal thigh while the peroneal division courses laterally. The nerve runs lateral to the popliteal artery as it enters the popliteal fossa then crosses over the artery in the midpoint of the fossa, exiting distally just medial to the vessels [27]. The nerve runs distally between the two heads of the gastrocnemius and courses down to the ankle between the tibialis posterior muscle and the overlying gastrocnemius-soleus complex before entering the tarsal tunnel. As it is the primary innervation of the posterior compartment of the leg, tibial nerve deficits typically manifest as weakness or inability to plantarflex, loss of normal plantar sensation, and atrophy of associated muscle groups [111].

14.4.4 Peroneal Nerve

The peroneal nerve is the most commonly injured nerve in the lower extremity. This is likely due in part to its intraneural structure and its anatomic location. Relative to the tibial nerve, the peroneal nerve is characterized by increased density of nerve fascicles and decreased connective tissue per unit of cross-sectional area, which could increase its propensity for compression-related injury (Fig. 14.8). The course of the peroneal nerve is also more vulnerable to injury as it courses lateral to the tibial division in the thigh and is in near proximity to the posterolateral capsule of the knee as it travels around the fibular neck. At the fibular neck, the common peroneal nerve flattens beneath the two heads of the peroneus longus and bifurcates into superficial and deep branches. Bruzzone et al. noted that the nerve is vulnerable to direct injury during posterolateral capsular release as it was shown to course within 13 mm of the postero-

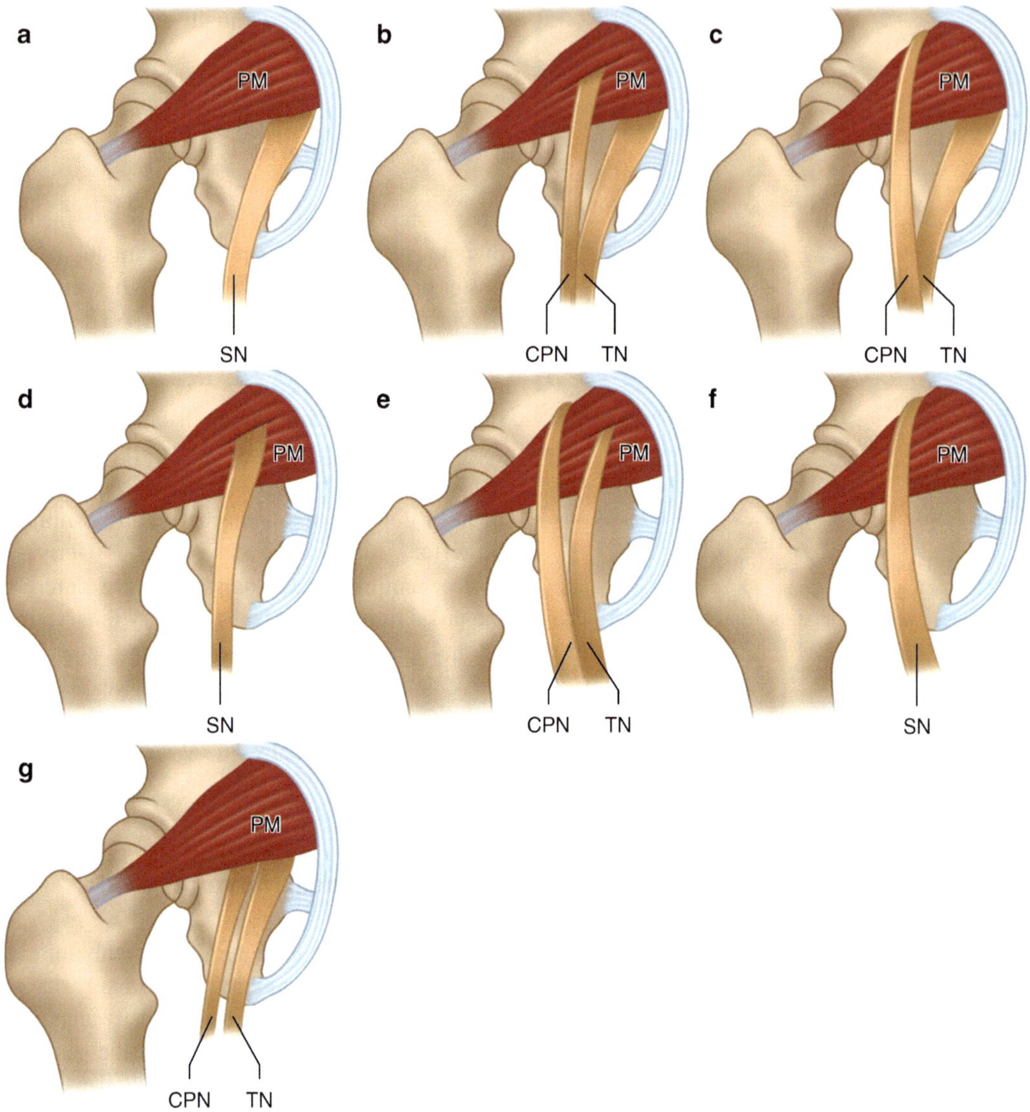

Fig. 14.5 Several variations in the anatomic relationship of the sciatic nerve to the piriformis muscle have been described as shown. (Adapted from Tomaszewski et al. 'Surgical Anatomy of the Sciatic Nerve: A Meta-Analysis')

lateral capsule at the level of the tibial cut surface in TKA [8]. The authors identified a "danger zone" for peroneal nerve injury defined as the triangle bound by the tibial cut surface inferiorly, the IT band anteriorly, and the popliteus tendon superiorly (Fig. 14.9). With regard to correction of deformity, the anatomic tethers at the level of the sciatic notch and the fibular neck have been postulated to increase the risk of traction-related injury as may be seen with correction of a significant flexion and valgus deformity. Finally, the superficial location of the peroneal nerve as it courses around the fibular neck may result in compression-related injury due to tight circumferential dressings, or uninterrupted rest of the leg against a bed rail.

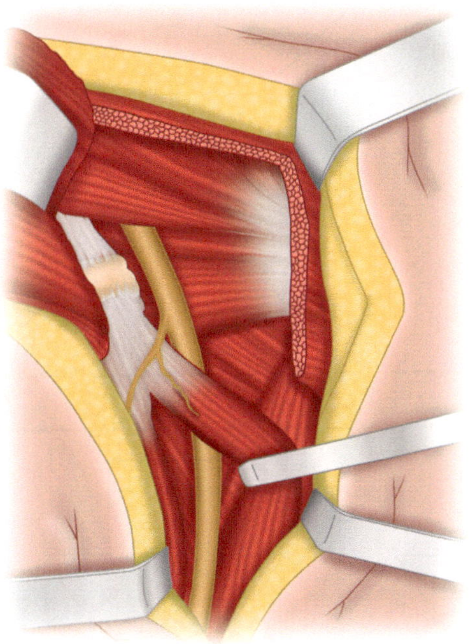

Fig. 14.6 The sciatic nerve in the posterior thigh runs between the lateral biceps femoris and semitendinosus muscles. (Adapted from Yarbrough et al. 'Nerve Injuries of the Lower Extremity')

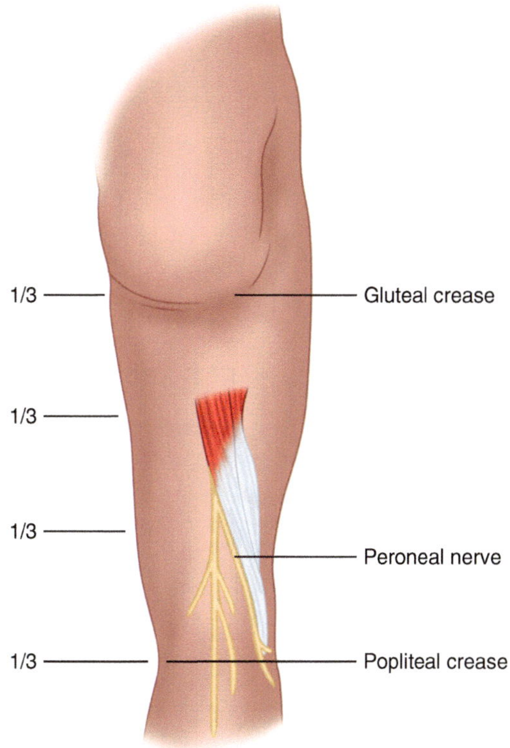

Fig. 14.7 The peroneal and tibial divisions of the sciatic nerve separate at the level of the junction of the middle and distal third of the thigh. (Adapted from Yarbrough et al. 'Nerve Injuries of the Lower Extremity')

Pearls and Pitfalls: Strategies for Prevention

- Understand risk factors, counsel patients appropriately, and exercise extreme caution in high-risk populations.
- Avoid repetitive strain injuries caused by repeated subluxations or retractions of the lateral tissues, particularly in higher risk patients.
- Maintain tourniquet times less than 120 minutes and pressure less than 350 mm Hg.
- In patients with valgus deformity requiring posterolateral capsular release, avoid deep penetration of the posterolateral capsule in the "danger zone" of maximal proximity to the nerve.
- Avoid overly exuberant lateral retraction or careless placement of lateral retractors, particularly in patients with known risk factors for injury.
- Long-acting neuraxial blockade should be used judiciously, particularly in cases with increased preoperative risk for nerve palsy given the challenges in obtaining an accurate postoperative exam. In cases where a deficit is identified, remove any circumferential dressings, flex the knee 30 degrees to relax the peroneal nerve, and ensure that the leg is positioned away from the bed railing or any other source of compression.

14.5 Natural History

The prognosis for recovery after injury varies by injury type and severity at initial presentation. With regard to IPBSN, the majority of patients do identify an area of inferolateral quadrant numbness, though longitudinal studies have reported that the area affected decreases over time and subjectively normal sensation may return in some patients [38, 57]. Mistry et al. noted that 100% of patients reported altered inferolateral quadrant sensation at 12 months; however, this decreased to 70% at 18 months and beyond.

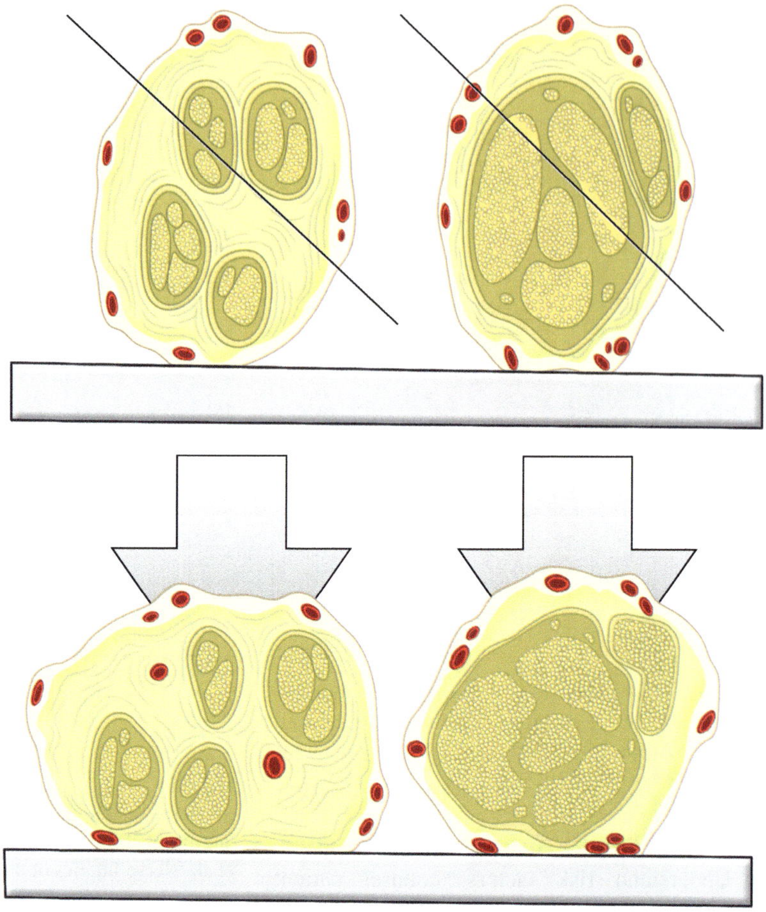

Fig. 14.8 The peroneal nerve (right side images) is characterized by increased density of nerve fascicles and decreased connective tissue per unit of cross-sectional area as compared to the tibial nerve (left side images). (Adapted from DeHart et al. 'Nerve Injuries in Total Hip Arthroplasty')

Postoperative foot drop related to peroneal nerve palsy is a far more commonly recognized injury and has thus been more extensively studied and reported on. Again the prognosis for recovery varies between reports. While Rose et al. reported a rather bleak 9.1% incidence of complete recovery [79], most other series have reported rates of complete recovery between 50% and 70% [3, 34, 81, 104]. In patients who fail to achieve complete recovery, mild to moderate improvement is typically seen [81]. The prognosis for recovery has also been shown to vary based upon the severity of initial presentation. For patients presenting initially with complete deficit and dense numbness, there is an increased possibility of incomplete recovery. Park et al. reported that among five patients noted upon initial evaluation to have a complete deficit, four went on to partial recovery while only one experienced complete recovery. By comparison, among the 32 patients who presented with an incomplete deficit, 24 went on to experience complete recovery and 8 had a partial recovery [67]. As a general rule of thumb, one-half to two-thirds of patients can be expected to make a full recovery, and the remaining one-third to one-half of patients may have a partial recovery. The prognosis is best if the initial presentation is an incomplete palsy and if some return of function is seen in the early postoperative period.

While they are rare, indirect injuries to the sciatic and posterior tibial nerves have a high rate of recovery, though as with many neurologic injuries, the time course for recovery can be protracted in some cases [90].

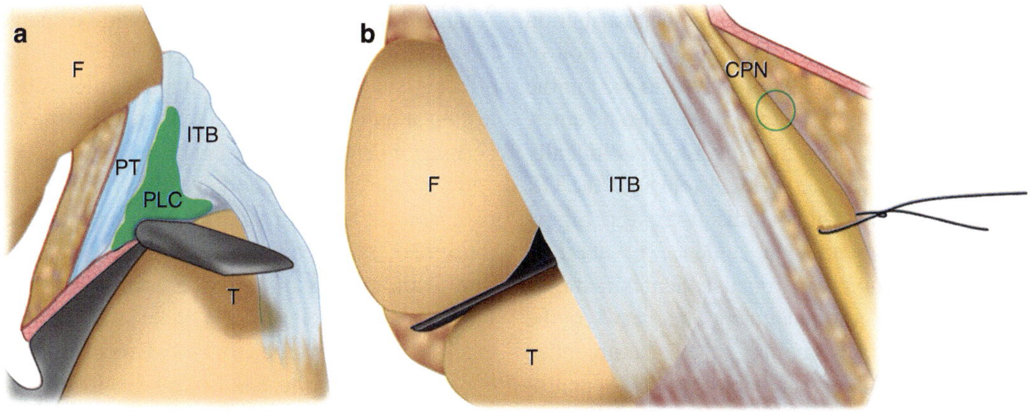

Fig. 14.9 The "danger zone" for peroneal nerve injury is defined as the triangle bound by the tibial cut surface inferiorly, the IT band anteriorly, and the popliteus tendon superiorly. (Adapted from Bruzzone et al. 'The Risk of Direct Peroneal Nerve Injury Using the Ranawat "Inside-Out" Lateral Release Technique in Valgus Total Knee Arthroplasty')

14.6 Initial Evaluation/Physical Exam/Diagnostic Testing

14.6.1 Peroneal Nerve

Early diagnosis is of paramount importance as interventions may be taken to reduce stress on the nerve, and, on rare occasion, early reoperation may be warranted. Furthermore, a thorough and accurate baseline examination is needed, as the degree of change provides clear insight into the magnitude of injury. For patients who have undergone neuraxial anesthesia, "persistence" of a neuromuscular blockade or sensory deficit beyond the typical time frame should be closely monitored. While time to resolution of spinal anesthesia or peripheral nerve blocks varies, early deficits which are felt to be attributable to residual anesthetic effects warrant close observation. While asymmetry between extremities can occasionally occur with spinal anesthetic, presence of symmetric bilateral weakness or anesthesia can be reassuring. Conversely, asymmetric numbness or weakness in the operative extremity should heighten awareness that an injury may have taken place. Similarly, numbness or weakness affecting both tibial and peroneal nerve distributions may be more likely related to resolving anesthesia, whereas deficits isolated to the peroneal nerve distribution, such as lack of dorsiflexion or numbness affecting only the dorsum of the foot, are more concerning for a peroneal nerve injury.

When a neurologic deficit is encountered during a routine postoperative check, if a spinal or nerve block was utilized, it is often helpful to discuss findings with the anesthesia team as the type of anesthetic used, dose, and location may impact the expected duration of neuromuscular blockade and thus an expected timeline for recovery can be established. Frequent follow-up examinations are warranted to establish whether early resolution is noted or there is a persistence of deficit suggestive of an injury. Early interventions to reduce strain on the peroneal nerve, including slight flexion of the knee and removal of any circumferential dressings, should be carried out as soon as a postoperative deficit is encountered. Close examination for any sign of expanding hematoma is also of critical importance, as this represents one of the few indications for emergent return to the operating room (OR) for exploration and evacuation of hematoma. Erickson reported two cases of nerve palsy following TKA with complete resolution following surgical evacuation of hematoma [19]. Apart from prominent and palpable swelling and ecchymosis, neurologic deficit related to expanding hematoma is generally characterized by pain radiating in the distribution of the affected nerve. Thus, the combination of neurologic deficit and painful dysesthesias in the distribution of the affected nerve warrant emergent axial imaging, or if hematoma is clinically apparent, may warrant a direct return to the OR for exploration. Other indications for urgent reoperation may include evidence of aberrant hardware position or extruded cement which may be causing direct impingement on a nerve. In the absence of these findings, the recommended management of an acute postoperative neurologic deficit is primarily supportive, including protective bracing, therapeutic stretching, and galvanic stimulation of affected muscle groups.

In the subacute setting, additional findings are likely to become apparent. Upon inspection, anterior and lateral compartment muscle atrophy may be noted [107]. Over time, a chronically plantarflexed ankle leads to stiffness and then contracture of the Achilles tendon; thus, flexibility of the foot and ankle should be evaluated and range of motion noted [5]. An equinovarus foot deformity can be the sequelae of a missed peroneal injury [5] and can make functional restoration more challenging A Silfverskiold test should be performed in order to assess the tightness of both the Achilles and gastrocnemius. This is done by passively dorsiflexing the ankle with the knee both fully extended and flexed to 90 degrees [39]. If attributable to gastrocnemius tightness, passive dorsiflexion should improve with the knee flexed due to relaxation of the calf muscles. If it does not improve with knee flexion, there is concern for Achilles tendon contracture.

Light touch and pain sensation can be checked both within the first webbed space and the dorsum of the foot to elicit deficits in the deep and superficial peroneal nerves, respectively [91]. Comparison to the opposite side is typically done, but may be impaired by baseline lumbosacral spine pathology, if present.

Peroneal injury results in loss of motor control of ankle and toe dorsiflexion, as well as subtalar eversion. Each individual muscle should have its strength graded 1–5 [44]. Hip abduction should be tested in order to differentiate an L5 radiculopathy from a peroneal nerve injury, as both have weakness of extensor hallucis longus [91]. A patient with a peroneal palsy should be unable to stand on his/her heel or do a "heel walk" on the affected side [107]. Patellar and Achilles reflex testing should show hyporeflexia in the case of a peripheral peroneal injury [91].

It is extremely important to scrutinize the patient's gait to identify the severity of dorsiflexion weakness. Specifically, one must pay attention to the phases of gait where dorsiflexion is vital to avoid tripping. During heel strike, tibialis anterior and the toe extensors eccentrically contract to hold the ankle slightly dorsiflexed past neutral. During midswing, these same muscles concentrically contracts so that the foot and toes can clear the ground without making contact through swing phase. Patients with a peroneal nerve palsy have a "steppage gait," as the foot slaps on the ground during heel strike due to lack of tibialis anterior control [44, 107]. Rather than the heel making first contact, the ankle is plantarflexed as the toes make first contact, followed by the lateral foot, with the heel coming down last [107]. The patient is able to avoid dragging the feet and toes during swing phase with increased hip flexion as if he/she was ascending a staircase [44, 88]. Therapy should be targeted to maintain foot and ankle flexibility, as bracing often cannot be tolerated in a rigid foot [5].

Electrodiagnostic studies can be an effective method in identifying an injury to a peripheral nerve, as well as identifying any baseline subclinical neuropathies complicating the patient's clinical picture [63]. Knutson reported electromyography (EMG) evidence of preoperative peroneal nerve palsy in 17% of rheumatoid arthritis undergoing TKA [63]. This suggests that if the EMG/NCS are performed early after surgery (when a palsy is noted, but prior to any Wallerian degeneration occurring), it can be used to establish baseline neuropathy. After Wallerian degeneration has occurred and can be detected on EMG (approximately 4 weeks), EMG can be used to identify reinnervation and shed light on prognosis for recovery [63, 109]. Serial EMG studies can be useful to observe improvement in motor unit recruitment patterns.

Magnetic resonance imaging (MRI) can be useful to identify entrapment and compressive neuropathy. This can be either as the common

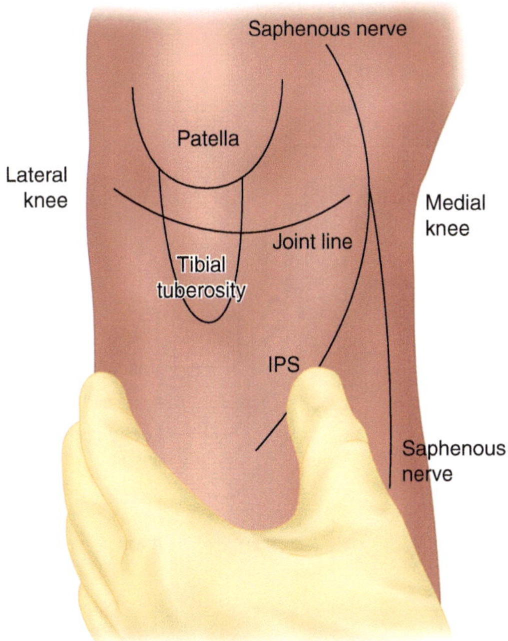

Fig. 14.10 The course of the saphenous nerve and its infrapatellar branch are depicted. (Adapted from Trescot et al. [98])

peroneal nerve crosses the fibular neck superficially, or as it dives beneath the origin of the peroneus longus [17]. Synovial cysts, aberrant musculature, compression via hematoma, or varicosities, all of which can be surgically released, can all be identified on MRI as well. Increased signal, size, and deviation can be seen within affected nerves on fluid-sensitive sequences [17]. Unfortunately, there are concerns about the sensitivity of MRI in this setting, as a recent study showed low correlation between MRI appearance and clinical symptoms [97].

14.6.2 Infrapatellar Branches of Saphenous Nerve

When evaluating a postoperative TKA patient, he/she will frequently mention numbness distal and lateral to the incision. Lee et al. performed a cadaveric study that showed there was no reproducible method to preserving these branches using a standard TKA incision [46]; therefore, it is important to educate patients both pre- and postoperatively that numbness in this region following TKA is normal and often expected.

As the infrapatellar branches of the saphenous nerve are small and purely sensory, physical exam maneuvers and nerve conduction studies must be used for diagnosis. Tinel's test can be performed medial and inferior to the tibial tuberosity, as well as using filaments to compare to the contralateral side [98] (Fig. 14.10). Sensory nerve conduction studies can demonstrate injury to the saphenous nerve [102] and differentiate it from the infrapatellar branches [98]. The nerve is stimulated with a surface electrode 2 cm medial and 2-2.5 cm distal to the inferior pole of the patella, and responses are measured proximally [4]. The infrapatellar branch can be differentiated from the main saphenous nerve via local anesthetic blockade [98].

14.7 Grading Nerve Injuries

In the context of TKA, there are two factors that determine the management of a nerve injury: (1) the degree of nerve injury, and (2) the nerve injured. A major stretch injury of the peroneal nerve, for example, requires different workup and treatment than a transection of the IPBSN. What follows in this section pertains primarily to the former, while management of the latter will be discussed separately.

The prognosis of a nerve injury varies widely depending upon the elements of neural tissue that are involved (Fig. 14.11). Seddon's 1943 system is the simplest and perhaps still the most clinically relevant, encompassing neurapraxia, axonotmesis, and neurotmesis [82].

Neurapraxia is a demyelinating injury that results from a mild stretch or crush. There is no disruption to the intraneural contents (Fig. 14.12). Although transient sensory and/or motor deficits will be seen, there is no Wallerian degeneration, and recovery is spontaneous and complete, usually within a few hours to a few weeks. Electrodiagnostic studies—if obtained prior to recovery—would show conduction distal to (but not across) the injured segment, and no fibrillation (denervation) potentials in the target muscle.

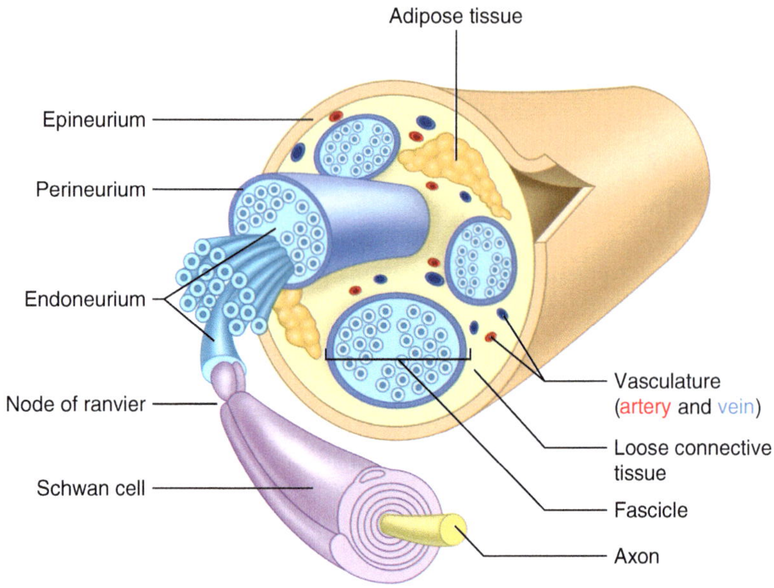

Fig. 14.11 Nerve layers in cross section. (Adapted from Kuliasha et al "Robust and scalable Tissue-Engineered Electronic Nerve Interfaces (TEENI)" https://www.researchgate.net/publication/330757070_ROBUST_AND_SCALABLE_TISSUE-ENGINEERINED_ELECTRONIC_NERVE_INTERFACES_TEENI)

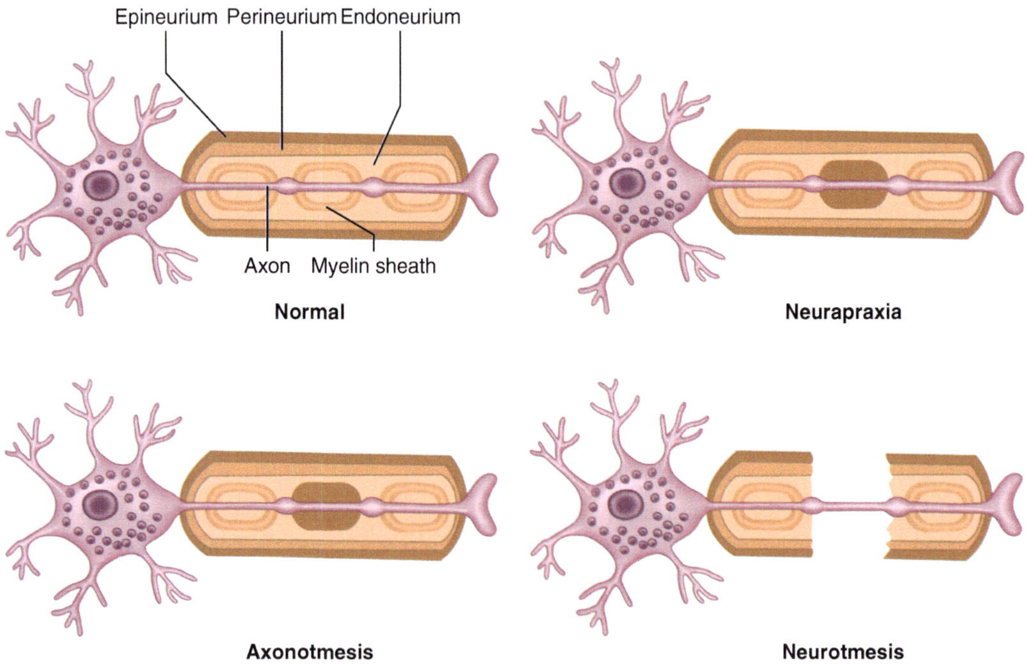

Fig. 14.12 Seddon system for grading nerve injury. (Adapted from Poage et al "Peroneal Nerve Palsy: Evaluation and Management" https://insights-ovid-com.ezproxy.lib.utexas.edu/article/00124635-201601000-00001)

Axonotmesis results from a moderate injury, with disruption of the axon and myelin, but preservation of the perineurium and epineurium. Wallerian degeneration occurs in these injuries after 3-4 days, leading to a lack of nerve conduction beyond the injured segment with fibrillation potentials in the target muscle. In lower grade axonotmetic injuries, the stromal scaffold remains intact and axons can regenerate to their target, proceeding at a rate of roughly 1 mm per day. This usually results in spontaneous recovery, although the speed and completeness of recovery can vary depending on the patient's age and overall health, as well as scarring in and around the nerve [82]. Moreover, the target muscle will gradually undergo denervation changes, which after about a year will be irrevocable, so if the nerve injury is far enough from the motor target (approximately 30 cm), motor function will be permanently impaired even if the regenerating axons eventually reach their target—hence the maxim, "time is muscle" [52]. Although uncommon after TKA, higher grade axonotmetic injuries have more severe scarring within the neural tissue and have a poorer prognosis for recovery [51, 92]. If there is a lack of recovery on serial physical examination and EMG studies, surgical reconstruction may be necessary. Neurotmesis, in Seddon's system, is complete disruption of the nerve [82]. Recovery is generally impossible without surgical intervention.

These categories reflect an inconvenient truth in grading nerve injuries—the axon is the most delicate structure within a nerve, and each successive stromal layer around the axon is more resilient. Thus, at least initially, the outward appearance of the nerve is identical in first-through fourth-degree injuries. Therefore, it is impossible to diagnose the degree of injury with the currently available methods of MRI or ultrasound, or even direct intraoperative inspection. Instead, the staging of nerve injury is reliant upon the clinical and electrophysiologic evidence of recovery. Given the challenges of timely neural reinnervation, this sets up the dilemma of not being able to determine higher stages of nerve injury until it may be too late to successfully intervene. Deciding whether and when to intervene is therefore a great challenge in the management of many nerve injuries.

14.8 Treatment Options

Intertwined with the ambiguity of whether and when to operate is the decision of what operation to perform. There are many options—direct repair, conduit, autograft/allograft, and nerve transfer—but not all are viable in all circumstances. For example, if a nerve were lacerated 5 cm from its neuromuscular junction, repair directly or with a short graft or conduit should yield a positive outcome, even if undertaken 9 months post-injury, as the regenerating fibers would reach the muscle before atrophy is irreversible. If the laceration occurred 15 cm away from the muscle, repair should be completed within 6 months, or there will be no muscle left to reinnervate. If 35 cm away (a highly unlikely scenario in TKA), even immediate direct repair will likely result in a poor outcome, and an alternative strategy—such as nerve or tendon transfer—should be employed.

14.8.1 Transection Injuries

Transection of a major nerve, such as the peroneal or tibial nerve, is a rare event in TKA. If it occurs and is immediately recognized, early intervention with immediate repair at the time of injury would be ideal. If this cannot be performed at the time of recognition due to lack of availability of equipment or personnel, repair within a few weeks can be performed with a similar outcome expectation. If the transected nerve is not repaired immediately, our preference is that the referring surgeon should place a distinctive suture, such as 3-0 polypropylene, from the epineurium of the nerve stumps to the surrounding fascia in order to facilitate identification at the subsequent surgery and to minimize retraction of the nerve ends.

With the exception of a nerve cut cleanly with a knife and repaired immediately, most transections, as from a wayward saw blade, will require trimming back of the nerve stumps to healthy, pouting fascicles, which—combined with the nerve's elastic recoil—will leave a gap. Rather than advancing the nerve stumps and repairing them under tension, which renders the repair site ischemic and induces neuroma formation, a gap should be bridged with a graft or conduit. Autologous nerve graft, usually obtained from the sural nerve, is the standard against which all other techniques have been compared, and none have been shown to be superior [47, 75]. Although the supporting literature is limited to small case series, nerve allografts have the potential to produce comparable outcomes while sparing donor site morbidity [23, 69]. Conduits can be adequate in conducting regeneration across short (less than 3 cm) gaps, but in the author's opinion, the handling properties of nerve allograft are far superior, especially for large-diameter nerves [76].

14.8.2 Stretch Injuries

Much more common than a transection would be a stretch injury. In the setting of TKA, this is typically an injury to the peroneal nerve from overzealous retraction or correction of valgus deformity. Because all neurapraxia and most axonotmesis injuries will recover spontaneously, observation alone is appropriate for at least 3 months. During that time, the patient should be assessed monthly for recovery of motor and sensory function, as well as passive range of motion. An advancing Tinel sign is a good prognostic indicator. If there has been no meaningful recovery at the 3-month mark, baseline electrodiagnostic studies should be obtained. These will generally not be prognostic but will serve as a comparison study if another 6–12 weeks pass without clinical improvement, at which point a second electrodiagnostic study should be obtained. If there is no electrodiagnostic evidence of improvement on the second study, surgical intervention should be considered.

As mentioned above, precisely localizing the zone of injury can be challenging. A discrete, non-advancing Tinel sign could pinpoint a neuroma or neuroma-in-continuity, as could a high-resolution ultrasound. A skilled electrodiagnostician, using an "inching" technique, can sometimes identify a relatively narrow zone at which conduction is blocked. If there is a focal conduction block at a known constriction point (e.g., the posterior crural septum at the fibular neck) during the nerve conduction studies, CPN decompression should be considered. Upon exposure, a compressed but not severely injured nerve will have an enlarged appearance proximal to the constriction point. For more severely injured nerves, upon exposure the scarred segment will often have a bulbous appearance with loss of normal fascicular striations and will feel firm on palpation. If the entire diameter of the nerve is involved, the scarred segment is excised and the stumps are trimmed back serially until the fascicles appear totally normal—not just to pouting fascicles, but to the point where no scar tissue is evident between fascicles.

The resulting gap will typically be several centimeters long, precluding the use of a conduit-assisted repair. If the distance from the proximal stump to the muscle is traversable by regenerating axons within the timeframe of muscle salvageability, repair with a graft should result in at least partial motor recovery. If the distance is too great, or the repair is undertaken too late, a nerve or tendon transfer should be considered.

If surgery is undertaken in the absence of localizing signs, the surgeon would need to expose the nerve widely. If no scarring can be identified within the nerve, the procedure may be limited to neurolysis, releasing scar tissue and any points of compression along the nerve, most likely around the fibular neck in the case of the peroneal nerve.

14.9 Surgical Techniques

14.9.1 Direct Repair

The prerequisite to direct repair is the ability to coapt the trimmed nerve stumps without tension. Nerves are very delicate, so the tissue must be handled very gently with microsurgical instruments, ideally under a microscope or other high-level magnification. A sharp pair of iris scissors, a scalpel, or a neurotome is used to freshen the nerve stumps. Perineurial or other internal sutures will obstruct regenerating fibers and should be avoided. Instead, only epineurial sutures are placed, aligning fascicles by matching surface landmarks, vessels, and striations between fascicular groups (Fig. 14.13). The author prefers 8-0 nylon. Fascicles that pout beyond the epineurial cuff should be trimmed so that they are completely contained within the epineurial cuff, ensuring that all regenerating fibers are channeled into the distal stump.

In an effort to minimize neural trauma and foreign body reaction, one should place as few sutures as possible to maintain epineurial alignment and contain the fascicles. For high-caliber nerves, this could require a large number of sutures. To minimize foreign material, some surgeons place just 2–3 sutures to establish alignment, then seal the coaptation site with fibrin glue. However, one should be aware that fibrin glue contributes almost no tensile strength to the repair but does add significant cost. Furthermore, this is an "off label" use based on United States Food and Drug Administration recommendations.

14.9.2 Conduit

Nerve conduits are simply hollow tubes made from collagen or absorbable material that guide regenerating axons toward the distal stump (Fig. 14.14). They can be effective for short gaps (<3 cm). Although experimental outcomes are inferior to grafts, conduits do have the undeniable advantages of off-the-shelf availability and obviation of donor site morbidity [76]. They are also technically simple—the stumps are intubulated within the conduit, which is secured to the epineurium with 2–3 sutures. However, long conduits may collapse or fill with scar tissue and are not recommended by the author.

14.9.3 Autograft/Allograft

The most common source of autograft is the sural nerve, which can provide ample length (up to 30 cm) with minimal morbidity—a small, noncritical area of numbness on the lateral foot and a scar on the leg [75]. The nerve is first found in the groove between the lateral malleolus and Achilles tendon. It is well camouflaged by the surrounding fat; it is helpful to look for the lesser saphenous vein, along which the nerve runs closely (Fig. 14.15). The nerve can be harvested with a longitudinal incision, small transverse skip incisions (which tend to heal with finer scars), or an endoscope. Compared to the peroneal nerve, the

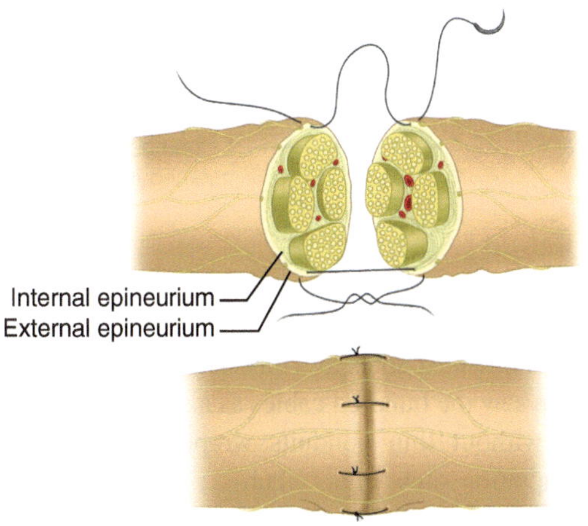

Fig. 14.13 Epineurial repair illustrated first with two-suture approximation (180 degree placement) (**a**) and reinforcement with additional sutures (**b**). (Adapted from Siemionow "Chapter 8 Current Techniques and Concepts in Peripheral Nerve Repair" in "International Review of Neurobiology" https://www.sciencedirect.com/science/article/pii/S0074774209870086)

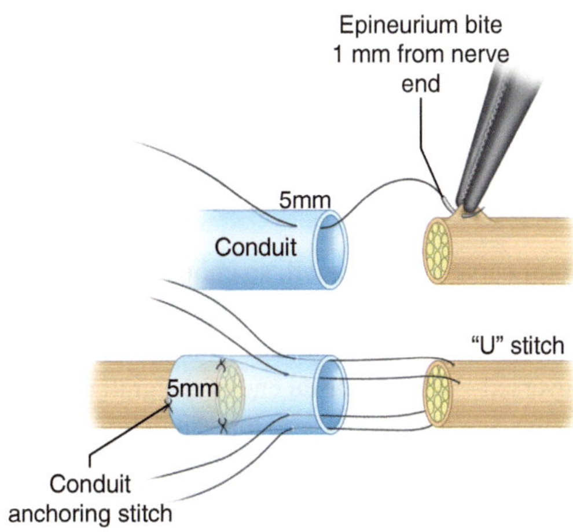

Fig. 14.14 Nerve conduit between regenerating axons with two suture closures. (Adapted from Houschyar et al "The Role of Current Techniques and Concepts in Peripheral Nerve Repair." https://www.hindawi.com/journals/psi/2016/4175293/)

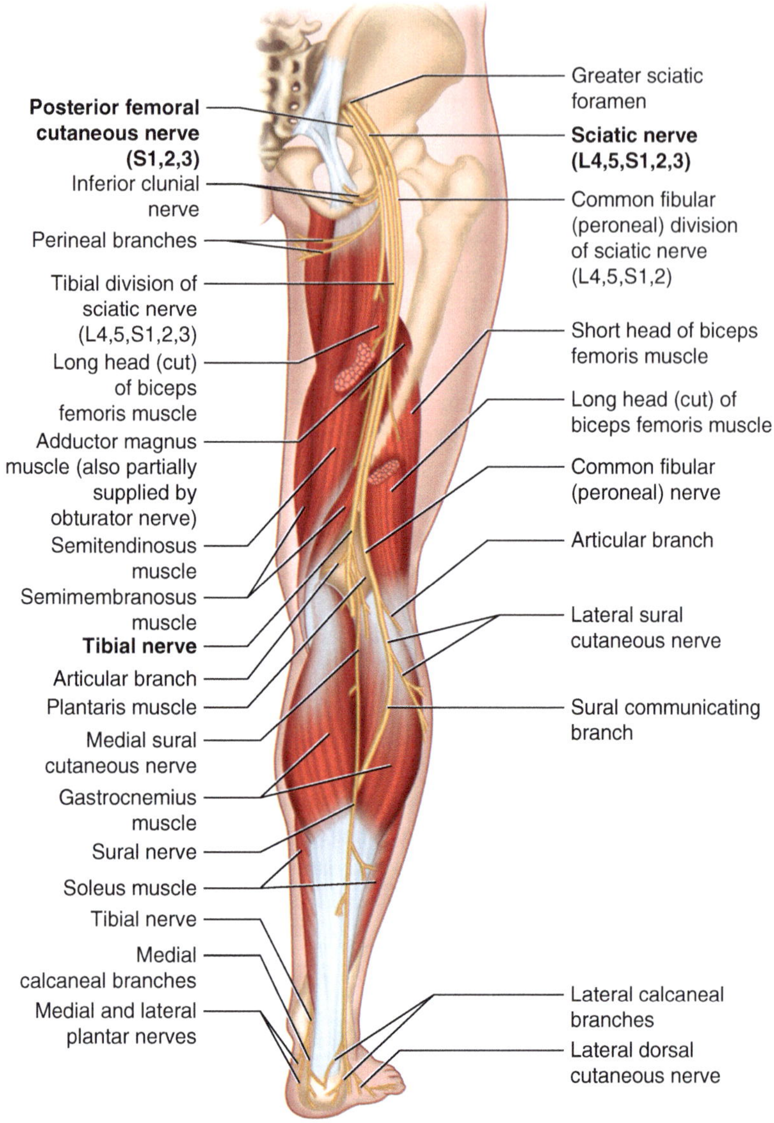

Fig. 14.15 The sural nerve runs between the gastrocnemius muscle proximally and translates laterally just superior to the lateral malleolus where it can be found between the lateral malleolus and the Achilles tendon. (Adapted from Frank Netter "Lower Limb" from "Atlas of Human Anatomy", 6th Ed, 2014)

sural nerve is quite small, so enough length must be harvested to provide 3–4 cable grafts.

Nerve grafts should theoretically be reversed—with the distal end of the graft coapted to the proximal stump—so that small branches of the graft do not divert regenerating axons away from the target. In reality, the sural nerve is essentially devoid of branches proximal to the foot, so this probably makes little difference.

The cable grafts can be sewn individually to the proximal and distal stumps, as in direct nerve repair, but this can be quite tedious when coapting several cables (Fig. 14.16a). An alternative is to bundle the cables together with fibrin glue, and then sew the bundled cables as a single unit, with or without thin conduits wrapped around the coaptation sites (Fig. 14.16b).

Nerve allografts lack the Schwann cells of autograft but maintain much of the internal scaffolding that provides support for regenerating axons. The literature regarding the use of acellular nerve allografts for mixed and motor nerve reconstruction is limited to case series, but has yielded promising results [45, 53, 93].

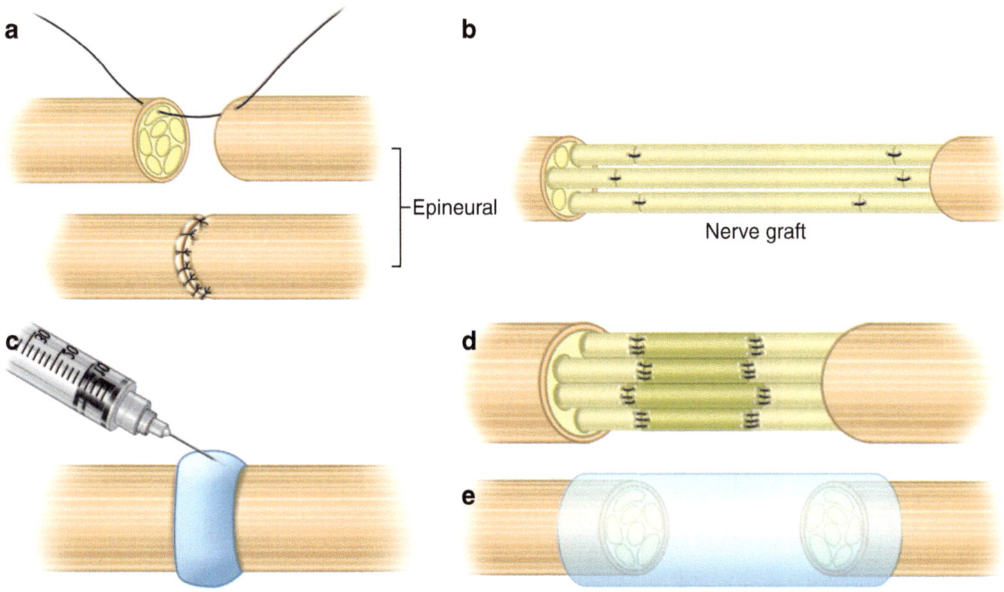

Fig. 14.16 (**a**) epineural coaptation; (**b**) coaptation of individual fascicles; (**c**) supplementation of repair with fibrin glue; (**d**) grouped fascicular coaptation; (**e**) conduit repair (Adapted from Linda Luca, in Hand and Upper Extremity Rehabilitation (Fourth Edition), 2016 https://www.sciencedirect.com/topics/medicine-and-dentistry/nerve-regeneration)

Like conduits, allografts are readily available and avoid donor site morbidity. They are available in calibers that match the major peripheral nerves about the knee, eliminating the need for cables. Allograft handles are much like autograft and can be sewn and/or glued similarly. In addition to the paucity of the published literature, a major offset to these many advantages is the cost of allograft, which can be quite substantial.

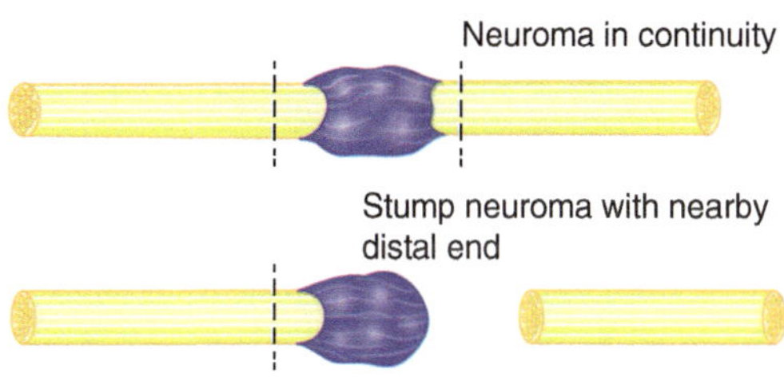

Fig. 14.17 Separation of neuroma in continuity from healthy fascicles. (Adapted from Eberlin "Surgical Algorithm for Neuroma Management: A Changing Treatment Paradigm" https://www.researchgate.net/publication/328361236_Surgical_Algorithm_for_Neuroma_Management_A_Changing_Treatment_Paradigm)

14.9.4 Neuroma-in-Continuity

In the case of a neuroma-in-continuity, the surgeon will first need to separate the intact fascicles from those blocked by scar (Fig. 14.17). This can be quite tedious and is best performed under a microscope. The fascicular gaps created after excising the scar can be managed according to the principles outlined above, although direct repair is usually precluded by both tension and interference from the preserved fascicles.

14.9.5 Nerve Transfer

In general, nerve transfer is utilized when a nerve is injured far away from its target, and/or when the decision to operate is made relatively late, such that repair/grafting is unlikely to result in reinnervation before the muscle is irreversibly atrophic. The former should be an

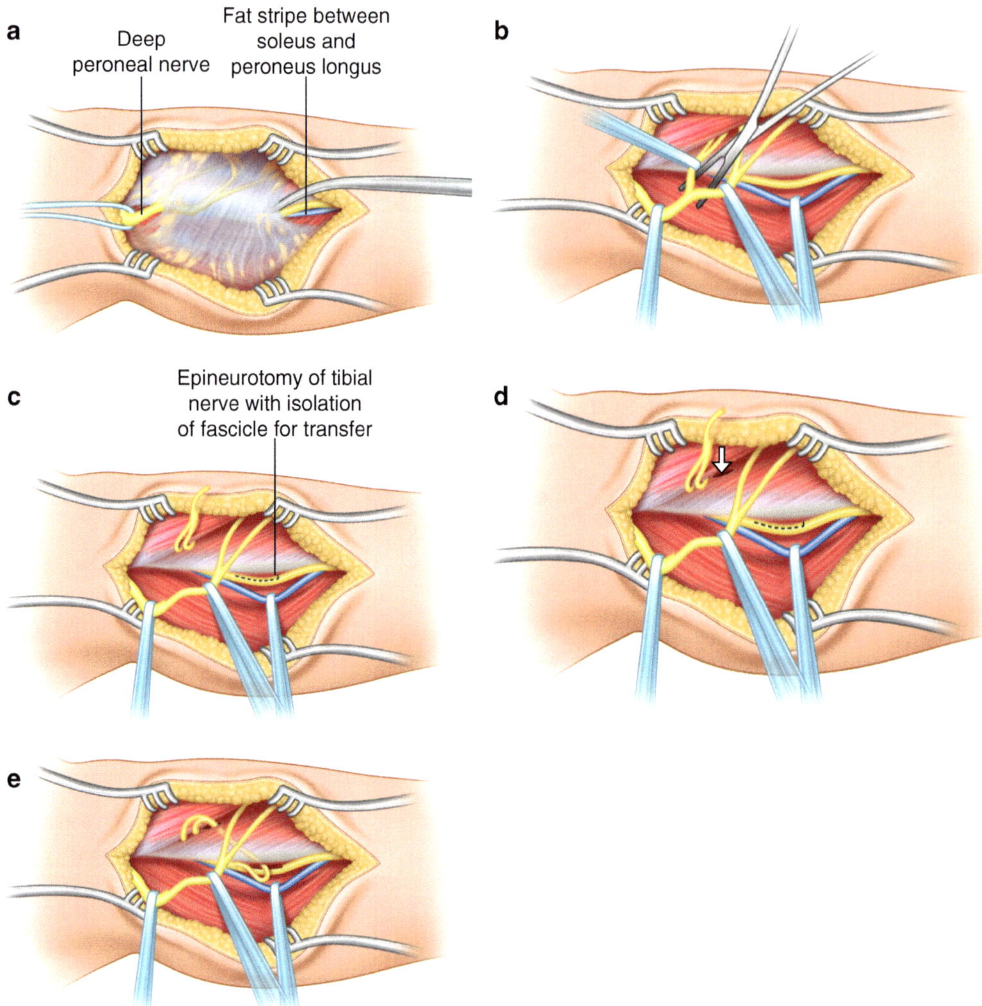

Fig. 14.18 Identify the deep peroneal nerve proximal to the fat stripe separating the soleus and peroneus longus (**a**). With the fat stripe divided, the tibialis anterior nerve branch can be isolated, (**b**) and a motor fascicle identified and cut distally (**c**). The tibial nerve fascicle is then fed through the interosseous membrane (**d**, **e**) and coapted to the tibialis anterior nerve. (Adapted from Giuffre et al "Partial Tibial Nerve Transfer to the Tibialis Anterior Motor Branch to Treat Peroneal Nerve Injury After Knee Trauma" https://www.ncbi.nlm.nih.gov/pmc/articles/PMC3270157/)

uncommon scenario in TKA, but the latter is possible if the nerve injury is not initially managed in a timely manner. Unfortunately, meaningful recovery of dorsiflexion from nerve transfer does not appear to be consistently obtainable, particularly if performed more than 6 months after injury. Thus, the role for nerve transfer after TKA is unclear.

The procedure is performed through a lateral approach (Fig. 14.19). The deep peroneal nerve is traced into the lateral compartment (Fig. 14.18a), and the branch to tibialis anterior is identified and cut *proximally*. The tibial nerve is then identified in the plane between soleus and peroneus longus (Fig. 14.18b). Internal neurolysis is performed to separate the fascicles of the tibial nerve, and a nerve stimulator is used to identify a motor fascicle, usually one producing movement in the flexor hallucis longus or flexor digitorum longus. This fascicle is cut *distally* (Fig. 14.18c), transposed through the interosseous membrane, and coapted to the tibialis anterior branch (Fig. 14.18d, e).

Reinnervation of the target muscle typically takes 3–6 months after nerve transfer, so if this procedure is to be performed, it should be done within 6 months of injury. Clinical results are mixed, and superiority to tendon transfers has not been shown. Given the lack of synergism and the need for extensive cortical re-education, the rehabilitation process is challenging and may influence ultimate functional outcomes.

Pearls and Pitfalls: Nerve Repair

- Identifying the degree of nerve injury is critical in determining *whether and when* to intervene. However, distinguishing first- through fourth-degree injuries can be largely impossible on gross visualization or imaging, creating a significant challenge for surgeons in nerve injury management.
- Stretch injuries in which the nerve is grossly intact should generally undergo a period of observation of at least 3 months prior to surgical intervention. However, waiting too long (greater than 9–12 months) risks irreversible atrophy of the target muscle.
- Transected nerves should be repaired directly only when trimmed nerve stumps can be coapted without tension. Sutures should be placed only in the epineurial layer to avoid obstruction of regenerating fibers.
- Nerve gaps resulting from trauma, stump retraction/debridement, or neuroma resection can be bridged with autograft, allograft, or conduit, although the latter perform adequately only for short gaps (less than 3 cm).
- Very long nerve gaps and nerve injuries far from the target muscle generally recover poorly. Nerve transfers can sometimes be a good alternative in such cases.
- Results of nerve transfers for peroneal nerve deficits are equivocal and should be considered with caution, particularly given the reliability of tendon transfers.

14.10 Postoperative Management of Nerve Repair/Reconstruction

Nerves are supposed to glide along tissue planes and should not be repaired or reconstructed under tension; for these reasons, postoperative splinting should be unnecessary, and may be detrimental [26, 31, 36, 49, 83]. Physical therapy may be indicated for recovery from arthroplasty but has a fairly minor role following nerve repair. There is no therapeutic intervention that speeds nerve regeneration or slows muscle degeneration. It is important to maintain passive range of motion, but this is a fairly simple task that can usually be patient-directed. Once the muscle begins to regain function, strengthening exercises become very important; however, simple ambulation is highly effective and probably adequate in most cases.

14.11 Management of Subcutaneous Neuromas

Anatomic studies have shown that it is nearly impossible to predictably avoid injury to the IPBSN in TKA [25, 40, 46]. Preoperative patient education should therefore include an expectation of some level of anesthesia or paresthesia in the infrapatellar region. In most cases, IPBSN injury poses nothing more than an annoyance, but occasionally a painful neuroma will arise. This may not be evident immediately but develop over several weeks. The patient will typically be able to localize the neuroma, as there is usually a distinctive radiation of paresthesias to the infrapatellar region. The patient may report this sensation and the surgeon typically elicits this with a Tinel sign. If a subcutaneous injection of 1–2 cc of 1% lidocaine produces complete (but transient) relief, the diagnosis and site are confirmed. Ultrasound can also be confirmatory and can be used to target the diagnostic injection.

Nonoperative treatment usually begins with subcutaneous corticosteroid injection [20]. Triamcinolone 40 mg, mixed with lidocaine to provide early confirmation of accurate placement, can be repeated every 4–6 months if temporarily effective, although soft tissue atrophy and cutaneous hypopigmentation are potential consequences.

Lidocaine patches can be quite effective and avoid systemic effects of oral medications such as opioids, gabapentin, and pregabalin.

The decision to operate on a subcutaneous neuroma should not be made lightly given the risk of recurrence even after initial improvement in symptoms. With that in mind, the surgery can be highly gratifying to patients, with 70–80% of patients having improvement after surgical treatment of neuroma [15, 37, 71, 108]. Truly eradicating a neuroma is an unrealistic goal; rather, the strategy is to resect the neuroma and transpose the fresh nerve stump to a less stimulable site, so that the new neuroma that inevitably forms will be less symptomatic.

In the case of the IPBSN, a neuroma entrapped in the skin closure will be repeatedly irritated with movement of the knee. Freeing the neuroma from the midline scar, trimming it back, and allowing it to retract into relatively unscarred subcutaneous fat can ameliorate movement-induced pain. Multiple studies addressing neuroma after TKA indicate neurectomy provides effective pain resolution [16, 24, 62, 86, 112]. However, given the risk of painful neuroma recurrence if the nerve end is exposed to continued mechanical stimuli after retracting into subcutaneous fat, the author prefers mobilization and transposition of the nerve stump into muscle, which has been shown to reduce neuroma size and scar formation [15, 18, 72]. Admittedly, however, the scientific evidence supporting this or any other method is limited and highly confounded.

14.12 Salvage Techniques

Once specific nerve procedures are ruled out, treatments to mitigate the functional deficits can be considered based on patient goals. Conservative measures including bracing and physical therapy are aimed at managing deficits and optimizing function in spite of them, whereas operative salvage techniques such as tendon transfers can restore specific movements and stability lost by lack of peroneal innervation. If EMG and nerve conduction studies show no signs of reinnervation, salvage tendon transfer can be attempted as early as 3 months [109]. If studies look favorable but dorsiflexion strength remains weak at 1 year following the injury, tendon transfer could still be attempted to maximize function [109].

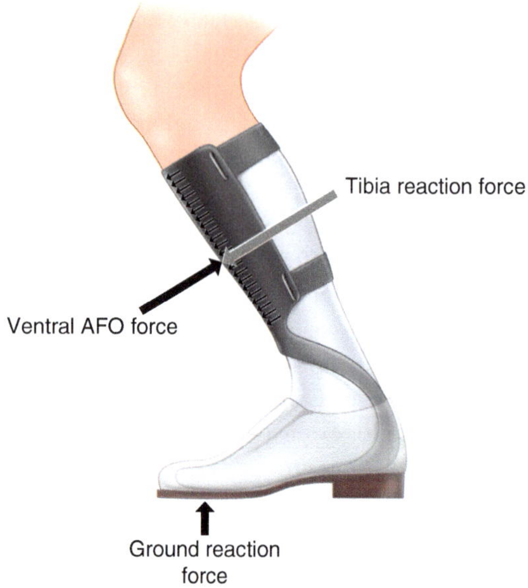

Fig. 14.19 Ankle foot orthosis. In this version, the larger contact area of the ventral AFO allows less pressure placed on the tibia. (Adapted from van der Wilk D, Dijkstra PU, Postema K, Verkerke GJ, Hijmans JM. Effects of ankle foot orthoses on body functions and activities in people with floppy paretic ankle muscles: a systematic review. Clin Biomech (Bristol, Avon). 2015)

14.12.1 Conservative Measures

Nonoperative treatments can be successful in improving symptoms of foot drop. Ankle foot orthoses can improve mobility by keeping the foot out of a plantar-flexed state during the swing phase of walking [70], thus preventing foot drag resulting in mechanical tripping (Fig. 14.19).

However, they can limit ankle range of motion when performing activities needing an increased ankle range of motion, such as walking up or down stairs or walking uphill/downhill [73]. In the setting of common peroneal injury as seen in TKA, a stiffer AFO is preferred [5]. As peroneal nerve injury during total knee arthroplasty affects the primary motor neurons, a flaccid paresis typically results. D. van der Wilk et al. conducted a systematic review assessing the effects of AFOs on body functions and activities in individuals with flaccid paresis of the ankle musculature [106]. When looking at dorsal paresis alone, AFOs increased exercise tolerance in two or three studies [21, 54, 55, 106]. Energy and oxygen expenditure decreased in elastic AFOs compared with shoes [54, 55, 106]. Dorsal, elastic, and circular AFOs increased dorsiflexion 4-6 degrees during gait [74, 106]. The added weight, cosmetic appearance, and increased pressure on specific soft tissue areas are considered negatives of the devices [10]. Although they can improve gait effort, pattern is not normal compared to those with an intact peroneal nerve [10].

Regardless of treatment with surgical or nonsurgical options, target physical therapy is vital to improvement of foot drop. The goals should focus on reducing atrophy, preserving range of motion, promoting reinnervation after nerve repair/decompression, maintaining central control following tendon transfer procedures, and developing gait control [10].

14.12.2 Tendon Transfers

Tendon transfers are a reliable option to treat foot drop associated with peroneal nerve injury. If the motor palsy persists for 1 year or more, there is slim chance for recovery, and a tendon transfer maintaining a plantigrade foot is indicated [11]. The posterior tibial tendon is transferred anteriorly to the dorsum of the foot [11]. Putti pioneered this procedure in 1914 [39], and it was successfully reproduced with good outcomes in 1954 by Watkins [39, 77]. Multiple modifications have since been made to this procedure [11, 30, 39, 59, 77]. Prior to surgical intervention, an Achilles lengthening or a gastrocnemius recession should be performed to allow the ankle to passively dorsiflex 5 degrees past neutral [39, 44]. In all modifications of the tendon transfer, the foot is casted in neutral and made non-weight bearing for a period of time, slowly advancing weight bearing after several weeks [39]. Complications include acquired pes planus deformity [11]. In the Hsu modification, the tendon is harvested from its insertion on the navicular and brought proximally through a skin incision at the middle/distal third junction of the leg. It is then passed through the interosseous membrane at this level and then subcutaneously tunneled to the base of the middle or lateral cuneiform [30]. The Bridle procedure was developed to control for iatrogenic coronal plane deformity caused by insertion of the tibialis posterior attachment in the midfoot [39]. The tibialis anterior tendon is longitudinally split at the middle/distal third junction of the leg. Here, the tibialis posterior tendon passes through the tibialis anterior on its way to anchor in the midfoot. The peroneus longus is identified through a separate incision and transected. Its distal end is transposed anterior to the malleolus and attached to the tibialis posterior as it comes anteriorly, forming a tri-tendon anastomosis. The peroneus longus and tibialis anterior are tensioned equally to control coronal plane motion (Fig. 14.20). The proximal end of peroneus longus is sewn to the peroneus brevis [39, 77]. By controlling forces within the coronal plane, there is no need for a triple arthrodesis to maintain a neutral plantigrade foot [39]. Newer procedures address the toes as well, including the Movahedi modification that transfers FDL and FHL to the toe extensors [59]. Cho et al. retrospectively compared 17 patients who had a tibialis posterior tendon transfer using the Hsu method to matched controls for a minimum of 3 years postoperatively. They found mean AOFAS, FAOS, and FAAM scores all had significant improvement. Active dorsiflexion significantly improved from −32.5 degrees to +12.1 degrees, while plantarflexion remained the same. Muscle strength significantly improved from a grade of 1.1 to 3.9. All radiographic measures assessing longitudinal arch,

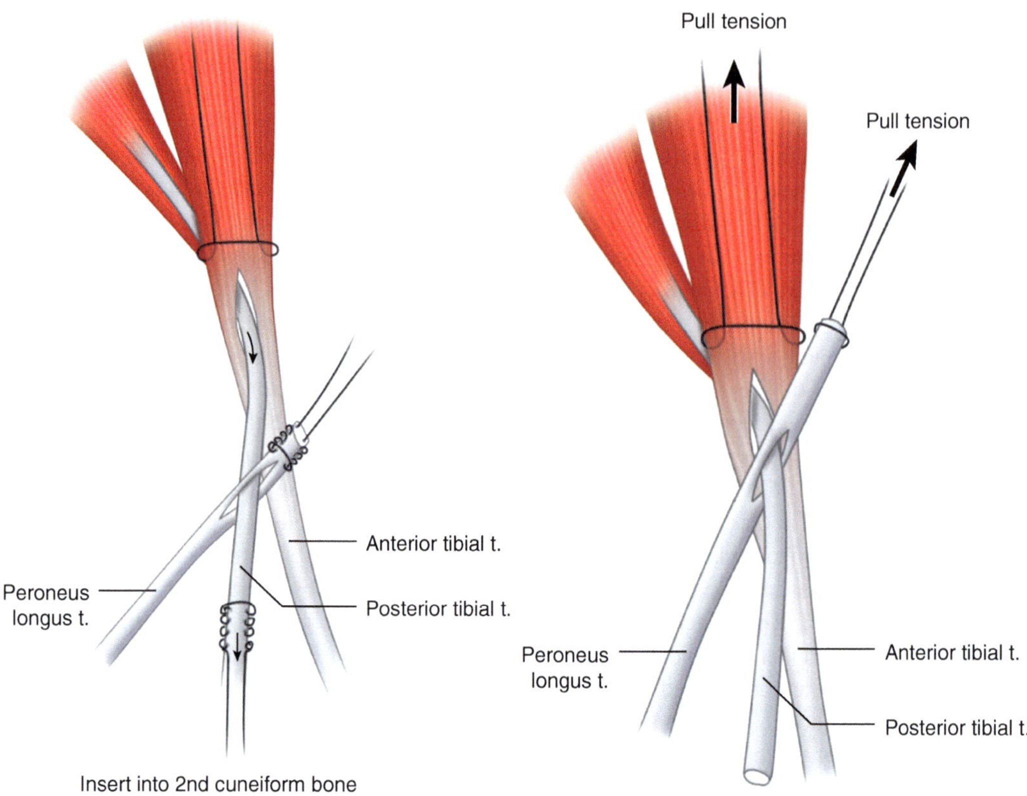

Fig. 14.20 The tri-tendon anastomosis of the Bridle procedure. The peroneus longus and tibialis anterior tendons are tensioned equally. (Adapted from Johnson et al., Outcomes of the Bridle Procedure for the Treatment of Foot Drop. Foot Ankle Int. 2015)

including Meary angle, calcaneal pitch, hindfoot alignment angle, and navicular height were unchanged. Although these results were significantly improved, all functional evaluation scores, active range of motion, and muscle strength were significantly less than the control group. Only 1 of the 17 patients needed an AFO [11]. A similar study looking at the Bridle procedure achieved similar results [39]. Thus, anterior transfer of the tibialis posterior tendon is a viable, but not a perfect option for treatment of peroneal nerve palsy.

Pearls and Pitfalls: Salvage Techniques

- Conservative management, including physical therapy and bracing, should first be attempted prior to any surgical intervention.
- Tendon transfers may permit restoration of ankle dorsiflexion.
- Percutaneous tendoachillies lengthening or gastrocnemius recession should accompany transfer procedures to ensure that contractures do not compromise surgical outcome.
- Care should be taken to achieve appropriate coronal plane balance though careful and symmetric tensioning of the tibialis anterior and the peroneus longus.

14.13 Summary

Nerve injury after TKA can be a significant source of morbidity and patient dissatisfaction. For peroneal nerve injuries, the prognosis for spontaneous recovery is variable but limited, and thus extreme care should be taken to ensure prevention where possible. Early diagnosis and supportive measures can improve the ultimate prognosis, and in the rare case of an expanding hematoma, may allow for emergent reoperation that could avoid permanent injury. Most cases will be managed more subacutely with supportive bracing, physical therapy, and monitoring for return of function. In those cases where deficits persist beyond 3 months, nerve exploration, neurolysis, and repair may be considered in consultation with a peripheral nerve expert. Tendon transfers represent an alternative salvage technique aimed at achieving a plantigrade foot and improved gait mechanics and may be an appropriate consideration for some patients.

References

1. Arthornthurasook A, Gaew-Im K. Study of the infrapatellar nerve. Am J Sports Med. 1988;16(1):57–9. https://doi.org/10.1177/036354658801600110.
2. Asp JP, Rand JA. Peroneal nerve palsy after total knee arthroplasty. Clin Orthop. 1990;261:233–7.
3. Asp JP, Rand JA. Peroneal nerve palsy after total knee arthroplasty. Clin Orthop. 1990;261:233–7.
4. Bademkiran F, Obay B, Aydogdu I, Ertekin C. Sensory conduction study of the infrapatellar branch of the saphenous nerve. Muscle Nerve. 2007;35(2):224–7. https://doi.org/10.1002/mus.20682.
5. Baima J, Krivickas L. Evaluation and treatment of peroneal neuropathy. Curr Rev Musculoskelet Med. 2008;1(2):147–53. https://doi.org/10.1007/s12178-008-9023-6.
6. Beaton LE, Anson BJ. The relation of the sciatic nerve and of its subdivisions to the piriformis muscle. Anat Rec. 1937;70(1):1–5. https://doi.org/10.1002/ar.1090700102.
7. Berry M, Bannister LH, Standring SM. Nervous system. In: Gray's anatomy. New York: Churchill Livingstone; 1995. p. 1279–82.
8. Bruzzone M, Ranawat A, Castoldi F, Dettoni F, Rossi P, Rossi R. The risk of direct peroneal nerve injury using the Ranawat "inside-out" lateral release technique in valgus total knee arthroplasty. J Arthroplast. 2010;25(1):161–5. https://doi.org/10.1016/j.arth.2008.08.016.
9. Bryan RS, Peterson LF, Combs JJ. Polycentric knee arthroplasty. A preliminary report of postoperative complications in 450 knees. Clin Orthop. 1973;94:148–52.
10. Carolus AE, Becker M, Cuny J, Smektala R, Schmieder K, Brenke C. The interdisciplinary management of foot drop. Dtsch Arztebl Int. 2019;116(20):347–54. https://doi.org/10.3238/arztebl.2019.0347.
11. Cho BK, Park KJ, Choi SM, Im SH, SooHoo NF. Functional outcomes following anterior transfer of the tibialis posterior tendon for foot drop secondary to peroneal nerve palsy. Foot Ankle Int. 2017;38(6):627–33. https://doi.org/10.1177/1071100717695508.
12. Christ AB, Chiu Y-F, Joseph A, Westrich GH, Lyman S. Incidence and risk factors for peripheral nerve injury after 383,000 total knee arthroplasties using a New York State Database (SPARCS). J Arthroplast. 2019;34(10):2473–8. https://doi.org/10.1016/j.arth.2019.05.008.
13. Christ AB, Chiu Y-F, Joseph A, Westrich GH, Lyman S. Incidence and risk factors for peripheral nerve injury after 383,000 total knee arthroplasties using a New York State Database (SPARCS). J Arthroplast. 2019;34(10):2473–8. https://doi.org/10.1016/j.arth.2019.05.008.
14. Cohen DE, Van Duker B, Siegel S, Keon TP. Common peroneal nerve palsy associated with epidural analgesia. Anesth Analg. 1993;76(2):429–31.
15. Dellon AL, Mackinnon SE. Treatment of the painful neuroma by neuroma resection and muscle implantation. Plast Reconstr Surg. 1986;77(3):427–36. https://doi.org/10.1097/00006534-198603000-00016.
16. Dellon AL, Mont MA, Krackow KA, Hungerford DS. Partial denervation for persistent neuroma pain after total knee arthroplasty. Clin Orthop. 1995;316:145–50.
17. Donovan A, Rosenberg ZS, Cavalcanti CF. MR imaging of entrapment neuropathies of the lower extremity. Part 2. The knee, leg, ankle, and foot. Radiographics. 2010;30(4):1001–19. https://doi.org/10.1148/rg.304095188.
18. Ducic I, Mesbahi AN, Attinger CE, Graw K. The role of peripheral nerve surgery in the treatment of chronic pain associated with amputation stumps. Plast Reconstr Surg. 2008;121(3):908–14; discussion 915–917. https://doi.org/10.1097/01.prs.0000299281.57480.77.
19. Erickson BJ, Brown N, Fernandez J, Della Valle CJ. Acute decompression for peroneal nerve palsy following primary total knee arthroplasty: a report of two cases. JBJS Case Connect. 2015;5(1):e16–e4. https://doi.org/10.2106/JBJS.CC.N.00134.
20. Shi GG, Schultz Jr DS, Whalen J, Clendenen S, Wilke B. Midterm outcomes of ultrasound-guided local treatment for infrapatellar saphenous neuroma following total knee arthroplasty. Cureus. 2020;12(1). https://www.cureus.com/articles/26118-midterm-outcomes-of-ultrasound-guided-local-treatment-for-infrapatellar-saphenous-neuroma-following-total-knee-arthroplasty. Accessed February 17, 2020.
21. Geboers JF, Wetzelaer WL, Seelen HA, Spaans F, Drost MR. Ankle-foot orthosis has limited effect on walking test parameters among patients with peripheral ankle dorsiflexor paresis. J Rehabil Med. 2002;34(2):80–5. https://doi.org/10.1080/165019702753557872.
22. Girolami M, Galletti S, Montanari G, et al. Common peroneal nerve palsy due to hematoma at the fibu-

lar neck. J Knee Surg. 2013;26(Suppl 1):S132–5. https://doi.org/10.1055/s-0032-1330055.
23. Griffin J, Hogan M, Chhabra A, Deal D. Peripheral nerve repair and reconstruction. J Bone Jt Surg. 2013;95(23):2144–51. https://doi.org/10.2106/JBJS.L.00704.
24. Harris JD, Fazalare JJ, Griesser MJ, Flanigan DC. Infrapatellar branch of saphenous neurectomy for painful neuroma: a case report. Am J Orthop Belle Mead NJ. 2012;41(1):37–40.
25. Henry BM, Tomaszewski KA, Pękala PA, et al. The variable emergence of the infrapatellar branch of the saphenous nerve. J Knee Surg. 2017;30(6):585–93. https://doi.org/10.1055/s-0036-1593870.
26. Henry SL, Hubbard BA, Concannon MJ. Splinting after carpal tunnel release: current practice, scientific evidence, and trends. Plast Reconstr Surg. 2008;122(4):1095–9. https://doi.org/10.1097/PRS.0b013e31818459f4.
27. Hoppenfeld S, deBoer P. The knee. In: Surgical exposures in orthopedics: the anatomic approach. Philadelphia: Lippincott Williams and Wilkins; 2003. p. 494–568.
28. Horlocker TT, Cabanela ME, Wedel DJ. Does postoperative epidural analgesia increase the risk of peroneal nerve palsy after total knee arthroplasty? Anesth Analg. 1994;79(3):495–500. https://doi.org/10.1213/00000539-199409000-00016.
29. Horlocker TT, Cabanela ME, Wedel DJ. Does postoperative epidural analgesia increase the risk of peroneal nerve palsy after total knee arthroplasty? Anesth Analg. 1994;79(3):495–500. https://doi.org/10.1213/00000539-199409000-00016.
30. Hsu JD, Hoffer MM. Posterior tibial tendon transfer anteriorly through the interosseous membrane. Clin Orthop. 1978;131:202-4. https://doi.org/10.1097/00003086-197803000-00031.
31. Huemer GM, Koller M, Pachinger T, Dunst KM, Schwarz B, Hintringer T. Postoperative splinting after open carpal tunnel release does not improve functional and neurological outcome. Muscle Nerve. 2007;36(4):528–31. https://doi.org/10.1002/mus.20839.
32. Hunter LY, Louis DS, Ricciardi JR, O'Connor GA. The saphenous nerve: its course and importance in medial arthrotomy. Am J Sports Med. 1979;7(4):227–30. https://doi.org/10.1177/036354657900700403.
33. Idusuyi OB, Morrey BF. Peroneal nerve palsy after total knee arthroplasty. Assessment of predisposing and prognostic factors. J Bone Joint Surg Am. 1996;78(2):177–84. https://doi.org/10.2106/00004623-199602000-00003.
34. Idusuyi OB, Morrey BF. Peroneal nerve palsy after total knee arthroplasty. Assessment of predisposing and prognostic factors. J Bone Joint Surg Am. 1996;78(2):177–84. https://doi.org/10.2106/00004623-199602000-00003.
35. Insall J, Scott WN, Ranawat CS. The total condylar knee prosthesis. A report of two hundred and twenty cases. J Bone Joint Surg Am. 1979;61(2):173–80.
36. Isaac SM, Okoro T, Danial I, Wildin C. Does wrist immobilization following open carpal tunnel release improve functional outcome? A literature review. Curr Rev Musculoskelet Med. 2010;3(1-4):11–7. https://doi.org/10.1007/s12178-010-9060-9.
37. Ives GC, Kung TA, Nghiem BT, et al. Current state of the surgical treatment of terminal neuromas. Neurosurgery. 2018;83(3):354–64. https://doi.org/10.1093/neuros/nyx500.
38. Johnson DF, Love DT, Love BR, Lester DK. Dermal hypoesthesia after total knee arthroplasty. Am J Orthop Belle Mead NJ. 2000;29(11):863–6.
39. Johnson JE, Paxton ES, Lippe J, et al. Outcomes of the bridle procedure for the treatment of foot drop. Foot Ankle Int. 2015;36(11):1287–96. https://doi.org/10.1177/1071100715593146.
40. Kalthur SG, Sumalatha S, Nair N, Pandey AK, Sequeria S, Shobha L. Anatomic study of infrapatellar branch of saphenous nerve in male cadavers. Ir J Med Sci. 2015;184(1):201–6. https://doi.org/10.1007/s11845-014-1087-2.
41. Kartus J, Ejerhed L, Eriksson BI, Karlsson J. The localization of the infrapatellar nerves in the anterior knee region with special emphasis on central third patellar tendon harvest: a dissection study on cadaver and amputated specimens. Arthrosc J Arthrosc Relat Surg Off Publ Arthrosc Assoc N Am Int Arthrosc Assoc. 1999;15(6):577–86. https://doi.org/10.1053/ar.1999.v15.015057001.
42. Knutson K, Leden I, Sturfelt G, Rosén I, Lidgren L. Nerve palsy after knee arthroplasty in patients with rheumatoid arthritis. Scand J Rheumatol. 1983;12(3):201–5. https://doi.org/10.3109/03009748309098533.
43. Knutson K, Leden I, Sturfelt G, Rosén I, Lidgren L. Nerve palsy after knee arthroplasty in patients with rheumatoid arthritis. Scand J Rheumatol. 1983;12(3):201–5. https://doi.org/10.3109/03009748309098533.
44. Krishnamurthy S, Ibrahim M. Tendon transfers in foot drop. Indian J Plast Surg. 2019;52(1):100–8. https://doi.org/10.1055/s-0039-1688105.
45. Leckenby JI, Furrer C, Haug L, Juon Personeni B, Vögelin E. A retrospective case series reporting the outcomes of avance nerve allografts in the treatment of peripheral nerve injuries. Plast Reconstr Surg. 2020;145(2):368e–81e. https://doi.org/10.1097/PRS.0000000000006485.
46. Lee SR, Dahlgren NJP, Staggers JR, et al. Cadaveric study of the infrapatellar branch of the saphenous nerve: can damage be prevented in total knee arthroplasty? J Clin Orthop Trauma. 2019;10(2):274–7. https://doi.org/10.1016/j.jcot.2018.03.005.
47. Lin MY, Manzano G, Gupta R. Nerve allografts and conduits in peripheral nerve repair. Hand Clin. 2013;29(3):331–48. https://doi.org/10.1016/j.hcl.2013.04.003.
48. Logigian EL, Berger AR, Shahani BT. Injury to the tibial and peroneal nerves due to hemorrhage in the

popliteal fossa. Two case reports. J Bone Joint Surg Am. 1989;71(5):768–70.
49. Logli AL, Bear BJ, Schwartz EG, Korcek KJ, Foster BJ. A prospective, randomized trial of splinting after minicarpal tunnel release. J Hand Surg. 2018;43(8):775.e1–8. https://doi.org/10.1016/j.jhsa.2018.01.016.
50. Lundborg G, Rydevik B. Effects of stretching the tibial nerve of the rabbit. A preliminary study of the intraneural circulation and the barrier function of the perineurium. J Bone Joint Surg Br. 1973;55(2):390–401.
51. Mackinnon SE, Dellon AL. Surgery of the peripheral nerve. New York: Thieme Medical Publishers; 1988.
52. Maroko PR, Kjekshus JK, Sobel BE, et al. Factors influencing infarct size following experimental coronary artery occlusions. Circulation. 1971;43(1):67–82. https://doi.org/10.1161/01.CIR.43.1.67.
53. Mauch JT, Bae A, Shubinets V, Lin IC. A systematic review of sensory outcomes of digital nerve gap reconstruction with autograft, allograft, and conduit. Ann Plast Surg. 2019;82(4S Suppl 3):S247–55. https://doi.org/10.1097/SAP.0000000000001851.
54. Menotti F, Laudani L, Damiani A, Mignogna T, Macaluso A. An anterior ankle-foot orthosis improves walking economy in Charcot-Marie-Tooth type 1A patients. Prosthetics Orthot Int. 2014;38(5):387–92. https://doi.org/10.1177/0309364613506250.
55. Menotti F, Laudani L, Damiani A, Orlando P, Macaluso A. Comparison of walking energy cost between an anterior and a posterior ankle-foot orthosis in people with foot drop. J Rehabil Med. 2014;46(8):768–72. https://doi.org/10.2340/16501977-1837.
56. Mistry D, O'Meeghan C. Fate of the infrapatellar branch of the saphenous nerve post total knee arthroplasty. ANZ J Surg. 2005;75(9):822–4. https://doi.org/10.1111/j.1445-2197.2005.03532.x.
57. Mistry D, O'Meeghan C. Fate of the infrapatellar branch of the saphenous nerve post total knee arthroplasty. ANZ J Surg. 2005;75(9):822–4. https://doi.org/10.1111/j.1445-2197.2005.03532.x.
58. Mochida H, Kikuchi S. Injury to infrapatellar branch of saphenous nerve in arthroscopic knee surgery. Clin Orthop. 1995;320:88–94.
59. Movahedi Yeganeh M. Triple tendon transfer for correction of foot deformity in common peroneal nerve palsy. Foot Ankle Int. 2016;37(6):665–9. https://doi.org/10.1177/1071100716629779.
60. Nagai K, Muratsu H, Matsumoto T, Fujibayashi I, Kuroda R, Kurosaka M. Early-onset severe neuromatous pain of the infrapatellar branch of the saphenous nerve after total knee arthroplasty. Asia-Pac J Sports Med Arthrosc Rehabil Technol. 2014;1(3):102–5. https://doi.org/10.1016/j.asmart.2013.11.002.
61. Nagai K, Muratsu H, Matsumoto T, Fujibayashi I, Kuroda R, Kurosaka M. Early-onset severe neuromatous pain of the infrapatellar branch of the saphenous nerve after total knee arthroplasty. Asia-Pac J Sports Med Arthrosc Rehabil Technol. 2014;1(3):102–5. https://doi.org/10.1016/j.asmart.2013.11.002.
62. Nahabedian MY, Johnson CA. Operative management of neuromatous knee pain: patient selection and outcome. Ann Plast Surg. 2001;46(1):15–22. https://doi.org/10.1097/00000637-200101000-00004.
63. Nercessian OA, Ugwonali OFC, Park S. Peroneal nerve palsy after total knee arthroplasty. J Arthroplast. 2005;20(8):1068–73. https://doi.org/10.1016/j.arth.2005.02.010.
64. Ochoa J, Fowler TJ, Gilliatt RW. Anatomical changes in peripheral nerves compressed by a pneumatic tourniquet. J Anat. 1972;113(Pt 3):433–55.
65. Olivecrona C, Blomfeldt R, Ponzer S, Stanford BR, Nilsson BY. Tourniquet cuff pressure and nerve injury in knee arthroplasty in a bloodless field: a neurophysiological study. Acta Orthop. 2013;84(2):159–64. https://doi.org/10.3109/17453674.2013.782525.
66. Park JH, Restrepo C, Norton R, Mandel S, Sharkey PF, Parvizi J. Common peroneal nerve palsy following total knee arthroplasty: prognostic factors and course of recovery. J Arthroplast. 2013;28(9):1538–42. https://doi.org/10.1016/j.arth.2013.02.025.
67. Park JH, Restrepo C, Norton R, Mandel S, Sharkey PF, Parvizi J. Common peroneal nerve palsy following total knee arthroplasty: prognostic factors and course of recovery. J Arthroplast. 2013;28(9):1538–42. https://doi.org/10.1016/j.arth.2013.02.025.
68. Pedowitz RA, Nordborg C, Rosenqvist AL, Rydevik BL. Nerve function and structure beneath and distal to a pneumatic tourniquet applied to rabbit hindlimbs. Scand J Plast Reconstr Surg Hand Surg. 1991;25(2):109–20. https://doi.org/10.3109/02844319109111270.
69. Pedrini FA, Boriani F, Bolognesi F, Fazio N, Marchetti C, Baldini N. Cell-enhanced acellular nerve allografts for peripheral nerve reconstruction: a systematic review and a meta-analysis of the literature. Neurosurgery. 2019;85(5):575–604. https://doi.org/10.1093/neuros/nyy374.
70. Perry J, Davids JR. Gait analysis: normal and pathological function. J Pediatr Orthop. 1992;12(6):815.
71. Poppler LH, Parikh RP, Bichanich MJ, et al. Surgical interventions for the treatment of painful neuroma: a comparative meta-analysis. Pain. 2018;159(2):214–23. https://doi.org/10.1097/j.pain.0000000000001101.
72. Prasetyono TOH, Permatasari E, Soetrisno E. Implantation of nerve stump inside a vein and a muscle: comparing neuroma formation in rat. Int Surg. 2014;99(6):807–11. https://doi.org/10.9738/INTSURG-D-13-00184.1.
73. Radtka SA, Oliveira GB, Lindstrom KE, Borders MD. The kinematic and kinetic effects of solid, hinged, and no ankle-foot orthoses on stair locomotion in healthy adults. Gait Posture. 2006;24(2):211–8. https://doi.org/10.1016/j.gaitpost.2005.09.005.
74. Ramdharry GM, Day BL, Reilly MM, Marsden JF. Foot drop splints improve proximal as well as distal leg control during gait in Charcot-Marie-tooth

disease. Muscle Nerve. 2012;46(4):512–9. https://doi.org/10.1002/mus.23348.
75. Ray WZ, Mackinnon SE. Management of nerve gaps: autografts, allografts, nerve transfers, and end-to-side neurorrhaphy. Exp Neurol. 2010;223(1):77–85. https://doi.org/10.1016/j.expneurol.2009.03.031.
76. Rebowe R, Rogers A, Yang X, Kundu SC, Smith TL, Li Z. Nerve repair with nerve conduits: problems, solutions, and future directions. J Hand Microsurg. 2018;10(2):61–5. https://doi.org/10.1055/s-0038-1626687.
77. Rodriguez RP. The bridle procedure in the treatment of paralysis of the foot. Foot Ankle. 1992;13(2):63–9. https://doi.org/10.1177/107110079201300203.
78. Rose HA, Hood RW, Otis JC, Ranawat CS, Insall JN. Peroneal-nerve palsy following total knee arthroplasty. A review of the Hospital for Special Surgery experience. J Bone Joint Surg Am. 1982;64(3):347–51.
79. Rose HA, Hood RW, Otis JC, Ranawat CS, Insall JN. Peroneal-nerve palsy following total knee arthroplasty. A review of the Hospital for Special Surgery experience. J Bone Joint Surg Am. 1982;64(3):347–51.
80. Schinsky MF, Macaulay W, Parks ML, Kiernan H, Nercessian OA. Nerve injury after primary total knee arthroplasty. J Arthroplast. 2001;16(8):1048–54. https://doi.org/10.1054/arth.2001.26591.
81. Schinsky MF, Macaulay W, Parks ML, Kiernan H, Nercessian OA. Nerve injury after primary total knee arthroplasty. J Arthroplast. 2001;16(8):1048–54. https://doi.org/10.1054/arth.2001.26591.
82. Seddon HJ, Medawar PB, Smith H. Rate of regeneration of peripheral nerves in man. J Physiol. 1943;102(2):191–215. https://doi.org/10.1113/jphysiol.1943.sp004027.
83. Shalimar A, Nor-Hazla MH, Arifaizad A, Jamari S. Splinting after carpal tunnel release: does it really matter? Malays Orthop J. 2015;9(2):41–6. https://doi.org/10.5704/MOJ.1507.011.
84. Shetty T, Nguyen JT, Sasaki M, et al. Risk factors for acute nerve injury after total knee arthroplasty. Muscle Nerve. 2018;57(6):946–50. https://doi.org/10.1002/mus.26045.
85. Shetty T, Nguyen JT, Sasaki M, et al. Risk factors for acute nerve injury after total knee arthroplasty. Muscle Nerve. 2018;57(6):946–50. https://doi.org/10.1002/mus.26045.
86. Shi S-M, Meister DW, Graner KC, Ninomiya JT. Selective denervation for persistent knee pain after total knee arthroplasty: a report of 50 cases. J Arthroplast. 2017;32(3):968–73. https://doi.org/10.1016/j.arth.2016.09.043.
87. Shin Y-S, Hwang Y-G, Savale AP, Han S-B. Popliteal artery pseudoaneurysm following primary total knee arthroplasty. Knee Surg Relat Res. 2014;26(2):117–20. https://doi.org/10.5792/ksrr.2014.26.2.117.
88. Simonsen EB, Moesby LM, Hansen LD, Comins J, Alkjaer T. Redistribution of joint moments during walking in patients with drop-foot. Clin Biomech. 2010;25(9):949–52. https://doi.org/10.1016/j.clinbiomech.2010.06.013.
89. Speelziek SJA, Staff NP, Johnson RL, Sierra RJ, Laughlin RS. Clinical spectrum of neuropathy after primary total knee arthroplasty: a series of 54 cases. Muscle Nerve. 2019;59(6):679–82. https://doi.org/10.1002/mus.26473.
90. Speelziek SJA, Staff NP, Johnson RL, Sierra RJ, Laughlin RS. Clinical spectrum of neuropathy after primary total knee arthroplasty: a series of 54 cases. Muscle Nerve. 2019;59(6):679–82. https://doi.org/10.1002/mus.26473.
91. Stevens F, Weerkamp NJ, Cals JW. Foot drop. BMJ. 2015;350:h1736. https://doi.org/10.1136/bmj.h1736.
92. Sunderland S. A classification of peripheral nerve injuries producing loss of function. Brain. 1951;74(4):491–516. https://doi.org/10.1093/brain/74.4.491.
93. Tang P, Whiteman DR, Voigt C, Miller MC, Kim H. No difference in outcomes detected between Decellular nerve allograft and cable autograft in rat sciatic nerve defects. J Bone Joint Surg Am. 2019;101(10):e42. https://doi.org/10.2106/JBJS.18.00417.
94. Tennent TD, Birch NC, Holmes MJ, Birch R, Goddard NJ. Knee pain and the infrapatellar branch of the saphenous nerve. J R Soc Med. 1998;91(11):573–5. https://doi.org/10.1177/014107689809101106.
95. Tifford CD, Spero L, Luke T, Plancher KD. The relationship of the infrapatellar branches of the saphenous nerve to arthroscopy portals and incisions for anterior cruciate ligament surgery. An anatomic study. Am J Sports Med. 2000;28(4):562–7. https://doi.org/10.1177/03635465000280042001.
96. Tomaszewski KA, Graves MJ, Henry BM, et al. Surgical anatomy of the sciatic nerve: a meta-analysis. J Orthop Res Off Publ Orthop Res Soc. 2016;34(10):1820–7. https://doi.org/10.1002/jor.23186.
97. Tran TMA, Lim BG, Sheehy R, Robertson PL. Magnetic resonance imaging for common peroneal nerve injury in trauma patients: are routine knee sequences adequate for prediction of outcome? J Med Imaging Radiat Oncol. 2019;63(1):54–60. https://doi.org/10.1111/1754-9485.12840.
98. Trescot AM, Brown MN, Karl HW. Infrapatellar saphenous neuralgia - diagnosis and treatment. Pain Physician. 2013;16(3):E315–24.
99. Tsukada S, Kurosaka K, Nishino M, Hirasawa N. Cutaneous Hypesthesia and kneeling ability after total knee arthroplasty: a randomized controlled trial comparing anterolateral and anteromedial skin incision. J Arthroplast. 2018;33(10):3174–80. https://doi.org/10.1016/j.arth.2018.06.010.
100. Upton AR, McComas AJ. The double crush in nerve entrapment syndromes. Lancet Lond Engl.

1973;2(7825):359–62. https://doi.org/10.1016/s0140-6736(73)93196-6.
101. Varenika V, Lutz AM, Beaulieu CF, Bucknor MD. Detection and prevalence of variant sciatic nerve anatomy in relation to the piriformis muscle on MRI. Skelet Radiol. 2017;46(6):751–7. https://doi.org/10.1007/s00256-017-2597-6.
102. Wainapel SF, Kim DJ, Ebel A. Conduction studies of the saphenous nerve in healthy subjects. Arch Phys Med Rehabil. 1978;59(7):316–9.
103. Watanabe M, Yamaga M, Kato T, Ide J, Kitamura T, Takagi K. The implication of repeated versus continuous strain on nerve function in a rat forelimb model. J Hand Surg. 2001;26(4):663–9. https://doi.org/10.1053/jhsu.2001.24142.
104. Webster DA, Murray DG. Complications of variable Axis total knee arthroplasty. Clin Orthop. 1985;193:160–7.
105. Weingarden SI, Louis DL, Waylonis GW. Electromyographic changes in postmeniscectomy patients. Role of the pneumatic tourniquet. JAMA. 1979;241(12):1248–50.
106. van der Wilk D, Dijkstra PU, Postema K, Verkerke GJ, Hijmans JM. Effects of ankle foot orthoses on body functions and activities in people with floppy paretic ankle muscles: a systematic review. Clin Biomech. 2015;30(10):1009–25. https://doi.org/10.1016/j.clinbiomech.2015.09.013.
107. Wiszomirska I, Blazkiewicz M, Kaczmarczyk K, Brzuszkiewicz-Kuzmicka G, Wit A. Effect of drop foot on spatiotemporal, kinematic, and kinetic parameters during gait. Appl Bionics Biomech. 2017;2017:3595461. https://doi.org/10.1155/2017/3595461.
108. Wolvetang NHA, Lans J, Verhiel SHWL, Notermans BJW, Chen NC, Eberlin KR. Surgery for symptomatic neuroma: anatomic distribution and predictors of secondary surgery. Plast Reconstr Surg. 2019;143(6):1762–71. https://doi.org/10.1097/PRS.0000000000005664.
109. Woodmass JM, Romatowski NP, Esposito JG, Mohtadi NG, Longino PD. A systematic review of peroneal nerve palsy and recovery following traumatic knee dislocation. Knee Surg Sports Traumatol Arthrosc. 2015;23(10):2992–3002. https://doi.org/10.1007/s00167-015-3676-7.
110. Xiang Y, Li Z, Yu P, Zheng Z, Feng B, Weng X. Neuroma of the infrapatellar branch of the saphenous nerve following total knee arthroplasty: a case report. BMC Musculoskelet Disord. 2019;20(1):536. https://doi.org/10.1186/s12891-019-2934-0.
111. Yarbrough C, Godzik J, Filler A, Ray W. Nerve injuries of the lower extremity. In: Winn R, editor. Youmans and Winn neurological surgery. 7th ed. Elsevier; 2017. p. 2089–102. https://www--clinicalkey-com.ezproxy.lib.utexas.edu:2444/#!/content/book/3-s2.0-B9780323287821002574?scrollTo=%23top. Accessed January 16, 2020.
112. Zhong G, Liang Z, Kan J, Muheremu A. Selective peripheral nerve resection for treatment of persistent pain around the knee joint after total knee arthroplasty. J Int Med Res. 2018;46(6):2301–6. https://doi.org/10.1177/0300060518764184.

15 Nerve Injury After Knee Arthroscopy, ACL Reconstruction, Multiligament Knee, and Open Knee Surgery

J. Ryan Hill, John M. Apostolakos, Christopher J. Dy, and Moira M. McCarthy

15.1 Introduction

Traction injury of the common peroneal nerve is a devastating, well-described issue following multiligamentous knee injury. Additionally, other injuries to the common peroneal nerve, tibial nerve, and saphenous nerve may occur due to a variety of traumatic causes, including fractures of the proximal tibia, sharp penetrating injury, gunshot injury, or direct impact.

The overall complication rates after knee arthroscopy, ligament reconstruction, and other sports medicine procedures are relatively low. Iatrogenic injury to the nervous structures about the knee is possible if care is not taken with surgical approaches and technique. Injuries to the saphenous nerve and peroneal nerve in particular have been described in association with routine arthroscopic procedures, meniscal repair, ligamentous reconstructions, high tibial osteotomies, and total knee arthroplasty.

J. R. Hill
Department of Orthopedic Surgery, Washington University School of Medicine, St. Louis, MO, USA
e-mail: hillryan@wustl.edu

J. M. Apostolakos · M. M. McCarthy
Department of Orthopaedic Surgery, Hospital for Special Surgery, New York, NY, USA
e-mail: apostolakosj@hss.edu; mccarthymo@hss.edu

C. J. Dy (✉)
Department of Orthopedic Surgery, Washington University, St. Louis, MO, USA
e-mail: dyc@wustl.edu

Understanding the injury mechanisms, diagnosis, and management of these injuries begins with a detailed familiarity with the neural anatomy about the knee. Prompt identification of nerve injury is important and requires a discerning sports medicine practitioner to maintain a high index of suspicion in the appropriate situations. Awareness of structures at risk when performing surgical procedures about the knee reduces incidence of iatrogenic injury. Appropriate management of nerve injury is determined by a variety of factors, including the nerve involved, nature of the injury, concomitant bony or soft tissue injuries, and timing of presentation.

15.2 Neural Anatomy of the Distal Thigh, Knee, and Proximal Leg

15.2.1 Detailed Neural Anatomy

15.2.1.1 Peroneal Nerve

The common peroneal nerve (CPN) is formed from posterior divisions of the anterior rami of the L4-S2 spinal nerves [1]. It has a mean diameter of 3.8–4.6 mm [2, 3] along its course through the distal thigh and proximal leg. Distal to the knee, the CPN divides into three terminal branches: the anterior tibial recurrent nerve (ATRN), the deep peroneal nerve (DPN), and the superficial peroneal nerve (SPN). The CPN gives off additional

C. J. Dy et al. (eds.), *Peripheral Nerve Issues after Orthopedic Surgery*,
https://doi.org/10.1007/978-3-030-84428-8_15

sensory fibers via the lateral sural cutaneous nerve, which join with fibers from the tibial nerve to form the sural nerve in the distal leg. Distinct DPN and SPN fibers can be identified along the entire length of the nerve, even proximal to the sciatic bifurcation [3]. The fascicular anatomy is arranged such that the compound nerve fascicles of the DPN lie adjacent and immediately lateral to those of the SPN, with sural sensory fibers located at the periphery (Fig. 15.1). At the level of the popliteal fossa, motor fibers to the tibialis anterior are located at the most anteromedial portion of the CPN [4].

The vascular supply to the CPN is robust in the proximal half of the popliteal fossa, arising directly from the popliteal artery. However, at the level of the knee joint and near the fibular neck, asymmetric branching of vasa nervorum arising from anastomoses with the anterior tibial recurrent artery leads to a tenuous blood supply along a large segment of the CPN, averaging 11.6 cm in length [5].

The CPN traverses the posterior compartment of the thigh in a common perineural sheath with fibers of the tibial nerve, together comprising the sciatic nerve [6, 7]. While rare variants demonstrate bifurcation of these two distinct components in the pelvis, the CPN typically separates from the tibial nerve 50–80 mm proximal to the popliteal fossa, with a reported mean pooled distance of 65.4 mm [6–9]. Within the thigh, the CPN provides a motor branch to the short head of the biceps. This branch can aid in distinguishing between CPN and sciatic nerve injuries.

The nerve travels obliquely along the superolateral margin of the popliteal fossa, between the tendon of biceps femoris and the lateral head of the gastrocnemius [2, 10]. The CPN then exits the fossa by passing over the lateral head of the gastrocnemius, emerging superficially 20–60 mm from the apex of the fibular head [11, 12]. The CPN gives off the lateral sural cutaneous nerve, which itself branches to provide cutaneous sensation to the lateral leg via the lateral cutaneous nerve of the calf and sural communicating branches [13]. As it courses from posterior to anterior across the lateral aspect of the knee, the CPN gives off small articular branches which innervate the lateral knee capsule. The posterior branch travels lateral to the popliteal vein and terminates in the superolateral posterior capsule at the level of the lateral femoral condyle [14]. The anterior branches accompany the superior and inferior retinacular arteries, terminating in the anterolateral capsule [2, 15].

At the lateral aspect of the knee joint, the CPN is within 2 cm of the posterolateral tibia and posterolateral joint capsule [16, 17] and moves closer

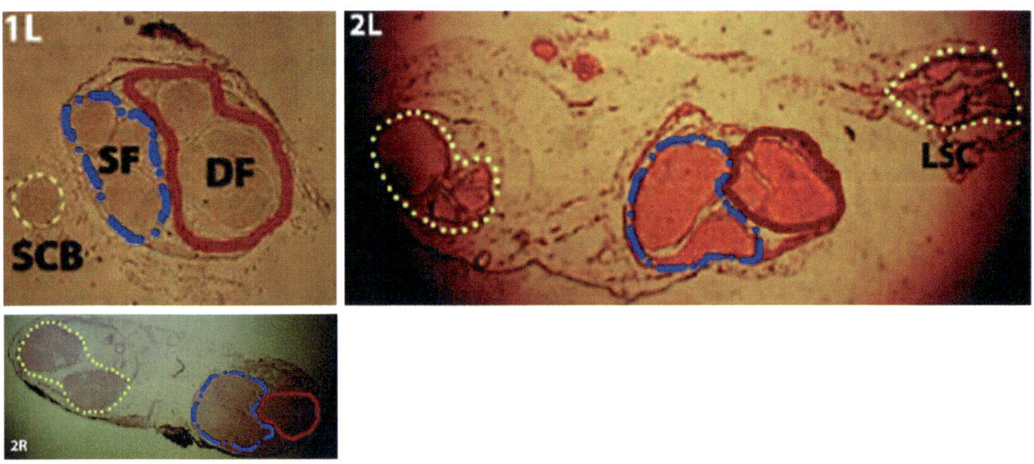

Fig. 15.1 Representative cross sections of human common peroneal nerves. Anterior is oriented at the top of the image and lateral is to the right. Dotted yellow outlines indicate the sural communicating branch (SCB) and lateral sural cutaneous (LSC) nerves. Solid red lines indicate deep peroneal nerve (DF) fibers. Dot-dash blue lines indicate superficial peroneal nerve (SF) fibers. Adapted from Gustafson et al. [3]

to these structures with the knee in full extension. Higher degrees of flexion bring the nerve further from the joint capsule and closer to the fibular head [12].

At its emergence from the deep fascia, the CPN is angled 10–32° anterior to the fibular axis [11, 18]. The CPN crosses the posterior border of the fibula on average 24.5 mm posterior and distal to the insertion of the fibular collateral ligament on the anterior fibular head [19]. At the level of the fibular neck, 22–42 mm distal to the fibular apex, the CPN passes between the two heads of the peroneus longus muscle through the fibular tunnel, the boundaries of which include the fibular neck (floor), and a musculoaponeurotic arch comprised of fibrous bands from the soleus and peroneus longus [10, 18–21]. The latter is also referred to as the posterior crural septum and is a commonly recognized point of compression of the common peroneal nerve. Within or just distal to the fibular tunnel, the CPN divides into its three terminal branches – the anterior tibial recurrent nerve (ATRN), deep peroneal nerve (DPN), and superficial peroneal nerve (SPN) (Fig. 15.2) [10]. In the vast majority of patients, this division occurs 22–47 mm distal to the fibular apex [11, 18, 20, 22, 23] and 42–52 mm from Gerdy's tubercle [11]. However, the branch point may be located proximal to the fibular neck, or even proximal to the knee joint in a subset of patients [24].

The ATRN is the most proximally oriented terminal branch, curving medially and proximally toward the knee joint approximately 4–5 cm distal to Gerdy's tubercle (Fig. 15.2) [11]. In some patients, it may branch from the DPN instead of the CPN [10]. It courses with the anterior recurrent tibial artery and terminates in the proximal muscle belly of tibialis anterior [2, 10].

The DPN travels distally and medially at an angle of 20–27° to the fibular axis in the coronal plane (Fig. 15.2). It enters the anterior compartment, passing deep to the proximal muscle belly of extensor digitorum longus, and continuing distally along the anterior aspect of the interosseous membrane [23]. The DPN provides motor innervation to the tibialis anterior, extensor hallucis longus and brevis, extensor digitorum longus and brevis, peroneus tertius as well as sensation to the first dorsal webspace of the foot.

The SPN enters the lateral compartment and courses directly distal, either immediately deep to the investing fascia or within the peroneus longus muscle belly (Fig. 15.2) [25]. It then pierces the deep fascia of the leg, becoming superficial at variable distances above the ankle and with several described superficial branching patterns [18]. The SPN provides motor innervation to the peroneus longus and peroneus brevis muscles as well as sensation to the anterolateral leg and dorsum of the foot. There are typically multiple branches from the SPN to the peroneus longus

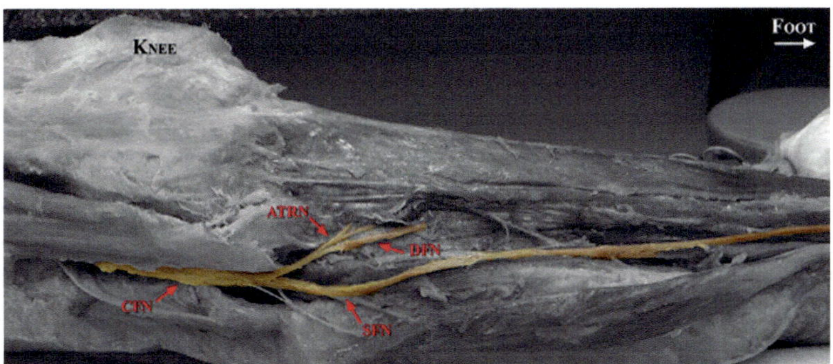

Fig. 15.2 Cadaveric dissection of the common peroneal nerve (CFN), anterior tibial recurrent nerve (ATRN), superficial peroneal nerve (SFN), and deep peroneal nerve (DFN). View is of the lateral aspect of the limb, with proximal oriented to the left of the image and distal to the right. (Adapted from Watt et al. [10] and reprinted with permission)

and brevis muscles. The area of highest density is located 7–13 cm distal to the head of the fibula, primarily comprised of branches to the peroneus longus. Branches to the peroneus brevis arise just distal to those of peroneus longus [26].

15.2.1.2 Saphenous Nerve

The saphenous nerve is composed of sensory fibers from the L3 and L4 spinal cord levels, providing sensory innervation to the medial aspect of the knee, leg, and foot [1, 27]. It arises from the medial aspect of the femoral nerve within the femoral triangle, approximately 6.5–9.3 cm distal to the inguinal crease [27]. The nerve then courses distally and posteromedially with the femoral vessels and the nerve of the vastus medialis to enter the adductor canal near the mid-thigh, on average 25 cm from the anterior superior iliac spine [28]. The adductor canal is approximately 10.5 cm in length [28], and terminates at the adductor hiatus, located 7–9.5 cm proximal to the base of the patella [27, 28]. Within the canal, the nerve travels from lateral to medial, crossing the vessels anteriorly [27]. In most cases, the nerve separates into its terminal branches – the infrapatellar branch and the sartorial branch – near the distal extent of the canal; however, the branch point may also occur after the main trunk exits the canal [29]. The terminal branches exit the adductor canal with the saphenous branch of the inferior geniculate artery, 7.4–14.1 cm proximal to the medial epicondyle of the femur [30, 31], and can be localized by dissecting within 5.6 cm distally from a consistent vascular leash formed by the artery [30].

The sartorial branch of the saphenous nerve provides sensation to the medial leg, ankle, and foot (Fig. 15.3) [30]. After the bifurcation, it continues on a vertical trajectory, passing superficial to the gracilis muscle belly approximately 12.6 mm from the musculotendinous junction and 11.8 cm from the distal insertion. It subsequently courses along the posteromedial aspect of the tendon, piercing the sartorial fascia 6.4–9.3 cm from the distal gracilis insertion [33, 34] and anywhere from 3.7 cm proximal to 3 cm distal to the knee joint line [30]. At its emergence superficially, the nerve lies at an average distance of 3.3 cm from the center point of the medial epicondyle of the femur [35]. In the majority of patients, the nerve travels deep to the sartorius fascia, deep or just posterior to the sartorius tendon, and superficial to the gracilis and semitendinosus at the level of the joint line [31]. The trajectory of the nerve then takes a slightly anterior curve, approximately 4.8 cm posterior to the anterior border of the superficial medial collateral ligament at 2 cm distal to the joint line, and 3.8 cm posterior to the ligament at its distal insertion on the proximal tibia, located 6 cm distal to the knee joint line [32]. Along its course through the posteromedial aspect of the limb, it is intimately associated with the great saphenous vein. Proximally, a fat stripe separates the two structures. Distally in the leg, however, they may be adherent to one another [27]. At the level of the proximal tibia, the sartorial branch can be found 5.3–9 cm posteromedial from the tibial tubercle [27].

The infrapatellar branch of the saphenous nerve provides sensation to the anterior knee, anterolateral proximal leg, anteroinferior knee capsule (Fig. 15.3) [36]. The path of the infrapatellar branch is highly variable. After separating from the main trunk of the saphenous nerve 7.4–14.1 cm proximal to the medial epicondyle of the femur [30, 31], it may pass anterior or posterior to the sartorius muscle belly, through the muscle belly, or through the sartorius tendon [27, 36–39]. It becomes subcutaneous near the posterior aspect of the medial femoral condyle, approximately 6.5–9 cm from the medial border of the superior pole of the patella [39, 40] and 4.5–5.6 cm from the medial border of the patellar tendon at the apex of the patella [36]. It splays into three to six branches, which curve laterally on the sartorius fascia, reaching or crossing the midline between the apex of the patella and the tibial tubercle in the vast majority of cases [33, 36, 39–41]. The course of these branches encompasses the entirety of the medial aspect of the knee and proximal tibia, and with specific locations highly variable [41]. Several "low risk" zones have been identified as containing a relatively low density of infrapatellar branches [41]. Medially, the infrapatellar neve takes a nearly vertical course, which transitions to nearly 45°

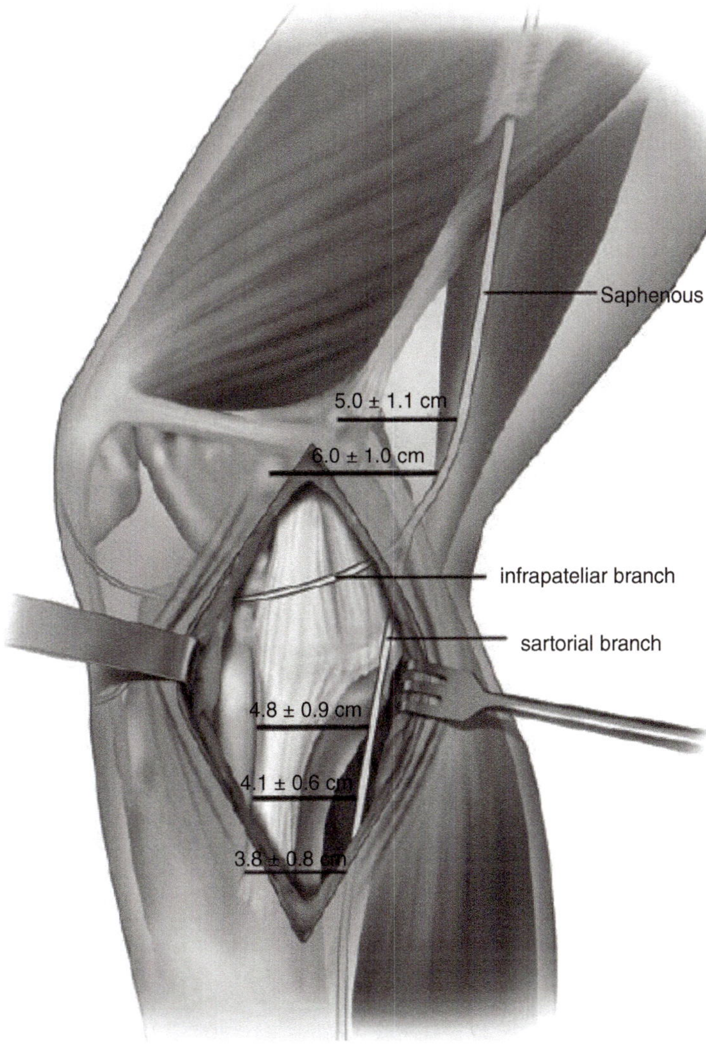

Fig. 15.3 Course of the saphenous nerve and its terminal branches – the infrapatellar and sartorial nerves. Distances represented as (mean ± SD). (Adapted from Wijdicks et al. [32] and reprinted with permission)

distal-lateral over the anteromedial knee, becoming nearly horizontal at the midline [41]. These branches communicate with terminal branches from the medial femoral cutaneous nerve to form the infrapatellar subsartorial plexus [36].

15.2.1.3 Tibial Nerve

The tibial nerve is derived from the anterior divisions of the anterior rami of spinal nerves from L4 to S3 [1]. Distal to the bifurcation of the sciatic nerve, the tibial nerve takes a vertical midline course through the popliteal fossa and deep compartment of the leg, traveling posterior to the medial malleolus to enter the plantar foot, where it gives off its terminal branches – the medial and lateral plantar nerves. It provides motor innervation to the entire posterior compartment of the leg and the entire plantar compartment of the foot, as well as sensation to the posterior aspect of the leg, posterior knee capsule, and plantar aspect of the foot. The fascicular anatomy is not as reproducible as that of the CPN; however, fascicles to the gastrocnemius and soleus as well as to the medial sural cutaneous nerve are consistently located in the posterolateral quadrant of the nerve (Fig. 15.4) [3].

Unlike the CPN, the tibial nerve has a consistent and robust vascular supply throughout its course, receiving symmetric vasa nervorum

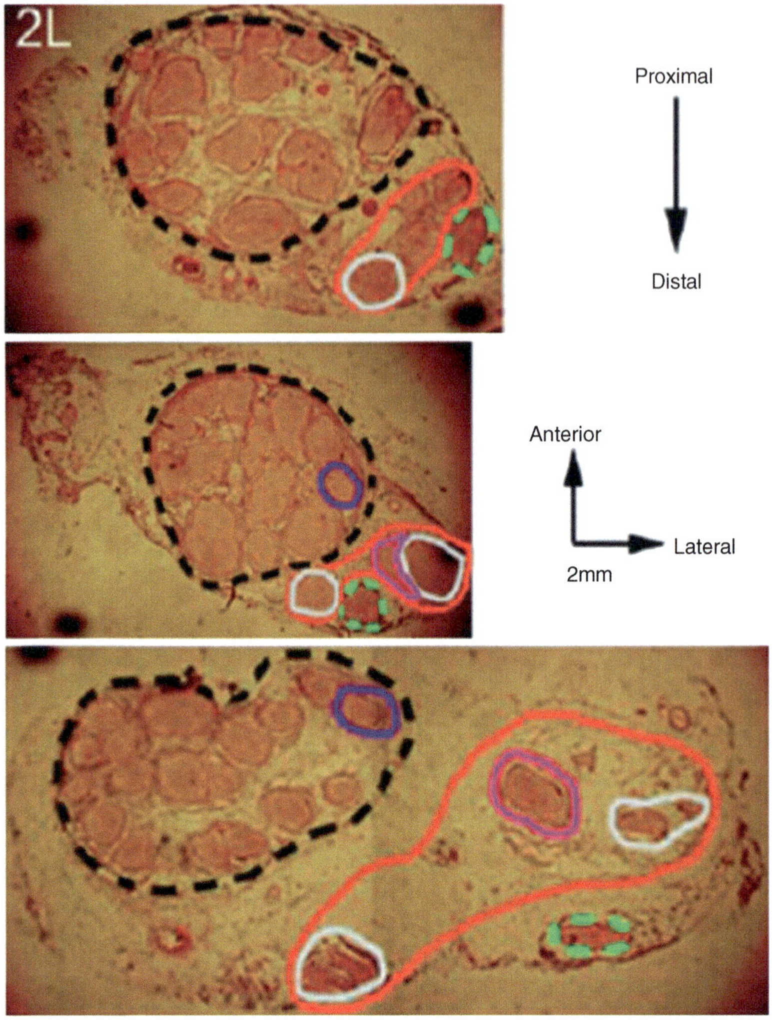

Fig. 15.4 Fascicular organization of the tibial nerve. Three sequential sections from the tibial nerve of a single specimen are displayed from proximal (top) to distal (bottom). Each individual image is oriented such that anterior is to the top and lateral is to the right. Sections were taken from a 6.5-cm segment of nerve distal to the sciatic bifurcation and proximal to the knee joint. Fascicles to the gastrocnemius and soleus muscles, as well as the medial sural cutaneous nerve are outlined with the solid orange line. Other fascicles are outlined by the dashed black line. (Adapted from Gustafson et al. [3])

branches from both the popliteal and posterior tibial arteries at 4 cm intervals [5].

The tibial nerve and the common peroneal nerve (CPN) traverse the posterior compartment of the thigh in a common perineural sheath, together comprising the sciatic nerve [6, 7]. While rare variants demonstrate bifurcation of these two distinct components in the pelvis, the CPN typically will separate from the tibial nerve 50–80 mm proximal to the popliteal fossa, with a reported mean pooled distance of 65.4 mm [6–9]. The tibial nerve continues distally in a vertical path, emerging in the popliteal fossa between the distal semitendinosus and biceps femoris muscle bellies and continuing distally to bisect the fossa along with the popliteal artery and vein [1]. While the nerve is the most superficial structure of the popliteal neurovascular bundle, it lies in a fairly deep position, providing protection from external blunt and penetrating trauma [1]. Within this region, nerve is surrounded by the interstitial adipose tissue that fills the popliteal fossa [1]. The location of the tibial nerve in this anatomic space varies with changes in position of the knee joint – flexion draws the neurovascular bundle away from the posterior knee structures in a posterolateral direction [42]. At 1 cm proximal to the joint line, the nerve can be found an average of 10.3 mm posterior to the distal aspect of the femoral condyles with the knee in extension and 26.2 mm in 90° of flexion. At the joint line, the nerve is located 13.1 and 21.5 mm from the posterior tibial cortex and 15.1 and 29.4 mm from the posterolateral border of the posterior cruciate ligament in extension and flexion, respectively [42]. At 1 cm distal to the joint line, the nerve is 8.7 and 16.6 mm from the posterior cortex in extension and flexion, respectively [42]. At the level of the fibular neck, the tibial nerve is typically 3.3–5.5 cm from the deep peroneal nerve [8].

In its course through the popliteal fossa, the tibial nerve gives off several motor and sensory branches, with many described branching patterns [43]. The most proximal branch is the medial sural cutaneous nerve, which originates on average 2.5 mm proximal to the superior aspect of the femoral condyles [43]. This branch takes a highly variable course to join either the peroneal communicating branch or lateral sural cutaneous branch of the CPN, forming the sural nerve in the leg [1]. The nerves to the medial and lateral heads of the gastrocnemius follow, branching at an average of 5.7 and 14 mm distal to the superior aspect of the femoral condyles, respectively [43]. The first muscular branch point is typically located 2–3.3 cm directly medial from the common peroneal nerve and 8.9–10.1 cm proximo-medial from the bifurcation of the common peroneal nerve at the fibular neck [8, 44]. These branches are typically 1.5–2 mm in diameter and can be neurolysed 5.5–10.9 cm proximal to the popliteal crease [45]. Further distally, the nerve gives off two branches to the soleus muscle, arising an average of 2.2 and 3.3 cm distal to the superior aspect of the femoral condyles. The proximal branch takes a superficial course, while the distal branch is located deep to the soleus muscle belly [43]. Within the popliteal fossa, the tibial nerve also gives off small motor branches to the plantaris and popliteus muscles. In addition, the nerve provides one to five posterior articular branches that emanate from the main trunk 10–25 cm proximal to the joint line [46], traveling to innervate the posterior capsule and contribute to the popliteal plexus [46]. As it exits the popliteal fossa, the nerve travels between the heads of the gastrocnemius, lying deep to the plantaris and superficial to the popliteus before coursing beneath the tendinous arch of the soleus to enter the posterior compartment of the leg [1].

15.2.1.4 Sural Nerve

The sural nerve is composed of fibers originating from the S1 and S2 spinal levels. It is formed in the leg by a confluence of sensory fibers from the tibial and common peroneal nerves. In 51.5% of patients, the medial sural cutaneous nerve (MSCN) from the tibial nerve joins the peroneal communicating nerve from the CPN, and in 13.8% of patients it joins the lateral sural cutaneous nerve from the CPN [47]. The junction typically occurs in the distal half to one-third of the leg, 9.0–20.4 cm proximal to the lateral malleolus [47–49]. In 31.2% of patients, no junction occurs, and the branches from the tibial nerve and CPN travel independently. Other uncommon branching patterns, including the sural nerve arising directly from the peroneal communicating nerve, lateral sural cutaneous nerve, or sciatic nerve, are present in 3.6% of patients [47]. When formed, the nerve has a mean diameter of 0.28 cm and courses in the distal posterolateral leg with the small saphenous vein along its medial border [47, 48]. It crosses the lateral border of the Achilles tendon 8–10 cm proximal to the calcaneal tuberosity in approximately 50% of patients [48, 50, 51]. The nerve then passes 1–2 cm posterior to the lateral malleolus in nearly all patients, finally terminating in the lateral aspect of the foot [50, 51]. Regardless of the branching pattern, this group of nerves provides cutaneous innervation to the posterolateral aspect of the leg and the lateral border of the foot, and in 6.2% of patients may also provide motor innervation to the intrinsic muscles of the foot [52].

15.2.2 Surgical Anatomy for the Sports Medicine Surgeon

15.2.2.1 Considerations During Arthroscopy

During standard arthroscopic portal placement in the knee, the anterolateral portal is created in the recess palpated by the surgeon between the lateral joint line and the lateral edge of the patellar tendon in the "soft-spot" [53, 54]. A stab incision is then made within this "soft-spot" to enter the joint. Similarly, during placement of the anteromedial portal the surgeon palpates a soft-spot between the medial joint line and the medial edge of the patella tendon aging making a stab incision into the joint [53]. While terminal portions of the infrapatellar branch of the saphenous nerve are in proximity, there are no other major neurovascular structures at risk during anteromedial portal placement.

Additional superolateral and superomedial portals can also be placed based on preference. Placement of these portals are made at the intersection of a line drawn transversely across the superior pole of the patella and a vertical line made along the medial or lateral aspect of the patella for superomedial and superolateral portals, respectively [54]. The risks for these portals are more related to soft tissue injury and chondral injury as opposed to neurological injury [54]. Each of these portals risks injury to the quadriceps insertion, and, more specifically, the superomedial portal risks injury to the vastus medialis oblique muscle, while the superolateral portal has a high risk of chondral injury based on the proximal extension of the lateral chondral surfaces [54]. These portal placements are considered safe from a neurological perspective.

Most concerning to the surgeon are accessory portals which can be made posteriorly. These portals may be beneficial for synovectomies, removal of loose bodies, or during posterior cruciate ligament reconstructions [54]. The posteromedial portal can be established along the posteromedial joint line, just posterior to the medial femoral condyle. With the arthroscope aimed between the PCL and medial femoral condyle through an anterior portal for direct visualization, a spinal needle is placed posteromedially to localize correct placement of the portal [54]. Once verification of placement under direct visualization is confirmed, skin incision can be made and blunt dissection is performed with special care to avoid iatrogenic injury to the saphenous nerve and vein [54]. During establishment of the posterolateral portal, again the placement is made under direct visualization. For this portal, the scope is placed between the anterior cruciate ligament and the medial femoral condyle. A spinal needle is placed along the posterolateral joint line just posterior to the lateral femoral condyle and is directly visualized to be posterior to the lateral collateral ligament and anterior to the biceps femoris [54]. As discussed in the previous anatomical description of the posterolateral knee, the common peroneal nerve travels posterior to the biceps femoris and therefore ensuring placement of this portal anterior to the biceps protects the CPN.

15.2.2.2 Considerations During Open Surgery

Medial Incisions

The medial parapatellar approach to the knee is an extensive incision to allow access to the suprapatellar pouch, patella, and the medial knee joint. This approach is commonly used for procedures including total knee arthroplasty, synovectomy, medial menisectomy, removal of loose bodies, ligamentous reconstructions, drainage of the knee joint, and open reduction and internal fixation of the distal femur [53]. Following a midline skin incision extending from the superior aspect of the patella to the medial aspect of the tibial tubercle, the superficial surgical dissection courses through the quadriceps tendon, the medial border of the patella, and the border of the patellar tendon extending through the underling joint capsule, finally gaining entry into the joint [53]. During this approach, the infrapatellar branch of the saphenous nerve is at risk and is often sacrificed during exposure [53]. While the frequency of painful neuromas of the infrapatellar branch is unknown, it is believed to be of minimal impact in the vast majority of patients.

An additional, however less commonly used, open approach is the anteromedial incision used for medial menisectomy, partial menisectomy, removal of loose bodies, and treatment of medial-sided OCD lesions [53]. The incision is made by identifying the inferomedial corner of the patella and angling inferiorly and posteriorly ending around 1 cm inferior to the joint line, as extending the incision most distally places the inferomedial branch of the saphenous nerve at risk [53]. The surgical incision is then carried deeper, through the anteromedial capsule, in order to gain entry into the medial aspect of the joint.

A direct medial approach to the knee joint can also be utilized to visualize the medial collateral ligament (MCL) and gain access to the medial joint [53]. The skin incision is made 2 cm proximal to the adductor tubercle of the distal femur and is extended anteroinferiorly along the medial aspect of the knee to roughly 6 cm distal to the medial joint line ending at the anteromedial aspect of the tibia [53]. During superficial dissection, the infrapatellar branch of the saphenous nerve will cross the operative field and is at risk for injury. The sartorial branch of the saphenous nerve, however, should be protected and preserved as it courses from between the gracilis and sartorius muscles [53].

Lateral/Posterolateral Incisions

The open lateral approach to the knee is less commonly utilized; however, it provides access to the lateral-sided ligamentous structures as well as intra-articular access. The skin incision begins proximally in line with the femur and extends distally roughly 3 cm lateral to the mid-portion of the patella further extending 4–5 cm distally aimed over Gerdy's tubercle [53]. This approach utilizes an internervous plane between the iliotibial band (an extension of muscular origins of the gluteus maximus and tensor fascia latae, supplied by the inferior gluteal and superior gluteal nerves, respectively) and the biceps femoris (sciatic nerve) [53]. The superficial dissection is carried down between the IT band and the biceps femoris. The CPN is posterior to the biceps femoris tendon and is protected by retracting the biceps posteriorly. Identification of the CPN in the proximal aspect of the approach can minimize risk of iatrogenic injury.

Posterior Incisions

The posterior approach to the knee is commonly used for repair of neurovascular structures, repair of posterior cruciate ligament avulsion fractures, recession of the gastrocnemius muscle heads, and excision of cysts in the back of the knee [53]. A curved skin incision is made beginning proximally over the lateral aspect of the biceps femoris, coursing obliquely across the popliteal fossa, and extending distally over the medial head of the gastrocnemius [53]. As the subcutaneous dissection is performed, the medial sural cutaneous nerve (a small branch of the tibial nerve) can be visualized just lateral to the small saphenous vein [53]. As this superficial dissection is continued through the fascia of the popliteal fossa, the medial sural nerve is traced proximally back to the tibial nerve [53]. In the proximal aspect of the approach, the apex of the popliteal fossa is developed between the semi-membranosus muscle medially and the biceps femoris laterally. This is an important landmark, as the sciatic nerve bifurcates into the common peroneal nerve and tibial nerve at this level [53]. The CPN can then be carefully dissected out by the surgeon from proximal to distal along the posterior border of the biceps femoris. At this time, the surgeon performs a careful dissection of the popliteal vascular structures to safely gain access to the posterior knee capsule, the posterolateral corner, and several muscular attachments.

15.3 Prevention Strategies

15.3.1 General Arthroscopic Considerations

- Establish portals under direct visualization, when possible, utilizing a spinal needle.
- After incising skin, proceed next with blunt dissection to minimize trauma to terminal cutaneous nerve branches.
- Consider moving the arthroscope and instrumentation to alternative portals prior to establishing new portals in an attempt to improve visualization and decrease the number of portals created.
  - An additional tool to consider would be a 70-degree scope which can improve visualization especially to the posteromedial and posterolateral compartments.

15.3.2 Meniscal Repair

15.3.2.1 Inside-Out

- The inside-out technique as described by Henning and others [55–57] combines arthroscopic suture management and open tensioning/knot tying [54]. This technique requires the use of accessory portals made posteromedially or posterolaterally based on the side of injury in order to retrieve the repair needles and accompanying sutures during repair. As described previously in this chapter, these posterior-placed portals risk injury to the CPN on the lateral side and saphenous nerve on the medial side. A popliteal tissue retractor (or spoon) can be placed in the posterior accessory portal to protect from iatrogenic injury during needle placement.
- Transillumination – using the light from the scope directed to the medial aspect of the knee, the surgeon can attempt to visualize the saphenous nerve by transilluminating the skin leaving a dark streak which reveals the saphenous nerve.
- Flexing the knee to 90 degrees moves the saphenous nerve posteriorly.

15.3.2.2 Outside-In

The outside in technique, as described by Rodeo et al. [58] is used most commonly in tears of the middle to anterior third of the meniscus [54]. A spinal needle is placed percutaneously from outside the joint to inside, through the meniscus. For anterior tears of the medial meniscus, there is potential risk to the infrapatellar branch of the saphenous nerve during spinal needle placement. Attempting the outside-in approach for a posterior tear, however, does place a significant risk to the CPN laterally and the saphenous medially. Palpating the biceps tendon and staying anterior to it will protect the CPN laterally, while flexing the knee will move the saphenous nerve posteriorly.

15.3.3 Anterior Cruciate Ligament Reconstruction

An additional risk for nerve injury exists during hamstring graft harvesting during ACL reconstructions. There is risk for iatrogenic injury to the saphenous nerve during hamstring autograft harvest [56, 57]. Damage to this structure can lead to hypoesthesia, dysaesthesia, and painful neuroma formation [56, 58]. Both infrapatellar and sartorial branches of the saphenous nerve are at risk. From an anatomical perspective, the two branches most at risk are the sartorial terminal branch and the infrapatellar branch [56]. The saphenous nerve branches into these two structures as it exits the adductor canal with the sartorial terminal branch traveling down the medial knee behind the sartorius before piercing between the fascia layers of the sartorius and gracilis tendons [56]. The infrapatellar branch travels more anteriorly and supplies sensation over the anterior knee.

The infrapatellar branch is at risk during the initial surgical approach for the hamstring harvest, as it takes an oblique course through the operative field [56]. Identification and protection of the infrapatellar branch can minimize the risk of injury. Injury to the infrapatellar branch can lead to anterior knee discomfort especially when kneeling and painful sensitivity over the anteromedial knee [56]. Iatrogenic damage to the sartorial branch of the saphenous nerve is believed to occur during passage of the tendon stripper at the time of graft harvest [56]. Injury to branches of the saphenous nerve is best avoided by utilizing an incision through the level of the skin only. This is followed by careful blunt dissection of the subcutaneous tissue down to the sartorial fascia [59].

15.4 Initial Evaluation and Physical Exam

15.4.1 Timing

Nerve injuries can present in both the pre- and/or postoperative periods. Traumatic knee injuries including dislocation and fibular head fracture may present with neurological deficit, especially to the CPN. In the immediate postoperative period, the surgeon should examine the causes of nerve injury including direct injury (cut), traction injury, or implant-related injury (e.g., suture from meniscal repair incorporating CPN) [54]. If there is reason to believe injury may be related to implant/suture, an immediate surgical evaluation should be initiated. Timely referral is particularly important for motor and mixed motor-sensory nerves, given the risk of irreversible denervation-related atrophy. However, referral for evaluation of sensory nerve injury should not be delayed given the often debilitating nature of neuropathic pain.

15.4.2 History and Physical Exam

A thorough history into timing and quality of any perceived deficit is critical. Patients may complain of a wide variety of clinical symptoms including burning, electric, sharp, or dull/achy pain. The discomfort may present acutely at the time of injury or may be perceived as intermittent or positional. These symptoms may also be perceived in isolation or in combination with a motor deficit.

Physical examination of patients with suspected peripheral nerve injuries should be as systematic as possible. Grading of muscle strength is subject to high intra- and inter-rater reliability, even when using standard scales. Sensation is assessed with a combination of light touch, temperature, pin prick, and vibratory sensation. For both motor and sensory testing, comparison to the contralateral side (provided it is uninjured) is essential to discern subtle grades of injury. Assessment of Tinel sign by percussing over the presumably injured nerve is important to delineate the advancing/regenerative front of nerve regeneration. Furthermore, it is important to examine for potential contributions from the lumbosacral spine.

15.5 Diagnostic Tests and Imaging

15.5.1 Imaging

15.5.1.1 Radiographs

Routine workup for pain about the knee should always include plain radiographs. This allows for basic evaluation of nonconcentric joint reduction, abnormalities in limb alignment, fractures, or bony avulsions as the source of a patient's symptoms [60]. It may also elucidate the underlying etiology of a peripheral nerve injury, such as a fibular neck fracture leading to common peroneal nerve injury [61]. Stress radiographs may serve as a supplement to the clinical examination or advanced imaging in determining ligamentous laxity [60]. Postoperatively, radio-opaque implants can be assessed for changes in position, breakage, or failure.

15.5.1.2 Advanced Imaging

In the evaluation of patients with suspected peripheral nerve injury, both computed tomography (CT) and magnetic resonance imaging (MRI) can be used to determine the presence of a hematoma or other fluid collections adjacent to a peripheral nerve. In addition to localizing injury and determining continuity of peripheral nerves, MRI can be used to assess severity of nerve injury. This may include disruption or contusion of nerve fibers, localized edema, or perineural hematoma [62]. It is important to note that the utility of MRI is variable, with some institutions and radiologists able to provide a more detailed assessment of nerve injury than others.

In the acute setting, nerve injury is represented by increased signal on T2-weighted images – not only at the site of trauma, but distally as well. Findings associated with subacute or chronic nerve dysfunction may be more subtle and include edema or fatty infiltration in muscles innervated by the affected nerve [63]. Neuromata can be identified as a nerve terminating in a fusiform mass with fascicular discontinuity and intermediate signal intensity on T1- and T2-weighted sequences. Other characteristic findings include the target sign – a peripheral ring of high intensity surrounding a central area of hypointensity on T2-weighted images, and split-fat sign – a peripheral ring of fat visualized on T1-weighted images [64].

When concern for peripheral nerve injury is high, magnetic resonance neurography (MRN) is an emerging modality that may aid in the diagnosis. Using short tau inversion recovery (STIR) sequences, MRN is able to provide improved anatomical detail of nervous tissue [65]. MRN can be used to complement information from the physical examination and electrodiagnostic studies, especially when traditional workup and imaging are inconclusive. It is also useful for discerning residual mass effect from unresolved inflammation or fibrosis in a postoperative patient. However, the utility of MRN is limited if symptoms have been present for greater than one year [65].

15.5.1.3 Ultrasonography

As a noninvasive modality with lower cost and increased convenience relative to the aforementioned imaging studies, ultrasonography is a useful tool in the evaluation of peripheral nerve injuries that provides the surgeon with immediate diagnostic information. It is best used in concert with electrodiagnostic studies [66]. Some data suggest that, when utilized appropriately, ultrasonography is more sensitive than MRI in the evaluation of peripheral nerves [67]. Similarly, some consider ultrasonography as first-line imaging for evaluation of neuromata [64]. However, it is highly dependent on a skilled and experienced practitioner using updated equipment [67–69]. Additional advantages include the ability to make real-time adjustments in data acquisition, ease with which the contralateral limb can be used as a control, and ability to perform dynamic evaluations [66]. High resolution ultrasonography has demonstrated accuracy not only in identifying the presence of nerve injury, but also providing information regarding the character of the injury. It is possible to determine if a nerve remains in continuity, measure the cross-sectional area of an injured but intact nerve, quantify the size of the zone of injury, and detect the presence of an encroaching structure such as adjacent muscles, tendons, vessels, hematoma, or fibrosis [69, 70]. Defined cut-offs for the diagnosis of nerve injury or entrapment for lower extremity peripheral nerves remain elusive due to a variety of factors [66]. Despite this, irregularities in other parameters such as echotexture, fascicle diameter, vascularity, and clarity of epineural margins strongly indicate the presence of pathology [71]. Neuromata typically will be visualized as a fusiform or cylindrical hypoechoic mass with hyperechoic internal bands, and a "target-sign" appearance similar to MRI [64].

15.5.2 Electrodiagnostic Studies

Nerve conduction velocity (NCV) and electromyography (EMG) studies are useful tools in the evaluation of peripheral nerve injuries. Neurapraxic (demyelinating) injuries will demonstrate slowed motor or and/or sensory conduction velocities. Axonotmetic injuries will demonstrate decreased amplitudes on motor and sensory conduction studies, while neurotmetic injuries (with complete nerve discontinuity) will show complete absence of amplitudes on nerve conduction studies. On EMG, acute injury is indicated by the presence of fibrillation potentials and positive sharp waves. The findings of acute nerve injury will not be detectable until 2–3 weeks from the time of injury, as the process of Wallerian degeneration occurs. For this reason, early nerve studies are not particularly helpful except to evaluate for the presence of baseline lumbosacral spine pathology or small fiber neuropathy. Chronic injury – and associated muscle denervation – is evidenced by complex repetitive discharges and fasciculations [72]. Baseline NCV and EMG studies are recommended approximately 4 to 6 weeks after the suspected insult. For neurapraxic and axonotmetic injuries, follow-up studies are useful for 3 to 6 months to evaluate for neurologic recovery [60]. For suspected neurotmetic injuries, earlier intervention is recommended.

15.5.3 Diagnostic Nerve Block

When evaluating for neuroma formation, nerve block with local anesthetic (typically lidocaine and/or bupivacaine) is a helpful diagnostic tool [64]. This affords greater clarity regarding the specific anatomic distribution of the zone of injury, which helps confirm the diagnosis, aids in surgical planning, and improves patient counseling regarding postoperative expectations. The diagnostic injection also confirms that the patient's pain can be modified with peripheral nerve-based intervention [64, 73]. Furthermore, the diagnostic nerve injection can help differentiate symptoms attributable to the nerve injury versus those associated with musculoskeletal causes. The primary limitation of diagnostic injection is the potential for false-positive results due to local anesthetic effects on surrounding nociceptors. This can be minimized by administering the block proximal to the area of interest [64, 74]. The negative predictive value of diagnostic nerve blocks has been reported at 83.3% [64].

15.6 Management of Peripheral Nerve Injuries

15.6.1 Peroneal Nerve

15.6.1.1 Background

While compressive neuropathy is the most common cause of peroneal nerve dysfunction, the peroneal nerve and its branches are vulnerable to both blunt and penetrating trauma due to their superficial location and proximity to bony structures about the knee [20, 61, 75, 76]. Peroneal nerve injuries encompass approximately 30% of lower-extremity nerve injuries [77] and are present in up to 40% of knee dislocations [75]. Tethering by fibrous soft tissue structures proximal and distal to the knee places the peroneal nerve at particular risk of stretch injury during posterolateral corner and multiligamentous knee injuries [75]. The zone of neural injury in these cases can be expansive, potentially spreading past the visible lesion-in-continuity as far as the myoneural junction [78]. Neurovascular injuries can occur even without gross knee instability, such as in bi-cruciate or isolated posterior cruciate ligament injuries [79, 80] – thus suspicion must remain high when evaluating any ligamentous injury. While uncommon during routine knee arthroscopic procedures, iatrogenic injuries are a known complication of lateral meniscus repairs [81]. Additionally, peroneal nerve compromise may accompany up to 10% of total knee arthroplasties and up to 20% of high tibial osteotomies [2].

Unlike compressive peroneal palsy, in which many patients will regain partial or full function over time, the outcomes for traumatic peroneal injury are notably worse [61, 82]. Spontaneous recovery occurs in only 14–56% of cases of peroneal nerve injury associated with multiligamentous knee injury [83, 84]. As a result, the majority of these patients will require surgical intervention to regain any significant function. Still, nonoperative modalities remain an essential component of a comprehensive treatment program. Any patient with motor deficits should receive an ankle-foot orthosis to prevent equinus contracture and to help with foot clearance during ambulation. These patients should begin therapy early in the post-injury period. Primary goals include strengthening the surrounding functional muscles, maintaining a supple ankle joint, and preventing Achilles tendon contractures [75].

Decisions regarding surgical intervention are influenced by several factors: time course of nerve injury (i.e., acute traumatic or iatrogenic injury vs. subacute or chronic palsy), acuity of nerve injury (i.e., complete motor and/or sensory deficit vs. subacute weakness, paresthesias, neuropathic pain), degree of injury (i.e., nerve discontinuity vs. traumatic or compressive neurapraxia), and relation of nerve injury to other structural injuries about the knee (i.e., associated with multiligamentous knee injury, iatrogenic injury discovered intraoperatively, iatrogenic injury discovered postoperatively, delayed presentation after injury, and/or knee surgery) [60, 61]. In the setting of acute traumatic injury, deficits in sensory and motor function should be carefully assessed to determine if the degree of neural injury is a simple neurapraxia or something of greater severity. When sensory or motor loss occurs in the setting of knee trauma, exploration of the nerve should be strongly considered in conjunction with procedures addressing the underlying structural injury. Subacute simultaneous ligamentous and nerve reconstruction within 3–6 weeks of the injury is preferred, as staged nerve reconstruction is made more difficult due to postoperative scarring. If no other procedures are planned for the knee, surgical intervention for the peripheral nerve should occur within 3 months if no clinical or electrodiagnostic improvement is seen. Cases involving complete motor or sensory loss should be treated earlier [61]. If sharp iatrogenic nerve injury to a nerve is identified during the index orthopedic procedure, all efforts should be made to carry out primary nerve repair immediately or soon thereafter, providing that a surgeon with microsurgical capabilities is available. Nerve palsies that develop postoperatively should undergo an initial trial of observation for at least 3 months with serial physical examination and electrodiagnostic testing. If there is no improvement on motor and sensory testing, no advancement of Tinel sign, and no signs of recovery on electrodiagnostic studies by the 3-month mark (or if plateau is seen in subsequent serial exams), surgical intervention is recommended. While we recognize that spontaneous recovery may occur with continued observation, the potential downsides of further delay (e.g., an increasing likelihood of irreversible denervation-related atrophy) shift our preference toward surgical intervention.

15.6.1.2 Nerve Exploration, Decompression, and Neurolysis

The goals of surgical exploration and decompression are improvement in function and reduction in pain [85]. Concomitant surgical exploration with peripheral nerve assessment and possible reconstruction should be considered in all patients with evidence of nerve injury who will be undergoing a procedure to address associated structural injuries about the knee, such as posterolateral corner or multiligamentous reconstruction. In cases of traumatic neural injury with no other surgical indications, exploration is indicated if no improvement is seen within 3 to 6 months from the inciting event. External neurolysis can be performed to address compression by hematoma or fibrous tissue, or incarceration by fracture fragments [60]. In patients with motor deficits following multiligamentous knee injuries, neurolysis of the CPN at the time of ligament reconstruction has demonstrated improvement in function, even when performed greater than 5 to 7 months after the injury [60, 86, 87]. In these settings, intraoperative ultrasonography may be valuable to identify nerve lesions when the nerve remains in continuity [88]. Open injuries involving suspected or confirmed sharp peroneal injury (e.g., a laceration) should be explored within 72 h. Nerve intervention for open injuries with known peripheral nerve discontinuity from blunt/blast mechanisms should be delayed for 2–3 weeks to allow the zone of injury within the nerve to declare itself. When there is concern for iatrogenic traction injury after surgery, surgical exploration should be considered in the absence of clinical or electrodiagnostic evidence for improvement by 3 to 6 months [89]. Decompression of a peripheral nerve at a known area of entrapment in the setting of a recent surgery (e.g., compression of the CPN at the posterior crural septa after an open knee surgery) can be considered earlier if there are signs and symptoms of acute compression.

Decompression of the common peroneal nerve can be performed in the lateral decubitus position or with the patient lying supine and the operative knee flexed to approximately 60° (Fig. 15.5). The fibular head is identified and the CPN is palpated just distal to this landmark. An oblique incision is created over the fibular neck, following the palpated trajectory of the nerve from posterosuperior to anteroinferior. Dissection is carried down to the fascia posterior to the fibular neck, taking care to protect the lateral sural cutaneous neve and branches of the posterior femoral cutaneous neve. The fascia can then be opened, either directly over the palpated nerve at the fibular neck, or more proximally where the nerve exits the popliteal fossa, posterior to the biceps femoris tendon (Fig. 15.5a). With careful dissection, the nerve is exposed along its course around the fibular neck to its entry into the lateral compartment. The fascia overlying the peroneus longus muscle is then incised in line with the skin incision and the muscle belly retracted anteriorly and distally (Fig. 15.5b–c). The CPN can then be further exposed as it courses deep to the peroneus longus and makes a sharp turn anteriorly to pass through three muscular septae. The first fibrous plane encountered is the posterior crural intermuscular septum, which is considered to be the main site of CPN compression. Once this is released, the nerve can be traced along its course through

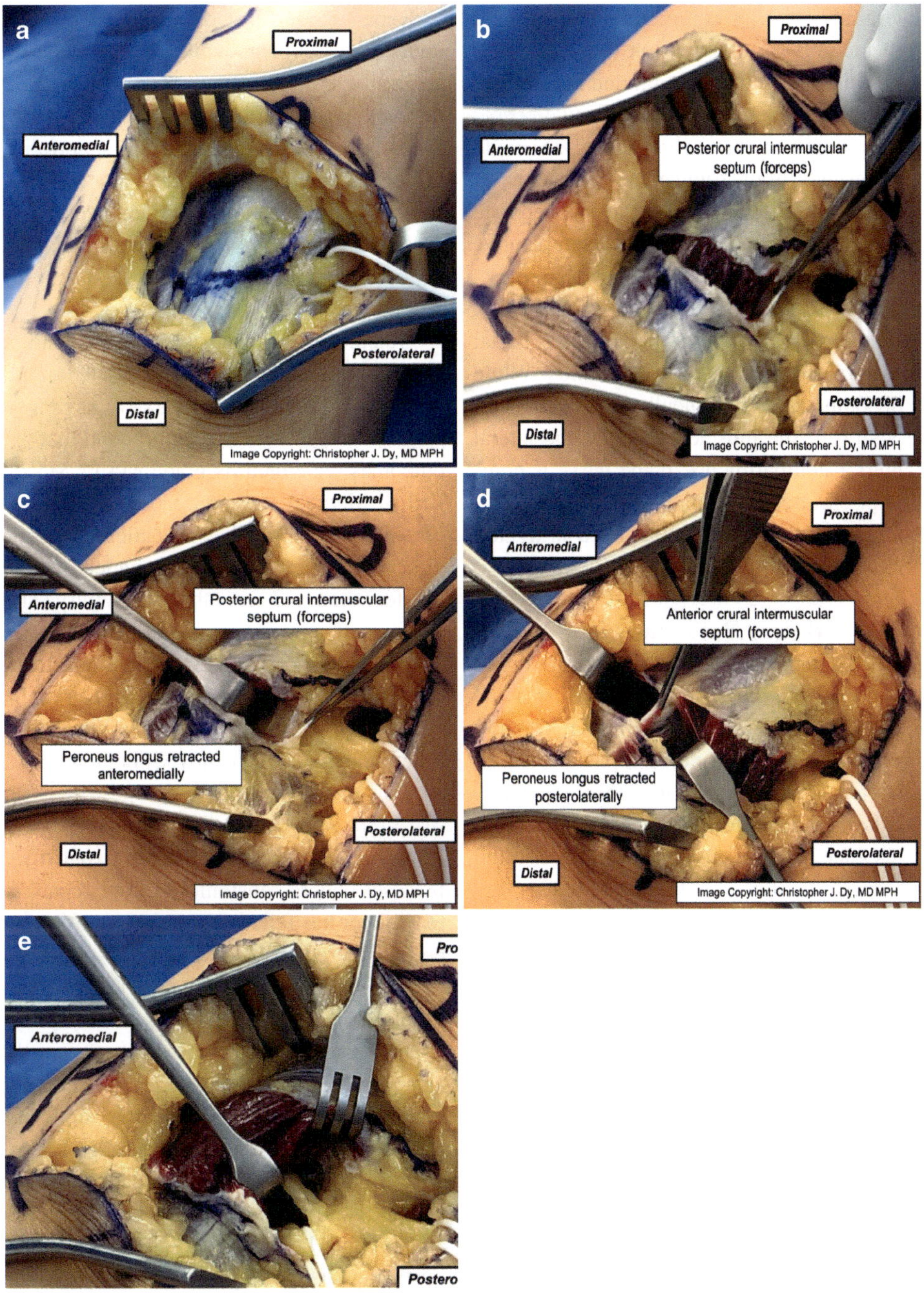

Fig. 15.5 Decompression of the common peroneal nerve (CPN) at the fibular neck. (**a**) The fascia is opened just posterior and proximal to the fibular neck. (**b**) The incision is carried along the fascia overlying the peroneus longus and the posterior crural intermuscular septum is identified. (**c**) The peroneus longus muscle belly is retracted anteriorly to reveal its deep fascia. (**d**) Release of the posterior crural intermuscular septum and deep fascia allows identification of the nerve as it courses deep to the peroneus longus and makes a sharp turn anteriorly. The nerve can be traced through the lateral and anterior compartments to address any other points of compression, such as the anterior crural intermuscular septum and innominate septum between the tibialis anterior and extensor digitorum longus muscle bellies. (**e**) The superficial and deep aspects of the septa are released, as well as the intervening "vertical" fascia that separate the muscle bellies. Images copyright Christopher J. Dy MD MPH and used with permission

the lateral and anterior compartments to address any other points of compression (e.g., the anterior crural intermuscular septum and innominate septum between the tibialis anterior and extensor digitorum longus muscle bellies). The superficial and deep aspects of the septa are released, as well as the intervening "vertical" fascia that separate the muscle bellies (Fig. 15.5c–e). It is imperative to confirm that the nerve is completely free distally, past its bifurcation into the SPN and DPN, as well as proximally where it passes superficial to the lateral head of the gastrocnemius. While CPN decompression is typically performed with preservation of the muscle bellies of the lateral and anterior compartments, if the nerve is compressed or elevated proximally, a bed can be created in the muscle belly to allow for a straighter, tension-free course [21, 61].

15.6.1.3 Primary Nerve Repair

If the CPN is not in continuity, direct nerve repair is the optimal treatment. This requires that the zone of injury be small, with minimal gapping of the nerve ends. Basic nerve repair principles call for a tension-free coaptation at the repair site. Due to the significant force involved in multiligamentous knee injuries, the zone of injury is often large enough that this is not achievable [75, 90]. However, sharp injuries secondary to penetrating trauma or iatrogenic insult may result in a discontinuity that is amenable to direct repair. If proper techniques are employed to remove tension from the coaptation site, gaps of 5 mm or less can easily be overcome [85, 91]. Generous mobilization of the nerve proximally and distally, as described above for CPN decompression, will increase the excursion of the proximal and distal ends. Flexion of the knee can also provide additional length, but must be done judiciously as the leg must be immobilized in the chosen position to protect the repair. This may lead to knee stiffness and flexion contractures, and the coaptation may still fail as the leg is gradually brought back into extension [85]. If a nerve coaptation is performed with the knee in flexion, a combination of a hinged knee brace and ultrasound monitoring of the nerve repair can be used to allow gradual increases in knee extension.

Repair is performed with 8-0 or 9-0 nylon under microscopic magnification. The nerve ends should be carefully inspected; sequential resection or "bread-loafing" may be required to expose clean fascicles [91]. Given that superiority has not been established between epineural and fascicular repair techniques [61], epineural repair is preferred by the senior author, using topographical cues such as epineural blood vessels to help align the nerve ends.

Outcomes following direct end-to-end repair of CPN injuries have demonstrated moderate success. A recent comprehensive review of 28 studies and 1577 CPN repairs found that "good" outcomes – defined as grade M4 or M5 on the British Medical Research Council Scale – were obtained in only 37% of patients undergoing direct suture repair. Patients undergoing repair greater than 12 months post-injury showed significantly worse outcomes [92]. In a large single-center cohort, Kim et al. found that 84% of patients undergoing direct repair achieved strength of at least grade M3, which enables functional gait mechanics without need for an orthosis [60, 93].

15.6.1.4 Intercalary Nerve Grafting

In cases where tensionless direct repair is not feasible or has failed, intercalary grafting should be considered. Options for nerve grafting continue to expand, but autograft remains the gold standard. Autogenous grafts serve not only as a structural template to guide axonal growth, but also provide viable Schwann cells, neurotrophic factors, and extracellular matrix substrates to support neuronal regeneration [60, 91, 94, 95]. Disadvantages include additional operative time and a second operative site at which hematomas and wound healing complications may arise. Further, patients may experience distal sensory abnormalities and persistent pain at the site of harvest due to neuroma formation [96, 97]. Two well-described sources for donor tissue are the sural nerve and the medial antebrachial cutaneous nerve. In cases of peroneal nerve injury, the sural nerve is most commonly used due to its size and proximity to the surgical field [60]. Preoperative assessment (either clinically or with electrodiagnostic studies) should be performed to confirm viability of the sural nerve. This is especially important if harvesting from the ipsilateral limb in cases of knee injury, as the nerve may have sustained damage during the initial trauma [60].

Autogenous nerve grafting has demonstrated fair success in the treatment of CPN injury, with up to 75% of patients achieving M3 motor strength and 36% reaching grade M4 or M5. However, outcomes decline sharply when the nerve gap exceeds 6 cm [92, 93]. In cases with larger nerve gaps, VSNGs have produced positive results. Terzis et al. reported on a cohort of patients receiving VSNG and found that all patients treated within 6 months of injury and with graft lengths up to 20 cm achieved M4 motor strength [98].

15.6.1.5 Nerve Transfer and Motor/Sensory Nerve Reconstruction

Nerve transfers provide another option to restore distal function, but these are indicated only in select cases of CPN injury. The primary advantage of nerve transfers lies in the ability to provide donor axons closer to the target motor endplate, reducing the time before regenerative axons reach the muscle of interest [99]. In cases where surgical intervention must be delayed, this can be invaluable, as a more proximal nerve repair or grafting procedure may not provide regenerated axons to the target motor endplate before the optimal window for muscle reinnervation closes around the 1-year mark [100]. The provision of donor axons at a more distal point is also advantageous in cases where a proximal nerve stump is not available for repair or grafting, where other factors preclude surgical intervention at the site of nerve injury, when a large zone of injury with segmental nerve loss is present, when the location of the level of nerve injury is not clearly defined, or simply for a proximal lesion with a long regeneration distance [61, 100]. However, nerve transfers for CPN injury can be difficult to re-educate and have a long recovery period. Patients may not be willing or able to endure this lengthy and intense rehabilitation, particularly in the context of having an alternative (tendon transfers) that can provide more immediate recovery of function.

When considering a nerve transfer, careful donor nerve selection is crucial. For motor transfers, the donor nerve should be located relatively close to the target muscle, and either be comprised exclusively of motor axons or contain motor axons that can be easily identified and neurolysed in sufficient quantity to appropriately match the injured nerve and its motor endplate. A nerve that innervates an expendable but synergistic muscle will enhance postoperative rehabilitation and motor re-education. Selection for sensory transfers is slightly more simple, requiring a branch located close to the target that provides nonessential sensation [68, 100].

Selection of an appropriate donor must take several factors into account. The length and branch point of the donor nerve will impact its ability to reach the coaptation site and achieve a tensionless repair, ideally done without use of an intercalary graft. The cross-sectional area and axon count should approximate that of the recipient nerve. Finally, collateral damage should be minimized – harvesting nerves that have reciprocal or dual innervation is ideal.

In the treatment of peroneal nerve injuries, a variety of potential donors from the tibial nerve exist, including motor branches to the tibialis posterior, popliteus, gastrocnemius, soleus, flexor hallucis longus, and flexor digitorum longus [8, 101–103]. Alternatively, others have described the harvest of motor axons directly from the proximal portion of the tibial nerve [4, 103, 104]. Donor nerves can be coapted to either the DPN or directly to the tibialis anterior (TA) motor branch. Based on branch point and branch length measurements taken from all proximal motor branches of the tibial nerve, Bodily et al. suggested that the branches to the flexor digitorum longus and flexor hallucis longus were adequate for transfer to the DPN in all cases. They also reported that motor branches to the soleus and lateral head of the gastrocnemius may be adequate for lesions proximal to the trifurcation of the CPN if intramuscular dissection is performed during harvest [102]. Pirela-Cruz et al. evaluated the branches to the medial gastrocnemius, lateral gastrocnemius, and soleus for transfer to TA motor branches through an interosseus window. They concluded that the branch to the soleus was best suited for this transfer based on its short distance from the coaptation site and its similarity to the TA branches in axonal count and cross-sectional area [101]. Morphometric analyses performed by White et al. suggest that the motor branches to the popliteus and tibialis posterior also closely match the axon count and cross-sectional area of the TA motor branches [105]. Table 15.1 provides a summary of branch length, cross-sectional area, and axon count values for the various potential donors to the common peroneal nerve.

Giuffre et al. [103] described a surgical window centered over the proximal one-third of the lateral aspect of the leg. The longitudinal incision begins at the fibular head and extends 10–12 cm distally. The CPN is identified at the level of the fibular neck, and dissection is carried out along the distal course of the nerve into the lateral compartment to identify the branch point of the DPN, as described above in the "Nerve Exploration" section. A reproducible fat stripe identifies the interval between the peroneus longus and soleus. The interval is opened and the soleus elevated from the posterolateral fibula, allowing identification of the tibial nerve and posterior tibial vessels lying deep in the surgical bed, posteromedial from the fibula. The peroneal muscles are then elevated subperiosteally from the anterior fibula to expose the proximal tibialis anterior motor branch, typically arising from the ATRN. This branch is then divided proximally and sectioned with the "bread-loafing" technique to expose clean fascicles. A nerve stimulator is then applied to the exposed tibial nerve to localize branches or fascicles innervating the FHL or FDL. Selection of the optimal donor is based upon location, length, and branching pattern of the tibial nerve as well as by the diameter of the recipient nerve. If no branches meet the appropriate criteria, donor fascicles can be harvested from the tibial nerve via intraneural dissection. The donor is then tunneled through an opening in the interosseous membrane to allow for protected, tensionless coaptation with the proximal tibialis anterior motor branch. Postoperatively, the patient should be made non-weightbearing on the operative extremity, and the ankle should be immobilized in a bulky plaster splint.

The peroneal nerve itself can also serve as a donor. Fascicles can be harvested from the proximal CPN (Fig. 15.6) or from the motor branch to the short head of the biceps (Fig. 15.7). Additionally, while isolated palsy of the DPN as a result of knee injury is uncommon, in these cases, the uninjured SPN can also be harvested as a donor. This can be accomplished through the same initial exposure as described above. The SPN should be stimulated to confirm adequate function of its motor innervation to the lateral

Table 15.1 Potential motor donors for transfer to the common peroneal nerve

Motor branch	Branch length (mm)		Cross-sectional area (mm^2)	Axon count (n)
Deep peroneal nerve				
Tibialis anterior	–		0.255 (0.111)	3363 (1997)
Extensor hallucis longus	–		0.197 (0.302)	2062 (2314)
Tibial nerve				
Popliteus	47.5 (5.1)		0.425 (0.421)	3317 (1467)
Lateral gastrocnemius	36.2 (3.8)		0.256 (0.105)	2352 (1249)
Medial gastrocnemius	39.5 (5.0)		0.309 (0.101)	2834 (718)
Soleus	46.8 (17.5)	[Anterior]	0.700 (0.222)	4941 (1994)
	51.7 (8.4)	[Posterior]		
Tibialis posterior	44.5 (15.4)		0.348 (0.253)	3039 (1528)
Flexor hallucis longus	139.0 (30.2)		0.234 (0.147)	1557 (735)
Flexor digitorum longus	121.7 (41.6)		–	–

Data presented as mean (standard deviation)
Adapted from Bodily et al. [102] and White et al. [105]

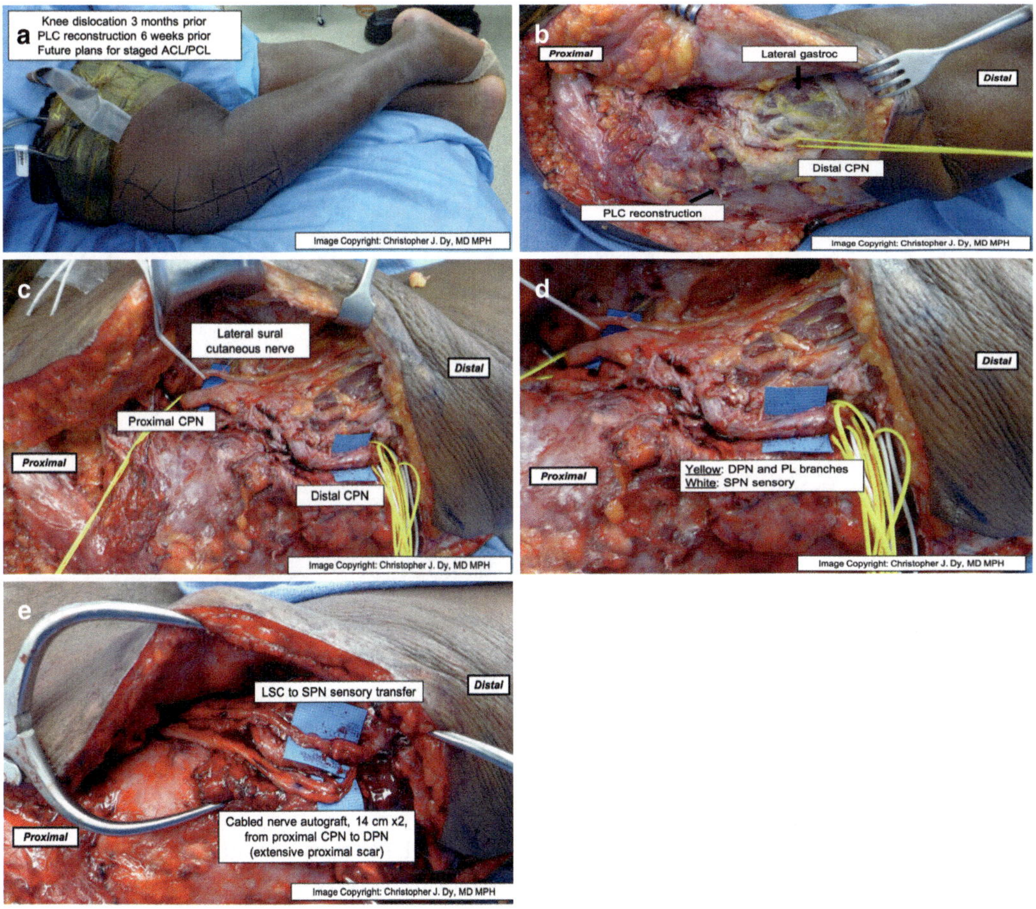

Fig. 15.6 Common peroneal nerve (CPN) to deep peroneal nerve (DPN) transfer, along with lateral sural cutaneous (LSC) nerve to superficial peroneal nerve (SPN) transfer. (**a**) Patient positioning and planned incision. (**b**) Exposure of the CPN distal to the knee. (**c**) Exposure of the CPN and LSC proximal to the knee. (**d**) Separation of the DPN from the sensory and peroneus longus (PL) motor branches of the SPN. (**e**) Final reconstruction. Images copyright Christopher J. Dy MD MPH and used with permission

compartment. The motor branch of the DPN to the tibialis anterior is approximately one-third the size of the SPN, allowing for group fascicle intraneural dissection of the SPN and partial transfer to the DPN tibialis anterior motor branch while maintaining innervation to the lateral compartment and preservation of clinical eversion [4].

Several technical points are critical to the success of a nerve transfer. First, injury to the recipient nerve should be verified through intraoperative stimulation in order to avoid unnecessary procedures on a regenerating nerve. Once this has been confirmed, the donor nerve should be dissected and stimulated to assess for appropriate function. Donor and recipient nerves are then generously mobilized. The donor is resected as far distal as possible, and the recipient resected as far proximal as possible to create the best opportunity for a tension-free coaptation. Motor transfers should always be performed in an end-to-end fashion. This is the preferred method for sensory transfers as well, but end-to-side coaptation can be used to regain basic protective sensation when donor options are limited. Use of long-acting paralytics and local anesthetics should be avoided. Tourniquet use beyond 30 min will limit the use of peripheral nerve stimulators to assess neuromas-in-

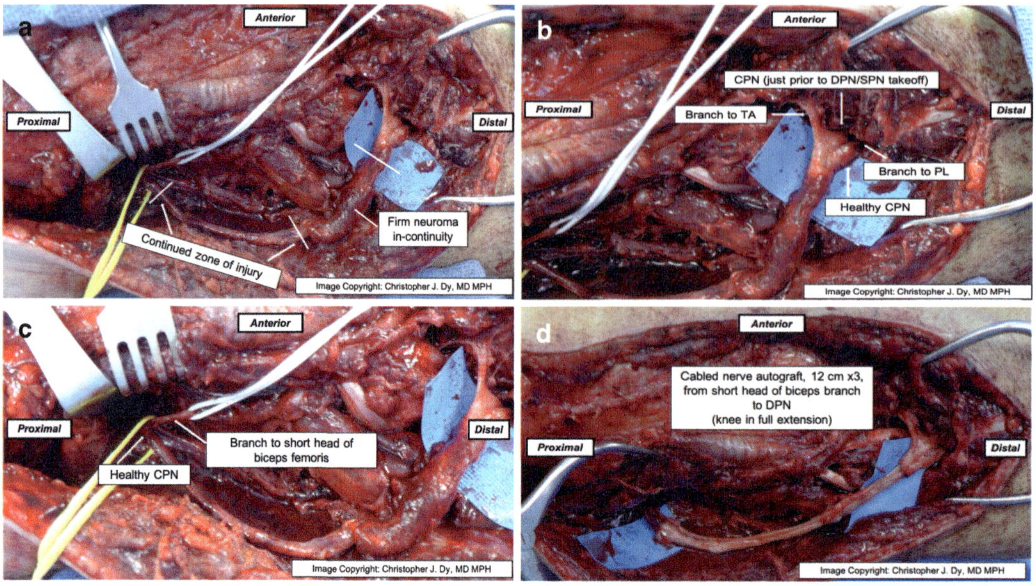

Fig. 15.7 Short head of biceps branch transfer to the deep peroneal nerve (DPN). The patient is positioned supine, with images depicting the lateral aspect of the right distal thigh and proximal leg with the knee in extension. (**a**) Initial exposure of the common peroneal nerve (CPN), demonstrating an extended zone of injury just proximal to a large neuroma in-continuity. (**b**) Distal exposure of the CPN to identify the terminal branches (SPN, superficial peroneal nerve; PL, peroneus longus; TA, tibialis anterior). (**c**) Proximal exposure to identify the branch to the short head of biceps femoris. (**d**) Final reconstruction. Images copyright Christopher J. Dy MD MPH and used with permission

continuity and potential donor nerves due to tourniquet-related ischemia.

While the popularity of nerve transfers has grown immensely for a variety of nerve conditions in the upper extremity [100], the true efficacy of nerve transfers for the treatment of CPN injury remains unclear [61]. There are mixed results from the limited short-term follow-up data available from a few small cohorts [106]. The first clinical study on the subject by Nath et al. in 2008 reported postoperative strength of grade M3 or higher in 12 of 14 patients at an average of 16 months utilizing motor fibers either from the SPN or tibial nerve. Two patients experienced no restoration of motor function [4]. In the cohort treated by Giuffre et al., 9 of 11 patients were able to ambulate and 7 of those were able to do so without an AFO at an average of 18 months postoperatively. However, only 4 of 11 patients regained M3 or greater strength, and 4 patients experienced no return of motor function [103]. The most recent clinical outcomes reported in 2015 by Leclère et al. showed mixed results for tibial to DPN transfer, with three of six patients achieving a good to excellent outcome and two of six patients experiencing poor outcomes [107]. A recent meta-analysis of the four available studies showed a bimodal distribution of postoperative dorsiflexion strength, which was not associated with injury site, injury mechanism, donor nerve, or recipient nerve [106]. This suggests that patient factors must be carefully evaluated, and indications for nerve transfers must be decided on a case-by-case basis. Further research investigating which patients respond well to these procedures will be essential.

15.6.1.6 Tendon Transfers

Tendon transfer procedures address the challenges of foot drop and equinovarus deformity when spontaneous nerve recovery has not occurred and nerve repair, grafting, or transfer procedures either have failed or are not feasible [60, 61]. Transfer of the posterior tibialis tendon (PTT) through the interosseous membrane (IOM) to the dorsum of the foot converts it to an ankle dorsiflexor, improving gait mechanics and decreasing reliance on orthoses [60]. While the literature suggests that tendon transfers do not allow patients to return to activities beyond simple ambulation [108], we have anecdotally noted remarkable function recovery (including return to some sports) in patients who have had tendon transfer.

15.6.2 Saphenous Nerve

15.6.2.1 Background

The superficial trajectory of the saphenous nerve across the anteromedial aspect of the knee places its terminal branches at high risk for injury during any orthopedic procedure requiring a midline or medial incision. While direct trauma or entrapment is fairly uncommon [38], iatrogenic injury to the infrapatellar branches has been described in up to 100% of patients after total knee arthroplasty [109, 110], up to 77% after anterior cruciate ligament reconstruction [111] – both with bone-patella-tendon-bone and hamstring autograft harvest [39], and up to 28% after meniscectomy [112]. Some studies have indicated that patient comfort after these procedures is inversely related to the presence of injury to the infrapatellar branches [38]. Although less frequently discussed, injury to the sartorial branch has been reported following meniscal repair, hamstring harvest for anterior cruciate ligament reconstruction, and fracture fixation [30]. Even in the absence of true injury, up to three-fourths of patients undergoing hamstring harvest for anterior cruciate ligament reconstruction will experience some degree of paresthesias or numbness following the procedure [34].

15.6.2.2 Saphenous Nerve Decompression and Neuroma Excision

In the preoperative holding area, the patient should be examined and the location of positive Tinel's sign marked on the skin. In the operating suite, the patient is placed in the supine position

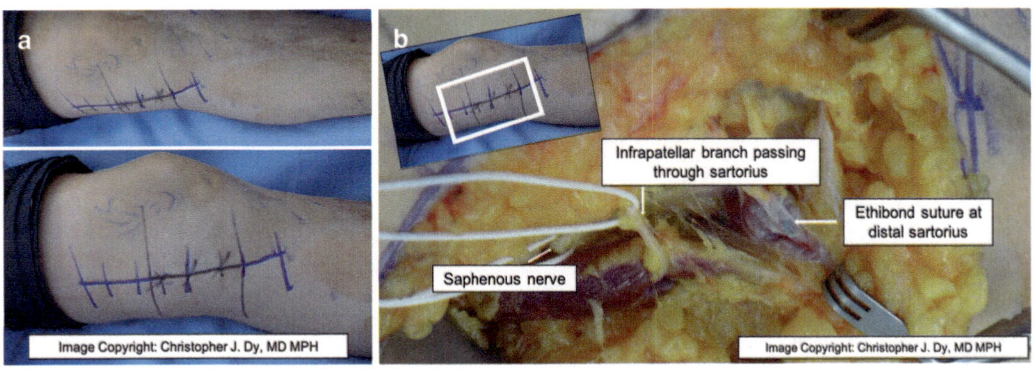

Fig. 15.8 Saphenous nerve decompression and infrapatellar branch neuroma excision with burying. (**a**) In the preoperative holding area, the location of positive Tinel's sign, pain, and paresthesias should be marked on the skin. In this case, a black "X" indicates locations of positive Tinel's sign, and blue dashes indicate areas of pain and paresthesias. The patient is placed on the operating table in the supine position. The limb is then positioned with the knee flexed and the hip in slight flexion, abduction, and external rotation. An 8–10-cm longitudinal incision is marked over the medial aspect of the distal thigh, centered over the sartorius muscle belly. The previously marked symptomatic area should be in the central or distal third. (**b**) Dissection is carefully carried to the sartorius fascia, where the infrapatellar and sartorial branches of the saphenous nerve can be identified. (**c**, **d**) Once localized and isolated, the branches should be carefully inspected for neuromata. If a lesion is identified, the proximal and distal segments of the nerve should be mobilized several centimeters. (**e**) Neurectomy is performed with a proximal crush injury, sharp transection just proximal to the neuroma end, and cautery ablation of the distal stump. A small opening is then made in the fascia and underlying muscle belly of the sartorius, and the proximal nerve end is buried. The entry site of the nerve into the muscle is loosely approximated with an absorbable suture and sealed with fibrin glue. Note the redundancy of the nerve as it lies in a tensionless loop. Images copyright Christopher J. Dy MD MPH and used with permission

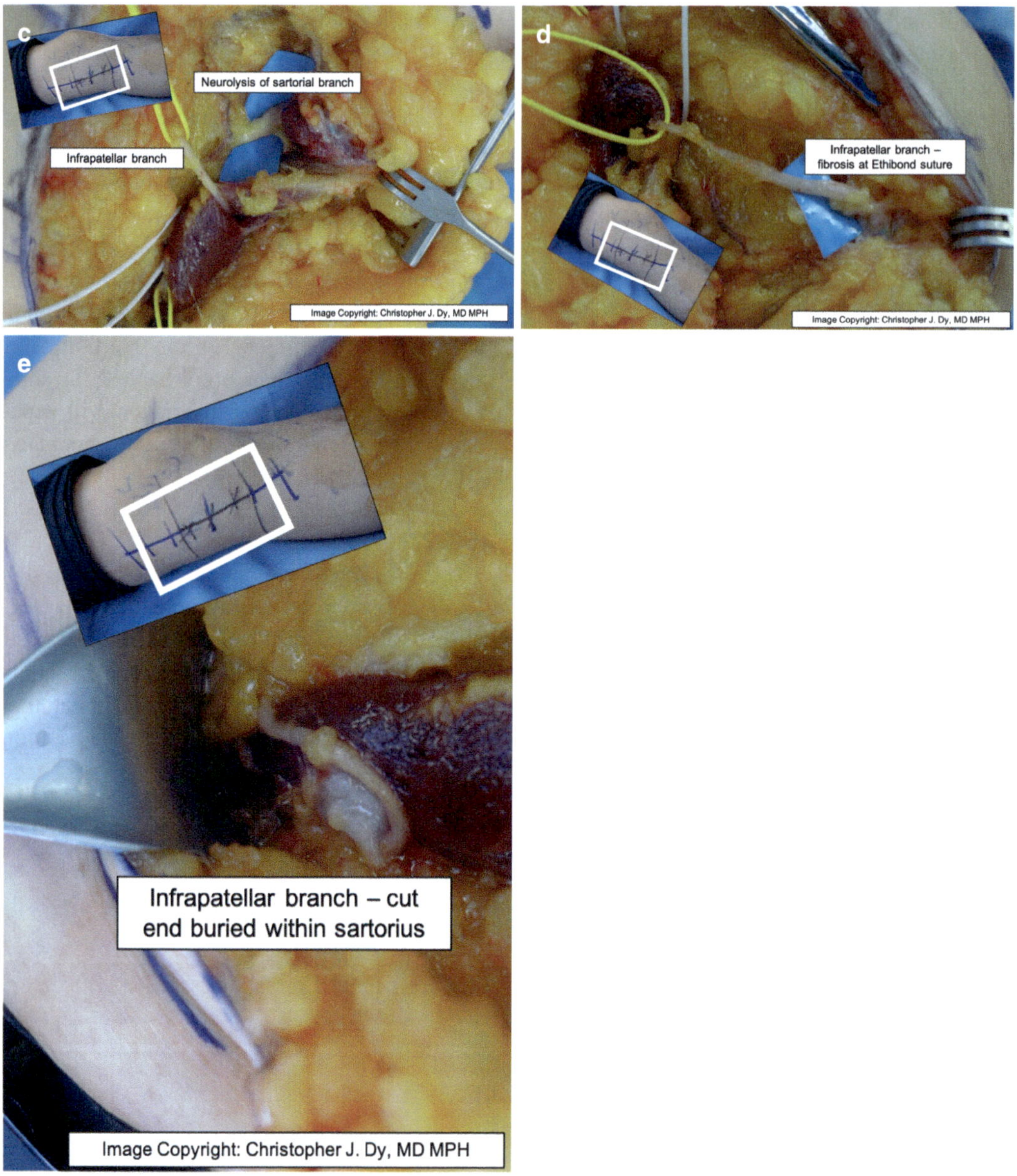

Fig. 15.8 (continued)

with the knee flexed and the hip slightly flexed, abducted, and externally rotated (Fig. 15.8a). Securing a firm object such as a sandbag to the operating table near the foot can help maintain this position during the procedure. To aid with hemostasis, a sterile tourniquet can be placed at the upper thigh. Alternatively, a small amount of dilute epinephrine can be injected at the surgical site. An 8–10 cm longitudinal incision is made over the medial aspect of the distal thigh. This incision should be centered over the sartorius muscle belly and should include the previously marked symptomatic area in its central or distal third. Dissection is then carefully carried to the sartorius fascia. As described previously, the infrapatellar and sartorial branches of the saphenous nerve take variable paths in relation to the distal sartorius muscle belly and may be found near its anterior border, posterior border, or piercing the muscle itself (Fig. 15.8b). Once localized and isolated, the branches should be carefully inspected for neuromata. If a lesion is identified, the proximal and distal segments of the nerve should be mobilized several centimeters (Fig. 15.8c, d). The decision is then made to perform intercalary nerve grafting (with autograft or acellular nerve allograft) or to perform neuroma excision and intramuscular relocation. For the latter, neurectomy is performed with a proximal crush injury, sharp transection just proximal to the neuroma end, and cautery ablation of the distal stump. A small opening is then made in the fascia and underlying muscle belly of the sartorius or vastus medialis, and the proximal nerve end is buried (Fig. 15.8e). There should be sufficient redundancy such that the nerve lies in a tensionless loop within the muscle [113]. The entry site of the nerve into the muscle is loosely approximated with an absorbable suture and sealed with fibrin glue. The knee joint is taken through passive motion to ensure that the nerve end does not displace from within the muscle. If no neuroma is identified, or if the appearance of the nerve indicates proximal compression, the infrapatellar and sartorial branches can be traced proximally and released from common compression points at the vastoadductor septum and adductor canal.

Descriptions of painful saphenous neuromas in the literature are limited largely to case reports. However, outcomes with excision of the neuroma are uniformly positive, with no complications and most reports describing complete pain relief postoperatively [114–118]. Ducic et al. followed a cohort of 35 consecutive patients undergoing neuroma excision or nerve decompression for suspected saphenous nerve pathology, reporting significant improvements in pain with an overall success rate of 83% for effective pain resolution and a 77% recovery of baseline quality of life [119].

15.6.3 Tibial Nerve

15.6.3.1 Background

Isolated injury to the tibial nerve is rare, accounting for 4% of significant peripheral nerve injuries [76, 120, 121]. This may be due in part to a more robust blood supply, greater number of fascicles, increased amount of surrounding connective tissue, and absence of tethering [76]. It has been reported in association with fractures of the tibia and distal femur, penetrating injuries about the knee, as well as knee arthroscopic and arthroplasty procedures [76]. In one of the more comprehensive reports on tibial nerve trauma conducted by Kim et al., 41% occurred about the knee and the remaining 59% occurred about the ankle. Two-thirds of the cases with injury about the knee did not improve with observation and were indicated for surgical intervention. Of these, 32% were due to laceration, 26% were contusions due to fractures, 18% were contusions due to blunt trauma, 16% were due to iatrogenic injury, and the remaining 8% were caused by gunshot wounds [120]. In general, direct trauma is a more common mechanism than iatrogenic injury, and inadvertent injury during surgical procedures is more commonly reported about the ankle than the knee [122–125]. The reported incidence of tibial nerve injury with tibial fractures is 0.5%, whereas the incidence with knee arthroscopy is <0.004% [76, 126].

15.6.3.2 Nerve Exploration, Decompression, and Repair

In cases of sharp laceration with minimal gapping, direct suture repair of the injured nerve can be considered. The incision can follow that of the standard approach to the posterior knee, with longitudinal limbs over the distal lateral thigh and proximal medial leg connected by a gently curving oblique incision across the popliteal fossa. Alternatively, a midline longitudinal incision can be made over the distal thigh with a large Brunner zig-zag to cross the popliteal crease. Repair principles are the same as those detailed in the *Peroneal Nerve* section. Decompression of the tibial nerve at the soleus sling can be considered, as that is a known point of compression of the tibial nerve. As recovery occurs, subsequent decompression of the tarsal tunnel may aid in alleviating paresthesia and pain in the tibial nerve distribution.

There is little description of the outcomes following surgical management of tibial nerve injuries about the knee. In their retrospective cohort, Kim et al. identified two patients who underwent suture repair of laceration injuries. Both of these patients achieved a minimum of Grade 3 function, defined by the authors as gastrocnemius contraction against moderate resistance, trace or better inversion, and minimum plantar sensation "response to touch and pin in autonomous zones, not localized, but normal with some over-response." Operative candidates with a discontinuous injury, or with a lesion in continuity but no intraoperative nerve action potentials, underwent nerve grafting procedures. Of these 16 patients, 15 recovered to Grade 3 or higher. Patients with lesions in continuity and positive intraoperative action potentials were treated with simple neurolysis. All of these patients experienced pain relief and returned to Grade 3 or higher [120]. Despite these encouraging results, return of protective plantar sensation often remains a significant challenge in treating these injuries with simple neurolysis or nerve repair [127].

15.6.3.3 Nerve Transfers

Due to the rarity of tibial nerve injuries, descriptions of nerve transfer procedures are limited, with many of the interventions originally designed to treat more proximal injuries to the sciatic nerve or sacral plexus. However, for similar reasons to those listed in the *Peroneal Nerve* section, nerve transfers may provide a superior alternative to nerve repair or reconstruction due to the proximal nature of these injuries.

Moore et al. [45] described the transfer of femoral nerve branches to address motor and sensory deficits in two patients with sciatic nerve palsy. The procedure first involves exposure and proximal division of the medial and lateral gastrocnemius branches of the tibial nerve as well as the sural nerve through a posterior approach with the patient supine. The medial gastrocnemius branch and sural nerve are passed through a medial soft tissue tunnel, and the lateral gastrocnemius branch is passed through a lateral soft tissue tunnel. The patient is then flipped supine, allowing anterior exposures to access branches of the femoral nerve. Through a proximal anterolateral incision, terminal motor branches of the femoral nerve are identified in the interval between the rectus femoris and vastus lateralis and neurolysed proximally. The previously tunneled lateral gastrocnemius branch is transposed anteriorly and coapted to these femoral nerve branches. Subsequently, a distal anteromedial incision is made, allowing identification of terminal femoral motor branches and the saphenous sensory branch posterior and deep to the vastus medialis muscle. These branches are divided distally, transposed posteriorly, and coapted to the previously tunneled medial gastrocnemius branch and sural nerve. In some cases, an interpositional nerve grafts may be necessary to create tensionless coaptations. Both patients treated with this procedure returned to grade M3 plantarflexion strength with moderate improvements in distal sensation and no deficits in quadriceps muscle strength.

Yin et al. [128] described the transfer of obturator nerve branches to reanimate the medial head of the gastrocnemius. In the supine position, the nerve to the gracilis muscle is first identified on the deep side of the muscle through a proximal medial incision just posterior to the mid-axis of the thigh. The anterior branch of the nerve is neurolysed and divided distally. The branch of the tibial nerve to the medial head of the gastrocnemius is then identified through a longitudinal incision over the posteromedial aspect of the distal boundary of the popliteal fossa. This branch is neurolysed and divided proximally. The two nerves are then coapted under a subcutaneous bridge using a sural nerve graft. Three of the five patients treated with this procedure returned to grade M3 strength or better. There were no complications and no deficits in hip adduction.

Koshima et al. [127] described the transfer of terminal sensory fibers from the deep peroneal nerve to the medial plantar branch of the tibial nerve to restore plantar sensation. The deep peroneal nerve is exposed through an incision between the first and second ray on the dorsum of the foot and neurolysed proximally to the level of the tarsometatarsal joints. The medial plantar branch of the tibial nerve is exposed through an incision along the medial arch of the foot and divided proximally. These two nerves are then coapted under a subcutaneous tunnel at the medial aspect of the foot. Both patients treated with this procedure experienced return of protective sensation and light touch of Semmes-Weinstein values 4.31–6.65.

Agarwal et al. [129] described the transfer of terminal branches of the saphenous nerve to the distal aspect of the tibial nerve to restore plantar sensation. Through a single inverted "V" incision centered over the medial malleolus, the terminal saphenous nerve is exposed, neurolysed, and divided distally. The tibial nerve is then carefully exposed posterior to the medial malleolus and the epineurium opened. Sensory fascicles are identified as those which do not cause muscle contraction with intraoperative stimulation. These fascicles are then coapted with fascicles from the previously divided saphenous nerve. All patients who returned for follow-up demonstrated improved light touch, discriminatory, temperature, vibratory, and pressure sensation. This technique is limited by the difficulty of identifying tibial nerve sensory fascicles via intraoperative stimulation in patients with proximal tibial nerve injuries who have no distal sensory or motor function.

References

1. Fallis A. Moore – clinically oriented anatomy. 7th ed. Lippincott Williams & Wilkins; 2014.
2. Reebye O. Anatomical and clinical study of the common fibular nerve. Part 1: anatomical study. Surg Radiol Anat. 2004;26(5):365–70.
3. Gustafson KJ, Grinberg Y, Joseph S, Triolo RJ. Human distal sciatic nerve fascicular anatomy: implications for ankle control using nerve-cuff electrodes. J Rehabil Res Dev. 2012;49(2):309–21.
4. Nath RK, Lyons AB, Paizi M. Successful management of foot drop by nerve transfers to the deep peroneal nerve. J Reconstr Microsurg. 2008;24(6):419–27.
5. Kadiyala RK, Ramirez A, Taylor AE, Saltzman CL, Cassell MD. The blood supply of the common peroneal nerve in the popliteal fossa. J Bone Jt Surg. 2005;87(3):337–42.
6. Tomaszewski KA, Graves MJ, Henry BM, Popieluszko P, Roy J, Pękala PA, et al. Surgical anatomy of the sciatic nerve: a meta-analysis. J Orthop Res. 2016;34(10):1820–7.
7. Vloka JD, Hadžić A, April E, Thys DM. The division of the sciatic nerve in the popliteal fossa: anatomical implications for popliteal nerve blockade. Anesth Analg. 2001;92(1):215–7.
8. Flores LP. Proximal motor branches from the tibial nerve as direct donors to restore function of the deep fibular nerve for treatment of high sciatic nerve injuries: a cadaveric feasibility study. Neurosurgery. 2009;17(3):201–5.
9. Silverman ER, Vydyanathan A, Gritsenko K, Shaparin N, Singh N, Downie SA, et al. The anatomic relationship of the tibial nerve to the common peroneal nerve in the popliteal fossa: implications for selective tibial nerve block in total knee arthroplasty. Pain Res Manag. 2017;2017:7250181.
10. Watt T, Hariharan AR, Brzezinski DW, Caird MS, Zeller JL. Branching patterns and localization of the common fibular (peroneal) nerve: an anatomical basis for planning safe surgical approaches. Surg Radiol Anat. 2014;36(8):821–8.
11. Labronici PJ, Teixeira TM, de Medeiros FB, Franco JS, Hoffmann R, Fonseca Passos MA, et al. Clinical and anatomical comparison of the fibular nerve in gerdy's safe zone. Rev Bras Ortop. 2010;45(1):23–7.
12. Hildebrand G, Tompkins M, Macalena J. Fibular head as a landmark for identification of the common peroneal nerve: a cadaveric study. Arthroscopy. 2015;31(1):99–103.
13. Kim GY, Ryou CH, Kim KH, Kim D, Rhyu IJ, Kim DH. Branching patterns and anatomical course of the common fibular nerve. Ann Rehabil Med. 2019;43(6):700–6.
14. Tran J, Peng PWH, Lam K, Baig E, Agur AMR, Gofeld M. Anatomical study of the innervation of anterior knee joint capsule: implication for image-guided intervention. Reg Anesth Pain Med. 2018;43(4):407–14.
15. Franco CD, Buvanendran A, Petersohn JD, Menzies RD, Menzies LP. Innervation of the anterior capsule of the human knee: implications for radiofrequency ablation. Reg Anesth Pain Med. 2015;40(4):363–8.
16. Jenkins MJ, Farhat M, Hwang P, Kanawati AJ, Graham E. The distance of the common peroneal nerve to the posterolateral structures of the knee. J Arthroplast. 2016;31(12):2907–11.
17. Jia Y, Gou W, Geng L, Wang Y, Chen J. Anatomic proximity of the peroneal nerve to the posterolateral corner of the knee determined by MR imaging. Knee. 2012;19(6):766–8.
18. Ryan W, Mahony N, Delaney M, O'Brien M, Murray P. Relationship of the common peroneal nerve and

its branches to the Head and neck of the fibula. Clin Anat. 2003;16(6):501–5.
19. Dearden P, Lowery K, Sherman K, Mahadevan V, Sharma H. Fibular head transfixion wire and its relationship to common peroneal nerve: cadaveric analysis. Strateg Trauma Limb Reconstr. 2015;10:73–8.
20. Rausch V, Hackl M, Oppermann J, Leschinger T, Scaal M, Müller LP, et al. Peroneal nerve location at the fibular head: an anatomic study using 3D imaging. Arch Orthop Trauma Surg. 2019;139(7):921–6.
21. Humphreys DB, Novak CB, Mackinnon SE. Patient outcome after common peroneal nerve decompression. J Neurosurg. 2007;107(2):314–8.
22. Aydoğdu S, Yercan H, Saylam C, Sur H. Peroneal nerve dysfunction after high tibial osteotomy. An anatomical cadaver study. Acta Orthop Belg. 1996;62(3):156–60.
23. Takeda A, Tsucbiya H, Mori Y, Tanaka S, Kikuchi S, Tomita K. Anatomical aspects of biopsy of the proximal fibula. Int Orthop. 2001;24(6):335–7.
24. Deutsch A, Wyzykowski RJ, Victoroff BN. Evaluation of the anatomy of the common peroneal nerve: defining nerve- at-risk in arthroscopically assisted lateral meniscus repair. Am J Sports Med. 1999;27(1):10–5.
25. Franco MJ, Phillips BZ, Lalchandani GR, Mackinnon SE. Decompression of the superficial peroneal nerve: clinical outcomes and anatomical study. J Neurosurg. 2017;126(1):330–5.
26. Lee JH, Lee BN, An X, Chung RH, Kwon SO, Han SH. Anatomic localization of motor entry point of superficial peroneal nerve to peroneus longus and brevis muscles. Clin Anat. 2011;24(2):232–6.
27. Ghosh A, Chaudhury S. Morphology of saphenous nerve in cadavers: a guide to saphenous block and surgical interventions. Anat Cell Biol. 2019;52(3):262–8.
28. Thiayagarajan M, Kumar S, Venkatesh S. An exact localization of adductor canal and its clinical significance: a cadaveric study. Anesth Essays Res. 2019;13(2):284–6.
29. Anagnostopoulou S, Anagnostis G, Saranteas T, Mavrogenis AF, Paraskeuopoulos T. Saphenous and infrapatellar nerves at the adductor canal: anatomy and implications in regional anesthesia. Orthopedics. 2016;39(2):e259–62.
30. Patterson DC, Cirino CM, Gladstone JN. No safe zone: the anatomy of the saphenous nerve and its posteromedial branches. Knee. 2019;26(3):660–5.
31. Dunaway DJ, Steensen RN, Wiand W, Dopirak RM. The sartorial branch of the saphenous nerve: its anatomy at the joint line of the knee. Arthroscopy. 2005;21(5):547–51.
32. Wijdicks CA, Westerhaus BD, Brand EJ, Johansen S, Engebretsen L, LaPrade RF. Sartorial branch of the saphenous nerve in relation to a medial knee ligament repair or reconstruction. Knee Surg Sports Traumatol Arthrosc. 2010;18(8):1105–9.
33. Roussignol X, Bertiaux S, Rahali S, Potage D, Duparc F, Dujardin F. Minimally invasive posterior approach in the popliteal fossa for semitendinosus and gracilis tendon harvesting: an anatomic study. Orthop Traumatol Surg Res. 2015;101(2):167–72.
34. Sanders B, Rolf R, McClelland W, Xerogeanes J. Prevalence of saphenous nerve injury after autogenous hamstring harvest: An anatomic and clinical study of sartorial branch injury. Arthroscopy. 2007;23(9):956–63.
35. Arthornthurasook A, Gaew-Im K. The sartorial nerve: its relationship to the medial aspect of the knee. Am J Sports Med. 1990;18(1):41–2.
36. Henry BM, Tomaszewski KA, Pekala PA, Ramakrishnan PK, Taterra D, Saganiak K, et al. The variable emergence of the infrapatellar branch of the saphenous nerve. J Knee Surg. 2017;30(6):585–93.
37. Natsis K, Konstantinidis G, Geropoulos G, Totlis T, Lazaridis N, Tegos T. Transtendinous course of the infrapatellar branch of saphenous nerve. A contribution to the aetiology of entrapment neuropathy and modification of the existing classification. Folia Morphol (Warsz). 2016;75(4):481–5.
38. Riegler G, Jengojan S, Mayer JA, Pivec C, Platzgummer H, Brugger PC, et al. Ultrasound anatomic demonstration of the infrapatellar nerve branches. Arthroscopy. 2018;34(10):2874–83.
39. Walshaw T, Karuppiah SV, Stewart I. The course and distribution of the infra patellar nerve in relation to ACL reconstruction. Knee. 2015;22(5):384–8.
40. Kartus J, Ejerhed L, Eriksson BI, Karlsson J. The localization of the infrapatellar nerves in the anterior knee region with special emphasis on central third patellar tendon harvest: a dissection study on cadaver and amputated specimens. Arthroscopy. 1999;15(6):577–86.
41. Kerver ALA, Leliveld MS, Den Hartog D, Verhofstad MH, Kleinrensink GJ. The surgical anatomy of the infrapatellar branch of the saphenous nerve in relation to incisions for anteromedial knee surgery. J Bone Jt Surg. 2013;95(23):2119–25.
42. Keyurapan E, Phoemphunkunarak W, Lektrakool N. Location of the neurovascular bundle of the knee during flexed and extended position: An MRI study. J Med Assoc Thail. 2016;99(10):1102–9.
43. Zhong S, Li G, Yang L, Yan Q, Wang Y, Zhao G, et al. Anatomic and ultrasonic study based on selective tibial neurotomy. World Neurosurg. 2017;99:214–25.
44. Hwang K, Jin S, Hwang JH, Han SH. Proximity of the common peroneal nerve to the tibial nerve entering the gastrocnemius muscle: the implications for calf reduction. Aesthet Plast Surg. 2008;32(1): 116–9.
45. Moore AM, Krauss EM, Parikh RP, Franco MJ, Tung TH. Femoral nerve transfers for restoring tibial nerve function: An anatomical study and clinical correlation: a report of 2 cases. J Neurosurg. 2018;129(4):1024–33.
46. Horner G, Dellon AL. Innervation of the human knee joint and implications for surgery. Clin Orthop Relat Res. 1994;301:221–6.

47. Ramakrishnan PK, Henry BM, Vikse J, Roy J, Saganiak K, Mizia E, et al. Anatomical variations of the formation and course of the sural nerve: a systematic review and meta-analysis. Ann Anat. 2015;202:36–44.
48. Eid EM, Hegazy AM. Anatomical variations of the human sural nerve and its role in clinical and surgical procedures. Clin Anat. 2011;24(2):237–45.
49. Jeon SK, Paik DJ, Hwang Y. Variations in sural nerve formation pattern and distribution on the dorsum of the foot. Clin Anat. 2017;30(4):525–32.
50. Kavyashree AN, Prabha Subhash L, Asha KR, Bindu Rani MK. Anatomical variations in formation of sural nerve in adult Indian cadavers. J Clin Diagnostic Res. 2013;7(9):1838–41.
51. Blackmon JA, Atsas S, Clarkson MJ, Fox JN, Daney BT, Dodson SC, et al. Locating the sural nerve during calcaneal (Achilles) tendon repair with confidence: a cadaveric study with clinical applications. J Foot Ankle Surg. 2013;52(1):42–7.
52. Amoiridis G, Schöls L, Ameridis N, Przuntek H. Motor fibers in the sural nerve of humans. Neurology. 1997;49(6):1725–8.
53. Hoppenfeld S, DeBoer P, Bucklet R. Surgical exposures in orthopaedics: the anatomic approach. 4th ed. Philadelphia: Lippincott Williams & Wilkins; 2009.
54. McGinty JB, Burkhart SS, editors. Operative arthroscopy. 4th ed. Philadelphia: Lippincott Williams & Wilkins; 2003.
55. Cannon WD, Vittori JM. The incidence of healing in arthroscopic meniscal repairs in anterior cruciate ligament-reconstructed knees versus stable knees. Am J Sports Med. 1992;20(2):176–81.
56. Scott GA, Jolly BL, Henning CE. Combined posterior incision and arthroscopic intra-articular repair of the meniscus. An examination of factors affecting healing. J Bone Jt Surg. 1986;68(6):847–61.
57. Henning CE, Lynch MA, Yearout KM, Vequist SW, Stallbaumer RJ, Decker KA. Arthroscopic meniscal repair using an exogenous fibrin clot. Clin Orthop Relat Res. 1990;252:64–72.
58. Rodeo SA. Arthroscopic meniscal repair with use of the outside-in technique. Instr Course Lect. 2000;49:195–206.
59. Frank RM, Hamamoto JT, Bernardoni E, Cvetanovich G, Bach BR, Verma NN, et al. ACL reconstruction basics: quadruple (4-Strand) hamstring autograft harvest. Arthrosc Tech. 2017;6(4):e1309–13.
60. Mook WR, Ligh CA, Moorman CT, Leversedge FJ. Nerve injury complicating multiligament knee injury: current concepts and treatment algorithm. J Am Acad Orthop Surg. 2013;21(6):343–54.
61. Poage C, Roth C, Scott B. Peroneal nerve palsy: evaluation and management. J Am Acad Orthop Surg. 2016;24(1):1–10.
62. Potter HG, Weinstein M, Allen AA, Wickiewicz TL, Helfet DL. Magnetic resonance imaging of the multiple-ligament injured knee. J Orthop Trauma. 2002;16(5):330–9.
63. Damarey B, Demondion X, Wavreille G, Pansini V, Balbi V, Cotten A. Imaging of the nerves of the knee region. Eur J Radiol. 2013;82(1):27–37.
64. Arnold DMJ, Wilkens SC, Coert JH, Chen NC, Ducic I, Eberlin KR. Diagnostic criteria for symptomatic neuroma. Ann Plast Surg. 2019;82(4):420–7.
65. Du R, Auguste KI, Chin CT, Engstrom JW, Weinstein PR. Magnetic resonance neurography for the evaluation of peripheral nerve, brachial plexus, and nerve root disorders: clinical article. J Neurosurg. 2010;112(2):362–71.
66. Bucklan JN, Morren JA, Shook SJ. Ultrasound in the diagnosis and management of fibular mononeuropathy. Muscle Nerve. 2019;60(5):544–8.
67. Zaidman CM, Seelig MJ, Baker JC, Mackinnon SE, Pestronk A. Detection of peripheral nerve pathology: comparison of ultrasound and MRI. Neurology. 2013;80(18):1634–40.
68. Dvali L, Mackinnon S. Nerve repair, grafting, and nerve transfers. Clin Plast Surg. 2003;30(2):203–21.
69. Gruber H, Peer S, Meirer R, Bodner G. Peroneal nerve palsy associated with knee luxation: evaluation by sonography – initial experiences. Am J Roentgenol. 2005;185(5):1119–25.
70. Bianchi S. Ultrasound of the peripheral nerves. Joint Bone Spine. 2008;24(3):254–8.
71. Gallardo E, Noto YI, Simon NG. Ultrasound in the diagnosis of peripheral neuropathy: structure meets function in the neuromuscular clinic. J Neurol Neurosurg Psychiatry. 2015;86(10):1066–74.
72. Geissler WB, Slade JF. Green's operative hand surgery. Elsevier Health Sciences; 2011.
73. Brogan DM, Kakar S. Management of neuromas of the upper extremity. Hand Clin. 2013;29(3):409–20.
74. Restrepo-Garces CE, Marinov A, McHardy P, Faclier G, Avila A. Pulsed radiofrequency under ultrasound guidance for persistent stump-neuroma pain. Pain Pract. 2011;11(1):98–102.
75. Johnson ME, Foster L, JC DL. Neurologic and vascular injuries associated with knee ligament injuries. Am J Sports Med. 2008;36(12):2448–62.
76. Immerman I, Price AE, Alfonso I, Grossman JA. Lower extremity nerve trauma. Bull Hosp Joint Dis. 2014;72(1):43–52.
77. Khan R, Birch R. Iatropathic injuries of peripheral nerves. J Bone Jt Surg. 2001;83(8):1145–8.
78. Prasad AR, Steck JK, Dellon AL. Zone of traction injury of the common peroneal nerve. Ann Plast Surg. 2007;59(3):302–6.
79. Bratt HD, Newman AP. Complete dislocation of the knee without disruption of both cruciate ligaments. J Trauma. 1993;34(3):383–9.
80. Cooper DE, Speer KP, Wickiewicz TL, Warren RF. Complete knee dislocation without posterior cruciate ligament disruption: a report of four cases and review of the literature. Clin Orthop Relat Res. 1992;284:228–33.

81. Rodeo SA, Forster RA, Weiland AJ. Neurological complications due to arthroscopy. J Bone Jt Surg. 1993;75(6):917–26.
82. Krych AJ, Giuseffi SA, Kuzma SA, Stuart MJ, Levy BA. Is peroneal nerve injury associated with worse function after knee dislocation? Clin Orthop Relat Res. 2014;472(9):2630–6.
83. Plancher KD, Siliski J. Long-term functional results and complications in patients with knee dislocations. J Knee Surg. 2008;21(4):261–8.
84. Peskun CJ, Chahal J, Steinfeld ZY, Whelan DB. Risk factors for peroneal nerve injury and recovery in knee dislocation. Clin Orthop Relat Res. 2012;470(3):774–8.
85. Spinner RJ, Kline DG. Surgery for peripheral nerve and brachial plexus injuries or other nerve lesions. Muscle Nerve. 2000;23(5):680–95.
86. Thoma A, Fawcett S, Ginty M, Veltri K. Decompression of the common peroneal nerve: experience with 20 consecutive cases. Plast Reconstr Surg. 2001;107(5):1183–9.
87. Seidel JA, Koenig R, Antoniadis G, Richter HP, Kretschmer T. Surgical treatment of traumatic peroneal nerve lesions. Neurosurgery. 2008;48(3):105–12.
88. Lee FC, Singh H, Nazarian LN, Ratliff JK. High-resolution ultrasonography in the diagnosis and intra-operative management of peripheral nerve lesions: clinical article. J Neurosurg. 2011;114(1):206–11.
89. Fabre T, Piton C, Andre D, Lasseur E, Durandeau A. Peroneal nerve entrapment. J Bone Jt Surg. 1998;1(2):147–53.
90. Vigasio A, Marcoccio I, Patelli A, Mattiuzzo V, Prestini G. New tendon transfer for correction of drop-foot in common peroneal nerve palsy. Clin Orthop Relat Res. 2008;466(6):1454–66.
91. Boyd K, Fox I. Nerve repair and grafting. In: Mackinnon S, editor. Nerve surgery. 1st ed. New York: Thieme; 2015.
92. George SC, Boyce DE. An evidence-based structured review to assess the results of common peroneal nerve repair. Plast Reconstr Surg. 2014;134(2):302e–11e.
93. Kim DH, Murovic JA, Tiel RL, Kline DC, Benzel EC, McGillicuddy JE, et al. Management and outcomes in 318 operative common peroneal nerve lesions at the Louisiana State University Health Sciences Center. Neurosurgery. 2004;54(6):1421–8.
94. Ray WZ, Mackinnon SE. Management of nerve gaps: autografts, allografts, nerve transfers, and end-to-side neurorrhaphy. Exp Neurol. 2010;223(1):77–85.
95. Siemionow M, Brzezicki G. Chapter 8 current techniques and concepts in peripheral nerve repair. Int Rev Neurobiol. 2009;87:141–72.
96. Weber RV, Boyd KU. Repair and grafting of peripheral nerves. In: Neligan PC, editor. Plastic surgery. Third ed. Elsevier; 2011.
97. Staniforth P, Fisher TR. The effects of sural nerve excision in autogenous nerve grafting. Hand. 1978;10(2):187–90.
98. Terzis JK, Kostopoulos VK. Vascularized nerve grafts for lower extremity nerve reconstruction. Ann Plast Surg. 2010;64(2):169–76.
99. Brown MC, Holland RL, Hopkins WG. Motor nerve sprouting. Annu Rev Neurosci. 1981;4:17–42.
100. Tung TH, Mackinnon SE. Nerve transfers: indications, techniques, and outcomes. J Hand Surg. 2010;35(2):332–41.
101. Pirela-Cruz MA, Hansen U, Terreros DA, Rossum A, West P. Interosseous nerve transfers for tibialis anterior muscle paralysis (foot drop): a human cadaver-based feasibility study. J Reconstr Microsurg. 2009;25(3):203–11.
102. Bodily KD, Spinner RJ, Bishop AT. Restoration of motor function of the deep fibular (peroneal) nerve by direct nerve transfer of branches from the Tibial nerve: an anatomical study. Clin Anat. 2004;17(3):201–5.
103. Giuffre JL, Bishop AT, Spinner RJ, Levy BA, Shin AY. Partial tibial nerve transfer to the tibialis anterior motor branch to treat peroneal nerve injury after knee trauma. Clin Orthop Relat Res. 2012;470(3):779–90.
104. Ferris S, Maciburko SJ. Partial tibial nerve transfer to tibialis anterior for traumatic peroneal nerve palsy. Microsurgery. 2017;37(6):596–602.
105. White CP, Cooper MJ, Bain JR, Levis CM. Axon counts of potential nerve transfer donors for peroneal nerve reconstruction. Can J Plast Surg. 2012;20(1):24–7.
106. Head LK, Hicks K, Wolff G, Boyd KU. Clinical outcomes of nerve transfers in peroneal nerve palsy: a systematic review and meta-analysis. J Reconstr Microsurg. 2019;35(1):57–65.
107. Leclère FM, Badur N, Mathys L, Vögelin E. Nerve transfers for persistent traumatic peroneal nerve palsy: the Inselspital Bern experience. Neurosurgery. 2015;77(4):572–9.
108. Levy BA, Giuseffi SA, Bishop AT, Shin AY, Dahm DL, Stuart MJ. Surgical treatment of peroneal nerve palsy after knee dislocation. Knee Surg Sports Traumatol Arthrosc. 2010;18(11):1583–6.
109. Sundaram RO, Ramakrishnan M, Harvey RA, Parkinson RW. Comparison of scars and resulting hypoaesthesia between the medial parapatellar and midline skin incisions in total knee arthroplasty. Knee. 2007;14(5):375–8.
110. Borley NR, Edwards D, Villar RN. Lateral skin flap numbness after total knee arthroplasty. J Arthroplast. 1995;10(1):13–4.
111. Gali JC, Resina AF, Pedro G, Neto IAM, Almagro MA, da Silva PA, et al. Importance of anatomically locating the infrapatellar branch of the saphenous nerve in reconstructing the anterior cruciate ligament using flexor tendons. Rev Bras Ortop. 2014;49(6):625–9.
112. Johnson RJ, Kettelkamp DB, Clark W, Leaverton P. Factors effecting late results after meniscectomy. J Bone Jt Surg. 1974;56(4):719–29.

113. Dellon AL, Mackinnon SE. Treatment of the painful neuroma by neuroma resection and muscle implantation. Plast Reconstr Surg. 1986;77(3):427–38.
114. Xiang Y, Li Z, Yu P, Zheng Z, Feng B, Weng X. Neuroma of the infrapatellar branch of the saphenous nerve following total knee arthroplasty: a case report. BMC Musculoskelet Disord. 2019;20(1):536.
115. Kim NH, Kang HJ, Hong SH, Park BK, Lee JH, Park JW, et al. A case of subcutaneous neuroma presenting with intractable pain and allodynia over the anteromedial aspect of the knee. Clin J Pain. 2012;28(7):635–8.
116. Heare A, Mitchell JJ, Bravman JT. Posttraumatic saphenous neuroma after open tibial fracture. Am J Orthop. 2015;44(11):E461–4.
117. Harris JD, Fazalare JJ, Griesser MJ, Flanigan DC. Infrapatellar branch of saphenous neurectomy for painful neuroma: a case report. Am J Orthop. 2012;41(1):37–40.
118. Nelissen E, van Arkel ERA, Hazelbag HM. Traumatic neuroma of the infrapatellar branch of the saphenous nerve after hamstring harvesting. J Knee Surg. 2010;23(4):233–6.
119. Ducic I, Levin M, Larson EE, Al-Attar A. Management of chronic leg and knee pain following surgery or trauma related to saphenous nerve and knee neuromata. Ann Plast Surg. 2010;64(1):35–40.
120. Kim DH, Cho YJ, Ryu S, Tiel RL, Kline DG, Huang JH, et al. Surgical management and results of 135 Tibial nerve lesions at the Louisiana State University Health Sciences Center. Neurosurgery. 2003;53(5):1114–24.
121. Rasulić L, Savić A, Vitošević F, Samardžić M, Živković B, Mićović M, et al. Iatrogenic peripheral nerve injuries—surgical treatment and outcome: 10 years' experience. World Neurosurg. 2017;103:841–51.
122. Kowalska J, Grabowski R, Pigonska J, Domzalski M. Management of an iatrogenic injury to the tibial nerve in a 24-year-old hurdle runner. J Int Med Res. 2018;46(8):3394–403.
123. Abdul-Jabar HB, Bhamra J, Quick TJ, Fox M. Iatrogenic posterior tibial nerve division during a combined anterior ankle arthroscopy with an additional posterolateral portal. J Surg Case Rep. 2016;2016(5):rjw097.
124. Freedman DM, Barron OA. Iatrogenic posterior tibial nerve division during ankle arthroscopy. Arthroscopy. 1998;14(7):769–72.
125. Wendt MC, Spinner RJ, Shin AY. Iatrogenic transection of the peroneal and partial transection of the tibial nerve during arthroscopic lateral meniscal debridement and removal of osteochondral fragment. Am J Orthop (Belle Mead NJ). 2014;43(4):182–5.
126. Murovic JA. Lower-extremity peripheral nerve injuries: a Louisiana State University Health Sciences Center literature review with comparison of the operative outcomes of 806 Louisiana State University Health Sciences Center sciatic, common peroneal, and tibial nerve. Neurosurgery. 2009;65(4 Suppl):A18–23.
127. Koshima I, Nanba Y, Tsutsui T, Takahashi Y. Deep peroneal nerve transfer for established plantar sensory loss. J Reconstr Microsurg. 2003;19(7):451–4.
128. Yin G, Chen H, Hou C, Xiao J, Lin H. Obturator nerve transfer to the branch of the tibial nerve innervating the gastrocnemius muscle for the treatment of sacral plexus nerve injury. Neurosurgery. 2016;78(4):546–51.
129. Agarwal P, Shukla P, Sharma D. Saphenous nerve transfer: a new approach to restore sensation of the sole. J Plast Reconstr Aesthetic Surg. 2018;71(12):1704–10.

16 Nerve Injury After Distal Tibia, Pilon, and Ankle Fractures

Jay T. Bridgeman and Kyle Schweser

16.1 Risks/Incidence/Mechanism of Injury

16.1.1 Sural Nerve

For surgical procedures around the ankle, the sural nerve is at greatest risk during any operation involving the posterolateral aspect of the ankle. Several surgical approaches are utilized; however, the most common is the posterolateral approach to the distal tibia. This approach is increasing in popularity as more literature is published in support of surgical fixation of posterior malleolar fractures [1–4]. No study has specifically examined sural nerve injuries during ankle fracture fixation; however, several have reported the incidence of sural nerve injury when examining outcomes from fracture fixation. In these studies, injury to the sural nerve occurs in 2.6–5.5% of patients during a posterolateral approach [1–3]. The relative risk during this surgical approach has been confirmed by anatomic studies. One anatomic study of 40 individuals utilized ultrasound to map the course of the nerve. At the level of the lateral malleolus, the risk of injury was high – damage to the nerve could occur anywhere from 66 to 100% of the time during surgical dissection, depending on the location of the incision [5]. A specific mechanism of injury to the nerve is rarely discussed; however, transection is a likely cause, especially in cases where the nerve was never directly visualized. Only one paper commented on the resolution of symptoms; however, in that paper three out of four patients had resolution of numbness at final follow-up [3]. This may indicate that neurapraxia is also a contributing factor to postoperative complications involving the sural nerve.

Minimally invasive/endoscopic procedures carried an ever higher risk of injury when compared to open techniques [6]. The incidence of sural injury with percutaneous Achilles tendon repair has been reported at 18% [7]; all injuries occurred in the group that did not undergo exploration of the nerve. Other studies examining Achilles tendon repair found an injury rate of anywhere from 0% to 40%, with most studies reporting some sural nerve complications. In a cadaveric study of 107 lower limbs, location of the nerve was examined as it crossed the lateral border of the Achilles tendon, where the nerve is at the highest risk for injury in Achilles tendon repair surgery. This study showed that the nerve reliably crossed the lateral border of the Achilles

J. T. Bridgeman (✉)
Division Chief Hand and Microvascular Surgery, Department of Orthopedic Surgery, University of Missouri, Columbia, MO, USA
e-mail: bridgemanj@health.missouri.edu

K. Schweser
Division Chief Foot and Ankle Surgery, Department of Orthopedic Surgery, University of Missouri, Columbia, MO, USA
e-mail: schweserk@health.missouri.edu

C. J. Dy et al. (eds.), *Peripheral Nerve Issues after Orthopedic Surgery*,
https://doi.org/10.1007/978-3-030-84428-8_16

tendon 8–10 centimeters proximal to the superior border of the calcaneal tuberosity [8].

16.1.2 Superficial Peroneal Nerve

The superficial peroneal nerve is unique compared to other nerves around the ankle as it is at high risk for injury at multiple locations, particularly in three common surgical approaches. These include the lateral approach to the fibula, the anterolateral approach to the distal tibia, and the creation of the anterolateral ankle arthroscopy portal. Despite these risks, the outcomes from injury are poorly documented in the literature.

A direct lateral approach to the fibula is commonly performed for fibular fracture fixation. During this approach, the superficial peroneal nerve is at greatest risk in the proximal aspect of the dissection. The data is limited on the overall risk during this approach. One retrospective review examined both operative and nonoperative treatment of ankle fractures, with 120 patients returning for final follow-up. Forty-three out of the 120 (36%) were found to have an injury to the superficial peroneal nerve. As expected, the operative group experienced a higher incidence of nerve injury (36%), but only 12 of these 20 patients were symptomatic. Interestingly, 13 of the nonoperative cases (20%) also had some form of nerve injury, 6 of which were symptomatic. No patient with a posterolateral approach to the fibula experienced superficial peroneal nerve injury; however, no comments were made regarding the sural nerve [9]. Overall, nerve injury following fibular fixation is likely underreported, or under recognized, as not all nerve injuries are symptomatic. Unlike the sural nerve, superficial peroneal nerve injury is not consistently reported in the literature describing outcomes for ankle fracture fixation. One study examining lateral plating of distal tibia fractures through a lateral fibular approach had a 5% incidence of nerve dysfunction [10]

The anterolateral approach also places the superficial peroneal nerve at risk. This approach is typically utilized for fixation of the distal tibia in pilon fractures or for reduction of the syndesmosis. Despite the fact that the nerve is identified during this approach, the incidence of injury is not well documented in the literature. No studies exist that examine the rate of injury, and nerve injury is rarely commented on during outcome studies following pilon fixation. The risk is often discussed in book chapters, but empirical evidence is lacking.

Finally anterolateral portal placement for ankle arthroscopy has a well-documented risk of injury to the superficial peroneal nerve. Injury to this nerve is the most common complication in ankle arthroscopy, with an incidence rate of 1–8% [11–19]. The branch at highest risk during portal placement is the medial branch of the superficial peroneal nerve [13]. A cadaveric study of 100 lower extremities found the nerve was present in the area of the anterolateral portal 82% of the time [20]. In another cadaveric study, almost 40% of ankles had branches of the nerve within 2 millimeters of the lateral border of peroneus tertius, a common landmark for portal placement [21].

16.1.3 Tibial Nerve

The tibial nerve is not typically directly visualized in surgeries around the ankle for fracture fixation. While some surgical approaches exist that utilize the tibial nerve as an interval landmark, for example, the modified posteromedial approach described by Assal et al., most do not involve directly identifying the nerve itself [22, 23]. Another instance of tibial nerve exposure would be during a release of the tarsal tunnel for tarsal tunnel syndrome. The typical approach to the posteromedial aspect of the ankle will either remain medial to the posterior tibial tendon or lateral to the flexor hallucis longus. In both of these approaches, the nerve is retracted with the associated muscles, depending on the approach. Due to this fact, retraction injuries to the tibial nerve are likely the most common. Similar to other nerves in this chapter, the injury rate is poorly documented in the literature. Single patient case reports exist regarding tibial nerve injury in ankle arthroscopy and ankle arthroplasty

[22–27]. Large case reports, case series, and even tibial nerve injury listed as a secondary complication in fracture fixation surgery are rare in the current literature. Authors who frequently utilize posteromedial approaches do discuss their experience with neuropraxia; however, specifically published literature on fixation through a posteromedial approach does not describe any neurological deficits [28–31]. In one retrospective review of total ankle arthroplasty, the authors found that 9 out of 150 total ankles experienced a tibial nerve injury [23]. Another anatomic study examining pin placement in total ankle arthroplasty found that almost all anterior to posterior pins placed in the proximal-medial aspect of the distal tibia came into contact with the neurovascular structures, most commonly the nerve [32].

While reported injuries are rare in the literature, the risk to this nerve can easily be inferred given its proximity to the other structures in the posteromedial ankle and its tethering between the posterior tibia and the flexor retinaculum. Surgical approaches in the area are rare, when compared to other surgical approaches around the ankle. This, combined with the close proximity to the artery, likely contribute to the low rate of reported injury as surgeons may tend to be more meticulous in this area or avoid it all together. The greatest risk to injury likely involves the sensory branches of the nerve, as this is the greatest variation in anatomy.

16.2 Deep Peroneal Nerve

The deep peroneal nerve is at greatest risk during any approach involving the anterior aspect of the ankle. Direct exposure of the nerve is utilized for ankle arthroplasty and ankle arthrodesis but limited data exists on nerve injury during these approaches [33, 34]. However, several studies exist regarding the risk of injury to the deep peroneal nerve during minimally invasive fracture fixation and arthroscopy. In one cadaveric study examining minimally invasive plate insertion for tibial plateau fractures, the authors found that the nerve was in direct contact with the plate between the 11th and 13th holes in 18 out of 18 legs. Of those 18 specimens, the nerve was actually interposed between the plate and bone in 6 legs [35]. This has relevance to this chapter as the 13-hole LISS plate frequently extends down to the distal tibia where the injury occurs. In another cadaveric study specifically looking at plate fixation of the distal tibia through an anterolateral approach, the deep peroneal nerve (along with the artery) is at risk during plate insertion. In ten legs, they found that the nerve was intimately associated with the anterior aspect of the plate as it crossed over the anterior aspect of the distal tibia [36]. In this study, they showed that neurovascular injury was at risk unless plate insertion is performed carefully with the plate in constant contact with the bone. A retrospective review of 150 primary total ankle arthroplasty cases found that nerve injury occurred in 23 patients (15%). Of those 23, 6 injuries occurred to the deep peroneal nerve [23]. Other literature involving total ankle arthroplasty reported the risk of deep peroneal nerve injury from 1.7% to 6% [37–40].

In ankle arthroscopy, several studies describe injury to the deep peroneal nerve. In 1 study of 79 ankles, 2 patients developed deep peroneal nerve neuropraxia [15]. In another study of 20 cadaver specimen, the arthroscope touched the neurovascular bundle and in some cases transected the deep peroneal nerve [41]. The nerve is at greatest risk during the antero-central portal placement [42].

16.2.1 Saphenous Nerve

The saphenous nerve is often at risk during medial approaches to the ankle for ankle fracture fixation. The nerve is not typically well visualized, as the terminal branches are relatively small. Because of this, there is a high rate of injury to branches of the nerve. In one cadaveric study, ten out of ten legs had an injury to the saphenous nerve with medial plate fixation of the tibia, consistently occurring 2–4.7 centimeters from the tip of the medial malleolus [43]. In another study looking at 612 ankle arthroscopy procedures, the saphenous nerve was injured 18% of the time [11].

16.3 Pertinent Anatomy

16.3.1 Sural Nerve

The sural nerve receives its innervation from both the common peroneal and tibia nerve (L5/S1). The anatomical location of the sural nerve varies around the ankle, to a degree. Several anatomic studies have been performed utilizing different methods. One cadaveric study of 17 lower limbs found that the nerve had a consistent course and was in close proximity to the Achilles tendon at 7 centimeters proximal to the tip of the lateral malleolus, crossing laterally to a point 14 millimeters posterior and 14 millimeters inferior to the tip of the lateral malleolus [44]. A second cadaveric study of 12 legs examined the location of the nerve with respect to the posterolateral incision. An incision was made at a point midway between the lateral malleolus and the Achilles tendon, starting at the tip of the lateral malleolus and extending proximally. They found that the sural nerve, along with the lesser saphenous vein, crossed the incision around 6–7 millimeters from the distal aspect of the incision. However, they noted that the nerve was at risk throughout the entire length of the incision [45]. Another study utilizing magnetic resonance imaging examined the position of the nerve from the posterior border of the fibula at three different heights along the lateral malleolus. At the level of the tip of the fibula, the nerve had an average location of 1.6 centimeters medial to the posterior border of the fibula. The nerve was within 2 centimeters of the posterior border of the fibula at a point 3 centimeters proximal to the tip of the fibula. This again highlights the close relationship of the nerve to the fibula and the risk for iatrogenic injury during the posterolateral approach [46].

One consistent finding of the sural nerve during the posterolateral approach is its location in the soft tissue layer. As seen in Fig. 16.1, the nerve can be found within the subcutaneous fat, in contrast to the superficial peroneal nerve that lies directly on the fascia during an anterolateral approach. The sural nerve can also be found in close proximity to the lesser saphenous vein; however, its location in relation to the vein can vary [47]. Unlike other approaches to the ankle, no tendinous landmarks will be directly visualized when attempting to locate the nerve; however, palpating the peroneal tendons and Achilles tendon can give the surgeon a clue to its potential anatomic location. As the incision is carried proximally and medially, the nerve is located deeper and more intimately associated with the crural fascia.

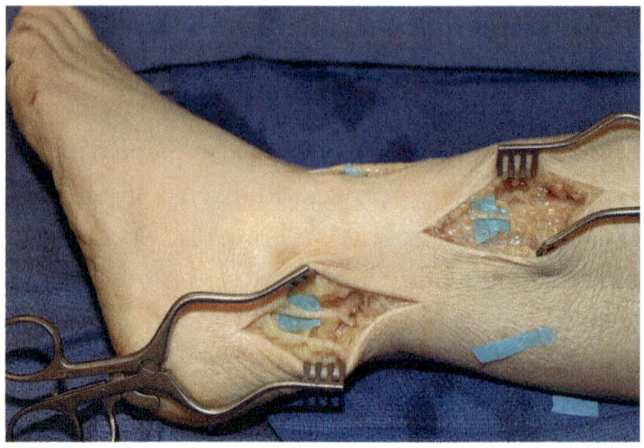

Fig. 16.1 Sural nerve shown through posterolateral approach to the ankle (in lower portion of figure). It is identified in relation to the lesser saphenous vein and the tip of the distal fibula

16.3.1.1 Superficial Peroneal Nerve

While the risk of injury is poorly documented in the literature, there are several anatomic studies regarding the superficial peroneal nerve. The nerve is a branch of the common peroneal nerve, which itself branches from the sciatic nerve (L4, L5, S1). The nerve is quite variable, both in its location around the ankle and in the number of branches, if any, that it gives off. In general, the nerve traverses the lateral aspect of the leg between the fibula and peroneus longus muscle before heading to the most anterior aspect of the lateral compartment – eventually piercing the fascia to cross anteriorly onto the anterolateral aspect of the lower leg and ankle as demonstrated in Fig. 16.2-. It typically has two terminal branches, the medial dorsal cutaneous and intermediate dorsal cutaneous nerve. One cadaveric study noted that 54 of the 66 legs had at least 1 branch and the location of the branching was variable, with 50 occurring prior to piercing the fascia. The nerve reached the ankle joint with no branches in 12 legs [48]. In another cadaveric study of 111 legs, it was noted that there were

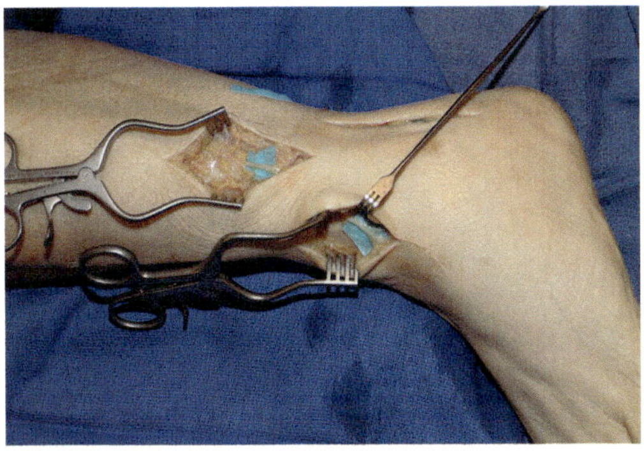

Fig. 16.2- Superficial peroneal nerve shown through lateral approach to the leg (shown in the two wounds with Weitlaner retractors). It is identified in relation to the fibula and the peroneus longus tendon at the lateral compartment

four distinct anatomic variations of the superficial peroneal nerve at the level of the ankle [49]. Despite the anatomic variation, the nerve tends to be located within the lateral compartment of the leg [49, 50]. This is the location that the nerve is at risk during the lateral approach to the fibula. The location where the nerve crosses the fibula, from a posterior to anterior direction, also varies. However, on average, it can be found 11 centimeters proximal to the tip of the fibula. There is a wide range of variation, with some studies documenting this location around 6 centimeters proximal to the tip [51, 52]. In general, the safe zone for full-thickness surgical approaches is from the tip of the fibula to 5 centimeters proximal; beyond that, careful attention should be paid for locating the nerve.

The termination of the superficial peroneal nerve varies, as well, and this is where the nerve is at highest risk during both the anterolateral approach and anterolateral arthroscopy. The branch at highest risk during the anterolateral approach is the intermediate dorsal cutaneous nerve, whereas both branches are at risk during portal placement. The termination of the nerve is divided into three different types. Type A, the most common, divides into two branches roughly 4 centimeters proximal to the ankle joint. Types B and C are similar in which the nerve divides into both branches independently in the calf, and the medial cutaneous branch assumes the typical anatomic course for the superficial peroneal nerve proper. The difference between the type B and type C is the location of the intermediate dorsal cutaneous nerve. In type B variants, the intermediate branch pierces the crural fascia posterior to the fibula and then crosses about 4.5 centimeters proximal to the ankle joint (not the tip of the fibula). In type C variants, the intermediate branch pierces the crural fascia anterior to the fibula [53]. Since this study, other anatomic variants have been described, but these three types remain the most common.

Unlike the sural nerve, the superficial peroneal nerve is typically found in close proximity, if not directly anterior, to the lower leg fascia. The nerve tends to pierce the crural fascia and stay in close proximity to the fascia. Even as the nerve moves anteriorly over the ankle, seen in Fig. 16.3, it lies in close proximity to the extensor retinaculum. The course of the nerve from the lateral compartment to the anterior compartment can be appreciated in Fig. 16.4. However, this should not provide a sense of comfort with surgical dissection, as the majority of structures in the lateral and anterior ankle are relatively subcutaneous. In fact, in the anterolateral aspect of the ankle, the nerve can be well visualized and even palpated under the skin.

16.3.1.2 Tibial Nerve

Unlike other nerves in the lower leg, the anatomy of the tibial nerve around the ankle is relatively constant. In the absence of distorted anatomy

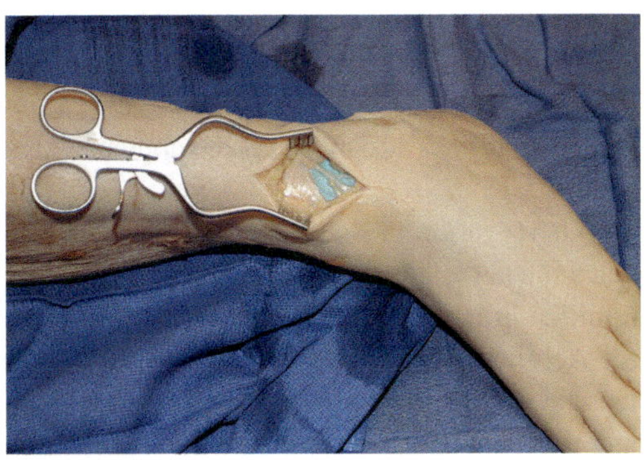

Fig. 16.3 Superficial peroneal nerve shown at the anterolateral ankle. It is identified in relation to the extensor retinaculum

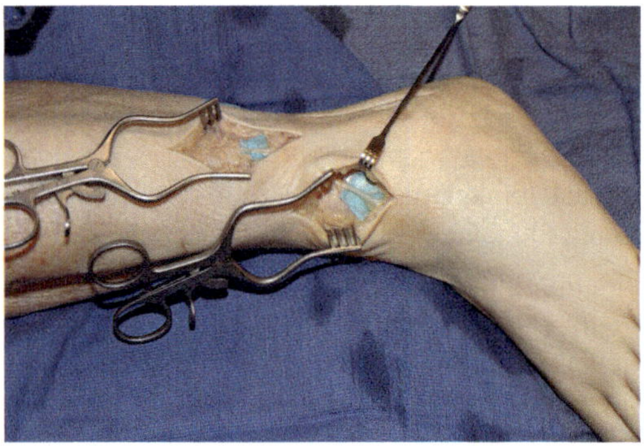

Fig. 16.4 Superficial peroneal nerve shown at the lateral ankle. It is identified as it transitions from the lateral compartment to the anterior compartment

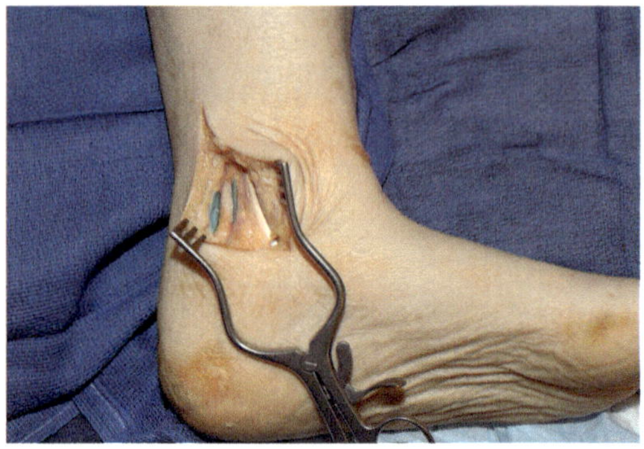

Fig. 16.5 Tibial nerve shown through the medial approach to the ankle. It is identified in relation to the posterior tibialis tendon, flexor digitorum longus tendon, posterior tibial artery, and vein which lie medial to the nerve. The flexor hallucis longus tendon is lateral to the nerve

(i.e., tumor, trauma), its location can be easily determined based on tendinous anatomy. The tibial nerve is a branch of the sciatic nerve (L4-S3). By the time the nerve reaches the level of the ankle, it has innervated the major muscles of the lower leg and foot. Its major function at the level of the ankle is to provide innervation to smaller intrinsic foot muscles (foot lumbricals/interossei, etc.) and plantar sensation. Little is known regarding variations of the nerve within the retromalleolar space, but the anatomy is thought to be generally constant, with the nerve lateral to the artery/vein (which itself is lateral to flexor digitorum longus) and medial to flexor hallucis longus. A common phrase regarding the anatomy of the medial ankle is "Tom, Dick, and A Very Nervous Harry." Each letter represents the location of an important structure, moving from medial to lateral: posterior tibialis (Tom), flexor digitorum longus (Dick), posterior tibial artery (A) and vein (Very), tibial nerve (Nervous), and flexor hallucis longus (Harry). The close proximity to the vascular and tendinous structures can be appreciated in Fig. 16.5.

Where variation does occur is in regard to when the nerve begins to branch into its separate terminal branches and its location in relation to the Achilles tendon. One cadaveric study of 50 legs found that the nerve bifurcated into medial and lateral plantar nerves inside the retinaculum 88% of the time, and there is extensive variation in the location of this bifurcation in relation to the joint[4747]. This important finding indicates additional tibial nerve branches may be at risk while mobilizing the tibial nerve and artery. Identification and release of the retinaculum requires caution as bifurcation of the nerve may have already occurred with nerve branches being superficial to the retinaculum. These branches become more superficial as they extend distally, with the lateral plantar nerve more superficial than the medial plantar nerve [54]. More reports regarding anatomic variation of the tibial nerve are found in the arthroscopy literature. Several studies attempt to identify where the nerve is in relation to palpable structures such as the Achilles tendon and medial malleolus, to allow for safe portal placement. According to these studies, the nerve can typically be found anywhere from 10–14 millimeters medial to the medial border of the Achilles tendon, at the level of the joint, with the average around 11 millimeters. That distance increases at the level of the medial malleolus to over 14 millimeters in one study [54–56].

16.3.2 Deep Peroneal Nerve

The deep peroneal nerve is a branch of the common peroneal nerve, which is a branch of the sciatic (L4-S1). The location of the deep peroneal nerve in the anterior aspect of the ankle is relatively constant. In one anatomic study of 17 specimens, the nerve was located superficial to the anterior tibia artery, lying between the tibialis anterior and extensor hallucis longus. It crossed deep to the extensor hallucis longus tendon to enter the interval between the extensor hallucis longus and extensor digitorum longus roughly 12.5 millimeters proximal to the ankle [57]. At the level of the ankle joint, the neurovascular bundle can reliably be found between the extensor hallucis longus and extensor digitorum brevis as seen in Fig. 16.6. In one study, the nerve was found in this interval in 76% of specimens. However, even when not situated in this interval, the nerve was either directly posterior to the extensor hallucis longus or extensor digitorum longus, making location of the nerve based on other anatomic landmarks relatively easy [42]. It is also typically associated with the anterior tibial artery, with one study noting that it was only not associated with the artery when no artery was present. In that same study, they found that the majority of the time the nerve was located lateral to the vascular structures [42]. The nerve does bifurcate, and this typically occurs distal to the ankle joint. However, in a cadaveric study of 34 limbs, 1 specimen (2.9%) bifurcated proximal to the ankle joint and 4 bifurcated at the level of the joint (11.8%). The remaining nerves either bifurcated distal to the ankle joint or did not bifurcate at all [58]. The nerve is in close contact with the bone, lying deep to the retinaculum and tendinous structures. Careful periosteal dissection is required on the anterior aspect of the tibia to avoid injury to this nerve.

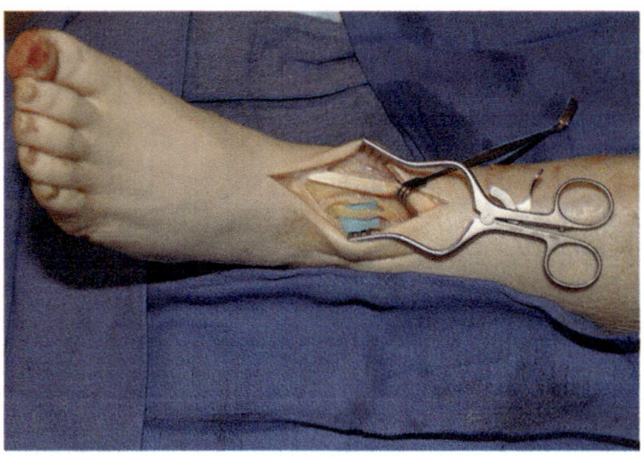

Fig. 16.6 Deep peroneal nerve shown through the anterior approach to the ankle. The nerve is identified between the extensor hallucis longus tendon medially and the extensor digitorum brevis tendon laterally

16.3.3 Saphenous Nerve

The nerve is the terminal extension of the femoral nerve (L3/4) and runs posterior to the greater saphenous vein in the lower leg. There are typically two branches in the distal leg, an anterior and posterior branch. These branches arise approximately 3 cm proximal to the medial malleolus with each branch terminating in their respective aspects of the medial malleolus. The anterior branch is typically associated with the greater saphenous vein. At the level of the medial malleolus, the nerve is not well visualized secondary to its size. In one cadaveric study, the average distance from the distal most visualized aspect of the nerve to the tip of medial malleolus measured 8 millimeters with only one specimen noted to have any visual branches of the nerve extending to the foot [59].

16.4 Prevention Strategies

Posterolateral approach to the ankle (sural nerve)

- While the anatomical location of the sural nerve varies, it can still predictably be found in the distal aspect of the incision at the level of the tip of the fibula.
- Preoperative measurements with markings on the skin are a helpful reminder of described nerve location. In this case, a measurement of roughly 15 millimeters proximal from the tip of the fibula, and 15 millimeters medial from the posterior border of the fibula, will give you a rough estimate of the location of the nerve as it crosses the field.
- The nerve is located in the subcutaneous fat, so careful incision of the dermal layer should be utilized with blunt dissection through the subcutaneous fat.
- In obese patients with excessive subcutaneous fat, locating the small saphenous vein may be a useful landmark. The vein has multiple

branches that cross the field and usually require ligation. Location of the main venous trunk can aid in locating the sural nerve.
- The nerve should be mobilized in order to prevent neurapraxia. Tenotomy scissors can be used to perform a neurolysis, thus mobilizing the nerve enough to allow for full exposure.
- Care must be taken when closing the distal aspect of the incision, especially in patients with little subcutaneous fat, in order to avoid tethering the nerve with suture.

Achilles tendon repair (sural nerve)
- For percutaneous repair, sutures should never be passed percutaneously from the lateral side. A nick-and-spread technique should be utilized.
- During any endoscopic treatment for Achilles pathology, a nick-and-spread technique should be utilized, and the endoscope should not be passed until the tendon is well visualized.
- When performing an open repair, the sural nerve should be identified as it crosses the lateral border of the Achilles and traced both proximally and distally.
- Small flaps can be raised laterally to ensure that the sural nerve is mobilized and completely free of the Achilles tendon.
- The nerve should be mobilized, with vessel loops used for identification and protection of the nerve.

Lateral approach to the fibula (superficial peroneal nerve)
- While anatomic variation occurs, the safe area typically extends from the tip of fibula proximally by about 5 centimeters. In this area, full-thickness flaps are generally safe.
- Once the fascia is encountered distally, blunt dissection can be safely performed as the incision is extended proximally. The superficial peroneal nerve is typically located in the anterior soft tissue flap.
- In general, if the fascia can be visualized, it can be safely incised. However, care should be taken to release only the fascia and nothing deep to it.
- The nerve is typically found crossing the fibula 11 centimeters proximal to the tip of the fibula. The nerve should be traced to where it pierces the fascia, and the fascia around the nerve should be released to allow for mobilization.
- It is important to remember that if the nerve is crossing the fibula, it is doing so in a posterior/proximal to anterior/distal direction, and dissection should occur in a similar direction when performing the neurolysis.
- If the nerve is not encountered, it does not have to be located and dissected in the anterior soft tissue flap.

Anterolateral approach to the distal tibia
- The incision for this approach is typically located in line with the fourth metatarsal.
- Prior to incision, plantarflex the ankle and fourth toe, while inverting the foot. This places the nerve on tension allowing visualization in the soft tissue, especially in patients with minimal swelling and subcutaneous fat [60].
- There is very little soft tissue in the anterior ankle, so dissection is minimal. When utilized for pilon fractures, full-thickness flaps are generally preferred, so a nick-and-spread technique may not be desirable.
- The authors' preferred method is to make a full-thickness incision through the dermis and then utilize a freer elevator to dissect through the fat, in line with the incision.
- Once the extensor retinaculum is located, the nerve is easily appreciated overlying it.
- Caution should be exercised once the nerve has been isolated secondary to the anatomic variation of the nerve. Identifying one branch does not mean it is the only branch within the surgical field.
- Once the nerve has been isolated, it should be freed both proximally and distally utilizing tenotomy scissors.
- The nerve should be completely untethered prior to extension of the approach with fascial incisions and muscle retraction in order to prevent a neurapraxia.
- Blunt, non-self-retraining retractors should be utilized, both for the nerve and soft tissue.

Anterolateral arthroscopy portals (superficial peroneal nerve)

- Prior to application of the ankle distractor, if applicable, a similar method of plantarflexion, as described in the previous section, should be utilized to identify the course of the nerve.
- If the peroneus tertius is palpable, then the portal should be placed 2 millimeters lateral to the tendon at the level of the joint. This has been shown to be the safest location in anatomic studies [21].
- Movement of the ankle can change the location of the nerve. When visualizing the nerve in plantarflexion, it has been shown to translate laterally when dorsiflexing the ankle. This should be kept in mind if the nerve is marked in a plantarflexed position, but the portal is made in neutral ankle position [61].
- Only the skin should be incised with the scalpel. The remainder of the dissection should be done with blunt technique.

Posteromedial approach to the ankle (tibial nerve)

- The posterior tibia can be exposed without direct visualization of the neurovascular bundle. However, excessive retraction should be avoided and exposure of the neurovascular bundle may be required to facilitate more extensive exposure [28].
- If dissection of the nerve is necessary, a good landmark is the posterior tibial vein and flexor digitorum longus tendon. The flexor digitorum longus can typically be palpated lateral to the posterior tibial tendon, allowing for a safe release of the retinaculum. The vein can be easily located after release of the retinaculum. The nerve is reliably lateral to the vein.
- Another landmark is the flexor hallucis longus muscle, which is readily identified as the most distal muscle belly in this location. The flexor hallucis longus can be safely retracted once the overlying fascia is released and the nerve is reliably medial to this structure.
- As the incision moves distally in the retromalleolar space, care should be taken to look for the cutaneous branches of the medial plantar nerve. These are very superficial and will not typically be encountered for an approach to the distal tibia for pilon and ankle fractures.
- While performing fracture fixation in this area, a vessel loop should be utilized to protect the neurovascular bundle.
- Arthroscopy portals should be placed with a nick-and-spread technique. As long as the portal remains in contact with bone along the medial malleolus, or within 10 millimeters of the medial aspect of the Achilles tendon, damage to the nerve can be limited.
- Retractors should always be placed along bone in the retromalleolar space when performing any osteotomy of the medial malleolus.

When utilizing an osteotome or saw blade to make a cut from an anterior to posterior direction, our preferred technique is to use fluoroscopy, guides that prevent penetration, and small posteromedial incisions with retractor placement to prevent injury to the nerve. Anterior approach **to the ankle (deep peroneal nerve)**

- When performing an anterior approach to the ankle, safe anatomic landmarks can guide you to the nerve.
  - Extensor digitorum longus
  - Extensor hallucis longus
- Between these two anatomic structures is typically where the nerve is located, and dissection lateral to the vascular structures will allow location of the nerve.
- When performing an anterolateral or anteromedial approach to the tibia and no identification of the nerve is required, then careful subperiosteal dissection is necessary to prevent injury to the nerve as it lies in intimate contact with the anterior tibia at the level of the ankle.
- When placing arthroscopy portals, a nick-and-spread technique should be utilized.
- Portal placement immediately lateral to the extensor hallucis longus should be avoided.

Medial approach to the tibia (saphenous nerve)

- While the saphenous nerve is not typically well visualized, the vein is. Preservation of the main branch of the greater saphenous vein will typically allow for indirect preservation of the nerve.
- Location of the main branch of the vein prior to incision can help preserve the nerve, which typically runs posterior to the vein.
- During arthroscopy portal placement, location of the vein, with a nick-and-spread technique anterior to the vein, will limit neurological injury.
- When performing percutaneous plate fixation on the medial tibia, careful dissection/mobilization of the saphenous vein proximally will allow for safer plate placement.
- Medial distal tibial plate placement should be performed subperiosteally when possible, and the soft tissue should be elevated prior to plate placement.

Natural History

At the ankle level, the sural, superficial peroneal, saphenous, and deep peroneal nerves are primarily sensory fibers with exception of the motor branches from the deep peroneal nerve to the extensor digitorum brevis muscle and extensor hallucis brevis [62]. Nerve injury leads to decreased sensation in the distal dermatomes of these nerves. Patients with tibial nerve injury at the ankle can develop morbidity from plantar insensate areas or a neuroma involving the weight bearing surface of the foot [62]. Denervated intrinsic musculature of the foot creates an imbalance with the extrinsic muscles leading to clawing of the toes. Deep peroneal nerve injury causes toe extension weakness which is well tolerated. Both the deep peroneal nerve and superficial peroneal nerve injury can lead to painful neuroma of the dorsal foot exacerbated with shoe wear. Sural and saphenous nerve injury can lead to neuroma formation as well. Prospective studies evaluating the sequelae of sural nerve autograft harvest as well as saphenous nerve symptoms after vein graft harvest have shown that many patients may do well in the long term [63, 64].

Initial Evaluation for Nerve Injury

- Timely and accurate diagnosis is crucial to good outcomes [65].
- Elicit a careful history of trauma or prior surgery that correlates to suspected site of nerve injury.
- Identify mechanism of injury.
- Identify timing of injury.
- Seek to understand prior treatment – obtain surgical reports.
- A positive Tinel's sign may identify the location of a suspected nerve injury.
- Document sensory deficits and motor weakness.
- Partial nerve deficits can indicate partial injury or resolving neurapraxia.

Diagnostic Tests/Imaging

- EMG/NCS should be obtained 6 weeks after an injury – consider serial studies if initial tests show signs of recovery.
- Ultrasound is an inexpensive and useful study when the diagnosis is unclear. Ultrasound can confirm the diagnosis and location of complete or partial nerve injury/neuroma. Diagnostic accuracy of ultrasound can be limited by edema and/or obesity [66].
- MRI can also aid in confirming the diagnosis of nerve injury and surgical planning but has not been found to be as sensitive compared to EMG/NCS [66].

Nerve Surgical Technique

Techniques to treat nerve injury at the ankle level include direct repair, neurolysis, and nerve grafting. There are no current reports of nerve transfer for nerve injury at the ankle level. The preoperative plan should include preparation for primary nerve repair or nerve grafting, depending on the length of damaged nerve. Knowledge of internal nerve fascicular topography is required for successful alignment of nerve ends. The sural nerve, superficial peroneal nerve, saphenous nerve, and deep peroneal nerve at the ankle level mostly contain sensory fibers (with exception of deep peroneal motor branches to the extensor digitorum brevis and extensor hallucis brevis muscles). The tibial nerve contains both motor and sensory fibers with predictable anatomy at this level including the lateral plantar nerve branch, medial plantar nerve branch, and calcaneal nerve branch as described by Lumsden et al. (Fig. 16.7) [67]. The position of the lateral plantar nerve branch in relation to the longitudinal axis of the tibial nerve changes along the course of the tibial nerve in the ankle. In the proximal ankle, the lateral plantar nerve branch lies posterior and lateral to the longitudinal axis of the tibial nerve. In the distal ankle, the lateral plantar nerve branch lies posterior and medial to the longitudinal axis of the tibial nerve. The medial plantar nerve branch is found most commonly anterior to the longitudinal axis of the tibial nerve. The calcaneal branch is found most commonly posterior and medial to the longitudinal axis of the tibial nerve. The preoperative plan should include reviewing both allograft and autograft options with the patient, patient positioning, and draping for appropriate access as needed. If autograft is required, access to the posterolateral leg for sural nerve harvest is mandatory.

- Identification of the injured nerve requires an incision long enough to visualize the uninjured portions of the nerve proximally and distally.
- Begin proximal and distal dissection outside of the scar zone surrounding the site of injury.
- Use nerve cutting forceps to debride back to healthy nerve fascicular anatomy.
- Measure the nerve gap (small gaps may be decreased with nerve mobilization).
- Assess whether primary repair is possible without undue tension (one study suggests that the maximum tensile strength of a 9–0 Nylon suture correlates to a satisfactory maximum tension level for nerve repair) [67].
- If possible, perform a primary repair. The repair should be without tension.
- Neuroma in continuity can be assessed with intraoperative electrodiagnostic testing or a handheld nerve stimulator.
- If nerve action potentials are present across the injury site, consideration can be given to external neurolysis.
- If there is no evidence of nerve action potential across the injury site, this likely represents a significant neuroma that requires excision and grafting.

Salvage Techniques

There are no described salvage techniques for sensory or motor nerve injury at the ankle level. Treatment for symptomatic toe clawing can range from flexor tendon release to arthrodesis. The location of the toe deformity, chronicity of the deformity, and whether the deformity is supple are important factors in deciding which treatment is best for symptomatic toe clawing.

Outcomes Reported outcomes for nerve repair at the foot and ankle level are limited, consisting mostly of descriptions of results from tibial nerve repair and graft reconstruction. An older series by Aldea et al. described 39–62% sensory recovery and 27–79% motor recovery after tibial nerve repair performed at or below the knee [68]. In 2003, Kim et al. included the results of treatment of 33 tibial nerve injuries at the foot and ankle level in a large series of tibial nerve injuries. Neurolysis resulted in good recovery in 74% in this group. They performed only two primary repairs with reported good results. Distal tibial nerve lesions that required graft reconstruction had 64% return of adequate sensation [69]. Dellon and Mackinnon reported good results with tibial nerve graft reconstruction at the ankle level with nerve grafts as long as 18 cm [70]. Nunley et al. reported five tibial nerve graft reconstruction procedures and found four good and one fair result for restoration of superficial sensation, resolution of plantar ulceration, and absence of neurogenic pain. They found that the improvement was slow with best results seen beyond 2 years [71]. In the past, described treatment of sensory nerve injury at the foot and ankle level centered on neuroma treatment. With the availability of processed nerve allograft, it is our practice to prevent neuromas by performing nerve repair or reconstruction with nerve graft. Prospective studies evaluating the sequelae of sural nerve autograft harvest as well as saphenous nerve symptoms after vein graft harvest have shown that many patients in these series had

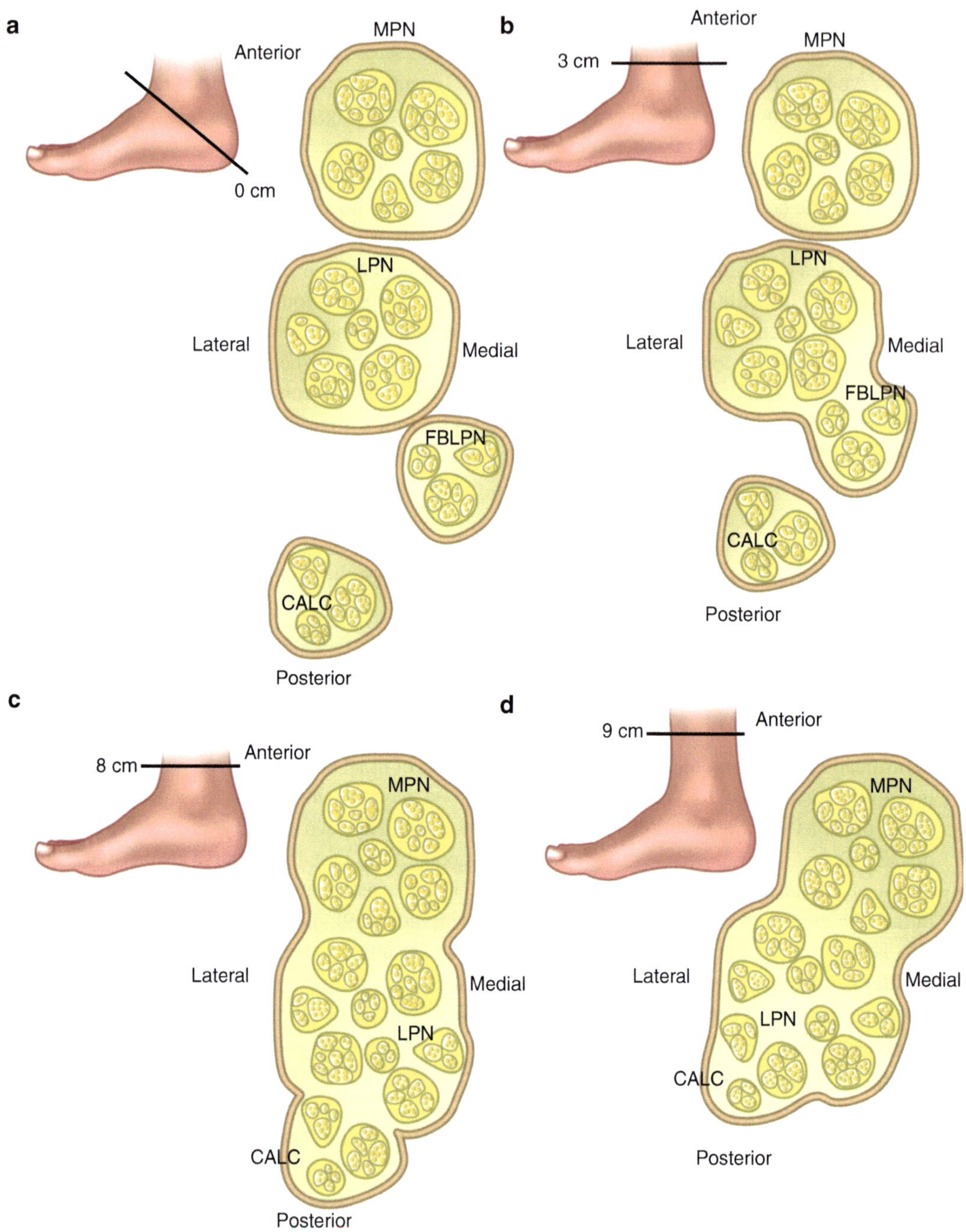

Fig. 16.7 Tibial nerve branches and group fascicular internal topography at the ankle and foot level (**a**–**f**)

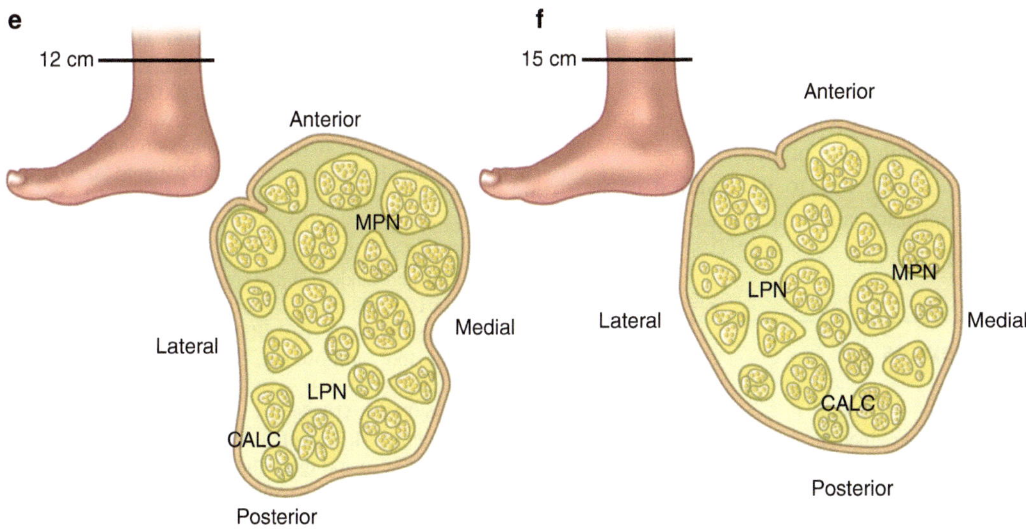

Fig. 16.7 (continued)

minimal donor site morbidity with resolution of symptoms at 1 year [63, 64].

Technical Pearls and Pitfalls

- When possible, perform primary repair for acute injury.
- Expect a nerve gap in most injuries (plan for possible autograft or allograft).
- Nerve reconstruction will be needed for patients with a delayed presentation.

Sural Nerve

- The sural nerve lies in close proximity to the lesser saphenous vein.
- Use "nick and spread" for percutaneous or endoscopic Achilles repair.
- Identify the sural nerve as it crosses the lateral Achilles tendon border for open repair.

Superficial Peroneal Nerve Use plantarflexion to help identify the location of the superficial peroneal nerve.

- The superficial peroneal nerve crosses from the posterior to the anterior fibula on average 11 cm proximal from the tip of the fibula.
- The "safe zone" for full-thickness flaps extends from the tip of the fibula to 5 cm proximal.

Saphenous Nerve

- Sensory only.
- Preservation of the greater saphenous vein will help to protect the saphenous nerve.
- Sural and saphenous nerves have variable rates of neuroma formation.

Deep Peroneal Nerve

- The deep peroneal nerve lies between the extensor hallucis longus and the extensor digitorum longus at the ankle.
- The deep peroneal nerve lies lateral to the vascular structures.
- Motor deficits at the ankle level are well tolerated.

Tibial Nerve

- Review internal topography preoperatively to facilitate anatomic alignment of fascicular groups (lateral plantar branch, medial plantar branch, calcaneal branch).
- Toe clawing due to denervation of intrinsic foot muscles can be addressed with flexor tendon releases.

References

1. Verhage SM, Boot F, Schipper IB, Hoogendoorn JM. Open reduction and internal fixation of posterior malleolar fractures using the posterolateral approach. Bone Joint J. 2016;98-B(6):812–7. https://doi.org/10.1302/0301-620X.98B6.36497.
2. Huber M, Stutz PM, Gerber C. Open reduction and internal fixation of the posterior malleolus with a posterior antiglide plate using a postero-lateral approach— a preliminary report. Foot Ankle Surg. 1996;2(2):95–103. https://doi.org/10.1046/j.1460-9584.1996.00012.x.
3. Tornetta P, Ricci W, Nork S, Collinge C, Steen B. The posterolateral approach to the tibia for displaced posterior malleolar injuries. J Orthop Trauma. 2011;25(2):123–6. https://doi.org/10.1097/BOT.0b013e3181e47d29.
4. Posterolateral Approach to the Displaced Posterior Malleolus: Functional Outcome and Local Morbidity - Jens Forberger, Philipp V. Sabandal, Michael Dietrich, Jan Gralla, Thomas Lattmann, Andreas Platz, 2009. https://journals.sagepub.com/doi/full/10.3113/fai.2009.0309. Accessed 31 Jan 2020.
5. Mizia E, Pękala PA, Chomicki-Bindas P, et al. Risk of injury to the sural nerve during posterolateral approach to the distal tibia: an ultrasound simulation study. Clin Anat. 2018;31(6):870–7. https://doi.org/10.1002/ca.23205.
6. Complications of the Treatment of Achilles Tendon Ruptures- ClinicalKey. https://www.clinicalkey.com/#!/content/playContent/1-s2.0-S1083751509000783?returnurl=https:%2F%2Flinkinghub.elsevier.com%2Fretrieve%2Fpii%2FS1083751509000783%3Fshowall%3Dtrue&referrer=https:%2F%2Fpubmed.ncbi.nlm.nih.gov%2F19857846-complications-of-the-treatment-of-achilles-tendon-ruptures%2F. Accessed 31 Jan 2020.
7. Majewski M, Rohrbach M, Czaja S, Ochsner P. Avoiding sural nerve injuries during percutaneous achilles tendon repair. Am J Sports Med. 2006;34(5):793–8. https://doi.org/10.1177/0363546505283266.
8. Blackmon JA, Atsas S, Clarkson MJ, et al. Locating the sural nerve during calcaneal (Achilles) tendon repair with confidence: a cadaveric study with clinical applications. J Foot Ankle Surg. 2013;52(1):42–7. https://doi.org/10.1053/j.jfas.2012.09.010.
9. Redfern DJ, Sauvé PS, Sakellariou A. Investigation of incidence of superficial peroneal nerve injury following ankle fracture. Foot Ankle Int. 2003;24(10):771–4. https://doi.org/10.1177/107110070302401006.
10. Manninen MJ, Lindahl J, Kankare J, Hirvensalo E. Lateral approach for fixation of the fractures of the distal tibia. Outcome of 20 patients. Arch Orthop Trauma Surg. 2007;127(5):349–53. https://doi.org/10.1007/s00402-006-0278-3.
11. Ferkel RD, Small HN, Gittins JE. Complications in foot and ankle arthroscopy. Clin Orthop Relat Res. 2001;391:89–104.
12. Carlson MJ, Ferkel RD. Complications in ankle and foot arthroscopy. Sports Med Arthrosc Rev. 2013;21(2):135–9. https://doi.org/10.1097/JSA.0b013e31828e5c6c.
13. Suzangar M, Rosenfeld P. Ankle arthroscopy: is preoperative marking of the superficial peroneal nerve important? J Foot Ankle Surg. 2012;51(2):179–81. https://doi.org/10.1053/j.jfas.2011.11.003.
14. Zengerink M, van Dijk CN. Complications in ankle arthroscopy. Knee Surg Sports Traumatol Arthrosc. 2012;20(8):1420–31. https://doi.org/10.1007/s00167-012-2063-x.
15. Amendola A, Petrik J, Webster-Bogaert S. Ankle arthroscopy: outcome in 79 consecutive patients. Arthroscopy. 1996;12(5):565–73. https://doi.org/10.1016/S0749-8063(96)90196-6.
16. Ferkel RD, Karzel RP, Del Pizzo W, Friedman MJ, Fischer SP. Arthroscopic treatment of anterolateral impingement of the ankle. Am J Sports Med. 1991;19(5):440–6. https://doi.org/10.1177/036354659101900504.
17. S H, AG. The role of ankle arthroscopy in acute ankle injuries of the athlete. Foot Ankle Clin. 2013;18(2):185–94. https://doi.org/10.1016/j.fcl.2013.02.001.
18. Young BH, Flanigan RM, DiGiovanni BF. Complications of ankle arthroscopy utilizing a contemporary noninvasive distraction technique. JBJS. 2011;93(10):963–8. https://doi.org/10.2106/JBJS.I.00977.
19. Zekry M, Shahban SA, El Gamal T, Platt S. A literature review of the complications following anterior and posterior ankle arthroscopy. Foot Ankle Surg. 2019;25(5):553–8. https://doi.org/10.1016/j.fas.2018.06.007.
20. Saito A, Kikuchi S. Anatomic relations between ankle arthroscopic portal sites and the superficial peroneal and saphenous nerves. Foot Ankle Int. 1998;19(11):748–52. https://doi.org/10.1177/107110079801901107.
21. Takao M, Uchio Y, Shu N, Ochi M. Anatomic bases of ankle arthroscopy: study of superficial and deep peroneal nerves around anterolateral and anterocentral approach. Surg Radiol Anat. 1998;20(5):317–20. https://doi.org/10.1007/bf01630612.
22. Jones. An iatropathic tibial nerve injury in a patient following total ankle replacement. http://www.journalmsr.com/article.asp?issn=2589-1219;year=2019;volume=3;issue=1;spage=169;epage=172;aulast=Jones. Accessed 3 Feb, 2020.

23. Primadi A, Xu H-X, Yoon T-R, Ryu J-H, Lee K-B. Neurologic injuries after primary total ankle arthroplasty: prevalence and effect on outcomes. J Foot Ankle Res. 2015;8 https://doi.org/10.1186/s13047-015-0112-7.
24. Retrouvey H, Silvanathan J, Bleakney RR, Anastakis DJ. A case of posterior tibial nerve injury after arthroscopic calcaneoplasty. J Foot Ankle Surg. 2018;57(3):587–92. https://doi.org/10.1053/j.jfas.2017.10.004.
25. Abdul-Jabar HB, Bhamra J, Quick TJ, Fox M. Iatrogenic posterior tibial nerve division during a combined anterior ankle arthroscopy with an additional posterolateral portal. J Surg Case Rep. 2016;2016(5) https://doi.org/10.1093/jscr/rjw097.
26. Kowalska J, Grabowski R, Pigonska J, Domzalski M. Management of an iatrogenic injury to the tibial nerve in a 24-year-old hurdle runner. J Int Med Res. 2018;46(8):3394–403. https://doi.org/10.1177/0300060518776061.
27. Freedman DM, Barron OA. Iatrogenic posterior tibial nerve division during ankle arthroscopy. Arthroscopy. 1998;14(7):769–72. https://doi.org/10.1016/s0749-8063(98)70109-4.
28. Meulenkamp B, Louati H, Morellato J, Papp S, Lalonde KA. Posterior malleolus exposure. OTA International. 2019;2(2):e021. https://doi.org/10.1097/OI9.0000000000000021.
29. Assal M, Ray A, Fasel JH, Stern R. A modified posteromedial approach combined with extensile anterior for the treatment of complex tibial pilon fractures (AO/OTA 43-C). J Orthop Trauma. 2014;28(6) https://doi.org/10.1097/01.bot.0000435628.79017.c5.
30. Amorosa L, Brown G, Greisberg J. A surgical approach to posterior Pilon fractures. J Orthop Trauma. 2010;24(3):188–93. https://doi.org/10.1097/BOT.0b013e3181b91927.
31. Wang Y, Wang J, Luo CF. Modified posteromedial approach for treatment of posterior pilon variant fracture. BMC Musculoskelet Disord. 2016;17:328. https://doi.org/10.1186/s12891-016-1182-9.
32. Reb CW, McAlister JE, Hyer CF, Berlet GC. Posterior ankle structure injury during total ankle replacement. J Foot Ankle Surg. 2016;55(5):931–4. https://doi.org/10.1053/j.jfas.2016.04.007.
33. Bibbo C. A modified anterior approach to the ankle. J Foot Ankle Surg. 2013;52(1):136–7. https://doi.org/10.1053/j.jfas.2012.10.010.
34. Dekker RGI, Kadakia AR. Anterior approach for ankle arthrodesis. JBJS Essential Surgical Techniques. 2017;7(2):e10. https://doi.org/10.2106/JBJS.ST.15.00066.
35. Pichler W, Grechenig W, Tesch NP, Weinberg AM, Heidari N, Clement H. The risk of iatrogenic injury to the deep peroneal nerve in minimally invasive osteosynthesis of the tibia with the less invasive stabilisation system. J Bone Joint Surg. 2009;91-B(3):385–7. https://doi.org/10.1302/0301-620X.91B3.21673.
36. Wolinsky P, Lee M. The distal approach for anterolateral plate fixation of the tibia: an anatomic study. J Orthop Trauma. 2008;22(6):404–7. https://doi.org/10.1097/BOT.0b013e31817614b2.
37. Perioperative Complications of Total Ankle Arthroplasty - Kenneth Mroczek, 2003. https://journals.sagepub.com/doi/full/10.1177/107110070302400102. Accessed 3 Feb, 2020.
38. Knecht SI, Estin M, Callaghan JJ, et al. The agility total ankle arthroplasty: seven to sixteen-year follow-up. JBJS. 2004;86(6):1161–71.
39. Lee K-B, Cho S-G, Hur C-I, Yoon T-R. Perioperative complications of HINTEGRA total ankle replacement: our initial 50 cases. Foot Ankle Int. 2008;29(10):978–84. https://doi.org/10.3113/FAI.2008.0978.
40. Krause FG, Windolf M, Bora B, Penner MJ, Wing KJ, Younger ASE. Impact of complications in Total ankle replacement and ankle arthrodesis analyzed with a validated outcome measurement. JBJS. 2011;93(9):830–9. https://doi.org/10.2106/JBJS.J.00103.
41. Buckingham R, Winson IG, Kelly AJ. An anatomical study of a new portal for ankle arthroscopy. J Bone Joint Surg. 1997;79(4):650–2. https://doi.org/10.1302/0301-620X.79B4.0790650.
42. ANATOMICAL STUDY OF THE ANKLE WITH VIEW TO THE ANTERIOR ARTHROSCOPIC PORTALS - Solomon - 2006 - ANZ Journal of Surgery - Wiley Online Library. https://onlinelibrary.wiley.com/doi/full/10.1111/j.1445--2197.2006.03909.x. Accessed 3 Feb 2020.
43. Mirza A, Moriarty AM, Probe RA, Ellis TJ. Percutaneous plating of the distal tibia and fibula: risk of injury to the saphenous and superficial peroneal nerves. J Orthop Trauma. 2010;24(8):495–8. https://doi.org/10.1097/BOT.0b013e3181cb584f.
44. Lawrence SJ, Botte MJ. The sural nerve in the foot and ankle: an anatomic study with clinical and surgical implications. Foot Ankle Int. 1994;15(9):490–4. https://doi.org/10.1177/107110079401500906.
45. Jowett AJL, Sheikh FT, Carare RO, Goodwin MI. Location of the sural nerve during posterolateral approach to the ankle. Foot Ankle Int. 2010;31(10):880–3. https://doi.org/10.3113/FAI.2010.0880.
46. Ellapparadja P, Husami Y, McLeod I. Safety profile of sural nerve in posterolateral approach to the ankle joint: MRI study. Eur J Orthop Surg Traumatol. 2014;24(4):615–9. https://doi.org/10.1007/s00590-013-1343-6.
47. Garagozlo C, Kadri O, Atalla M, et al. The anatomical relationship between the sural nerve and small saphenous vein: an ultrasound study of healthy participants. Clin Anat. 2019;32(2):277–81. https://doi.org/10.1002/ca.23302.
48. Zhou Q, Tan D-Y, Dai Z-S. The location of the superficial peroneal nerve in the leg and its relation to the surgical approach of the fibula. Zhongguo Gu Shang. 2008;21(2):95–6.
49. Ducic I, Dellon AL, Graw KS. The clinical importance of variations in the surgical anatomy of the superficial peroneal nerve in the mid-third of the lateral leg. Ann Plast Surg. 2006;56(6):635–8. https://doi.org/10.1097/01.sap.0000203258.96961.a6.

50. Adkison DP, Bosse MJ, Gaccione DR, Gabriel KR. Anatomical variations in the course of the superficial peroneal nerve. J Bone Joint Surg Am. 1991;73(1):112–4.
51. The superficial peroneal nerve: a review of its anatomy and surgical relevance. OA Anatomy. http://www.oapublishinglondon.com/article/1272#4. Accessed 3 Feb 2020.
52. Halm JA, Schepers T. Damage to the superficial peroneal nerve in operative treatment of fibula fractures: straight to the bone? Case report and review of the literature. J Foot Ankle Surg. 2012;51(5):684–6. https://doi.org/10.1053/j.jfas.2012.05.021.
53. Jm B, Mj B. Surgical Anatomy of the Superficial Peroneal Nerve in the Ankle and Foot. Clinical orthopaedics and related research. https://pubmed.ncbi.nlm.nih.gov/8050234/. Published August 1994. Accessed 3 Feb 2020.
54. Sora M-C, Jilavu R, Grübl A, Genser-Strobl B, Staykov D, Seicean A. The posteromedial neurovascular bundle of the ankle: an anatomic study using plastinated cross sections. Arthroscopy. 2008;24(3):):258.e1–7. https://doi.org/10.1016/j.arthro.2007.08.030.
55. Lijoi F, Lughi M, Baccarani G. Posterior arthroscopic approach to the ankle. Arthroscopy. 2003;19(1):62–7. https://doi.org/10.1053/jars.2003.50003.
56. Sitler DF, Amendola A, Bailey CS, Thain LMF, Spouge A. Posterior ankle arthroscopy : an anatomic study. JBJS. 2002;84(5):763–9.
57. Lawrence SJ, Botte MJ. The deep peroneal nerve in the foot and ankle: an anatomic study. Foot Ankle Int. 1995;16(11):724–8. https://doi.org/10.1177/107110079501601110.
58. Ucerler H, Ikiz ZAA, Uygur M. A cadaver study on preserving peroneal nerves during ankle arthroscopy. Foot Ankle Int. 2007;28(11):1172–8. https://doi.org/10.3113/FAI.2007.1172.
59. Mercer D, Morrell NT, Fitzpatrick J, et al. The course of the distal saphenous nerve: a cadaveric investigation and clinical implications. Iowa Orthop J. 2011;31:231–5.
60. Stephens MM, Kelly PM. Fourth toe flexion sign: a new clinical sign for identification of the superficial peroneal nerve. Foot Ankle Int. 2000;21(10):860–3. https://doi.org/10.1177/107110070002101012.
61. de Leeuw PAJ, Golanó P, Sierevelt IN, van Dijk CN. The course of the superficial peroneal nerve in relation to the ankle position: anatomical study with ankle arthroscopic implications. Knee Surg Sports Traumatol Arthrosc. 2010;18(5):612–7. https://doi.org/10.1007/s00167-010-1099-z.
62. Thordarson D, Shean C. Nerve and tendon laceration about the foot and ankle. JAAOS. 2005;13:186–96.
63. Martins R, et al. Morbidity following sural N. Harvest: a prospective study. Clin Neur N Surg. 2012;114:1149–52.
64. Reidl O, et al. Sural nerve harvesting beyond the popliteal region. Plast Rec Surg. 2008;3:798–805.
65. Immerman I, et al. Lower extremity nerve trauma. Bull Hospital for Jt Diseases. 2014;1:43–52.
66. Griffith J, et al. Peripheral nerve repair and reconstruction. JBJS. 2013;23:2144–51.
67. Lumsden D, et al. Topography of the distal tibial nerve and its branches. Foot Ankle Int. 2003;24:696–700.
68. Aldea P, Shaw W. Lower extremity nerve injuries. Clin Plast Surg. 1986;4:691–9.
69. Kim D, et al. Surgical Management and Results of 135 Tibial Nerve lesions at the Louisiana State University Health Science Center. Neurosurgery. 2003;5:114–24.
70. Dellon A, Mackinnon S. Results of posterior tibial nerve grafting at the ankle. J Recon Micro. 1991;2:81–3.
71. Nunley J, Gabel G. Tibial nerve grafting for restoration of plantar sensation. Foot Ankle Int. 1993;9:489–92.

Nerve Injury After Fractures of the Hindfoot, Midfoot, and Forefoot

17

Jared Bookman and Jacques Hacquebord

17.1 Risks/Incidence/Mechanism of Nerve Injury

Neurologic complications after foot and ankle fractures and fracture surgery are common and underreported. Many of these complications may initially go unrecognized and untreated. Fractures of the hindfoot, midfoot, and forefoot often necessitate operative fixation and place nerves of the foot at risk of injury. These are primarily cutaneous nerves and are at risk for traction injuries, compression, partial, or complete transection. While motor deficits are typically considered to be more debilitating, the severity and importance of sensory disturbances in the foot is often underestimated. Recovery is slow and unpredictable.

J. Bookman
Department of Orthopedic Surgery, New York University School of Medicine, New York, NY, USA
e-mail: Jared.Bookman@nyulangone.org

J. Hacquebord (✉)
Department of Orthopedic Surgery, Hansjörg Wyss Department of Plastic Surgery, New York University School of Medicine, New York, NY, USA

Hand Surgery Service, Bellevue Hospital Center, New York, NY, USA
e-mail: Jacques.Hacquebord@nyulangone.org

17.2 Pertinent Anatomy

Innervation to the foot and ankle is chiefly supplied by branches of the sciatic nerve that have divided at the knee in the popliteal fossa into the common peroneal nerve (CPN) and the tibial nerve (TN). The overall anatomy will be reviewed and discussed in further detail with regard to specific injuries [1, 2].

Plantar sensation is supplied by the tibial nerve and its terminal branches. The tibial nerve receives contributions from L4 to S3 at the lumbosacral plexus. After traveling through the two heads of the gastrocnemius at the level of the popliteal fossa and giving off a medial sural nerve branch, it runs deep to the soleus and innervates muscles of the posterior compartment of the leg. There it lies between the flexor digitorum longus and flexor hallucis longus, before traveling behind the medial malleolus and into the tarsal tunnel. The tibial nerve runs posterior to the tendons of the posterior tibialis and toe flexors and the tibial artery and deep to the flexor retinaculum, which form the tarsal tunnel.

At this point, the branching pattern of the distal tibial nerve is quite variable. The nerve bifurcates into a medial plantar nerve (MPN) and lateral plantar nerve (LPN), and additionally gives off terminal medial and inferior calcaneal branches. The medial plantar nerve is the larger terminal division responsible for innervating great toe and medial foot intrinsics. It courses deep to the

C. J. Dy et al. (eds.), *Peripheral Nerve Issues after Orthopedic Surgery*,
https://doi.org/10.1007/978-3-030-84428-8_17

abductor hallucis, gives off a medial proper digital nerve to the great toe, and then divides adjacent to the metatarsal bases to give off common digital nerves supplying sensory innervation to the toes. The sensory distribution of the MPN is somewhat analogous to the median nerve in the hand, providing sensation to the medial three and a half toes. Each common digital nerve has a cutaneous branch, an articular branch, and a muscular branch. Similarly, the LPN innervates lateral foot intrinsics and typically gives rise to the inferior calcaneal nerve branch. It similarly branches into common digital nerves, and its sensory distribution is somewhat analogous to the ulnar nerve in the hand, innervating the lateral sole and lateral one and a half toes.

Branching patterns and nomenclature of the medial and inferior calcaneal nerves is very inconsistent in the literature [3]. The first branch of the lateral plantar nerve (Baxter's nerve) typically provides motor innervation to the abductor digiti quinti. Either the entire nerve or just its sensory branch is known as the inferior calcaneal nerve which supplies cutaneous innervation to the anterior aspect of the calcaneus and sensory innervation to the anterior calcaneal periosteum. The medial calcaneal nerve (MCN) has a variable origin and branching patterns and typically provides cutaneous innervation to the plantar and medial aspects of the heel pad. A recent cadaver study demonstrated that the branching pattern is quite variable, and in their specimens 64% of medial calcaneal nerves branch off the tibial nerve proper, 9% split at the same time as the MPN and LPN, and 27% branched off the LPN. The inferior calcaneal nerve always branches off the lateral plantar nerve [3].

The lateral aspect of the foot is chiefly supplied by the sural nerve. Its proximal course in the leg is well described and well known from autograft harvesting; however, its distal anatomy is less consistent and less well described. The common sural nerve receives fibers from both the lateral sural nerve, a branch of the common peroneal nerve, and the medial sural nerve, a branch of the tibial nerve. Typically, these sensory nerves join to constitute the sural nerve in the posterior calf, which carries S1 sensory fibers and supplies cutaneous innervation to the lateral aspect of the foot up to the dorsolateral surface of the small toe. There is one contribution from each nerve in 80% of cases. The sural nerve then runs along the posterolateral leg, running midway between the Achilles tendon and the lateral malleolus. The nerve runs with the short saphenous vein for the majority of its course. Below the level of the ankle, the branching patterns of this nerve are variable and inconsistently described, with the nerve giving off lateral calcaneal branches and a terminal branch running as the lateral dorsal nerve of the foot.

The deep peroneal nerve is purely a sensory nerve at the level of the foot. It emerges from beneath the belly of the extensor hallucis longus muscle, lateral to its tendon approximately 2.5 cm above the ankle. The nerve passes under the extensor retinaculum and then divides into a medial and lateral branch underneath the extensor digitorum tendons. After emerging from under the retinaculum, the medial branch follows the dorsalis pedis artery and terminates to provide cutaneous innervation to the first webbed space. The lateral branch innervates the extensor digitorum brevis (EDB) muscle from its deep surface and travels distally as a terminal branch below the EDB tendon.

The superficial peroneal nerve begins at the bifurcation of the common peroneal nerve at the proximal fibula. Initially it runs deep to the peroneus longus and then passes between the peroneus longus and extensor digitorum longus (EDL) to pierce the deep fascia in the distal third of the leg. It then divides into a large medial dorsal cutaneous nerve and a smaller, more laterally placed intermediate dorsal cutaneous nerve, usually after piercing the crural fascia. The medial dorsal cutaneous nerve typically passes in front of the ankle joint, dividing into two dorsal digital branches, and supplies the medial side of the great toe and the dorsum of the second and third toes. The intermediate branch travels laterally along the dorsum of the foot and divides into dorsal digital branches that supply the contiguous sides of the third to fifth toes. Figure 17.1 depicts a laceration of the superficial peroneal nerve over the dorsum of the foot.

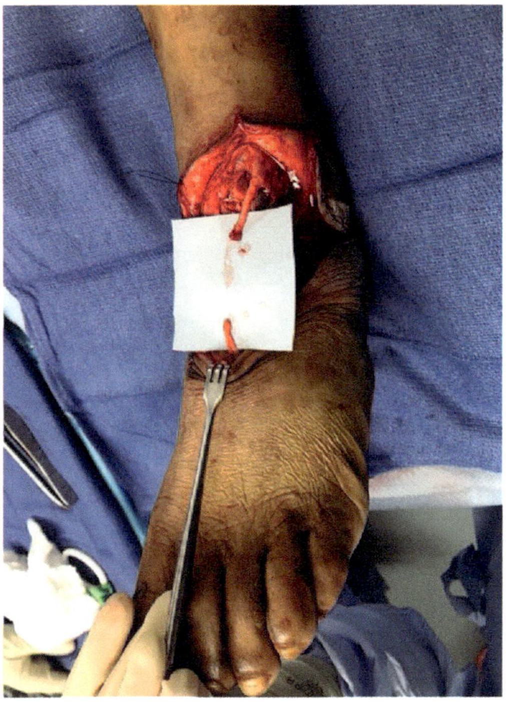

Fig. 17.1 Intraoperative photograph of superficial peroneal nerve laceration with a significant nerve gap noted in dorsal foot degloving injury

The saphenous vein is the largest purely sensory branch of the femoral nerve. Below the knee, the saphenous nerve runs with the greater saphenous vein until the medial side of the ankle and foot. Classically, its terminal branches are said to run as far as the medial aspect of the first metatarsal head. However, there is considerable variability in the terminal cutaneous branches, and a recent cadaveric study noted that in most specimens (15 of 16) the nerve terminated proximal to the tip of the medial malleolus and had minimal contribution to sensory innervation of the foot [4].

17.3 Prevention Strategies

17.3.1 Percutaneous Placement of External Fixator Pins in the Calcaneus

Placement of percutaneous pins into the calcaneus is a relatively common procedure. Management of ankle, hindfoot, and forefoot fractures, particularly high-energy fractures and dislocations, often necessitates provisional or definitive fixation in an external fixator. Additionally, use of the Ilizarov-type constructs require placement of multiple pins or wires into the hindfoot. These external fixation constructs often rely on medially placed pins placed into the calcaneus or a transcalcaneal pin from medial through to the lateral side. Techniques for safe pin placement have been studied extensively, but often recommendation for pin insertion is simply stated as medial-to-lateral insertion with careful avoidance of neurovascular structures.

On the medial side of the foot, pin placement risks injury to the medial neurovascular bundle and all terminal branches of the tibial nerve distal to the tarsal tunnel. Injuries to the medial and lateral plantar nerves and the medial calcaneal nerve have all occurred. Generally, the lateral plantar nerve branches and the medial calcaneal nerve branch are thought to be at the highest risk. Figure 17.2 depicts this anatomy and the relative safe zone.

There have been extensive efforts in cadaveric studies to delineate radiographic safe zones. Santi and Botte assessed calcaneal pins in the feet of cadaver specimens and found that the most reliable medial safe zone was a rectangle drawn in the posterior portion of the calcaneal tuberosity, posterior to the neurovascular bundle and posterior tibial tendon [5]. Within this region, they found that the first branch of the LPN was a mean of 5 mm away from the pin site. However, the medial calcaneal branch was still consistently at risk, with variable anatomy and inconsistent small, terminal branches spanning over the field.

Casey and Tornetta et al. revisited this concept in a similar study of cadaver specimens in an attempt to clarify more simple and reproducible landmarks [6]. They inserted pins in a safe zone defined by two lines. One was on the posterior half of a line drawn between the inferior medial malleolus and the posteroinferior medial calcaneus. The second was on the posterior third of a line between the navicular tuberosity and the posterior-inferior medial calcaneus. Even within this "safe zone" on their ten cadaver feet – the major-

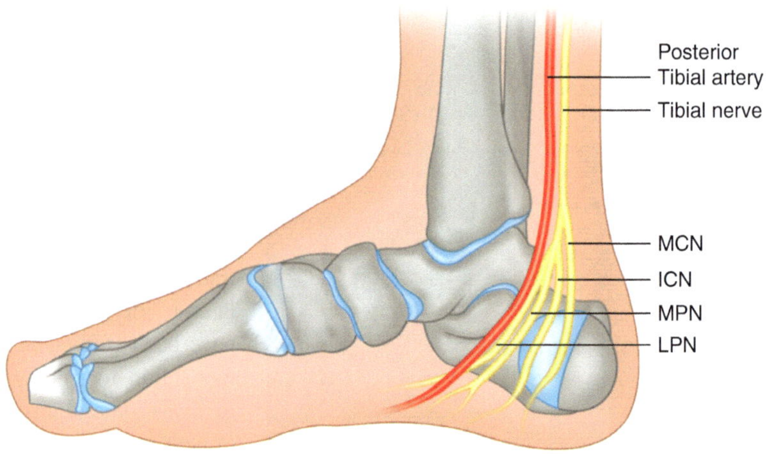

Fig. 17.2 Relative safe zone in placement of external fixator pins in the calcaneus

ity of the specimens had one of these branches (lateral plantar nerve, posterior branch of lateral plantar nerve, medial calcaneal nerve) impaled or within 3 mm of injury [7]. Multiple studies have found similar outcomes, essentially demonstrating that more posterior placement of a transfixation pin risks tuberosity fracture but is generally safer to avoid the LPN and its posterior branches, but iatrogenic injury to the MCN may be somewhat unavoidable given its location, inconsistent anatomy, and terminal branching pattern [8, 9].

On the lateral side of the calcaneus, the nerve structure most at risk is the sural nerve (in addition to the peroneal tendons). These same cadaveric studies demonstrated that the main trunk of the lateral sural nerve typically falls on the anterior aspect of this same relative safe zone. A pin placed parallel in the posterior aspect of the calcaneus should avoid the sural nerve; however, there are similarly variable and broadly branching patterns of small terminal lateral calcaneal branches which overlie the likely pin exit site.

Despite appropriate technique and best practices, there is no true safe zone for pin placement in the medial calcaneus. For the safest pin insertion in the calcaneus, the following steps can be used:

- Delineate relative safe zones using fluoroscopy, more posterior placement is generally safer for tibial nerve branches besides the MCN.
- Use a scalpel to incise the skin only, and bluntly dissect down to the bone.
- Drill and insert pins using drill sleeves or cannulas to protect soft tissue.

17.3.2 Open Reduction and Internal Fixation of Calcaneus Fractures

Fractures of the calcaneus are generally severe and debilitating injuries. Operative management of these complex, intra-articular fractures is often necessary and even with modern techniques commonly results in wound complications and posttraumatic arthritis. Importantly, there are significant nerve injuries that can occur during the surgical approach and operative fixation of calcaneus fractures. This can further complicate an already debilitating injury, leading to severe heel pain, hypersensitivity, and difficulty with walking and shoe wear [13].

The most commonly utilized surgical approach to the calcaneus is the extensile lateral approach. Recently, the less-invasive sinus tarsi approach has seen increased use as well. The primary nerve structures at risk in both of these approaches are the sural nerve and its lateral calcaneal branches. Sural nerve-related complications have been described in up to 10% of patients undergoing operative fixation of displaced intra-articular calcaneus fractures, and it is suspected that this condition has been significantly underreported [14–16].

The extensile lateral approach involves an "L-shaped" incision and full-thickness flap on the lateral heel raised without direct exposure of the sural nerve. In the landmark series on treatment of this injury using the extensile lateral technique, Sanders reported that 12 of his 120 patients had postoperative sural nerve symptoms [14]. Freeman et al. reported that 22% of patients had some sort of persistent nerve pain after operative fixation of calcaneus fracture, likely some combination of sural nerve and chronic regional pain syndrome (CRPS) cases [15, 16].

The sinus tarsi approach is a more recently described approach directed at improving wound complication rates. It is a less invasive technique that utilizes an incision running from the tip of the lateral malleolus to the calcaneocuboid joint in line with the fourth ray. The exposure continues deep between the peroneal tendons and the sinus tarsi fat pad, up to the fascia of the extensor hallucis brevis distally. The original series of 24 patients described no cases of sural nerve injury, potentially demonstrating its merits as a safer approach [17, 18]. It should be noted that there is a communicating branch (sometimes referred to as anastomotic branch) between the sural and the intermediate dorsal cutaneous branch of the superficial peroneal nerve, and this more dorsal incision may place that at risk.

A cadaveric study done by Smyth et al. reported on 17 cadaveric foot dissections done using both approaches with a focus on sural nerve anatomy and injury [19]. The main sural nerve did not cross the extensile lateral incision in any specimen; however, there was at least one lateral calcaneal branch crossing the incision in all specimens. The sinus tarsi approach intersected the path of the main trunk of the sural nerve in two specimens (12%), and the connecting/anastomotic branch was at risk in nine specimens (53%).

17.3.3 Midfoot Fractures

Injuries to the tarsometatarsal joints, the Lisfranc complex, are devastating injuries to the foot. These fractures and fracture-dislocations frequently prompt intervention on the midfoot, necessitating a dorsal approach requiring identification and dissection of the deep peroneal nerve. The deep peroneal nerve innervates the anterior compartment muscles of the leg and the extensor digitorum brevis and provides cutaneous innervation to the first webspace. Injury to the distal portion of the deep peroneal nerve primarily results in sensory deficits of this cutaneous distribution and painful neuroma. Midfoot surgical approaches have long been known to be associated with postoperative peroneal nerve complications, with Mann reporting in 1996 on a series of midfoot fusions for primary or posttraumatic osteoarthritis with a 7.5% rate (3/40) of dorsal incisional neuroma [20]. Similarly, in the same year Komenda and colleagues reported on their series of 32 patients requiring midfoot fusion for posttraumatic arthritis and similarly noted a 9% rate (3 patients) of symptomatic neuromas requiring excision [21]. Some component of the Lisfranc injury itself may even be responsible for DPN compression, as sensory nerve conduction studies of the DPN have been shown to be altered after Lisfranc injuries, even before any surgical intervention [22].

Typically, either a single or multiple longitudinal dorsal incisions on the midfoot are required for the surgical approach for open reduction of these injuries. Typically, to address the medial column of the foot, a longitudinal incision is placed between the first and second ray [23]. This dorsomedial incision is centered over the tarsometatarsal (TMT) area, between the extensor hallucis longus tendon (EHL) and extensor hallucis brevis (EHB) [23]. This incision allows access to the first TMT and the medial base of the second TMT. The plane between these two tendons is developed, and the deep peroneal nerve must be identified and protected [24, 25]. By this level, the deep peroneal nerve has bifurcated into a medial and lateral terminal branch, and it is the medial branch that is most at risk in this approach while exposing the proximal metatarsal bases and TMT joints for reduction and plate or screw fixation across the TMT joint.

An anatomic study of ten cadaver feet by Loveday et al. provides clarity on the anatomic relationships in this region [26]. They demonstrated that in all feet the DPN and dorsalis pedis artery run together along the lateral border of the EHL tendon. The relationship between the two is variable, in five specimens the artery was lateral, and in five the nerve was lateral. However, in all specimens, the bundle could be reliably identified at the obliquely oriented musculotendinous junction of the EHB. In nine of the ten specimens, it ran just below this EHB tendon, and in one of the ten specimens, it ran between two muscle bellies of a split EHB.

Given the degree of swelling and deformity that can be associated with these Lisfranc complex injuries, particular care must be taken to avoid damaging DPN branches during these approaches. Of note, one cohort reported by Meyerkort et al. actually showed a 11% rate of DPN injury during the index surgery for Lisfranc injuries and a 21% rate of DPN injury during hardware removal surgery [27]. This additionally underscores the elevated risk of DPN injury that comes with operating in a swollen, deformed, or scarred tissue plane.

17.3.4 Forefoot Fractures

Neurologic injuries due to fracture surgery on the forefoot are not commonly reported. Many fractures are treated nonoperatively, or using limited incisions. As with the midfoot, the majority of incisions are dorsal, primarily to avoid incisions placed on the plantar surface of the foot. The majority of reports of neurologic injury in forefoot fracture surgery can be extrapolated from reports of surgery on the first ray, often primarily done for reasons of arthritis or deformity.

Campbell reported on a series of 75 patients who had a dorsomedial skin incision and approach to the first ray for a variety of indications. In the series, it was noted that there was a 45% rate of postoperative symptoms due to injury of the medial dorsal cutaneous nerve branch of the superficial peroneal nerve [29]. Pont et al. performed a cadaveric model of multiple surgical approaches to the foot. In their approaches on ten cadaveric feet, using a medial approach to the first ray and the metatarsophalangeal joint of the great toe, four specimens had medial dorsal nerves of the foot in the path of the incision [30]. This is consistent with Campbell's reported rate, implying that there is likely a considerable chance of cutaneous nerve injury in approaches to the first ray.

17.4 Typical Course/Natural History

Observational natural history studies of patients with postoperative sensory nerve injuries after foot and ankle surgery have demonstrated that the majority of patients will go on to have incomplete recovery. Maximal recovery typically occurs within 6 months of surgery. A small proportion of patients form neuromas, which can cause debilitating pain, paresthesia, and limitations in shoe wear.

17.5 Initial Evaluation/Exam

17.5.1 Percutaneous Placement of External Fixator Pins in the Calcaneus

Injury to nerve branches during placement of an external fixator would present with persistent heel pain. Compression neuropathy of the terminal tibial nerve branches, in particular compression of the inferior or medial calcaneal branches between the quadratus plantae muscle and the deep fascia of the abductor hallucis muscle, is a described phenomenon which presents with chronic heel pain, especially with weight-bearing [10]. It may be occasionally possible to detect perineural scarring on magnetic resonance imaging or ultrasound. Injury to the first branch of the lateral plantar nerve, in particular, may demonstrate atrophy of the abductor digiti quinti on imaging. However, given the difficulty of reliably imaging these small, sensory branches, the diagnosis should be made clinically with an appropriate history accompanied by an affected sensory distribution on exam with local tenderness and possible Tinel's sign.

17.5.2 Open Reduction and Internal Fixation of Calcaneus Fractures

For the patient who presents with postoperative nerve symptoms after open reduction and internal fixation of the calcaneus, it first must be well localized and clinically differentiated from a healing fracture, planar fasciitis, tendinous scarring, or subtalar arthritis. Pain after this injury is difficult to diagnose and treat. Occasionally, neuromas may be palpable.

17.6 Diagnostic Tests/Imaging

Nerve conduction studies may demonstrate prolonged sensory latency in the case of peripheral nerve injury, when compared to the contralateral side. Imaging is not likely to be helpful, although ultrasound or magnetic resonance imaging may demonstrate some perineural scarring or neuroma formation. There is little evidence to guide treatment and prognosticate expected clinical outcomes. Nonoperatively there is a role for neurotrophic medications, local nerve blocks, and therapy. If patients have failed nonoperative measures, any surgical management could involve exploration with decompression and external neurolysis. This has the benefit of retaining sensory function. However, the area of anesthesia after loss of the sural nerve is not critical and can be well tolerated. Tibial nerve loss affecting plantar sensation is more critical and its loss poorly tolerated.

17.7 Surgical Techniques/Salvage Techniques/Outcomes

17.7.1 Percutaneous Placement of External Fixator Pins in the Calcaneus

Surgically, the primary treatment option for this nerve injury would be exploration with local decompression and external neurolysis of these terminal nerve branches. There is no meaningful literature to guide expected outcomes after these iatrogenic nerve injuries, and any pain relief would be expected to be inconsistent. Historically, heel neurectomy with division of these sensory fibers has been described, but concern for development of heel pad atrophy and ulceration would be significant [11, 12].

Open Reduction and Internal Fixation of Calcaneus Fractures

In the case of a painful sural neuroma, neurectomy with excision of the damaged nerve, with implantation of the proximal stump into muscle or bone well away from the zone of injury, would be our recommendation. There is a theoretical role for excision and repair with intercalary grafting; however, this carries the risk of donor site morbidity with autograft and cost of surgery, especially if allograft is used. Furthermore, the sensory deficit itself is of minimal importance, and surgery does not guarantee prevention of neuroma formation. For these reasons, our recommendation is resection of the painful neuroma.

17.7.2 Midfoot Fractures

Postoperative symptomatic neuroma has been shown to be treatable with neuroma excision in the few limited case series on these injuries. Similarly, we can extrapolate from the small case series of Dellon and colleagues, who have described a compressive nerve entrapment of the DPN under the EHB tendon [28]. In their series, they report good or excellent results with decompression by release and excision of this EHB slip in 80% of their cohort of 20 patients. It stands to reason that neurolysis of the nerve and release of this compressive EHB tendon would be a reasonable approach to a symptomatic DPN compression after a Lisfranc injury.

17.7.2.1 Crush Injury and Compartment Syndrome

Finally, one of the more common and devastating reasons for neurologic sequelae after forefoot trauma is a crush injury. This should be suspected when a high-energy, crush type mechanism is associated with disproportionate or uncontrollable pain in the presence of typical physical findings such as severe swelling, ecchymosis, pain with passive motion of the toes, and decreased sensation. While midfoot and hindfoot fractures are associated with this phenomenon as well, crush type injuries to the forefoot, especially when associated with multiple metatarsal fractures, is most predictive of development of compartment syndrome. Reporting of this clinical phenomenon varies, but it is generally established to be relatively uncommon, associated with less than 2% of foot injuries, and represents less than 5% of overall lower extremity compartment syndromes [31].

The reported number of compartments within the foot varies, with numbers that have ranged from 3 to 10 compartments [32]. The role of fasciotomy is similarly debated given the morbidity of multiple incisions on the already traumatized soft tissue of the foot. The most common technique involves three incisions, based on the nine compartment model of the foot. A medial 6 cm incision is made starting several centimeters anterior to the posterior aspect of the heel and superior to the plantar surface of the foot. Through this approach, the medial, superficial and deep central, and lateral compartments are released. Additionally, two dorsal incisions are used, one just medial to the second metatarsal and one just lateral to the fourth metatarsal to release the interosseous and adductor compartments.

While not strictly a peripheral nerve injury, foot compartment syndrome involves ischemic injury to multiple nerves of the foot that carry many of the same clinical sequelae of neuropathic pain. Stiffness, chronic disability, deformity, and pain are some of the complications associated with untreated foot compartment syndrome. Necrosis of the intrinsic muscles of the foot can lead to an intrinsic minus ischemic contracture. The most common associated deformity is multiple claw toes, due to intrinsic weakness and extrinsic overpull. Flexible claw toe deformities can be managed with flexor tenotomies and extensor tendon lengthening. Rigid deformities require proximal interphalangeal joint (PIP) fusion if sufficiently symptomatic. Additionally, an associated cavus deformity can result due to fibrosis of plantar fascia and plantar intrinsic muscles. This can necessitate plantar fascia release or possible osteotomies or selective fusions for more severe deformity.

Technical Pearls and Pitfalls

- Neurologic complications after foot and ankle fractures and fracture surgery are common and underreported.
- Operative fixation of fractures of the hindfoot, midfoot, and forefoot place the primarily sensory nerves of the foot at risk of injury.
- Hindfoot, midfoot, and forefoot fractures that involve nerve injuries typically represent a very large zone of injury in relation to the small, sensory distal nerve branches.
- The soft tissue envelope is typically poor, the zone of injury is large requiring a large nerve graft and decreased likelihood of recovering, and reconstruction is of limited benefit – sensory function is noncritical except in tibial nerve branches. Therefore, we generally recommend against nerve reconstruction and recommend resection of symptomatic neuromas.

References

1. Coughlin MJ, Saltzman CL, Anderson RB. Mann's surgery of the foot and ankle. 9th ed. Philadelphia, PA: Elsevier Saunders; 2014.
2. Mackinnon SE. Nerve surgery. New York: Thieme; 2015.
3. Kim BS, Choung PW, Kwon SW, Rhyu IJ, Kim DH. Branching patterns of medial and inferior calcaneal nerves around the tarsal tunnel. Ann Rehabil Med. 2015;39(1):52–5. https://doi.org/10.5535/arm.2015.39.1.52.
4. Mercer D, Morrell NT, Fitzpatrick J, et al. The course of the distal saphenous nerve: a cadaveric investigation and clinical implications. Iowa Orthop J. 2011;31:231–5.
5. Santi MD, Botte MJ. External fixation of the calcaneus and talus: an anatomical study for safe pin insertion. J Orthop Trauma. 1996;10(7):487–91. https://doi.org/10.1097/00005131-199610000-00007.
6. Casey D, McConnell T, Parekh S, Tornetta P. Percutaneous pin placement in the medial calcaneus: is anywhere safe? J Orthop Trauma. 2002;16(1):26–9. https://doi.org/10.1097/00005131-200201000-00006.
7. Mekhail AO, Ebraheim NA, Heck BE, Yeasting RA. Anatomic considerations for safe placement of cal-

caneal pins. Clin Orthop Relat Res. 1996;332:254–9. https://doi.org/10.1097/00003086-199611000-00033.
8. Gamie Z, Donnelly L, Tsiridis E. The "safe zone" in medial percutaneous calcaneal pin placement. Clin Anat. 2009;22(4):523–9. https://doi.org/10.1002/ca.20778.
9. Kwon JY, Ellington JK, Marsland D, Gupta S. Calcaneal traction pin placement simplified: a cadaveric study. Foot Ankle Int. 2011;32(6):651–5. https://doi.org/10.3113/FAI.2011.0651.
10. Rodrigues RN, Lopes AA, Torres JM, Mundim MF, Silva LLG, Silva BR de CE. Compressive neuropathy of the first branch of the lateral plantar nerve: a study by magnetic resonance imaging. Radiol Bras. 2015;48(6):368–72. https://doi.org/10.1590/0100-3984.2013.0028.
11. Tanz SS. Heel pain. Clin Orthop Relat Res. 1963;28:169–78.
12. Sallick MA, Blum L. Sensory denervation of the heel for persistent pain following fractures of the calcaneus. J Bone Joint Surg Am. 1948;30A(1):209–12.
13. Haugsdal J, Dawson J, Phisitkul P. Nerve injury and pain after operative repair of calcaneal fractures: a literature review. Iowa Orthop J. 2013;33:202–7.
14. Sanders R. Displaced intra-articular fractures of the calcaneus. J Bone Joint Surg Am. 2000;82(2):225–50. https://doi.org/10.2106/00004623-200002000-00009.
15. Freeman BJ, Duff S, Allen PE, Nicholson HD, Atkins RM. The extended lateral approach to the hindfoot. Anatomical basis and surgical implications. J Bone Joint Surg Br. 1998;80(1):139–42. https://doi.org/10.1302/0301-620x.80b1.7987.
16. Harvey EJ, Grujic L, Early JS, Benirschke SK, Sangeorzan BJ. Morbidity associated with ORIF of intra-articular calcaneus fractures using a lateral approach. Foot Ankle Int. 2001;22(11):868–73. https://doi.org/10.1177/107110070102201102.
17. Weber M, Lehmann O, Sägesser D, Krause F. Limited open reduction and internal fixation of displaced intra-articular fractures of the calcaneum. J Bone Joint Surg Br. 2008;90(12):1608–16. https://doi.org/10.1302/0301-620X.90B12.20638.
18. Park J-H, Chun D-I, Park K-R, et al. Can sural nerve injury be avoided in the sinus tarsi approach for calcaneal fracture?: a cadaveric study. Medicine (Baltimore). 2019;98(42):e17611. https://doi.org/10.1097/MD.0000000000017611.
19. Smyth NA, Zachwieja EC, Buller LT, Miranda AD, Steinlauf SD. Surgical approaches to the calcaneus and the sural nerve: there is no safe zone. Foot Ankle Surg. 2018;24(6):517–20. https://doi.org/10.1016/j.fas.2017.06.005.
20. Mann RA, Prieskorn D, Sobel M. Mid-tarsal and tarsometatarsal arthrodesis for primary degenerative osteoarthrosis or osteoarthrosis after trauma. J Bone Joint Surg Am. 1996;78(9):1376–85. https://doi.org/10.2106/00004623-199609000-00013.
21. Komenda GA, Myerson MS, Biddinger KR. Results of arthrodesis of the tarsometatarsal joints after traumatic injury. J Bone Joint Surg Am. 1996;78(11):1665–76. https://doi.org/10.2106/00004623-199611000-00005.
22. Pourcho AM, Liu YH, Milshteyn MA. Electrodiagnostically confirmed posttraumatic neuropathy and associated clinical exam findings with Lisfranc injury. Foot Ankle Int. 2013;34(8):1068–73. https://doi.org/10.1177/1071100713481454.
23. Kuo RS, Tejwani NC, Digiovanni CW, et al. Outcome after open reduction and internal fixation of Lisfranc joint injuries. J Bone Joint Surg Am. 2000;82(11):1609–18. https://doi.org/10.2106/00004623-200011000-00015.
24. Kanbe K, Kubota H, Shirakura K, Hasegawa A, Udagawa E. Entrapment neuropathy of the deep peroneal nerve associated with the extensor hallucis brevis. J Foot Ankle Surg. 1995;34(6):560–2. https://doi.org/10.1016/S1067-2516(09)80078-1.
25. Lawrence SJ, Botte MJ. The deep peroneal nerve in the foot and ankle: an anatomic study. Foot Ankle Int. 1995;16(11):724–8. https://doi.org/10.1177/107110079501601110.
26. Loveday DT, Nogaro M-C, Calder JDF, Carmichael J. Is there an anatomical marker for the deep peroneal nerve in midfoot surgical approaches? Clin Anat. 2013;26(3):400–2. https://doi.org/10.1002/ca.22173.
27. Meyerkort DJ, Gurel R, Maor D, Calder JDF. Deep peroneal nerve injury following hardware removal for Lisfranc joint injury. Foot Ankle Int. 2019;1071100719893699 https://doi.org/10.1177/1071100719893699.
28. Dellon AL. Deep peroneal nerve entrapment on the dorsum of the foot. Foot Ankle. 1990;11(2):73–80. https://doi.org/10.1177/107110079001100203.
29. Campbell DA. Sensory nerve damage during surgery on the hallux. J R Coll Surg Edinb. 1992;37(6):422–4.
30. Pont M-P, Assal M, Stern R, Fasel JH. Cutaneous sensory nerve injury during surgical approaches to the foot and ankle: a cadaveric anatomic study. Foot Ankle Surg. 2007;13(4):182–8. https://doi.org/10.1016/j.fas.2007.05.004.
31. Thakur NA, McDonnell M, Got CJ, Arcand N, Spratt KF, DiGiovanni CW. Injury patterns causing isolated foot compartment syndrome. J Bone Joint Surg Am. 2012;94(11):1030–5. https://doi.org/10.2106/JBJS.J.02000.
32. Dodd A, Le I. Foot compartment syndrome: diagnosis and management. J Am Acad Orthop Surg. 2013;21(11):657–64. https://doi.org/10.5435/JAAOS-21-11-657.

18

Nerve Injury After Open and Arthroscopic Surgery of the Ankle and Foot, Including Morton Neuroma

Jared M. Gopman, Steven Weinfeld, and Eitan Melamed

18.1 Risks/Incidence/Mechanism of Nerve Injury

Arthroscopic surgery of the ankle has continued to increase in popularity among foot and ankle surgeons in the past several decades as it allows for preservation of the soft tissue envelope, direct viewing of the internal joint structures, and earlier return to athletic activity compared to open approaches [1]. Prior to modern intraoperative distraction techniques, incidence of surgical complications with ankle arthroscopy in the literature was recorded as 24.6% [2]. However, a variety of invasive and noninvasive distraction techniques exist today which, in conjunction with standardization of portal placement and continued evolution of safe arthroscopic practices, has decreased the overall complication rate to 3–10% [3–5] Nevertheless, nerve injury following ankle arthroscopy remains the most common complication [6] and can have devastating consequences on postoperative outcome.

Anterior ankle arthroscopy is commonly performed for both diagnostic and therapeutic indications. Evaluation and treatment of ankle impingement from bony and soft tissue etiologies, removal of osteochondral lesions, assessment of ankle instability, and management of arthritis and chronic synovitis are all common conditions where anterior ankle arthroscopy use has been supported by literature [7]. The most common portal sites are the anteromedial (between the tibialis anterior and great saphenous vein) and anterolateral (lateral to the peroneal tertius tendon if present, or the extensor digitorum longus between the medial and lateral dorsal cutaneous branches of the superficial peroneal nerve) (Fig. 18.1). Injury to these branches of the superficial peroneal nerve are the most reported neurologic complication of anterior ankle arthroscopy [6], and great care during placement of the anterolateral portal is taken to prevent permanent neurologic sequelae. Injury to the saphenous nerve, which runs longitudinally with the greater saphenous vein, is at risk of injury during insertion of the anteromedial portal. A previously described anterocentral portal, which lies between the extensor hallucis longus and extensor digitorum longus, has fallen out of favor due to unacceptably high risk to the deep peroneal nerve and dorsalis pedis artery [8].

J. M. Gopman
Division of Plastic and Reconstructive Surgery, Department of Surgery, Icahn School of Medicine at Mount Sinai Hospital, New York, NY, USA

S. Weinfeld
Summit Medical Group, NJ, Berkeley, NJ, USA
e-mail: sweinfeld@smgnj.com

E. Melamed (✉)
Division of Plastic and Reconstructive Surgery, Department of Surgery, Icahn School of Medicine at Mount Sinai Hospital, New York, NY, USA

Elmhurst Hospital Center, Elmhurst, NY, USA
e-mail: melamede2@nychhc.org

C. J. Dy et al. (eds.), *Peripheral Nerve Issues after Orthopedic Surgery*,
https://doi.org/10.1007/978-3-030-84428-8_18

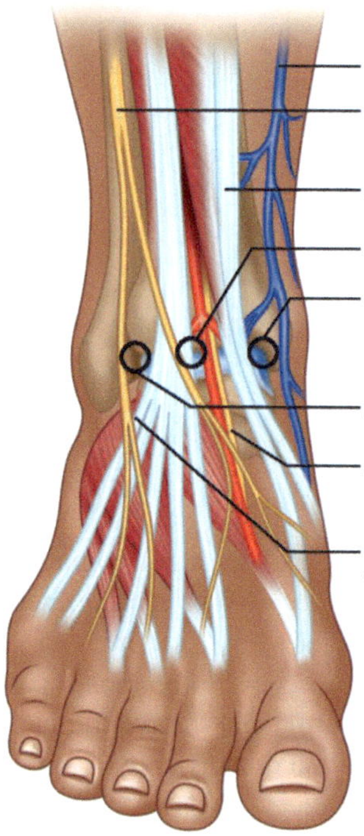

Fig. 18.1 Anterior ankle arthroscopy portals and critical nearby anatomic structures

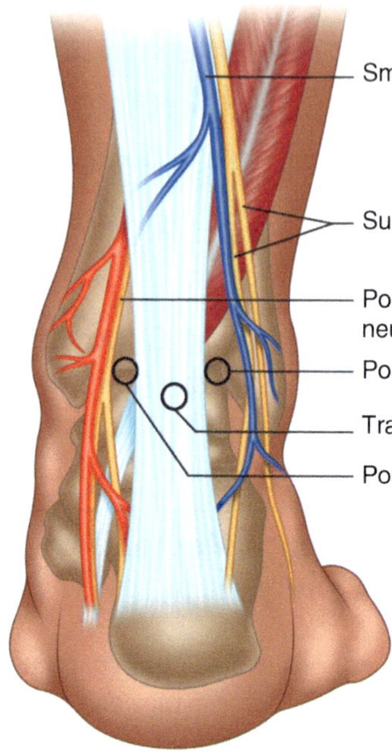

Fig. 18.2 Posterior ankle arthroscopy portals and nearby critical anatomic structures

Posterior ankle arthroscopy, first described by van Dijk et al. in 2000 [9], allows for greater viewing of the tibiotalar and subtalar joints and has gained increased support for diagnosis and treatment of causes of posterior ankle impingement and cartilage and soft tissue disorders of the posterior hindfoot. The two portals used in posterior arthroscopy are the posteromedial (medial to the Achilles tendon) and posterolateral (lateral aspect of Achilles tendon) (Fig. 18.2). The medial portal risks injury to the main posterior tibial neurovascular bundle to the foot, while the lateral portal can injure the sural nerve and lesser saphenous vein.

18.2 Pertinent Anatomy

18.2.1 Superficial Peroneal Nerve

The superficial peroneal nerve arises from the common peroneal nerve at the fibular head and runs longitudinally in the lateral compartment of the lower leg. As it descends, it becomes more superficial within the compartment until approximately 4–5 cm above the ankle joint where it pierces the crural fascia to enter the subcutaneous plane. At the ankle, the nerve has been described by Takao et al. to have five branching patterns [10]. The most common branching pattern is type 2, with division into a medial dorsal cutaneous nerve and intermediate or lateral dorsal cutaneous nerve at the ankle, with further divisions into the terminal branches occurring more distally. The intermediate dorsal cutaneous nerve runs over the lateral two rays in the direction of the third metatarsal space before dividing into the lateral dorsal digital branches (Fig. 18.3), while the medial dorsal cutaneous nerve passes over the common extensor digitorum longus tendon to run with the extensor hallucis longus tendon and divides into the medial dorsal digital branches (Fig. 18.4). The variability of the branching patterns at the level of the ankle joint places the nerve at risk during creation of the anterolateral portal.

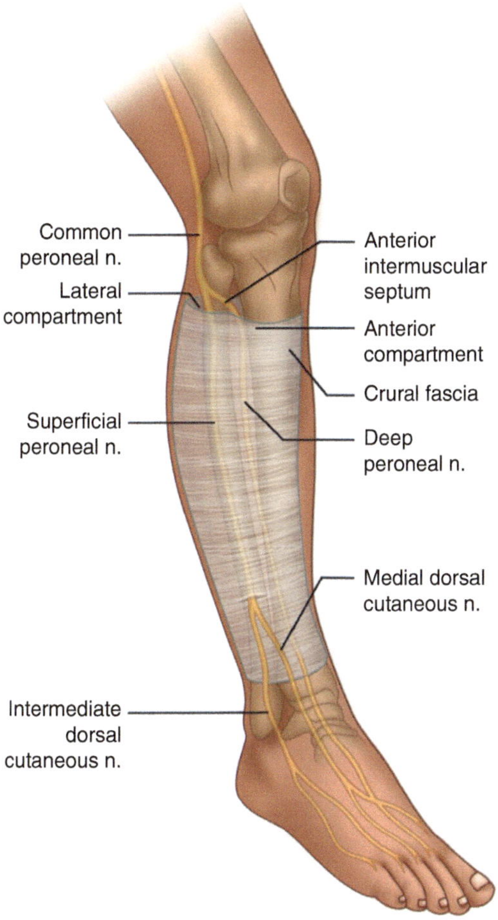

Fig. 18.3 Course of the peroneal nerve in the lower extremity

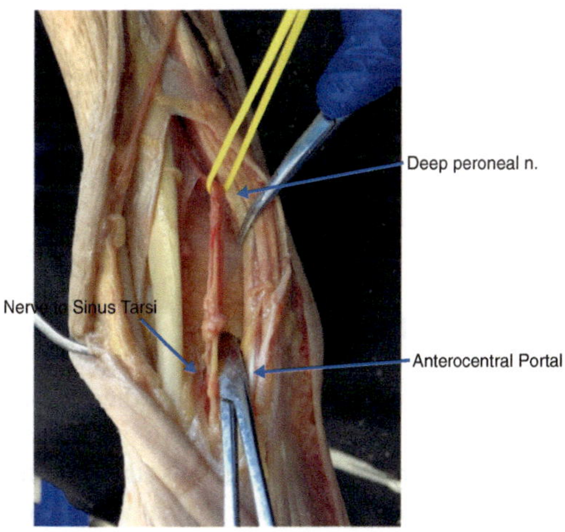

Fig. 18.4 Deep anterior ankle dissection demonstrating the deep peroneal nerve and its relationship to the anterocentral portal

18.2.2 Deep Peroneal Nerve

The deep peroneal nerve begins as a branch of the common peroneal nerve in the proximal leg and then courses through the anterior compartment between the fibula and peroneus longus, where it gives off several muscular branches as well as a branch to the articular surface of the ankle. At the ankle joint, it lies beneath the crural fascia, lateral to the dorsalis pedis artery between the extensor hallucis longus tendon and first tendon of the extensor digitorum longus. The previously described anterocentral portal places the deep peroneal nerve at great risk (Fig. 18.5). For this reason, the anteromedial portal, first described by Buckingham et al. [11], has replaced the anterocentral portal for general use.

18.2.3 Posterior Tibial Nerve

The tibial nerve arises as a branch of the sciatic nerve in the distal thigh, continues through the popliteal fossa, and then traverses the lower extremity on the deep surface of the soleus until it traverses posterior to the medial malleolus with the posterior tibial artery. At this point, the continuation of the tibial nerve is described as the posterior tibial nerve. The posterior tibial nerve then branches in the hindfoot to give rise to the medial and lateral plantar nerves, the main motor nerves of the foot musculature. Injury to the posterior tibial nerve is an uncommon complication of posteromedial portal insertion during posterior ankle arthroscopy.

18.2.4 Sural Nerve

The sural nerve is formed by fusion of the medial sural cutaneous nerve, a branch of the tibial nerve at the head of the lateral gastrocnemius, and the lateral sural cutaneous nerve, a cutaneous branch of the common peroneal nerve at the fibular head prior to division into its superficial and deep branches. The medial and lateral sural cutaneous nerves travel distally and join at the distal third of the gastrocnemius via the sural communicating branch where it pierces the muscular fascia and enters the subcutaneous

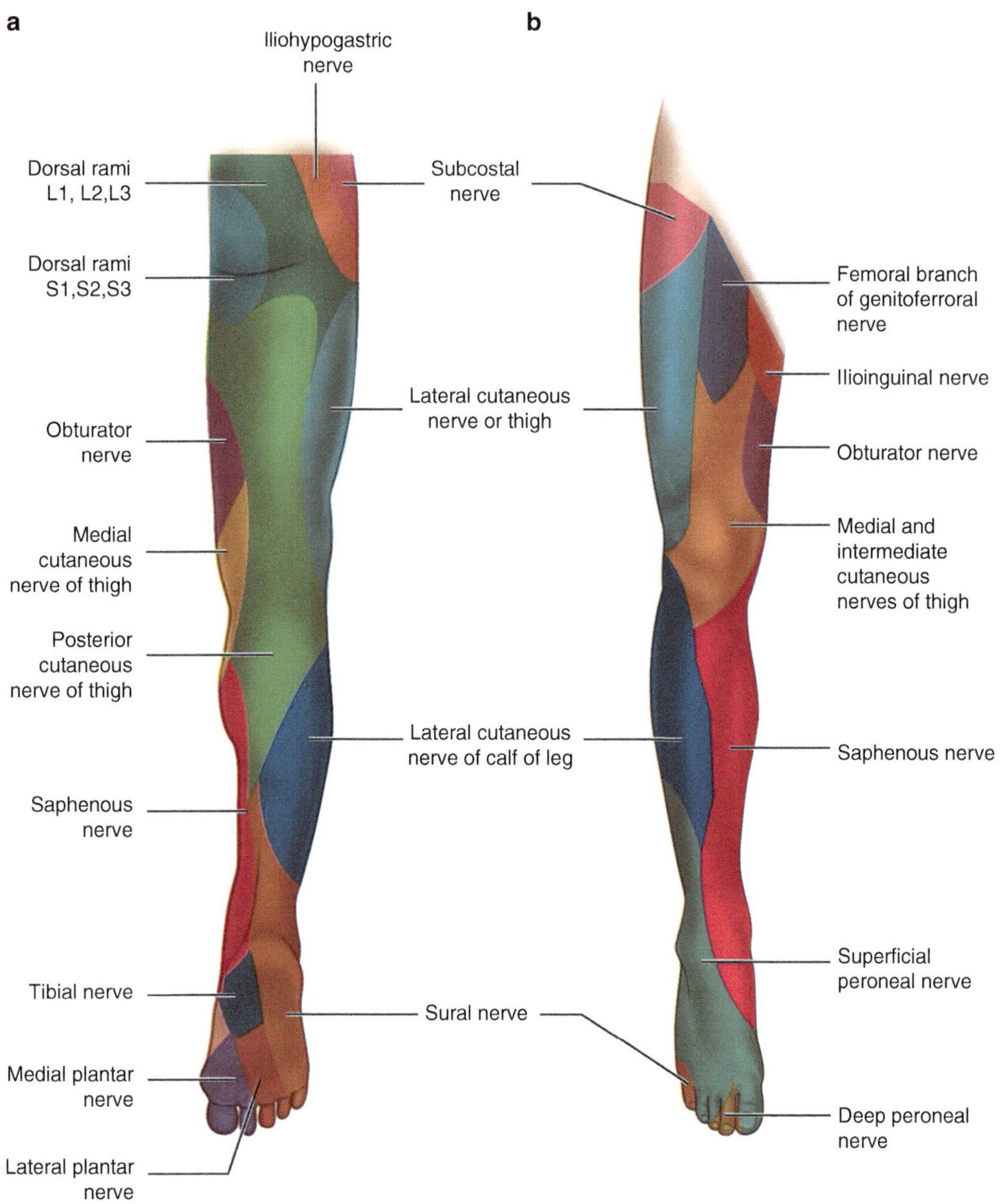

Fig. 18.5 Dermatome distribution of the anterior and posterior lower extremity

plane. It travels along this plane with the lesser saphenous vein and traverses the ankle 1.5 cm posterior to the lateral malleolus, posterior to the peroneal tendons. The nerve runs anterior to the short saphenous vein and then divides into the medial and lateral terminal branches at the base of the fifth metatarsal (Fig. 18.6). Insertion of the posterolateral portal places the sural nerve at risk during posterior ankle arthroscopy.

18.2.5 Saphenous Nerve

The saphenous nerve arises from the femoral nerve in the anterior thigh, where it passes deep to the sartorius muscle, travels through the adductor canal, and pierces the deep fascia 10 cm above the level of the knee between the tendons of the sartorius and gracilis where it enters the subcutaneous plane. The nerve then travels along the tibial side of the leg in close proximity to the great saphenous vein and then descends posterior to the medial border of the tibia where it gives off anterior and posterior branches approximately 3 cm proximal to the tip of the medial malleolus. These branches provide sensation to the medial leg and ankle (Fig. 18.6). The saphenous nerve may be injured from insertion of the anteromedial portal during anterior ankle arthroscopy, or loss of sensation could also occur following harvest as a donor nerve graft (Fig. 18.7).

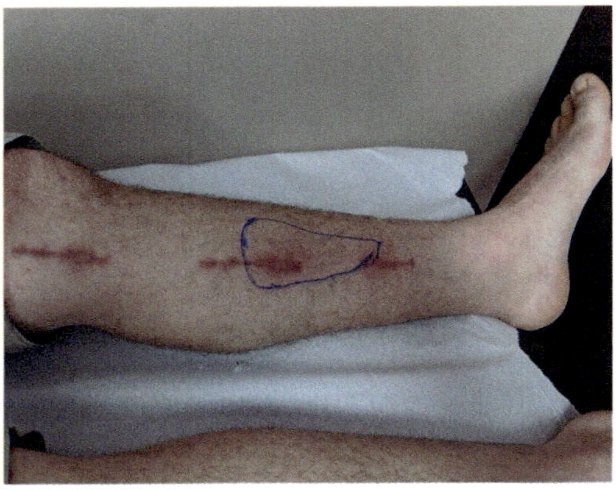

Fig. 18.6 Sensory deficit following saphenous nerve harvest for brachial plexus reconstruction. The marked area shows the resultant sensory deficit 2 years after donor harvest

18.3 Prevention Strategies

- A well-padded pneumatic tourniquet on the thigh, proper positioning of the extremity with the hip abducted, the knee flexed, and a knee holder for anterior ankle arthroscopy (removed for posterior ankle arthroscopy).
- Noninvasive ankle distractors using the dorsiflexion method or an ankle strap for longitudinal traction to widen the ankle joint space during surgery.
- Plantarflexion and inversion of the ankle can assist with surface identification of the intermediate dorsal cutaneous nerve, which can be marked preoperatively to prevent inadvertent injury.
- Placement of the anteromedial portal first and then placement of the anterolateral portal under inside-out visualization during anterior ankle arthroscopy.
- Placement of the posterolateral portal first and then placement of the posteromedial portal under inside-out visualization during posterior ankle arthroscopy.

18.4 Typical Course/Natural History

Injury to the superficial peroneal nerve or its branches during anterior ankle arthroscopy will

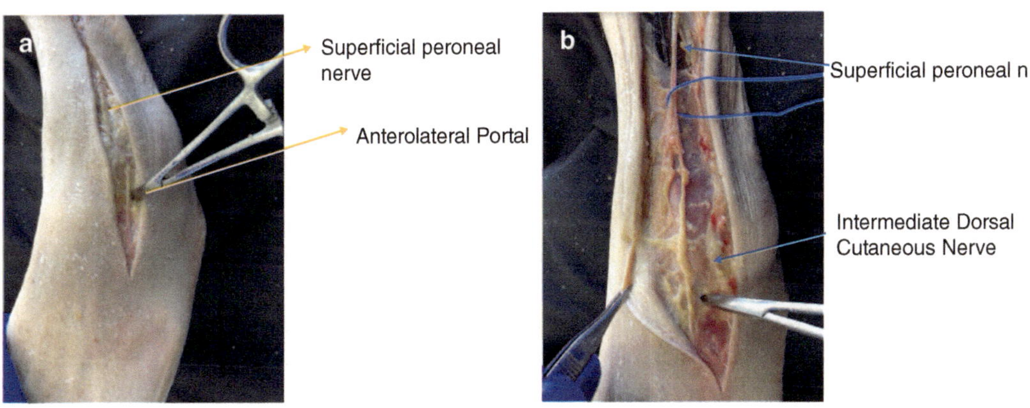

Fig. 18.7 Surface anatomy (**a**) and superficial dissection (**b**) showing the course of the superficial peroneal nerve and the relationship with the anterolateral portal

present immediately with loss of sensation within the affected dermatome on the lateral dorsal aspect of the foot and "wicked" neuroma pain. Severe axonotmesis or neurotmesis injury from portal placement will not allow for regeneration of normal sensation in this distribution, and permanent sensory loss will develop. Alternatively, aberrant nerve fibers may develop into a cutaneous neuroma over the subsequent months, which will present with paresthesia and palpable tenderness manifesting as a shock-like sensation at the neuroma site. Similar effects will be seen in the dermatome distribution for the other sensory nerves of the foot and ankle at risk during arthroscopy.

Damage to the posterior tibial nerve during posterior ankle arthroscopy is a much more devastating complication, as immediate loss of plantarflexion and the intrinsic motor function of the foot will occur. Patients will complain about inability to plant their foot during athletic activities and while driving an automobile. In addition, patients will exhibit sensory loss on the plantar surface of the foot, important for proprioception and protective movements.

18.5 Initial Evaluation/Exam

If a patient presents with concern for neurologic injury following anterior or posterior ankle arthroscopy, clinical examination with meticulous documentation is the key to determining the etiology of their symptoms and likelihood for improvement:

- Examination of surgical scars created from portal sites
- Tinel's sign at patient-directed affected areas to identify neuroma
- Sensation testing via light touch, two-point discrimination, proprioception, and monofilament threshold testing
- Motor testing of plantarflexion, inversion, and abduction/adduction of phalanges

18.6 Diagnostic Tests/Imaging

- Ultrasonography can be helpful to assist with identification of discontinuity at surgical site and surrounding scar tissue. If unable to visualize using ultrasound, magnetic resonance imaging can better identify areas of compression or neuroma locations.
- Diagnostic nerve blocks using lidocaine or bupivacaine can be beneficial to determine cause-effect alleviation of patient symptomology in nerve distribution and can rule out nerve injury as a potential cause of pain if the diagnosis of postoperative neurologic complication is unclear. Patients are encouraged to keep a diary documenting pain intensity at regular intervals to monitor pain relief. The diary is brought to the next consult and scanned into the medical record.
- Electromyography and nerve conduction studies can complement the physical examination, helping to localize the level of injury to the sensory nerves of the foot and ankle, as well as the posterior tibial nerve, and predict the likelihood of spontaneous recovery.

18.7 Surgical Techniques

Principles of peripheral nerve injury management have been largely elucidated as pertains to upper extremity injuries and similarly apply to foot and ankle surgery as well. If a peripheral nerve injury is recognized at the time of the index procedure, it is important to return to the operating room for re-exploration within 72 hours. Within this timeframe, the distal nerve ends contain neurotransmitters, and motor end plates can be stimulated intraoperatively, [12] critical for proper alignment of the posterior tibial nerve topography during repair. More often, iatrogenic nerve injuries go unnoticed during the immediate postoperative period and only become apparent when a painful neuroma has formed. Prior to surgical management of painful sensory neuroma, conservative measures such as desensitization protocols and neuropathic medications do no harm and may be occasionally beneficial. These should be employed for at least 6 weeks, depending on patient response [13].

When the decision to move forward with surgical intervention is made, careful preoperative planning of location to explore, modalities of repair, and likelihood of successful outcomes must be considered prior to entering the operating room. The first critical step in any nerve injury exploration is identification of the proximal and distal ends. Knowledge of nerve course is essential for this, as surgical planes will often be obfuscated by scar formation. Exploration should be performed under loupe magnification, and a well-padded tourniquet is preferred to provide a bloodless field during exploration. The primary goal is to reconnect the proximal and distal stumps whenever possible and allow the proximal axons to reach their targets. Once the proximal and distal stumps are identified and trimmed properly to healthy fascicles, tension-free coaptation may be attempted, to restore continuity. However often the resultant gap will demand a graft. Neurolysis from the surrounding scar tissue and anatomic positioning of the ankle (i.e., dorsiflexion for dorsal branches) can be helpful to decrease nerve gap; however, nerve gaps should not be directly repaired under tension as traction ischemia and contraction during healing will decrease likelihood of proper regeneration [14].

18.8 Salvage Techniques

In a delayed re-exploration, direct repair is usually not possible, as retraction of the proximal end and perineural scarring will make tension-free repair exceedingly difficult. In these cases, gap management using nerve substitutes must be considered. Nerve autograft is considered the gold standard for gap management, as it contains the necessary components for nerve regeneration including viable Schwann cells, endoneurial tubes, and extracellular matrix [15]. Commonly used autografts within the surgical field include the sural nerve and saphenous nerve, with the medial or lateral antebrachial cutaneous nerves easily harvested at a second surgical site. However, increased operative time along with sensory nerve loss and neuroma formation at the donor site preclude the use of autografts in small gaps <3 cm when other options are available [12].

Nerve substitutes include synthetic conduits and processed nerve allografts (PNAs). Both conduits and PNAs are appealing due to their “off-the-shelf” availability in a variety of lengths and diameters, ability to relieve tension off a direct repair, prevention of surrounding scar tissue formation, and support regeneration across a nerve gap without need for a donor site. Success of nerve regeneration with conduits and PNAs has been demonstrated in small sensory nerves such as the digital nerves of the hand; however, failed regeneration has been reported with larger diameter nerves and greater gap lengths. While nerve substitutes retain normal nerve architecture such as endoneurial tubes and extracellular matrix, [16]·they lack the Schwann cells and nerve vasculature that aid in nerve regeneration [17].

When approaching a patient with peripheral nerve injury, repair is commonly performed utilizing the following procedural steps:

- Identification of proximal and distal ends of the injured peripheral nerve, and neurolysis within the surgical field to allow for free movement of the severed ends.
- Resection of scar tissue until visualization of healthy fascicular bundles in the cut ends.
- Measurement of nerve diameter and gap length while under minimum tension.
- If direct repair can be performed (<1 cm gap), place two to three 9/0 or 10/0 nonabsorbable monofilament sutures in the epineurium to coapt the ends with minimal trauma. Then, use an appropriately sized nerve conduit to wrap the coaptation site and protect from sur-

rounding scar tissue infiltration and take the tension off the repair ("remote detensioning").
- If direct repair cannot be performed without tension and nerve gap measures <3 cm, then utilization of a conduit (for gap <5 mm) or PNA is warranted. Coaptation of the proximal and distal ends to the substitute should be performed similarly to direct repair, with the minimal number of epineural sutures needed to secure the substitute across the nerve gap.
- If a conduit is used, the proximal and distal ends can be telescoped into the conduit via 9/0 or 10/0 nonabsorbable monofilament sutures in order to decrease the nerve gap and take tension off the severed ends.

Neuroma formation occurs following any failure of nerve regeneration; therefore, neuromas may be seen following the index procedure or after failed nerve repair from the aforementioned methods. Upon exploration of the surgical field, the proximal end may be found to end in a "scar ball," or the proximal and distal ends may be joined by a thickened segment of scar tissue, known as a neuroma-in-continuity. Following identification of the neuroma, it should be resected back to healthy nerve fascicles. When resection length is in question, frozen sections of nerve margins have been utilized for histologic evaluation of the margin of resection, with 75% of axonal elements in the stump being the threshold for adequate repair [18].

After resection is performed, multiple management options exist, including nerve repair using autografts or nerve substitutes; placement of an acellular nerve allograft "cap"; transposition of the proximal end into surrounding tissue such as muscle, bone, or veins; use of regenerative peripheral nerve interfaces; or targeted muscle reinnervation [18, 19]. While the data for each of these methods are largely based on studies on neuromas of the upper extremity and following lower extremity amputations, each technique has shown good to excellent results, and at this time no head-to-head studies for iatrogenic foot and ankle neurologic injuries have confirmed benefit of one technique over others [20].

18.9 Outcomes

In the foot and ankle literature, Souza et al. used PNAs to treat iatrogenic painful neuromas in 22 patients, most commonly of the sural and superficial peroneal nerve branches. After excision of end-neuromas and neuromas-in-continuity, the average gap spanned by PNAs was 3.3 cm, and after a minimum of 6 months' follow-up, their average pain scores decreased by a statistically significant and clinically important proportion with decreased ordinal pain and less interference with activities of daily living. While this retrospective review was limited by its small sample size, inherent bias due to its retrospective nature, and lack of comparison treatment outcome, it validated the use of PNAs for treatment of neuromas following neurologic injury in foot and ankle surgery [21].

Alternatively, Bibbo et al. described a methodology for treatment of severe recalcitrant superficial peroneal neuromas following anterior ankle arthroscopy via nerve transfer to the deep peroneal nerve using an allograft conduit in the mid-leg. Upon dissection and neurolysis of the superficial and deep peroneal nerves, stimulation was used to ensure the motor branches of the deep peroneal nerve had emanated proximally to their planned recipient site. Once the deep peroneal nerve sensory branch was confirmed, both nerves were divided proximally to the neuroma site, and a PNA with nerve wrap was used to span the gap between them for neurorrhaphy. After performing this transfer in 11 patients with a mean follow-up of 31 months, a statistically significant decrease in neuropathic pain was recorded by each patient, with all patients responding that they would choose to undergo the procedure again [22].

18.10 Technical Pearls and Pitfalls

18.10.1 Tarsal Tunnel Syndrome

18.10.1.1 Risks/Incidence/Mechanism of Nerve Injury/Structures at Risk

The tarsal tunnel is a fibro-osseous space located posterior to the medial malleolus. It has a bony floor formed by the medial talar surface, the sustentaculum tali, and the medial calcaneal wall. The roof of the tarsal tunnel is formed by the flexor retinaculum which is the thin fibrous tissue that has its origin from the medial and inferior aspect of the medial malleolus and inserts into the periosteum of the medial tuberosity of the calcaneus. The base of the flexor retinaculum corresponds to the superior border of the abductor hallucis muscle [23] (Fig. 18.8).

The posterior tibial, flexor digitorum longus, and flexor hallucis longus tendons are located within the tarsal tunnel, each with its own syno-

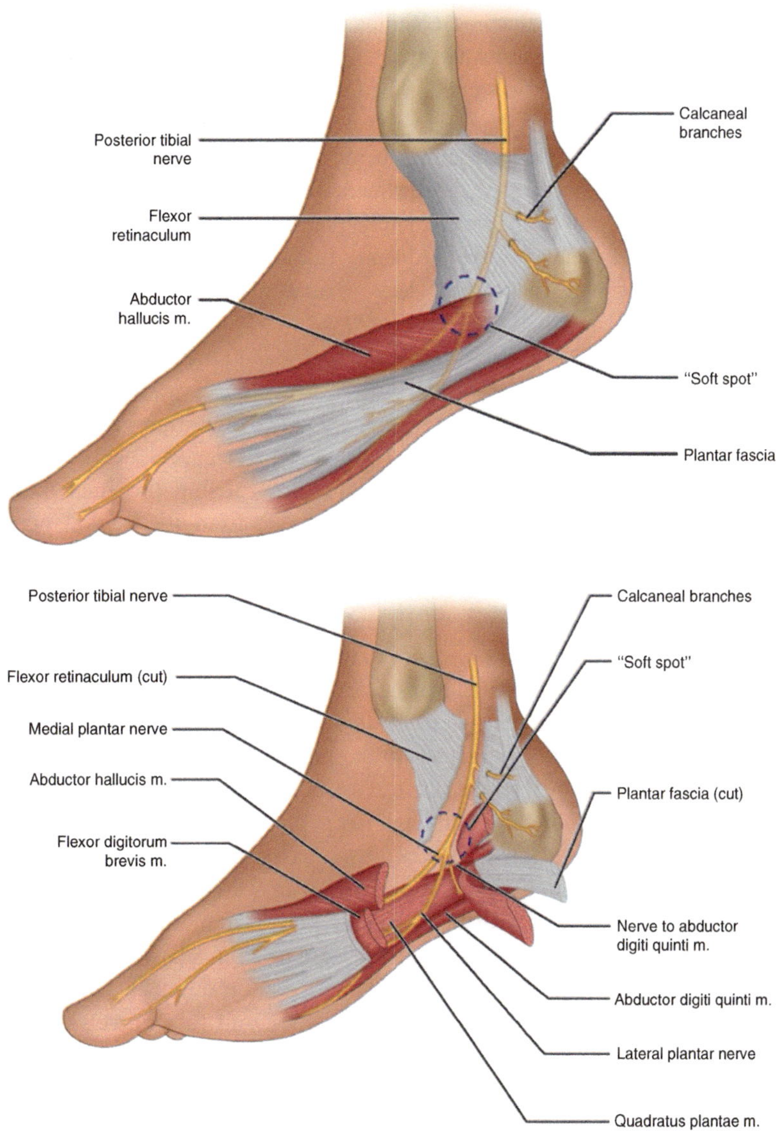

Fig. 18.8 Tarsal tunnel anatomy

vial sheath. The tendons are contained within a separate compartment formed by the fibrous projections from the undersurface of the flexor retinaculum. The tibial nerve enters the tarsal tunnel between the overlying flexor retinaculum and the underlying tendon sheath of the posterior tibial flexor digitorum longus and flexor hallucis longus muscles. The tibial nerve and artery are often attached to these sheets through surrounding areolar tissue. The tarsal tunnel is narrowest at its distal portion where it is conjoined with the fascia of the abductor hallucis longus muscle. The nerve at this level can become trapped causing tarsal tunnel syndrome, the most common entrapment neuropathy of the tibial nerve.

Tarsal tunnel syndrome was described in 1962 and was thought to be analogous to carpal tunnel syndrome with the flexor retinaculum being comparable to the transverse carpal ligament [24]. However, the medial plantar nerve, lateral plantar nerve, and the calcaneal nerve frequently reside in their own tunnels, making this analogy inaccurate [25].

18.11 Pertinent Anatomy

The tibial nerve arises from the medial half of the sciatic nerve, usually at the middle to distal one third of the thigh. The nerve is deep to the hamstring muscles, which are on either side of the posterior compartment of the thigh, and in the popliteal fossa the nerve lies posterior to the popliteal artery and vein. A medial hamstring branch occasionally leaves the tibial nerve at this level. More commonly, sensory branches to the proximal calf may arise before the nerve reaches its first major target as it courses through the popliteal fossa. The tibial nerve runs beneath the gastrocnemius soleus muscle group giving an abundance of branches to it and the plantaris, popliteus, and tibial muscles. Such branches begin to define themselves as separate tibial branches proximal to the superior edge of the gastrocnemius soleus complex [26].

A deeper posterior tibial branch accompanies the tibial artery and vein and runs through the leg medial and posterior to the tibia and posterior to the intermuscular septum, separating the anterior from the posterior compartments. The posterior tibial nerve carries fibers destined for the foot but gives off branches in the more proximal leg to supply the flexor digitorum longus and flexor hallucis longus muscle. As the posterior tibial nerve approaches the ankle, it courses inferior to the medial malleolus. At this level, it passes beneath the flexor retinaculum and branches into medial and lateral plantar nerves, although these nerves can also arise and be well defined proximal to the malleolus [27]. The lateral plantar nerve, which is comparable with the ulnar nerve at the hand, runs deep in the instep and supplies the second to fourth lumbricals, the adductor hallucis, and all interossei except that of the fourth metatarsal. It also supplies the skin of the fifth toe and the lateral half of the fourth toe.

The medial plantar branch provides sensation to the medial plantar surface of the foot and innervation to the abductor hallucis and flexor digitorum brevis muscles. A third branch – the calcaneal nerve – can usually be found either arising proximal to these nerves or branching from the medial plantar nerve. The calcaneal nerve can have numerous anatomic variations [28]. Injury to the medial and lateral plantar nerves may spare sensation on the heel of the foot as the calcaneal nerve provides cutaneous innervation to this region.

The tarsal tunnel may be divided into a proximal zone which extends from the retinaculum to the origin of the abductor muscle and a distal zone which begins at the fibrous origin of the abductor hallucis muscle and extends through this muscle. The distal zone may contain three additional separate tunnels: the medial plantar tunnel, the lateral plantar tunnel, and the calcaneal tunnel. The goal of surgery is to decompress all four tunnels: the tarsal tunnel and the three separate distal tunnels [29] (Fig. 18.9).

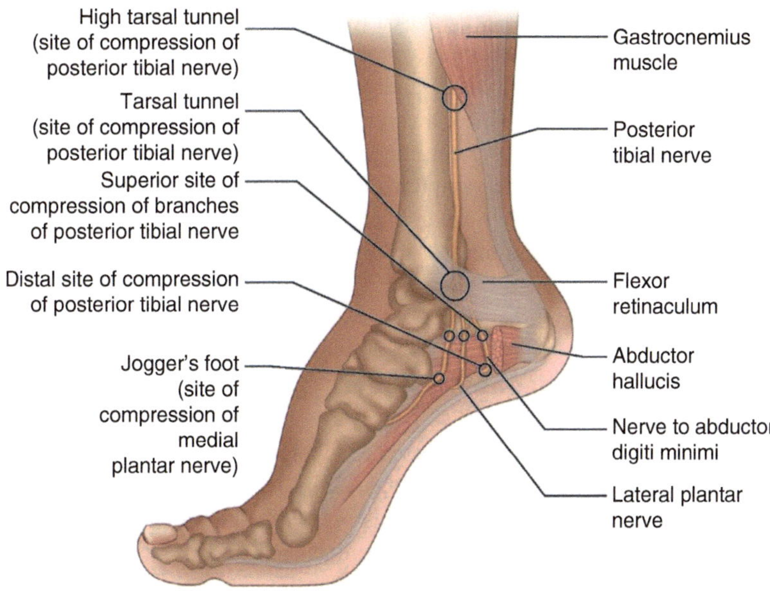

Fig. 18.9 Artist depiction of the four compression sites at tibial nerve branches

18.12 Typical Course/Natural History

Tarsal tunnel syndrome is a spontaneous and slowly progressive condition. Common associations include obesity, decreased elasticity of collagen, or a progressive flatfoot in an adult [23]. Other causes of the syndrome are a deep medial ganglion from the subtalar joint, an adjacent chronic tenosynovitis, or partial rupture of the posterior tibial tendon with secondary compression of the nerve [30].

18.13 Initial Evaluation

An accurate diagnosis depends on a detailed history and meticulous clinical examination, with adjunctive electrical studies and occasionally advanced imaging. Patients complain of burning plantar heel pain, often in the metatarsal area and occasionally radiating to the medial calf. This may be alleviated by rest and aggravated activity, although some patients report night pain [31]. The main physical examination finding is a Tinel sign producing paresthesias on the plantar surface of the foot and usually elicited inferior to the medial malleolus and sometimes proximally or distally in the region of the instep.

A positive Tinel sign test proximal to the point of compression usually means that the nerve is compressed about 2 cm distal to the enlarged tibial nerve. Sometimes there is either a mild hypoesthesia or mixed hypo- and hyperesthesia on the sole or heel of the foot. Toe flexion and foot intrinsic function are usually spared in the majority of cases unless there has been a prior operation, ankle or foot injury as a precipitating factor, or if symptoms have been long-standing. The presence of Tinel's sign is predictive of a positive response to nerve decompression [32].

18.14 Diagnostic Tests

Perineural infiltration of 1% lidocaine with or without cortisone via local injection may diminish paresthesias and pain with weight-bearing, and although anesthesia is only temporary, the relief of pain and discomfort provides diagnostic information [33]. Patients are advised to keep a "pain diary" and document pain symptoms following the injection. Pain relief after lidocaine injection may be therapeutic for a varying period of time and signals that surgical intervention in the future may resolve the symptoms. However partial response may signify different etiology or a second nerve compression at a different anatomical site.

18.14.1 Electrodiagnostic Studies

Electrodiagnostic studies may be used to supplement the clinical examination findings [23] but are not essential to make the diagnosis in every case. A recent review could not determine the sensitivity and specificity of electrodiagnostic studies in the diagnosis of tarsal tunnel syndrome [34]. As with other compression neuropathies, it is important to compare values from the involved foot with those in the contralateral unaffected limb. The normal reference limits are far less precisely defined for tibial nerve compression than they are for carpal tunnel studies.

Since nerve compression is dynamic in its early stages, it is not unusual to have a negative electrical study unless the patient undergoes 10–15 minutes of walking, standing, or tiptoeing before the tests are performed. Typically, if exercise causes paresthesias, compression is usually present [23, 35].

18.15 Surgical Techniques

Nonoperative treatment for tarsal tunnel syndrome includes ankle immobilization, anti-inflammatory medications, and frequent use of a wide comfortable shoe. An orthosis with a relief within the medial arch may be effective if distal tarsal tunnel is suspected or if symptoms are worsened by longitudinal arch support orthosis.

It is important to exclude diabetes and alcoholic neuropathies and to be certain that the foot has sufficient blood supply to heal the surgical wound before performing tarsal tunnel release. Metabolic neuropathy with secondary nerve compression is not a contraindication to surgery, as evidence supports the role of nerve decompression in this patient population as an adjunct to medical optimization [36, 37]. Contraindications for surgery include morbid obesity, severe venous stasis, and insufficient blood supply to heal surgical wounds. Caution should be exercised in patients older than 60 and those with no identifiable cause of the symptoms.

18.15.1 Tarsal Tunnel Release

The procedure begins with a curvilinear skin incision about 5 cm proximal and posterior to the medial malleolus, curving anteriorly to the heel. Alternatively, two incisions can be made – the one proximal to the malleolus and the second distal to the malleolus to expose the three tarsal tunnels. Magnification and the use of the tourniquet, medium-sized tenotomy scissors, microbipolar electrocautery, and Penrose drains or vessel loops for retraction are helpful. Stepwise and patient dissection is essential, especially as the dissection progresses distally. Initially, the posterior tibial nerve is found medial to the Achilles tendon and proximal to the medial malleolus. The nerve is then traced beneath the medial malleolus by dividing the overlying flexor retinaculum. Exposure of the posterior tibial nerve at this level is often compared with that of the median nerve, though the tarsal tunnel is much more complex, and dissection is more tedious. The tibial artery has a serpiginous course and arterial and venous branches are intertwined with the nerve as it forms the medial and lateral plantar and calcaneal nerves. The medial and lateral plantar nerves are traced distally as they reach the medial border of the abductor hallucis and continue plantarward deep to the muscle. As dissection continues distally, three fascial layers require release: superficial abductor fascia, deep abductor fascia, and septum anchoring the deep fascia of the muscle to the calcaneus (Fig. 18.10).

The lateral plantar nerve is identified first and followed into its separate tunnel by dividing the

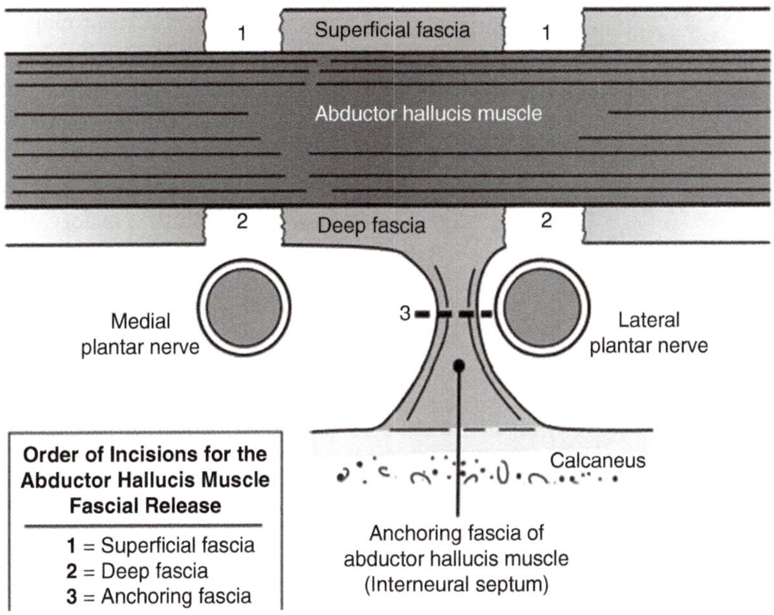

Fig. 18.10 Cross-sectional illustration of the medial and lateral plantar tunnels with interneural septum

fascial origin of the abductor hallucis brevis, which is the roof of the tunnel. The medial plantar nerve is more anterior and is unroofed in its separate tunnel as well. Care is taken to avoid injury to the little unnamed branch from the medial plantar nerve into the skin of the medial arch [38]. Injury to this nerve will lead to chronic pain at the distal aspect of the tarsal tunnel skin incision.

The branches are separated and must be entirely unroofed and exposed circumferentially to provide a bed for the nerves and branches free of scar or compressive tissue. This must include sectioning of the overlying muscle and its fascial edge in the instep portion of the foot. The septum between the medial and lateral plantar tunnels is longitudinally released. The calcaneal branch should be decompressed in its tunnel, especially in patients reporting heel pain (Fig. 18.11). Complete external neurolysis is performed at this stage. Successful release of the distal tunnels allows the surgeon's small finger to pass into the plantar aspect of the foot (Fig. 18.12). The wound is then closed in a standard fashion. The patient is encouraged to ambulate after surgery in order to prevent scarring of the nerve.

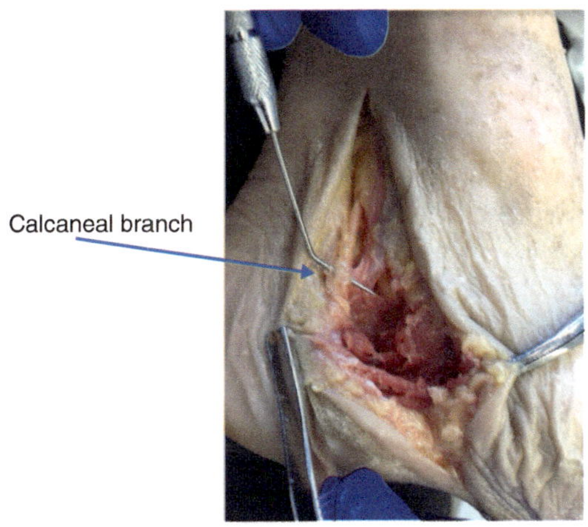

Fig. 18.11 Anatomic dissection of the calcaneal branch of the posterior tibial nerve. Isolated decompression of the calcaneal nerve should be performed especially in patients with heel pain. Unnamed proximal branches of this nerve (not shown) can lead to painful neuroma if cut unintentionally

18.16 Outcomes

Mullick and Dellon summarize their long-term outcomes after 87 release procedures with an average follow-up of 3.6 years. They reported

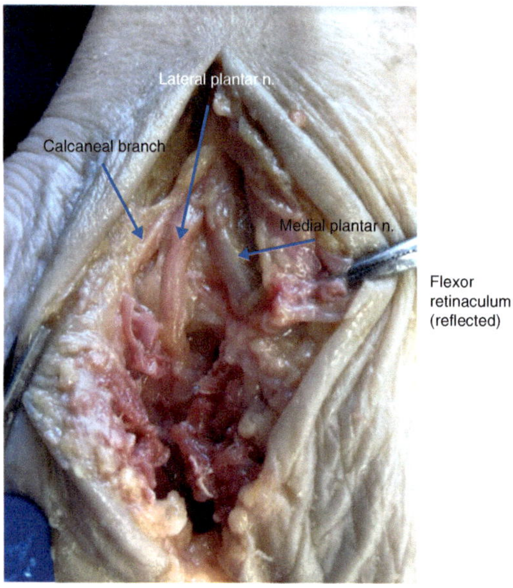

Fig. 18.12 Anatomic dissection demonstrating decompression and neurolysis of all branches of the posterior tibial nerve

resolution of symptoms in 82% of patients, with slight residual numbness and tingling in 11% of the patients who still were able to return to work [39]. Kim and Murovic reported their results in 46 feet from 43 patients with the diagnosis of tarsal tunnel syndrome who underwent decompression with complete external neurolysis, sectioning of the flexor retinaculum and origin of the abductor hallucis muscle, and splitting of the muscles of the instep. In 28 patients without prior surgery, the outcome following external neurolysis was excellent in 22 (79%) and fair to poor in 6 (21%) [40]. Lack of response following nerve decompression is well-described and may signify a second compression site or severe neuropathy. We tell our patients that decompressive surgery does not cure neuropathy, and regeneration may take up to 1 year. We encourage them to walk frequently postoperatively in order to prevent adhesions and mobilize the released nerves.

18.17 Technical Pearls

- Successful relief of symptoms may be offered to the patient with tibial nerve entrapment in the tarsal tunnel, using the same principles that were developed to treat the upper extremity nerves.
- Careful surgical technique can lead to successful outcomes even in patients with superimposed metabolic neuropathy predisposed to compression neuropathy.
- Clinical history, the presence of Tinel's sign, and response to local nerve blocks are the cornerstones of diagnosis.

Decompression of the proximal tarsal tunnel as well as the three distal tunnels is essential along with external neurolysis to separate the nerve from surrounding structures.

18.17.1 Hallux Valgus

18.17.1.1 Risks/Incidence/Mechanism of Nerve Injury

Hallux valgus or "bunion deformity" is one of the most common disorders of the forefoot. The hallmark of the condition is lateral deviation of the great toe phalanges (hallux) and medial deviation of the first metatarsal. The disease is progressive with multiple stages, eventually leading to progressive subluxation of the first metatarsophalangeal (MTP) joint [41]. As the disease progresses, symptoms such as poor fitting shoes, plantar foot, medial first MTP joint pain, decreased athletic performance from loss of propulsion and abnormal weight-bearing distribution, [42] and first MTP joint destruction are all seen. While the disease is commonly seen in adults, juvenile hallux valgus can occur. Furthermore, women are diagnosed more frequently than men, with some studies quoting a F:M ratio of 15:1; women are also more likely to have surgery. This disparity is theorized to be the consequence of more frequent use of tight fitting and high-heeled shoes [43]. While restrictive footwear is thought to play a role in development of the disorder, intrinsic factors such as genetics, pronation of the hindfoot, pes planus (flat foot), hypermobility, Achilles tendon contracture, cerebral palsy, and previous strokes have all been associated with hallux valgus onset [44].

Diagnosis of hallux valgus includes a thorough history, including duration of symptoms, footwear, activity modification, and family history. Physical examination should test observance of gait, alignment, range of motion of the first MTP joint, specific areas of tenderness, presence of calluses or bunions, and presence or absence of Achilles tightness. Weight-bearing radiographs are also necessary for diagnosis to view the angle between the longitudinal axis of the first metatarsal and first proximal phalanx, known as the hallux valgus angle, and the intermetatarsal angle between the longitudinal axis of the first and second metatarsal. Typically, a hallux valgus angle >15 degrees or an intermetatarsal angle >9 degrees has been defined as abnormal with varying degrees of severity as these angles increase [45]. The radiographic classification of hallux valgus divides the deformity into mild, moderate, and severe based on these angles and the degree of subluxation of the lateral sesamoid on anteroposterior view.

Management of hallux valgus always starts conservatively, with modalities such as avoidance of tight-fitting high-heeled shoes and use of wide-toed soft footwear, as well as various inserts/pads such as bunion shields and toe spacers for support and comfort. Physical therapy is prescribed for stretching and balance correction [46]. When patients fail nonoperative management and continue to have symptoms of the progressive deformity, surgical intervention is indicated to improve athletic performance and alleviate disruption of lifestyle and activities of daily living.

Over 100 options for surgical intervention of hallux valgus exist, with severity of disease dictating choice of treatment. Mild to moderate deformity is typically treated by distal procedures such as simple bunionectomy, the modified McBride procedure, or distal Chevron osteotomy. Severe deformity usually involves surgical treatment of the MTP joint, and procedures such as the proximal Chevron osteotomy, proximal oblique ("Ludloff") osteotomy, proximal crescentic osteotomy, and opening wedge proximal first metatarsal osteotomy all have been described and advocated by different surgeons. Additionally, minimally invasive percutaneous surgery has become increasingly popular, with proponents touting quicker surgical and recovery times with an overall decrease in morbidity [47]. The descriptions of the many individual operations are beyond the scope of this chapter, but at this time no consensus has been made as to which open surgical technique [48], or minimally invasive procedure [49], provides the best outcomes.

Neurologic injury following surgical correction of hallux valgus is a rare complication, as a recent systematic review by Bard et al. that evaluated 229 studies for outcomes analysis found only 3% of patients suffered intraoperative nerve injury [50]. The nerve most commonly injured in these cases was the dorsomedial cutaneous nerve (DMCN), which innervates the medial surface of the hallux (Fig. 18.13a, b). Despite the many operative techniques for correction of the deformity, exposure of the underlying anatomic structures typically requires a dorsomedial incision which places the DMCN at risk. Damage to this nerve can result in a very painful postoperative course following a relatively benign procedure and must be avoided at all costs.

18.17.1.2 Pertinent Anatomy

As described previously in this chapter, the superficial peroneal nerve divides into multiple branches that give sensation to the dorsum of the foot (Fig. 18.3). The medial most branch, termed the medial dorsal cutaneous nerve (MDCN), typically branches from the superficial peroneal nerve near the ankle. The MDCN then further branches and gives off the dorsomedial cutaneous nerve (DMCN), which travels superficial to the extensor hallucis longus (EHL) tendon, before terminating near the distal dorsomedial aspect of the first metatarsal [51]. Solomon et al. reported that the DMCN independently supplies the cutaneous innervation to the first metatarsal and medial aspect of the great toe in 100% of cadaver specimens [52]; thus, the DMCN is also referred to as the proper dorsal digital nerve to the great toe. Additionally, Solomon et al. determined the DMCN supplies sensation to the lateral aspect of the great toe and the medial aspect of the second digit in 41% and 47% of specimens, respectively, in conjunction with branches from the deep peroneal nerve. This emphasizes the

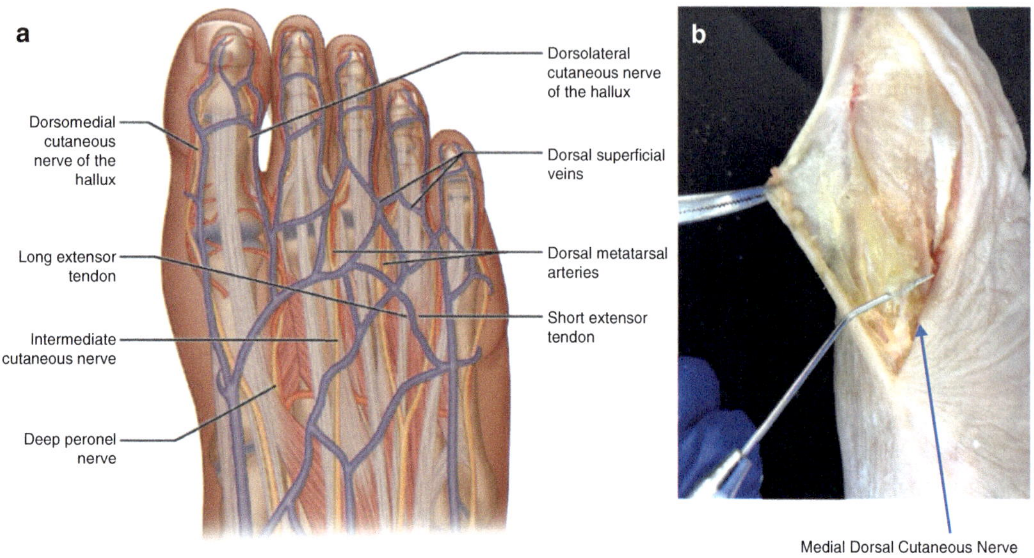

Fig. 18.13 (**a**) Artist depiction of superficial anatomy of the dorsal forefoot; (**b**) anatomic dissection of the dorsomedial cutaneous nerve

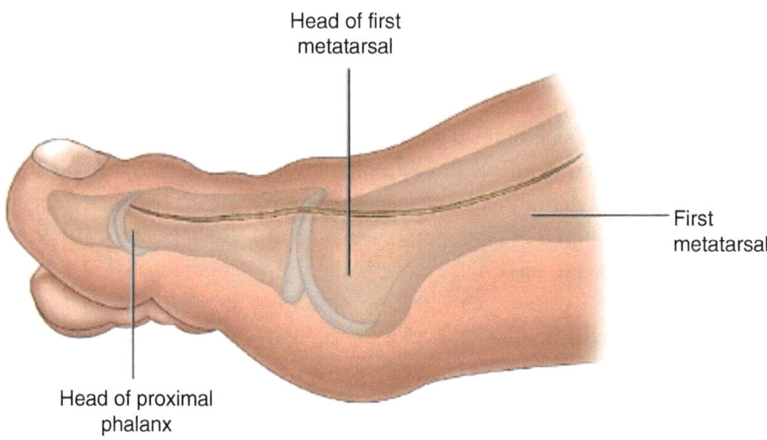

Fig. 18.14 Illustration demonstrating the dorsomedial incision with nearby bony landmarks

clinical importance of the DMCN during operations on the forefoot.

18.17.1.3 Prevention Strategies

- Use of a well-padded pneumatic tourniquet and loupe magnification to aid in visualization of neurovascular structures.
- A mid-dorsal incision should be made at the junction of the dorsal and plantar skin (Fig. 18.14).
- Identification of subcutaneous superficial veins and careful division under direct vision will avoid injury to the DMCN in the direct vicinity.
- When performing MTP arthroscopy, placement of dorsomedial and dorsolateral portals to the MTP joint should be approximately 0.5 cm from the margins of the EHL to avoid injury to the DMCN and terminal branches to the peroneal nerve [53] (Fig. 18.15).

18.17.1.4 Typical Course/Natural History

Intraoperative injury to the DMCN will lead to immediate numbness over the medial aspect of the hallux and in some patients may cause numbness of the lateral aspect of the hallux as well. Within subsequent weeks, sensation can

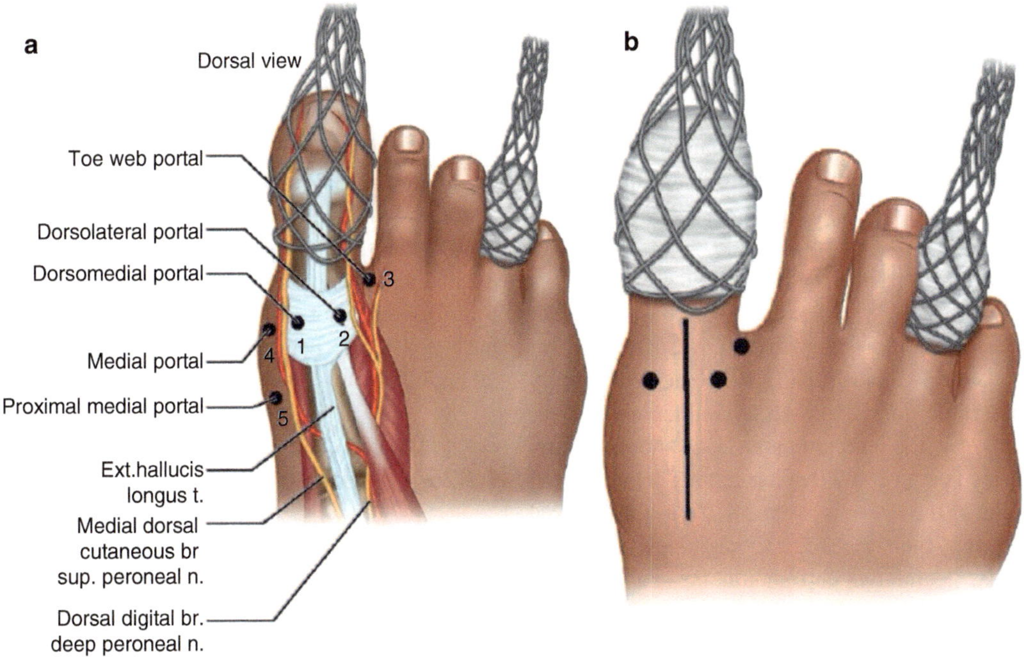

Fig. 18.15 (**a**) Underlying anatomic structures and (**b**) superficial skin landmarks for first MTP arthroscopy

remain absent or patients can begin to develop what's known as DMCN syndrome: neuropathic pain at the site of injury with numbness or paresthesia distally along the nerve innervation course. A Tinel sign may be present at the surgical scar line where the nerve injury occurred, with hyperesthesia and a shock-like sensation occurring from even minimal palpation. This can often cause difficulty with activities of daily living, as patients may be unable to wear shoes or place weight on the affected limb, leading to an overall useless limb secondary to pain intolerance.

18.17.1.5 Initial Evaluation

If a patient presents with concern for neurologic injury following surgical correction of hallux valgus deformity, clinical examination is the key to determining the etiology of their symptoms and likelihood for improvement.

- Examination of surgical scars
- Tinel's sign at patient-directed affected areas to identify neuroma
- Sensation testing via two-point discrimination, proprioception, and monofilament esthesiometer sensation (standard monofilament values 3.5–4.5 for feet) [54–56]

18.17.2 Diagnostic Tests/Imaging

- Ultrasonography can be helpful to assist with identification of discontinuity at surgical site and surrounding scar tissue. If unable to visualize using ultrasound, magnetic resonance imaging can better identify areas of compression or neuroma locations.
- Diagnostic nerve blockade using lidocaine can be beneficial to determine cause-effect alleviation of patient symptomology in nerve

distribution and can rule out nerve injury as a potential cause of pain if the diagnosis of postoperative neurologic complication is unclear.
- Electromyography and nerve conduction studies can assist with identification of injury to the sensory nerves of the foot and ankle.

18.18 Surgical Techniques

Identification of injury to the DMCN intraoperatively necessitates repair. If the ends are sharply transected during exposure, simple nerve repair with or without conduit assistance should be performed using 2–3 9/0 nylon sutures in the epineurium. If the nerve is injured via crush or thermal damage, then the affected segments should be excised, and the gap should be spanned with peripheral nerve allografts (PNAs) or nerve conduits. These products can be coapted to proximal and distal nerve ends in similar fashion with minimal amount of 9/0 or 10/0 nylon in the epineurium of the nerve ends.

More often, damage to the DMCN goes unnoticed during the index surgery, and discovery of nerve injury is recognized once patients present with medial hallux numbness or DMCN symptoms such as paresthesia and shock-like sensation from neuroma formation. Initial numbness should not immediately lead to re-exploration, as neurapraxia may resolve over the subsequent months. However, patients with persistent symptoms should undergo re-exploration if pain and sensitivity cause excessive morbidity and therefore unfavorable outcomes.

When approaching a patient with peripheral nerve injury, repair is commonly performed utilizing the procedural steps detailed previously in this chapter (see "Ankle Arthroscopy" section, "nerve repair").

18.19 Salvage Techniques

After neuroma resection is performed, multiple options of management exist, including nerve repair using autografts or nerve substitutes; placement of an acellular nerve allograft "cap"; transposition of the proximal end into surrounding tissue such as muscle, bone, or veins; use of regenerative peripheral nerve interfaces; or targeted muscle reinnervation [18, 19]. While the data for each of these methods are largely based on studies on neuromas of the upper extremity and following lower extremity amputations, each technique has shown good to excellent results, and at this time no head-to-head studies for iatrogenic foot and ankle neurologic injuries have confirmed benefit of one technique over others [20].

18.20 Outcomes

Miller [57] published his data of a small cohort of nine patients with DMCN syndrome following hallux valgus surgery which were treated with re-operation following a minimum of 4 months' symptom duration. After identification of the DMCN neuroma, the neuroma was resected, and the proximal end of the nerve was buried into nearby bone, preferably the base of the first metatarsal, but also the cuneiform or navicular bones if the neuroma was found more proximally. Nerve burial was performed by exposing a small area of denuded bone and drilling a 3.5 mm hole into the bone 1.5 cm in depth. After placement of the proximal end in this burial site without substantial tension, a 5/0 absorbable suture was used to secure the epineurium to nearby periosteum. Following closure of superficial tissue, the patient began weight-bearing in a hard-soled shoe at 2 days postoperatively, which they continued for 4 weeks.

At a mean follow-up of 20 months, all patients had a substantial decrease in pain symptoms, with all stating they could walk much better and would likely undergo the surgery again if given the choice. However, these results may be somewhat confounded as all patients underwent concurrent surgery at the time of nerve burial, most commonly bunionectomy or arthrodesis. At follow-up, patients felt confident that they could distinguish neuropathic pain from other pain sources. Furthermore, all postoperative pain scoring was performed by the operative surgeon, a potential source of bias. Nevertheless, this study proved the feasibility of nerve transection and osseous implantation in patients suffering from DMCN syndrome. Invariably, the end of the nerve will attempt to regrow (albeit in its new position inside the bone) and may then form a recurrent symptomatic neuroma. Although this is the surgical technique with the longest track record, it does not address the nerve end. Although there are no randomized trials comparing this technique to others, there is rationale to believe that it may be inferior to more active methods of neuroma treatment such as coaptation-based techniques.

18.21 Technical Pearls and Pitfalls

18.21.1 Interdigital Neuritis (Morton's Neuroma)

18.21.1.1 Risks/Incidence/Mechanism of Nerve Injury

The painful forefoot condition known as Morton's neuroma presents with sharp or burning pain in the second or third webspace, often radiating to one or two toes. As previously reported, this is a compression neuropathy of the common digital nerve involving the distal transverse metatarsal ligament (DTML), making terms like Morton's metatarsalgia or interdigital neuritis (IDN) more appropriate [58].

The terminology used to describe IDN and its treatment is replete with confusion.

Morton's neuroma is the most commonly used term despite the fact that the condition is not the neuroma per se, lacking the haphazard proliferation of axons seen in a neuroma. This leads to additional misleading terminology regarding treatment.

Neuroma excision is a misnomer and should be termed neuroma production; *recurrent Morton's neuroma* is the result of excision becoming a symptomatic neuroma and not a recurrence. The true meaning of these terms should be kept in mind while reading the literature and counseling patients.

18.21.2 Pertinent Anatomy

The medial plantar nerve enters the foot between the abductor hallucis and quadratus plantae and then continues distally to give off four digital branches (Fig. 18.16). The most medial branch is the proper digital nerve to the medial aspect of the big toe. The other three branches including the first, second, and third common digital nerves supply sensation to the first, second, and third interspaces. The lateral plantar nerve divides into the proper digital nerve to the lateral side of the fifth toe and the common digital nerve to the fourth interspace, which has a communicating branch that passes to the third digital branch of the medial plantar nerve in the third interspace. This makes the third interspace dually innervated from both medial and lateral plantar nerves.

18.21.3 Prevention Strategies

Nonoperative treatment should always be the first line in treatment of IDN, with the goal of avoiding surgery or delaying it as much as possible. Nonsurgical interventions to treat a compression neuropathy of a sensory nerve in the foot come in different varieties. These interventions may address the weight-bearing environment and the surrounding local irritation or modulate the production of pain. Orthosis to offload the forefoot, injections of different materials, and shockwave therapy are some common methods. Special attention should be given to calf muscle stretching to offload the forefoot and ameliorate the gait abnormalities associated with calf muscle tightness.

A recent literature review demonstrated corticosteroid injections to be effective for 12 months, with the response rate declining to 50% after 12 months, leading to surgical excision in 33% [63]. Alcohol injection resulted in pain relief in 29% of patients at 5 years but was also associated with burning pain. Shockwave therapy, botulinum toxin injection, capsaicin injection, and laser therapy had little or no evidence.

Since a satisfying surgical solution does not exist, surgery should be thought of as the final

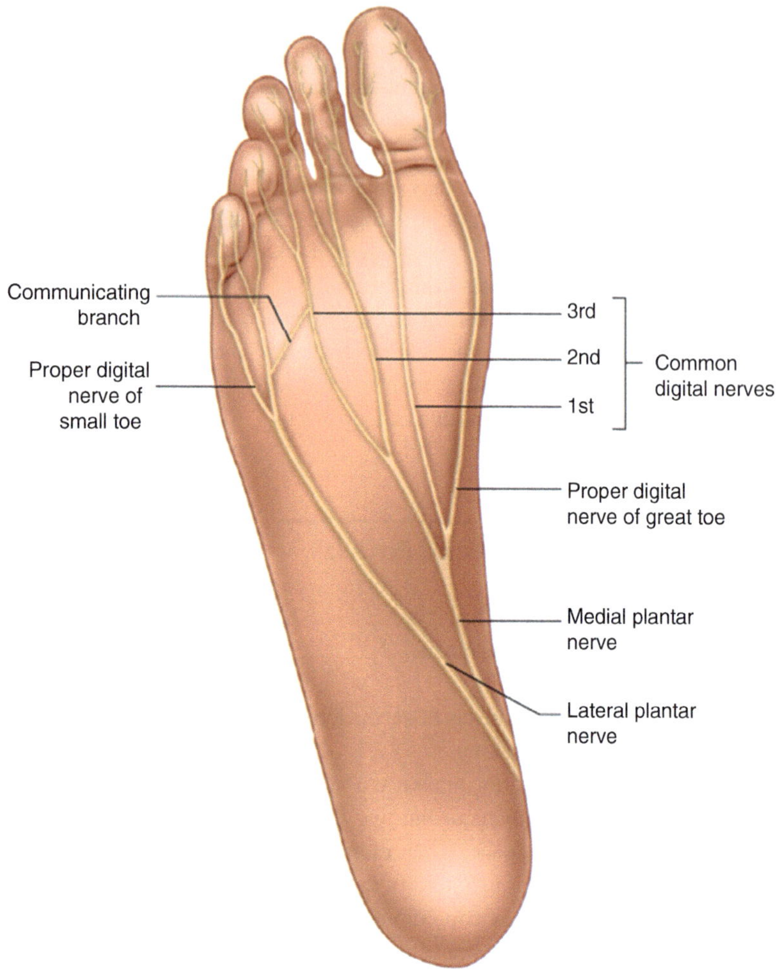

Fig. 18.16 Plantar nerve anatomy of the foot

resort in patients with persistent pain, and every effort should be made to maximize nonoperative treatment.

18.21.4 Typical Course/Natural History

The typical patient with Morton's neuroma will report footwear-related pain and frequent need to remove shoes and massage his or her foot. Nerve quality is sharp, with tingling in the toes. Women are more commonly affected than men.

18.21.4.1 Initial Evaluation/Exam Findings

The physical examination of Morton's neuroma begins with localizing tenderness and dorsal bulging of the affected webspace (typically the third) between the metatarsal heads but not at the heads themselves. Pain is induced with compression of the intermetatarsal space or with tightening the metatarsals to one another which may be associated with a painful click (Mulder's sign) [59]. The thumb and index finger squeeze test, which is simply squeezing the webspace between the thumb and index, has a

96% sensitivity for the diagnosis of Morton's neuroma [60].

Calf muscle tightness should be examined and every patient with forefoot pathology. This reduces the pressure in the heel and instead transfers pressure distally to the metatarsal heads. Gastrocnemius contracture is assessed using the Silfverskiold test: assessing ankle dorsiflexion with the knee in full extension and 90° of flexion, with the foot locked in subtalar neutral position. Equinus contracture is noted by lack of dorsiflexion past neutral.

18.21.5 Diagnostic Tests/Imaging

Although imaging is not indicated for diagnosis of Morton's neuroma, plain weight-bearing foot radiographs are helpful to exclude other causes of pain such as stress fractures and degenerative MTP changes or subluxation and in order to assess the relative length of the metatarsals (which may contribute to metatarsalgia). These diagnoses are not mutually exclusive and may coexist with IDN.

In cases of clinical uncertainty and multiple webspace involvement, ultrasound has been suggested as the imaging modality of choice [61].

A diagnostic block using 1–2 mL of local anesthetic with or without cortisone may be useful in equivocal cases; however, caution must be exercised in interpreting the results since the local anesthetic may diffuse toward neighboring structures such as joint capsule and can therefore limit its diagnostic utility [62].

18.22 Surgical Techniques

18.22.1 General Considerations

The mainstay of surgical treatment is sharp division of the nerve proximal to the enlarged nerve segment, such that the proximal stump retracts to the level of the muscle bellies. This converts a peripheral compression neuropathy into a true stump neuroma. For comparison, compression neuropathies in other locations are treated with decompression procedures alone and release of the offending structures. There are no other reports of compression neuropathy treated with nerve resection. This led to the development of alternative approaches to nerve resection and prevention of painful stump neuromas.

18.22.2 Decompression Alone

Decompression involves incision of the DTML and decompression of the common digital nerve [64], thereby interrupting the pathophysiology of the Morton entrapment process (Fig. 18.17).

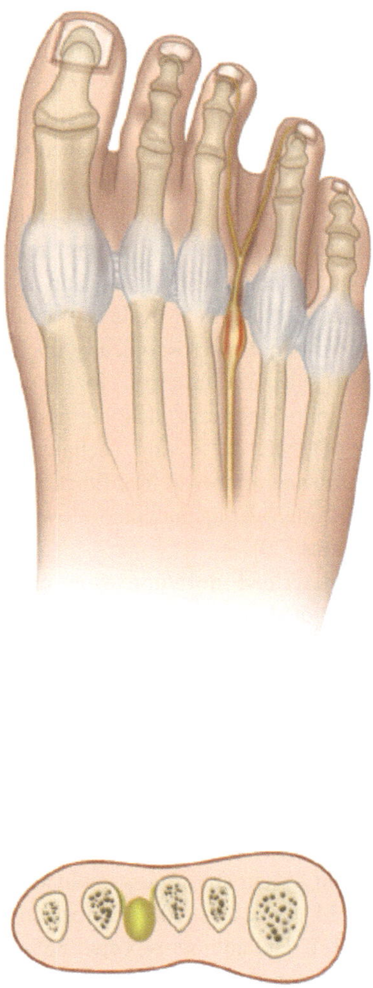

Fig. 18.17 Schematic of dorsal deep transverse metatarsal ligament division and nerve decompression. Note that the nerve crosses plantarward under the ligament

Dellon in 1992 performed decompression on five patients, with pain relief in 80% (four) of the patients. Earlier series suggested partial split of the DTML with good results in 83% of cases, improved results in 14.5%, and 2.5% failure rate [65].

Others have recommended against simple resection of the ligament due to recurrent compression from the regenerated soft tissue [66]; however, their study involved patients who underwent excision making that conclusion questionable. Although this consideration may be anatomically correct, this has not been demonstrated in clinical studies.

Okafor reported the results of neurolysis 1 cm distal to the DTML and 3 cm proximal to it, with patient satisfaction noted to be "extremely high," and complete pain relief in 17 out of 35 patients [67]. Zelent reported on the results of nerve decompression using a device designed for carpal tunnel release [68], resulting in absent symptoms in 11 of the 14 patients at 25 months' follow-up.

Villas [69] reported similar pain relief with neurolysis and neurectomy in a group of 69 feet. They concluded that neurolysis is a valid option if the nerve is not macroscopically thick, which was their selection criterion for neurectomy. Recent report on nerve decompression using Dellon's DTML sectioning technique in 12 patients showed improved foot functional scores and pain scores over the median follow-up period of 37 months [70].

Song described decompression and dorsal suspension of the nerve using the dorsal transverse ligament and compared it to standard neurectomy, with a mean follow-up of 34 months [72]. They showed comparable results with fewer complications of paresthesia and numbness in the dorsal suspension group, essentially relocating the nerve to a more dorsal position away from the weight-bearing surface.

A recent systematic review included neurectomy in 14 studies and decompression in four studies [72]. The authors reported 88% success rate for neurectomy versus 94% success rate for decompression, with no difference between dorsal and plantar approaches, over 46 months' follow-up.

Taken together, these studies demonstrate favorable outcomes for nerve decompression, supporting the notion that IDN is an entrapment neuropathy. The results are comparable with nerve resection, without the risk of creating a stump neuroma and sensory loss. Simple decompression is a straightforward and easy to master procedure with minimal risk to surrounding tissues and low morbidity. Cadaver study has demonstrated negligible and clinically undetectable widening of the intermetatarsal angle and metatarsal alignment [73].

18.22.3 Neurectomy

Resection of the common digital nerve is the most common procedure for interdigital neuritis although the procedure converts an irritated nerve into an inevitable stump neuroma (Fig. 18.18).

Nerve excision can be performed from plantar or dorsal approach. The dorsal approach (Fig. 18.19a) allows release of the DTML, as well as neurolysis. It is considered technically easy and does not involve a scar at the sensitive plantar surface. This approach is usually recommended for primary cases. Plantar incision is more direct as the common digital nerve is more superficial at this location. Its drawbacks include a sensitive plantar scar and delayed weight-bearing. This approach is usually reserved for revision or "recurrent" cases. The plantar longitudinal incision is designed proximally and between the metatarsal heads so that any scarring will not be directly under the weight-bearing area but instead over the intermetatarsal spaces (Fig. 18.19b, c).

18.22.4 Nerve Excision and Interpositional Nerve Grafting

Ratanshi reported their experience with nerve excision and interpositional nerve grafting in eight patients with nine neuromas, after failure of nonoperative treatment with a minimum of 1-year follow-up [77]. The neuroma was excised and a

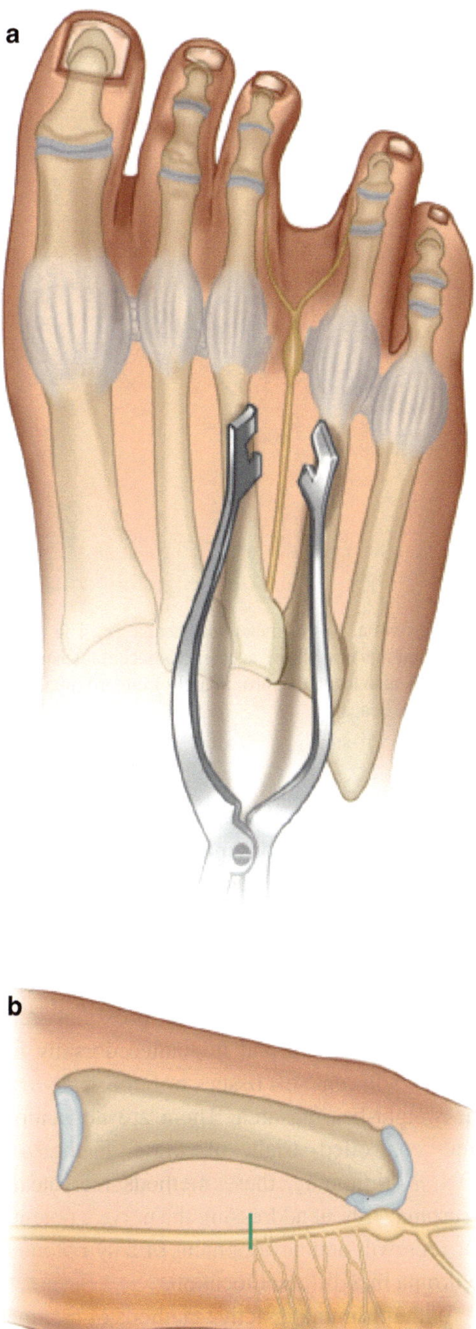

Fig. 18.18 (**a**) Exposure of the common digital nerve through the soft tissues between the metatarsal heads. A Weitlaner is placed between the metatarsal heads to gain optimal exposure. (**b**) Lateral view of the common digital nerve with the level of resection marked in green

segment of the proper digital nerve to one of the toes just distal to the excised neuroma was harvested, reversed, and interposed as a nerve graft between the common digital nerve stump and the adjacent distal proper digital nerve.

The authors reported pain relief in all patients with no recurrence as well as return of sensation. The authors recommended excision and nerve grafting as the primary treatment for cases that failed nonoperative treatment, given the above advantages.

18.22.4.1 Salvage Techniques

Nerve resection is associated with a 14%–21% failure rate [78]. In general, patients with symptoms following nerve resection can be classified into three groups: (1) Patients describe the same symptoms postoperatively with no period of relief; (2) the period of relief followed by recurrence of the same or worse symptoms; (3) patients describe new symptoms following surgery.

In the first group of patients where symptoms never subsided, the problem may have been initially thought to be IDN but is in fact a different condition that mimics the symptom complex (wrong diagnosis). In these patients, the correct diagnosis should be sought, such as tarsal tunnel syndrome, other causes of metatarsalgia, or IDN at an adjacent space (wrong interspace).

In the second group of patients, symptoms are related to the inevitable neuroma formed at the proximal stump by the excision of the common plantar digital nerve. This is erroneously termed "recurrent neuroma." The stump may have not retracted proximal enough, became adherent to the plantar plate or skin and irritated with cyclic weight-bearing.

The third group of patients is challenging to manage since they describe a new symptom complex: either hypersensitivity from disruption of the small plantar branches of the digital nerve or chronic regional pain syndrome (CRPS).

In patients with a symptomatic proximal stump neuroma, associated conditions such as tight calf muscles should be optimized. A local anesthetic injection with or without cortisone and

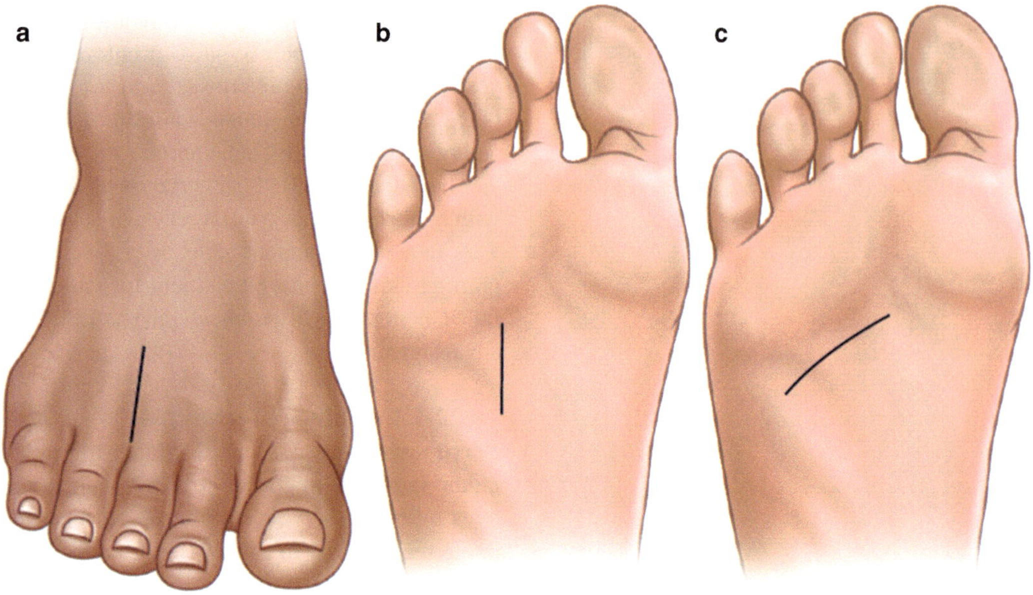

Fig. 18.19 Dorsal and plantar longitudinal incisions. (**a**) The dorsal incision is begun in the webspace and carried proximally and midline for about 3 cm to the level of the metatarsal heads. (**b**) The plantar longitudinal incision centered over the intermetatarsal space approximately 1 cm proximal to the metatarsal heads. (**c**) The plantar horizontal incision allows access to adjacent intermetatarsal space, also located approximately 1 cm proximal to the metatarsal heads

documentation of pain intensity using a pain diary reviewed at a follow-up consultation are essential in confirming the proximal stump as the offending agent. A trial of nonoperative treatment is appropriate before embarking on revision surgery. This will typically include medications such as pregabalin or nortriptyline that may be helpful in decreasing neuropathic pain. This group of patients is historically reported to do poorly with re-resection, with unsatisfactory results in 20–40% of patients [79].

Given the significant morbidity and unsatisfactory results of re-resection, alternative surgical techniques have been developed to alleviate pain with minimal morbidity and complications.

The approach to the symptomatic stump neuroma has been revolutionized in the past few years, incorporating new surgical approaches and techniques, which may be employed following IDN resection. The two major categories of stump neuroma management are passive-ablative and active-reconstructive interventions [19]. These are based on the presence or absence of the distal stump. If on exploration the distal proper digital nerve is available, autograft allograft or conduit reconstruction may be considered, to complete the nerve circuit. This potentially restores sensation to one or two toes. If however the distal end is unavailable, reconstruction is deemed unfeasible, or the distal nerve is extremely small or scarred, the proximal stump may be re-resected and implanted dorsally into muscle, adjacent soft tissues or bone, away from the weight-bearing area. There are no randomized controlled trials of these methods in IDN. Additionally, these methods relocate the neuroma without addressing the nerve's potential for regrowth and development of a symptomatic neuroma in a different location.

With this in mind, active methods of treatment have been developed, to provide a neural pathway for the regenerating axons, thereby decreasing the potential for regrowth and symptomatic neuroma formation. These include relocation nerve grafting using the long nerve graft, capping the nerve with a vein or conduit to ameliorate regrowth, or coapting the nerve stump to a nearby muscular branch. This last technique (targeted

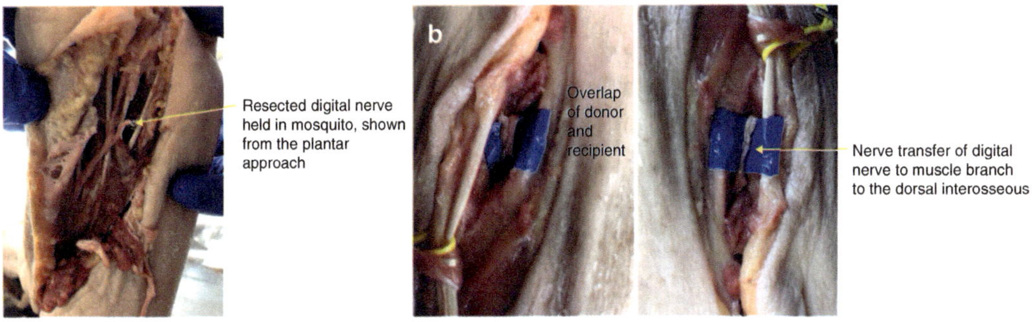

Fig. 18.20 (**a**) Nerve transfer for persistently painful neuroma stump, following primary nerve resection – plantar view. (**b**) Nerve transfer for persistently painful neuroma stump, following primary nerve resection – dorsal view

muscle reinnervation) provides the nerve with a denervated, vascularized target to grow into. Taking into account the unique local anatomy of the foot, nerve transfers to dorsal interossei motor branches can be designed to relocate the nerve away from the susceptible weight-bearing area and provide it with a target for regeneration. If a gap exists between the donor and recipient, due to the very proximal excision, nerve graft is necessary to overcome the segmental nerve loss. In this regard, commercially available cadaveric nerve allograft is ideal as it is available off the shelf, has good handling properties, and avoids creating a donor site neuroma as with autograft. However, its use is associated with increased cost.

Figure 18.20 shows a cadaver dissection with a simulated nerve transfer of the cut proximal stump of the third common digital nerve to a nearby dorsal interosseous motor branch. The motor nerves to the interossei foot muscles are of adequate size to facilitate nerve rotation to the common digital nerve. Further anatomic studies are underway to map the location of the motor entry points in the foot.

Alternatively, a muscle graft may provide a pathway for neural regeneration from the distal nerve stump into empty motor endplates of the denervated muscle graft. This technique is known as regenerative peripheral nerve interface (RPNI), found to be useful in reduction of neuroma pain and phantom limb pain in major limb amputations [80].

18.22.4.2 Outcomes

After a thorough and accurate diagnosis, nerve excision results in considerable improvement of IDN symptoms in the majority of patients, around 80% [58]. In Mann's series, 65% of patients still noted local plantar tenderness after surgery and 20% noted the improvement to be less than 50% [66]. Womack reported 51% good to excellent results, 10% failure results, and 40% poor results on long-term follow-up of 120 patients [74]. Other authors reported 15-year follow-up of nerve excision, with 76% good or excellent result, fair in 15%, and poor in 8% [75]. Finally, a prospective study reporting the pre- and postoperative patient-reported outcomes and satisfaction scores following nerve excision reported 9% poor and very poor results and pain relief in only 63% of patients. The authors concluded that patient-reported outcomes after nerve excision are acceptable but may not be as good as earlier studies suggested [76].

References

1. Epstein DM, Black BS, Sherman SL. Anterior ankle arthoscopy: indications, pitfalls, and complications. Foot Ankle Clin N Am. 2015:41–57.
2. Sprague NF III, Guhl JF, Olson DW. Specific complications: elbow, wrist, hip, and ankle. Complications in arthroscopy. 1st ed. New York: Raven Press; 1989. p. 199–224.
3. Ferkel RD, Heath DD, Guhl JF. Neurological complications of ankle arthroscopy. Arthroscopy. 1996;12:200–8.

4. Zengerink M, van Dijk CN. Complications in ankle arthroscopy. Knee Surg Sports Traumatol Arthrosc. 2012;20:1420–31.
5. Young BH, Flanigan RM, DiGiovanni BF. Complications of ankle arthroscopy utilizing a contemporary noninvasive distraction technique. J Bone Joint Surg Am. 2011;93:963–8.
6. Zekry M, Shahban SA, Gamal TE, Platt S. A literature review of the complications following anterior and posterior ankle arthroscopy. Foot Ankle Surg. 2019;25:553–8.
7. Hepple S, Guha A. The role of ankle arthroscopy in acute ankle injuries of the athlete. Foot Ankle Clin. 2013;18:185–94.
8. Ucerler H, Ikiz AA, Uygur M. A cadaver study on preserving peroneal nerves during ankle arthroscopy. Foot Ankle Int. 2007;28(11):1172–8.
9. van Dijk CN, Scholten PE, Krips R. A 2-portal endoscopic approach for diagnosis and treatment of posterior ankle pathology. Arthroscopy. 2000;16:871–6.
10. Takao M, Uchio Y, Shu N, Ochi M. Anatomic bases of ankle arthroscopy: study of superficial and deep peroneal nerves around anterolateral and anterocentral approach. Surg Radiol Anat. 1998;20(5):317–20.
11. Buckingham RA, Winson IG, Kelly AJ. An anatomical study of a new portal for ankle arthroscopy. J Bone Joint Surg. 1997;79-B:650–2.
12. Moore AM, Wagner IJ, Fox IK. Principles of nerve repair in complex wounds of the upper extremity. Semin Plast Surg. 2015;29(1):40–7.
13. Watson J, Gonzalez M, Romero A, Kerns J. Neuromas of the hand and upper extremity. J Hand Surg Am. 2010;35:499–510.
14. Bassilios Habre S, Bond G, Jing XL, et al. The surgical management of nerve gaps present and future. Ann Plast Surg. 2018;80(3):252–61.
15. Millesi H. Bridging defects: autologous nerve grafts. Acta Neurochir Suppl (Wien). 2007;100:37–8.
16. Moore AM, MacEwan M, Santosa KB, et al. Acellular nerve allografts in peripheral nerve regeneration: a comparative study. Muscle Nerve. 2011;44(2):221–34.
17. Moore AM, Kasukurthi R, Magill CK, et al. Limitations of conduits in peripheral nerve repairs. Hand (NY). 2009;4(2):180–6.
18. Regal S, Tang P. Surgical management of neuromas of the hand and wrist. J Am Acad Orthop Surg. 2019;27:356–63.
19. Eberlin KR, Ducic I. Surgical algorithm for neuroma management: a changing treatment paradigm. Plast Reconstr Surg Glob Open. 2018;6(10):e1952. Published 2018 Oct 16. https://doi.org/10.1097/GOX.0000000000001952.
20. Hendrickson NR, Cychsoz CC, Akoh CC, Phisitkul P. Treatment of postsurgical neuroma in foot and ankle surgery. Foot Ankle Orthopaed. 2018:1–8.
21. Souza JM, Purnell CA, Cheesborough JE, Kelikian AS, Dumanian GA. Treatment of foot and ankle neuroma pain with processed nerve allografts. Foot Ankle Int. 2016;37(10):1098–105.
22. Bibbo C, Rodrigues-Colazzo E, Finzen AG. Superficial peroneal nerve to deep peroneal nerve transfer with allograft conduit for neuroma in continuity. J Foot Ankle Surg. 2018;57(3):514–7.
23. Edwards WG, Lincoln CR, Bassett FH 3rd, Goldner JL. The tarsal tunnel syndrome. Diagnosis and treatment. JAMA. 1969;207(4):716–20.
24. LAM SJ. A tarsal-tunnel syndrome. Lancet. 1962;2(7270):1354–5.
25. Dellon AL. The four medial ankle tunnels: a critical review of perceptions of tarsal tunnel syndrome and neuropathy. Neurosurg Clin N Am. 2008;19(4):629–48, vii.
26. Kim DH, Hudson AR, Kline DG. Tibial nerve. Atlas of peripheral nerve surgery. Elsevier; 2013. Chapter 18,. p. 221–7.
27. Dellon AL, Mackinnon SE. Tibial nerve branching in the tarsal tunnel. Arch Neurol. 1984;41(6):645–6.
28. Davis TJ, Schon LC. Branches of the tibial nerve: anatomic variations. Foot Ankle Int. 1995;16(1):21–9.
29. Dellon AL. The Dellon approach to neurolysis in the neuropathy patient with chronic nerve compression. Handchir Mikrochir Plast Chir. 2008;40(6):351–60.
30. Henricson AS, Westlin NE. Chronic calcaneal pain in athletes: entrapment of the calcaneal nerve? Am J Sports Med. 1984;12(2):152–4.
31. Mann RA. Orthopedics: tarsal tunnel syndrome. West J Med. 1976;125(5):380–1.
32. Dellon AL, Muse VL, Scott ND, Akre T, Anderson SR, Barret SL, Biddinger KR, Bregman PJ, Bullard BP, Dauphinee DM, JM DJ, RA DJ, Ducic I, Dunkerly J, Galina MR, Hung V, Ichtertz DR, Kutka MF, Jacoby RP, Johnson JB, Mader DW, Maloney CT Jr, Mancuso PJ, Martin RC, Martin RF, BA MD, Rizzo VJ, Rose M, Rosson GD, Shafiroff BB, Steck JK, Stolarski RG, Swier P, Wellens-Bruschayt TA, Wilke B, Williams EH, Wood MA, Wood WA, Younes MP, Yuksel F. A positive Tinel sign as predictor of pain relief or sensory recovery after decompression of chronic tibial nerve compression in patients with diabetic neuropathy. J Reconstr Microsurg. 2012;28(4):235–40.
33. Kaplan PE, Kernahan WT Jr. Tarsal tunnel syndrome: an electrodiagnostic and surgical correlation. J Bone Joint Surg Am. 1981;63(1):96–9.
34. Patel AT, Gaines K, Malamut R, Park TA, Toro DR. Holland N; American Association of Neuromuscular and Electrodiagnostic Medicine. Usefulness of electrodiagnostic techniques in the evaluation of suspected tarsal tunnel syndrome: an evidence-based review. Muscle Nerve. 2005;32(2):236–40.
35. Oh SJ, Sarala PK, Kuba T, Elmore RS. Tarsal tunnel syndrome: electrophysiological study. Ann Neurol. 1979;5(4):327–30.
36. Ducic I, Felder JM 3rd, Iorio ML. The role of peripheral nerve surgery in diabetic limb salvage. Plast Reconstr Surg. 2011;127 Suppl 1:259S–26.
37. Dellon AL. Discussion. The role of peripheral nerve surgery in diabetic limb salvage. Plast Reconstr Surg. 2011;127 Suppl 1:270S–4S.

38. Kim J, Dellon AL. Neuromas of the calcaneal nerves. Foot Ankle Int. 2001;22(11):890–4.
39. Mullick T, Dellon AL. Results of decompression of four medial ankle tunnels in the treatment of tarsal tunnels syndrome. J Reconstr Microsurg. 2008;24(2):119–26.
40. Kim DH, Murovic JA. Lower extremity nerve injuries. In: Kim DH, Midha R, Murovic JA, editors. Kline and Hudson's nerve injuries. Philadelphia: Saunders; 2008. p. 209–78.
41. Mann RA, Coughlin MJ. Hallux valgus-etiology, anatomy, treatment and surgical considerations. Clin Orthop Relat Res. 1981;undefined:31–41.
42. Fournier M, Saxena A, Maffulli N. Hallux valgus surgery in the athlete: current evidence. J Foot Ankle Surg. 2019;58:641–3.
43. Pique-Vidal C, Sole MT, Antich J. Hallux valgus inheritance: pedigree research in 350 patients with bunion deformity. J Foot Ankle Surg. 2007;46:149–54.
44. Perera AM, Mason L, Stephens MM. The pathogenesis of hallux valgus. J Bone Joint Surg Am. 2011;93:1650–61.
45. Hardy RH, Clapham JC. Observations on hallux valgus; based on a controlled series. J Bone Joint Surg Br. 1951;33:376–91.
46. Hecht PJ, Lin TJ. Hallux valgus. Med Clin N Am. 2014;98(2):227–32.
47. Maffulli N, Longo UG, Marinozzi A, et al. Hallux valgus: effectiveness and safety of minimally invasive surgery. A systematic review. Br Med Bull. 2011;9:149–67.
48. Easley ME, Trnka H-J. Current concepts review: hallux valgus part II: operative treatment. Foot Ankle Int. 2007;28(6):747–58.
49. Malagelada F, Sahirad C, Dalmau-Pastor M, et al. Minimally invasive surgery for hallux valgus: a systematic review of current surgical techniques. Int Orthop. 2019;43:625–37.
50. Barg A, Harmer JR, Presson AP, et al. Unfavorable outcomes following surgical treatment of hallux valgus deformity. J Bone Joint Surg Am. 2018;100: 1563–73.
51. Miller RA, Hartman G. Origin and course of the dorsomedial cutaneous nerve to the great toe. Foot Ankle Int. 1996;17(10):620–2.
52. Solomon LB, Ferris L, Tedman R, Henneberg M. Surgical anatomy of the sural and superficial fibular nerves with an emphasis on the approach to the lateral malleolus. J Anat. 2001;199:717–23.
53. Sherman TI, Kern M, Marcel J, et al. First metatarsophalangeal joint arthroscopy for osteochondral lesions. Arthrosc Tech. 2016;5(3):e513–8.
54. Jeng C, Michelson J, Mizel M. Sensory thresholds of normal human feet. Foot Ankle Intl. 2000;21(60):501–4.
55. Holewski JJ, Stress RM, Graf PM, et al. Aesthesiometry: quantification of cutaneous pressure sensation in diabetic peripheral neuropathy. J Rehabil Res Dev. 1988;25:1–10.
56. Mueller MJ, Diamond JE, Delitto A, et al. Insensitivity, limited joint mobility, and plantar ulcers in patients with diabetes mellitus. Phys Ther. 1989;69:453–9.
57. Miller SD. Dorsomedial cutaneous nerve syndrome: treatment with nerve transection and burial into bone. Foot Ankle Int. 2001;22(3):198–202.
58. Weinfeld SB, Myerson MS. Interdigital neuritis: diagnosis and treatment. J Am Acad Orthop Surg. 1996;4(6):328–35.
59. Mulder JD. The causative mechanism in Morton's metatarsalgia. J Bone Joint Surg Br. 1951;33-B(1):94–5.
60. Mahadevan D, Venkatesan M, Bhatt R, Bhatia M. Diagnostic accuracy of clinical tests for Morton's neuroma compared with ultrasonography. J Foot Ankle Surg. 2015;54(4):549–53.
61. Pastides P, El-Sallakh S, Charalambides C. Morton's neuroma: A clinical versus radiological diagnosis. Foot Ankle Surg. 2012;18(1):22–4.
62. Hembree WC, Groth AT, Schon LC, Guyton GP. Computed tomography analysis of third webspace injections for interdigital neuroma. Foot Ankle Int. 2013;34(4):575–8.
63. Thomson L, Aujla RS, Divall P, Bhatia M. Nonsurgical treatments for Morton's neuroma: A systematic review. Foot Ankle Surg. 2019. pii:S1268-7731(19)30179-1
64. Dellon AL. Treatment of Morton's neuroma as a nerve compression. The role for neurolysis. J Am Podiatr Med Assoc. 1992;82(8):399–402.
65. Gauthier G. Thomas Morton's disease: a nerve entrapment syndrome. A new surgical technique. Clin Orthop Relat Res. 1979;142:90–2.
66. Mann RA, Reynolds JC. Interdigital neuroma--a critical clinical analysis. Foot Ankle. 1983;3(4):238–43.
67. Okafor B, Shergill G, Angel J. Treatment of Morton's neuroma by neurolysis. Foot Ankle Int. 1997;18(5):284–7.
68. Zelent ME, Kane RM, Neese DJ, Lockner WB. Minimally invasive Morton's intermetatarsal neuroma decompression. Foot Ankle Int. 2007;28(2):263–5.
69. Villas C, Florez B, Alfonso M. Neurectomy versus neurolysis for Morton's neuroma. Foot Ankle Int. 2008 Jun;29(6):578–80.
70. Mischitz M, Zeitlinger S, Mischlinger J, Rab M. Nerve decompression according to A.L. Dellon in Morton neuroma – a retrospective analysis. J Plast Reconstr Aesthet Surgry. 2020; https://doi.org/10.1016/j.bjps.2020.01.008.
71. Song JH, Kang C, Hwang DS, Kang DH, Kim YH. Dorsal suspension for Morton's neuroma: a comparison with neurectomy. Foot Ankle Surg. 2019;25(6):748–54.
72. Valisena S, Petri GJ, Ferrero A. Treatment of Morton's neuroma: a systematic review. Foot Ankle Surg. 2018;24(4):271–81.
73. Preston N, Peterson D, Allen J, Kawalec JS, Whitaker J. Deep transverse metatarsal ligament transection in

Morton's neuroma excision: a cadaveric study examining effects on metatarsal alignment. Foot Ankle Spec. 2018;11(4):342–6.
74. Womack JW, Richardson DR, Murphy GA, Richardson EG, Ishikawa SN. Long-term evaluation of interdigital neuroma treated by surgical excision. Foot Ankle Int. 2008;29(6):574–7.
75. Kasparek M, Schneider W. Surgical treatment of Morton's neuroma: clinical results after open excision. Int Orthop. 2013;37(9):1857–61.
76. Bucknall V, Rutherford D, MacDonald D, Shalaby H, McKinley J, Breusch SJ. Outcomes following excision of Morton's interdigital neuroma: a prospective study. Bone Joint J. 2016;98B(10):1376–81.
77. Ratanshi I, Hayakawa TE, Giuffre JL. Excision with Interpositional nerve grafting: an alternative technique for the treatment of Morton neuroma. Ann Plast Surg. 2016;76(4):428–33.
78. Di Caprio F, Meringolo R, Shehab Eddine M, Ponziani L. Morton's interdigital neuroma of the foot: a literature review. Foot Ankle Surg. 2018;24(2):92–8.
79. Johnson JE, Johnson KA, Unni KK. Persistent pain after excision of an interdigital neuroma. Results of reoperation. J Bone Joint Surg Am. 1988;70(5):651–7.
80. Woo SL, Kung TA, Brown DL, Leonard JA, Kelly BM, Cederna PS. Regenerative peripheral nerve interfaces for the treatment of postamputation neuroma pain: a pilot study. Plast Reconst Surg Glob Open. 2016;4(12):e1038. Published 2016 Dec 27. https://doi.org/10.1097/GOX.0000000000001038.

Lumbosacral Double Crush Syndrome

19

Christopher F. Dibble, Robert C. Bucelli, Jacob K. Greenberg, and Wilson Z. Ray

Abbreviations and Acronyms

DCS	Double crush syndrome
EDx	Electrodiagnostic studies
EMG	Electromyography
MEP	Motor evoked potentials
MRC	Modified Medical Research Council
MRI	Magnetic resonance imaging
NCS	Nerve conduction studies
NF	Neurofibromatosis
SSEP	Somatosensory evoked potentials
TTS	Tarsal tunnel syndrome

19.1 Introduction and Epidemiology

Double crush syndrome (DCS) is a clinical constellation of additive neurological dysfunction due to compressive pathology at multiple sites along the trajectory of a group of axons, classically at the level of a spinal nerve root with a concurrent peripheral lesion at the carpal or cubital tunnels. This phenomenon was first described by Upton and McComas in 1973 after they observed that there were a number of carpal tunnel patients who were worse or not improved following an apparent successful decompression surgery (i.e., a successful surgery that in other patients typically translated into symptomatic benefit). They also noted an increased frequency of cervical radiculopathy among patients with carpal tunnel syndrome [1]. They went on to demonstrate electrophysiological evidence of neuropathy in both the cervical spine and the carpal and/or cubital tunnel in many of these patients.

This led to the formation of the DCS hypothesis, i.e., that the proximal lesion may predispose the distal segment of the axon to subsequent damage (Fig. 19.1) [2]. In other words, a degree of compression that would otherwise be subclinical in a nerve with just one source of compression may manifest clinically in a nerve that is compressed at a second site. The pathophysiology was postulated as surpassing a critical obstruction of axoplasmic flow down neurons leading to motor or sensory neuropathy [2, 3]. Disrupted axoplasmic flow between the soma and the distal portions of the axon translates into degenerative changes and/or impaired function (Fig. 19.2). This mechanism has been supported by a number of translational and basic science studies, including studies performed by Dellon and Mackinnon in rat sciatic nerve [4–6]. Additional pathophysi-

C. F. Dibble (✉) · R. C. Bucelli · J. K. Greenberg · W. Z. Ray
Department of Neurological Surgery, Washington University School of Medicine, Saint Louis, MO, USA

Department of Neurology, Washington University School of Medicine, Saint Louis, MO, USA
e-mail: cdibble@wustl.edu; bucellir@wustl.edu; jacobgreenberg@wustl.edu; rayz@wustl.edu

C. J. Dy et al. (eds.), *Peripheral Nerve Issues after Orthopedic Surgery*,
https://doi.org/10.1007/978-3-030-84428-8_19

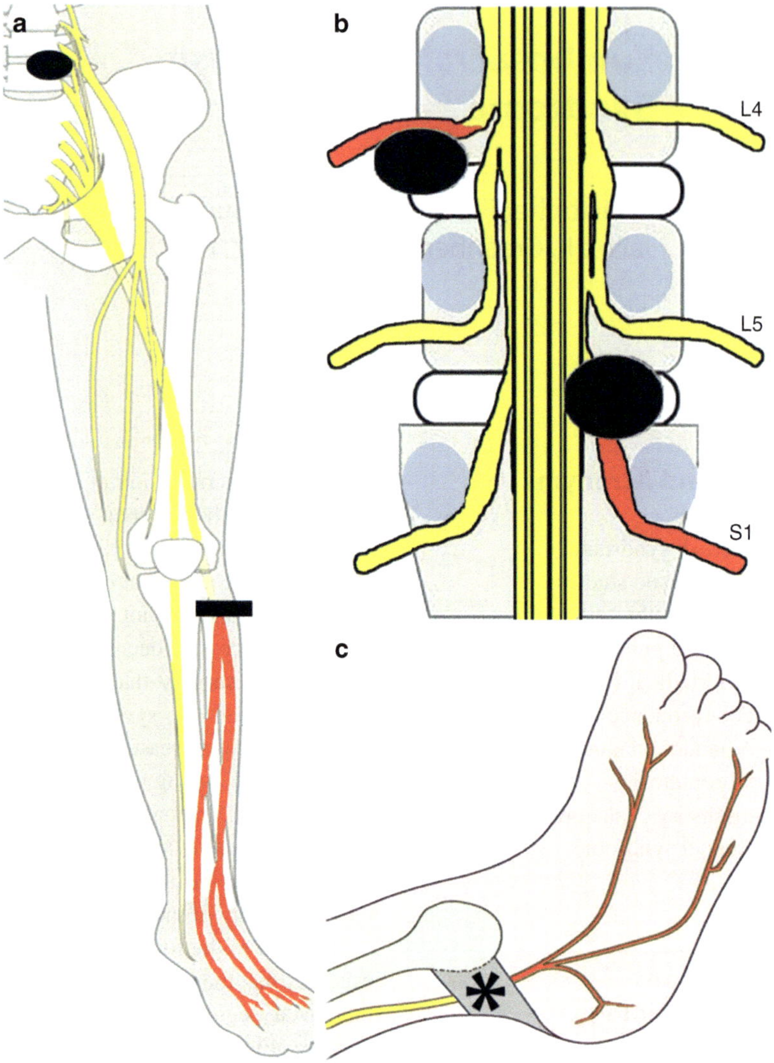

Fig. 19.1 Cartoon illustrating concepts of lumbosacral double crush syndrome. (**a**) A subclinical proximal lesion, often compression of a nerve root due to a disc bulge or foraminal stenosis, combines with a distal lesion to cause clinical manifestations of double crush syndrome. In this case, compression of the L5 nerve root is shown, with distal compression of the peroneal nerve at the fibular head, resulting in double crush syndrome. (**b**) AP view of the lumbosacral spine. The most common causes of a proximal lesion are compression of the traversing nerve root by a paramedian disc (in this diagram the S1 nerve root), followed by a lateral disc affecting the exiting nerve root (in this diagram the L4 nerve root). A central disc is least likely. Lateral discs, as well as bony stenosis, can sometimes be overlooked on initial imaging studies. (**c**) In double crush syndrome, distal nerves are affected by the additive neuropathy of a proximal and distal lesion. Here, the patient has proximal subclinical compression of the S1 nerve root combined with compression of the posterior tibial nerve at the flexor retinaculum (i.e., tarsal tunnel syndrome)

ologies for DCS were postulated in a Delphi study in 2011, including an immune and inflammatory response targeting the dorsal root ganglia, ion channel dysregulation, and neuroma in continuity [7]. Over time, the definition of DCS has evolved to include the concept of a systemic or metabolic "hit" from diseases such as diabetes or uremia, with some nerve surgeons calling the concurrent metabolic process the second "hit" in DCS [8]. Some authors have advocated for including these disorders and DCS under the umbrella of "multifocal neuropathy" [9]. Overall,

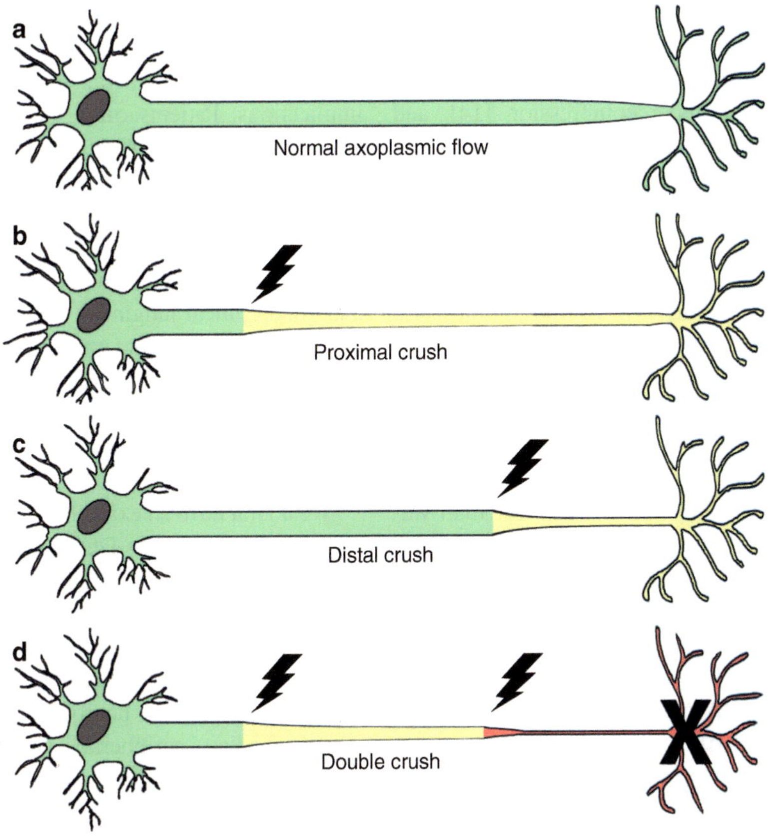

Fig. 19.2 Illustration of the proposed pathophysiological mechanism of double crush syndrome. (**a**) A normal upper motor neuron, with functional anterograde and retrograde axoplasmic flow. (**b**) A proximal lesion, e.g., at the exiting nerve root, causes compromise of axoplasmic flow, but the nerve is able to continue functioning. At this point, a patient may display mild or transient symptoms and have no abnormalities on electrodiagnostic testing. The same can be seen with a single distal lesion, as shown in (**c**). (**d**) However, a second distal compressive lesion causes additive axoplasmic flow disruption, resulting in clinically apparent neuropathy and end target dysfunction. Patients may complain of worsening pain or sensory disturbances, along with weakness that eventually leads to muscle wasting. Electrodiagnostic studies may be abnormal but remain relatively unimpressive relative to the symptoms

DCS remains a controversial and poorly understood phenomenon, with most attention focused on the cervical spine, thoracic outlet, and upper extremity peripheral nerves [10, 11].

While not originally described by Upton and McComas, it is logical that an analogous DCS hypothesis would exist for lumbosacral radiculopathy (LSR) and the lower extremity nerves. The first clinical report of lower extremity double crush was by Chodoroff and Ball in 1985 that described a patient with L5 radiculopathy that underwent an L5-S1 laminectomy and developed worsening postoperative foot pain. The patient was initially diagnosed with reflex sympathetic dystrophy before undergoing electrodiagnostic studies (EDx) that revealed findings compatible with tarsal tunnel syndrome (TTS) [12]. There was symptomatic relief following tarsal tunnel decompression surgery. From this report, evidence of lumbosacral DCS slowly accumulated, with three more cases of combined LSR and TTS published in 1992 [13] and a larger set of studies in 1998 and 2016 demonstrating a notable correlation between lower extremity peripheral nerve entrapment and LSR [14, 15]. Less common causes of lower limb DCS have been described, including sciatic neuropathy with concurrent L5/S1 radiculopathy [14], proximal sciatic nerve injury with distal peroneal involvement [17], multifocal tibial nerve compression [14], and multifocal proximal nerve root compression (paracentral and lateral recess disc) [16, 17].

Lower extremity DCS is likely under-appreciated and under-reported, impeding efforts to describe the true prevalence and epidemiology of this phenomenon [9]. In the lumbosacral spine, the most common causes of DCS are L5/S1 radiculopathy with TTS and L5 radiculopathy with peroneal entrapment at the fibular head. Based on current estimates, the prevalence of DCS in patients with lumbosacral pathology is approximately 5–10% [15, 18], lower than values reported for DCS of the upper limbs, which range from 10% to 70% across different studies [2, 19].

19.2 Evaluation and Initial Workup

The diagnosis of DCS is challenging, especially in patients with vague, multifocal, or complex symptoms. However, failure to diagnose DCS carries with it a high likelihood of persistent symptoms despite an apparently successful surgical intervention and contributes to patient dissatisfaction. A coordinated evaluation with a neurologist or neuromuscular specialist for a superimposed polyneuropathy, such as that seen with uremia and diabetes, may be indicated. Unfortunately, the nerve surgeon's usual diagnostic adjuncts are often less helpful in DCS, due to the additive effects of two sites, rather than one particularly diagnostically convincing lesion. In other words, the patient may not have a particularly impressive disc or particularly impressive EDx findings depending on which studies are sent first, whereas the symptoms are coming from the combination of both lesions. The lack of established diagnostic criteria for DCS contributes to missed diagnoses and patient frustration. Compounding this is that DCS can be misdiagnosed as a complex regional pain syndrome (CRPS) or reflex sympathetic dystrophy (RSD), which has different therapeutic and prognostic implications. Patients often describe feeling as though their reports of ongoing symptoms lack legitimacy or that they are not being heard. In the absence of an accepted standard, an effective diagnostic approach requires a comprehensive history and physical exam, judicious use of EDx, and good clinical judgment. Imaging studies are an important adjunct but must be interpreted cautiously given the high prevalence of lumbosacral pathology in asymptomatic individuals [20]. MRI or ultrasound of the extremity should be considered as well.

We do not have an exact algorithm for diagnosis of lower extremity DCS and differentiating these cases from more routing peripheral or central complaints. The surgeon must keep an open mind and broad differential, especially at the initial clinic encounter, and consider the possibility with any compressive neuropathy. Care must be taken to elicit peripheral symptoms through understanding of anatomy and exam maneuvers such as Tinel's sign or Lasègue's sign (straight leg raise test), but also radicular symptoms, and to understand pain and weakness patterns for common radiculopathies. Briefly, patients should be screened for back pain and specifically asked about radiating or dermatomal patterns of pain, weakness, or sensory disturbance. Classically, L3 is radiating into the groin, L4 into the anterior thigh, L5 into the lateral thigh and dorsum, and S1 into the buttock, back of the leg, and plantar (what some patients refer to as "sciatica"). A positive response should elicit further review, including obtaining a lumbar spine MRI. These are relatively sensitive in delineating lumbosacral causes of neuropathy. EDx are critical to obtain when there is clinical suspicion for DCS. It is important to communicate to the electrodiagnostician that you may suspect DCS so they screen appropriately. In cases with imaging localizing to the spine, it is appropriate to refer for pain management with targeted injections, or surgical consultation as warranted.

19.3 History and Physical Exam

As with cervical DCS, clinical manifestations in the lumbar spine are a function of the nerves compressed, sites of compression, and extent/severity of compression. DCS generally manifests as a combination of pain, weakness, and paresthesias in the distribution of a nerve root or a distal peripheral nerve. Patients may present with symptoms of radiculopathy, mononeuropathy, or both. Clinically, our experience with lower extremity DCS is that these patients usually present with persistent lower limb symptoms following spinal decompression and have often been through multiple office visits and numerous rounds of diagnostic testing before being referred to us. Many arrive frustrated and desperate for answers. A thorough spinal and peripheral nerve exam should be conducted. The motor exam should focus on focal wasting or loss of bulk, tone, and power. Noting limitations in sensitivity to using pinprick to assess for loss of sensation in specific dermatomes (i.e., given the overlapping coverage of individual roots across neighboring dermatomes), one should allow the patient to map out specific regions that "feel different" to them even in the absence of an objective deficit on exam. Asymmetric or absence of reflexes aids in localization. A thorough gait exam is warranted to look for evidence of an antalgic gait, an inability to walk on toes (posterior leg weakness), back-kneeing (excess knee hyperextension in the setting of knee extensor weakness), steppage (in the setting of foot drop), or a Trendelenburg sign (from hip abduction weakness) which are all beneficial. A Tinel sign and its relationship to any scars may aid in localization. The presence of low-back pain, especially radiating low-back pain, would indicate a radicular site of compression. A positive straight leg raise test would raise suspicion for a lumbosacral radiculopathy [21].

Literature describing physical exam findings specific to lumbosacral DCS is limited. Findings that help distinguish carpal and cubital tunnel syndrome from upper extremity DCS may also have relevance in the lower extremity. Upper extremity DCS patients typically have more proximal pain, higher rate of paresthesias, and lower rates of numbness [22–24]. In a large retrospective study of DCS with TTS, Tinel's was positive in 56% of patients [15], a value comparable to that reported in series of isolated TTS [25].

19.4 Diagnostic Studies

When confronted with complex physical exam findings and/or an exam limited by pain, EDx and imaging studies can be of great help. Electrodiagnosticians consider electromyography and nerve conduction studies as an extension of the physical exam. We find that having a good multidisciplinary relationship with our neurophysiologists is key to successful treatment of DCS. With respect to the proximal cause of lumbosacral DCS, lumbosacral spine MRI is the imaging modality of choice for delineating soft tissue pathology and foraminal stenosis. EDx can be fairly specific in localizing lesions to the lumbosacral roots, when abnormalities are detectable, but abnormalities won't always be detectable on EDx, even in the presence of a clear lumbosacral radiculopathy. Some reasons for normal EDx in the setting of radiculopathy include an acute lesion, a pure demyelinating lesion, a lesion with differential fascicular involvement, and/or a lesion preferentially involving the sensory nerve root. It is important to be aware of these limitations of EDx when reciprocating the results with the clinical context. Needless to say, EDx are operator dependent and should be both performed and interpreted by experienced, ideally board certified, practitioners. Please see our case example below for a detailed EDx scenario of DCS.

With respect to imaging the distal causes of DCS, MRI can be useful where higher resolution understanding of 3D anatomy is needed. MRI is also sensitive to edema based on diffusion tensor imaging and dimensional measurement of at least medium to large nerves [26, 27]. Advances in imaging capabilities, such as increasingly sensitive diffusion tensor sequences, may be able to reveal nerve damage at the level of the peripheral nerve [26]. Ultrasound can also be useful in identifying the distal DCS lesion. In addition to evaluating compressive lesions, ultrasound can diagnose the presence of edema in that symptomatic nerve roots often have larger cross-sectional areas than asymptomatic roots [28]. One can check a Tinel's with the ultrasound probe, which may aid in localization, and ultrasound, much like EDx, is a much more dynamic study relative to MRI in that the ultrasonographer can adjust the study based off their findings in real time. Furthermore ultrasound is a relatively inexpensive and noninvasive/nonionizing modality, although quality and interpretation is operator dependent [29].

19.5 Surgical Management

There is currently no high-level evidence about management of DCS, but like other compressive peripheral lesions, as well as spinal lesions, most cases warrant an initial conservative trial with multimodal nonsurgical measures. In the case of DCS, this means focusing on the unique pathology and symptomatology of each lesion. This typically includes directed physical or occupational therapy, orthotics, injections both peripherally and at the nerve root (which are both patient and operator dependent), pain management, and activity modification. If these measures fail, surgical strategies should be considered. In the case of patients who present with persistent symptoms after an initial decompression, treating their second lesion can be effective. However, a subset of these patients may also be predisposed to do less well after surgical treatment. For patients presenting with new-onset DCS, the decision regarding which lesion to address first is patient dependent, and we typically advise patients that a staged intervention may be needed. In situations where the cause is unclear, we err on treating the spine, because it is statistically more likely to be the cause of the problem. A counter-argument would be that a peripheral nerve procedure has lower morbidity, but we would argue that many spine surgeries we currently do are also same day and low morbidity. In complex cases, collaboration among multidisciplinary care teams is key to designing appropriate treatment strategies.

DCS represents multiple pathophysiological problems and therefore often requires multiple surgical treatments. Since both spine and peripheral nerve decompressions generally have low morbidity, we typically seek to intervene first on the lesion presumed to cause the greatest distress, based on diagnostic testing, history, and physical exam. It is critical to provide patients with appropriate expectations, and patients should understand that outcomes in DCS may be worse than in cases of isolated peripheral neuropathies [1, 22]. Likewise, surgeons should not expect the same degree of improvement typically observed after decompressing an entrapped peripheral nerve. It is our practice to counsel patients when we suspect DCS, in order to best educate them as well as set expectations. There is no hard evidence with which to counsel patients about relative improvement expected from treating each component, but we estimate the relative contributions based on our understanding of the Seddon-Sunderland nerve injury classification as well as principles of nerve regeneration. We also are relatively aggressive about obtaining EDx, and it is important for surgeons to either ask for or pay attention to peripheral as well as radicular findings.

According to the literature available to date, the most likely DCS scenarios the peripheral nerve surgeon will encounter are L5 radiculopathy with peroneal entrapment or S1 radiculopathy with anterior or posterior TTS (Fig. 19.3) [14, 15]. Surgical approaches for decompressing the common, superficial, and deep peroneal nerve, as well as the tarsal tunnel, are well known. Peripheral nerve surgeons may be less familiar, however, with the surgical treatment of lumbosacral radiculopathy.

In most cases of DCS, the proximal lesion is compression of the nerve root, either from a degenerative pathology, such as the facet, or soft tissue compression from disc extrusion or ligamentous hypertrophy. Treatment depends on decompression, both direct and indirect. The surgical approach chosen depends on the anatomy of the pathology. Most nerve root compression can be directly addressed through a posterior approach. Traditionally, nerve root compression

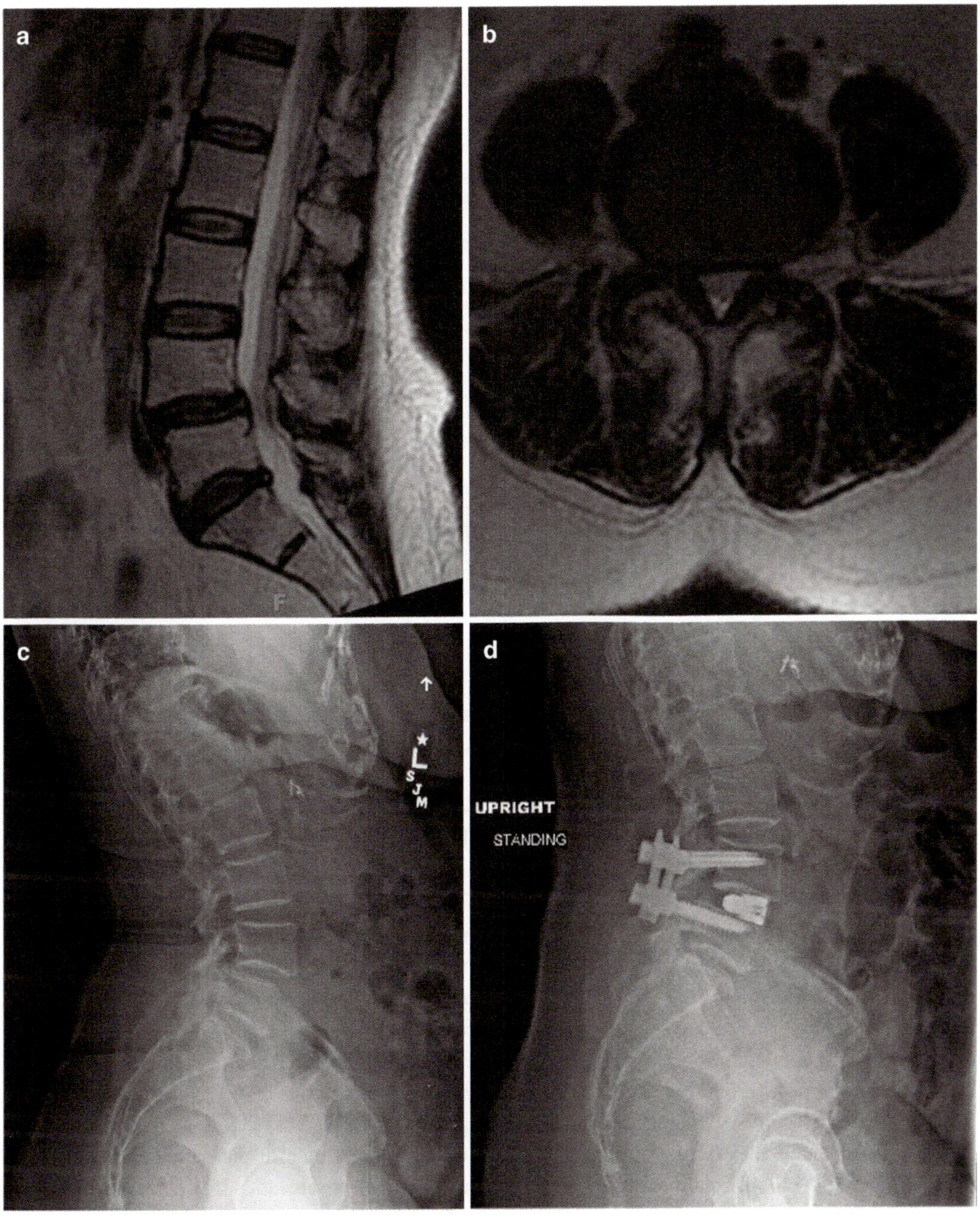

Fig. 19.3 Case example of a patient suffering from lumbosacral double crush syndrome. This patient is a 65-year-old male who presented with symptoms of bilateral L5 radiculopathy, left worse than right, with weakness in ankle dorsiflexion and eversion on the left. An MRI of the lumbar spine demonstrated grade 1 anterolisthesis of L4 on L5, with severe bilateral neuroforaminal stenosis (**a**, **b**). Because of this, he was offered an L4–L5 minimally invasive transforaminal lumbar interbody fusion, which he tolerated well, leaving the hospital POD 1 with notable relief of symptoms (**c**, **d**). At his 6-week postoperative visit, his radiating back pain was resolved but he continued to complain of pain and paresthesias in the dorsum of the foot and had little improvement in his foot drop on the left. Electrodiagnostic studies were obtained and were consistent with a mild-to-moderate peroneal neuropathy that localized to the fibular head. We offered him decompression, with exposure of the nerve shown in (**e**), and release of several compressive bands, including the leading edge of the peroneus longus (arrowheads) (**f**)

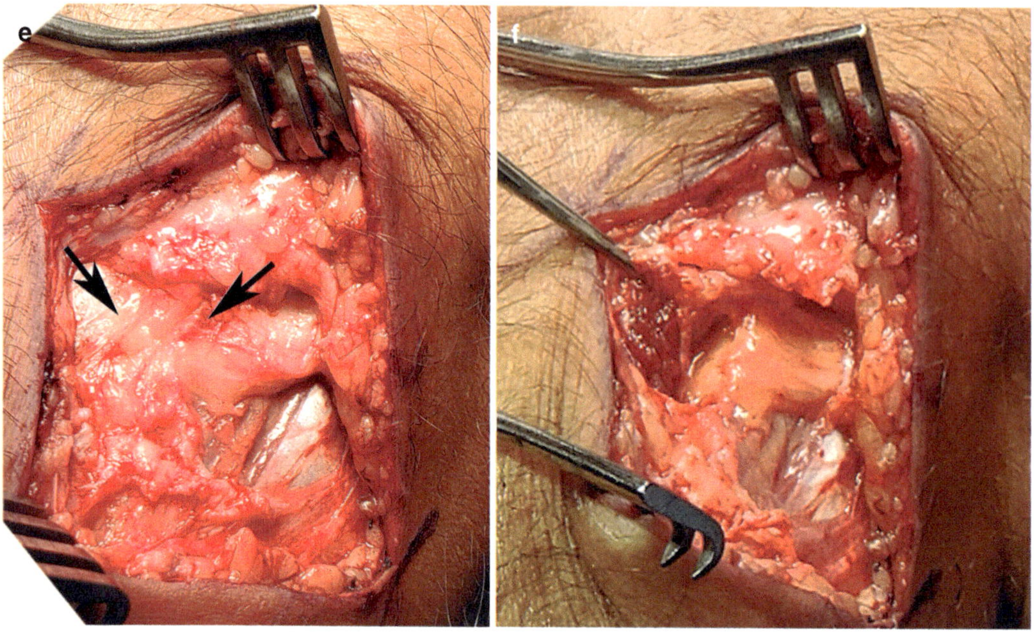

Fig. 19.3 (continued)

has been addressed through an open approach with hemilaminectomy and discectomy. Increasingly, "mini-open" and minimally invasive options are thought to be equally effective and associated with less morbidity. In either approach, patients can often go home the next day, with some cases being done as outpatient procedures (Fig. 19.4a–c).

Anterior and lateral approaches can be used when a fusion is indicated, such as mobile spondylolisthesis, and provide the added benefit of indirect nerve root decompression. The workhorse anterior approach for spine surgeons is the anterior lumbar interbody fusion, usually done with the assistance of a vascular surgeon for the approach. The levels that can be treated through an anterior approach depend on the patient's vascular anatomy, most importantly where the bifurcation of the great vessels. L5–S1 can reliably be addressed through this approach, often L4–L5 as well, and then L3–L4 more rarely. This procedure serves to decompress the lumbosacral nerve roots indirectly, by placing a large interbody spacer to restore disc and neuroforaminal height. We find that patients do well with this procedure and sometimes report immediate improvement of symptoms.

19.6 Discussion

Overall, lumbosacral DCS remains a challenging and important clinical entity for both spine and peripheral nerve surgeons. While rigorous data is lacking, estimates that 5–10% of patients with lumbosacral radiculopathy also have a peripheral entrapment suggest this phenomenon will be encountered and is likely under-recognized in clinical practice. Skilled judgment will be needed to determine which of these concomitant lesions are clinically relevant. If a patient has been referred for "failed" surgery or continues to have symptoms after what seems to be successful decompression of a suspected culprit lesion, a diagnosis of DCS should be entertained and further studies obtained. As expanded prospective clinical and translational science research improve our understanding of this disease, the diagnosis and effective treatment of DCS are likely to improve.

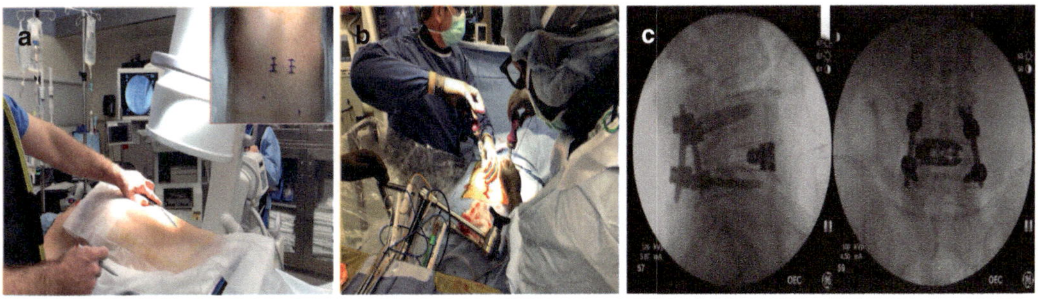

Fig. 19.4 Images from a typical minimally invasive transforaminal lumbar interbody fusion procedure, which we will perform as either a same day or single overnight stay. Our experience is patients do well with proper expectations and analgesia, as well as short-term help at home. (**a**) Preoperative markings, note the small paramedian incisions in the top right. (**b**) Intraoperative images, (**c**) postoperative radiographs showing good hardware placement and restoration of lordosis

To us, the major challenge in treating DCS is diagnosis or recognition of the second lesion, rather than the technical aspects of treatment. Indeed, once recognized, most peripheral nerve surgeons are experienced with common decompressive treatments of the peripheral nerves. There should be a high suspicion for DCS in cases of "failed back surgery syndrome" or "failed surgery" for peripheral neuropathy. When seeing these patients who "failed" surgery, the practitioner must keep an open mind and be willing to pursue additional diagnostic studies. Early recognition is also key to maintaining patient rapport and trust.

In patients presenting with ongoing symptoms after a surgical decompression, surgeons must weigh the benefit from a second decompression versus the risk of a second surgery. There is little published information to guide whether the procedures should be staged or the order in which the lesions should be addressed. Clearly, the surgeon must use judgment, collaboration with colleagues in other fields (e.g., radiologists, neurophysiologists, and neuromuscular experts), and diagnostic testing to understand which lesion is more severe or more likely to account for the symptoms present. In cases with clinical equipoise, some surgeons argue that spinal decompression should take precedence, since radiculopathy is neurologically "upstream" and affects more nerves and muscles, and with proximal injuries, there is often a longer distance for axons to cover in their regenerative paths to reinnervating target muscles. This would be congruent with the accepted theory of anterograde/retrograde axonal flow. It also may be difficult for a nerve to regenerate past a proximal area of injury or compression, if the distal lesion is addressed first. Finally, with modern MRI imaging, structural spine pathology can be diagnosed with high confidence. Others adopt a different perspective, arguing that peripheral decompression remains the lower morbidity procedure and should be tried first, reserving higher risk spinal surgery for cases of inadequate symptom relief [30]. The final decision in these cases should involve shared decision-making between the surgeon and patient. In our own practice, we typically stage procedures, usually treating the spinal lesions first in ambiguous cases. We then gauge response to this first intervention and discuss with patients whether a peripheral decompression should also be considered. The severity of deficits on EDx can also aid in the decision-making process as there is a likely a window of opportunity for successful reinnervation in the setting of very severe lesion, extrapolating from the literature on neurotization with trauma-related nerve injury.

For trainees, the most important lessons about DCS are to maintain a high index of clinical suspicion and remain open-minded in making a diagnosis. Of course, trainees are well served to ensure they use their training to develop a thorough understanding of peripheral nervous system anatomy to aid the diagnostic workup. Surgeons at all levels should remain compassionate with frustrated patients, some of whom may have been misdiagnosed by other providers. As mentioned earlier, some of these patients may have been incorrectly diagnosed with CRPS/RSD due to a perceived lack of benefit after "maximal" surgical treatment. This is a challenging situation, as some of these patients may have incompletely treated DCS, some may have DCS that did not respond as well as expected to intervention, and some may in fact have CRPS. Thorough understanding of the history and EDx and imaging studies are needed to make the proper diagnosis. Finally, given the broad range of knowledge needed to effectively diagnose and manage DCS, working within a multidisciplinary team will aid in ensuring the greatest likelihood of an accurate diagnosis and optimization of the therapeutic approach.

19.7 Key Points

- Lumbosacral DCS is a challenging clinical entity that requires a high index of clinical suspicion. Management should focus on ensuring an accurate diagnosis and identifying an appropriate treatment plan for all contributing pathologies.
- There may be a peripheral lesion in 5–10% of patients with lumbosacral radiculopathy. The most common cases are L5 or S1 radiculopathies with peroneal or tibial nerve entrapment(s), but other etiologies have been reported.
- Both clinical symptoms and electrodiagnostic studies can be misleading unless considered in the context of DCS. An accurate diagnosis of DCS requires a thorough physical exam, selective imaging, and electrodiagnostic tests. While controversial, it is worth considering whether systemic or metabolic etiologies, such as uremia or diabetes, are present that may place the patient at an increased risk of peripheral nerve entrapment.
- MRI without contrast is the imaging study of choice to screen for proximal spinal lesions, and ultrasound can be useful in evaluating peripheral nerves. Electromyography and nerve conduction studies also play an integral role in the diagnosis as well.
- Conservative measures should be trialed initially unless there are signs of acute neurological deterioration or severe motor deficits (as determined by exam or electrodiagnostic studies). These interventions include physical and occupational therapy, injections, behavior modification, and other forms of pain management, pharmacologic and nonpharmacologic.
- When determining which lesion to address first, a limited evidence base emphasizes the importance of surgeon judgment and shared decision-making with the patient. We generally favor a staged approach, allowing an opportunity to evaluate response to the first intervention.
- Surgeons should also temper patient expectations of experiencing full relief from a single procedure.

19.8 Case Example

A 75-year-old man with non-Hodgkin's lymphoma status post chemotherapy, now in remission, presented for evaluation of bilateral foot drop. Onset was 6 months prior to presentation and occurred in the setting of a 40-pound weight loss during chemotherapy. He frequently crossed his legs while sitting. The right foot drop had shown a great deal of spontaneous improvement over the 3 months leading up to his evaluation in clinic but the left side had not improved. Along with foot drop, he described a squeezing sensation over the dorsum of the left foot. Complicating his history was the presence of chronic low-back pain with intermittent radiation into his left ankle and foot, last treated with epidural steroid injections 3 years prior to presentation. His examination at the time of initial presentation was only notable for impaired toe extension and ankle dorsiflexion on the left (graded at 4-/5 and 4/5 by MRC scale).

Electrodiagnostic testing performed 3 months prior to presentation demonstrated bilateral peroneal neuropathies at the fibular head, left worse than right. NCSs were notable for a definite conduction block across the left fibular head and a possible conduction block across the right fibular head (Fig. 19.5a, b). Bilateral superficial peroneal sensory responses were preserved and within normal limits, a slightly atypical finding but compatible with a primary demyelinating process at the fibular heads (Fig. 19.5c). Electromyography showed abnormalities limited to the distribution of the bilateral common peroneal nerves with only equivocal chronic neurogenic changes evident in the left gluteus medius, but no other abnormalities to suggest a proximal lesion of the left sciatic nerve, lumbosacral plexus, or lumbosacral roots (Fig. 19.5d).

Neuromuscular ultrasound showed no structural abnormalities in either peroneal nerve, including no evidence of entrapment or compression at the fibular head on either side. The combination of the history of weight loss with spontaneous improvement on the right side and prior electrodiagnostic evidence of peroneal entrapment at the fibular heads resulted in a diagnosis of "slimmer's paralysis" [31, 32]. The patient opted to pursue a conservative approach with lifestyle modification and use of an ankle-foot orthotic in the hopes that the left side would eventually show a comparable degree of recovery to that experienced on the right.

He returned for follow-up 5 months later and endorsed new sensory deficits in the left leg, and his left ankle dorsiflexion weakness had progressed. His exam also showed new deficits in left hip abduction and ankle eversion and inver-

a

MNC

Nerve / Sites	Latency ms	Amplitude mV	Segments	Distance mm	Lat Diff ms	Velocity m/s
R Peroneal - EDB						
Ankle	5.47	2.1	Ankle - EDB	100		
Fib head	12.08	2.0	Fib head - Ankle	300	6.61	45.4
Pop fossa	15.10	1.5	Pop fossa - Fib head	100	3.02	33.1
			Pop fossa - Ankle		9.64	
L Peroneal - EDB						
Ankle	7.03	1.2	Ankle - EDB	100		
Fib head	14.22	1.4	Fib head - Ankle	300	7.19	41.7
Pop fossa	16.87	0.9	Pop fossa - Fib head	100	2.66	37.6
			Pop fossa - Ankle		9.84	
R Tibial - AH						
Ankle	5.10	4.4	Ankle - AH	100		
Pop fossa	14.48	3.3	Pop fossa - Ankle	380	9.37	40.5
R Peroneal - Tib Ant						
Fib head	3.49	2.6	Fib head - Tib Ant	120		
Pop fossa	6.20	1.7	Pop fossa - Fib head	100	2.71	36.9
L Peroneal - Tib Ant						
Fib head	3.96	3.7	Fib head - Tib Ant	100		
Pop fossa	6.61	1.8	Pop fossa - Fib head	100	2.66	37.6

b

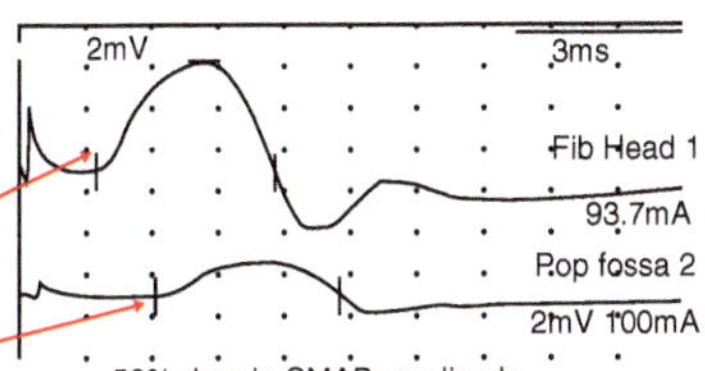

c

SNC

Nerve / Sites	Onset Lat ms	Peak Lat ms	Amplitude µV	Onset Diff ms	Distance mm	Cond Vel m/s
R Radial - Anatomical snuff box (Forearm)						
Forearm	1.7	2.4	25	1.7	100	58
R Sural - Ankle (Calf)						
Calf	3.0	3.6	5	3.0	140	47
L Sural - Ankle (Calf)						
Calf	3.2	4.0	6	3.2	140	43
R Superficial peroneal - Ankle						
Lat leg	1.9	2.4	10	1.9	100	53
L Superficial peroneal - Ankle						
Lat leg	1.6	2.6	7	1.6	100	64

d

EMG

Summary										
	Insertional	Spontaneous				MUAP				
Muscle	Activity	Fib	PSW	Fasc	Other	Dur.	Amp	Poly	Recruit	Activate
L. Tibialis anterior	Normal	None	None	None	-	Mod Incr	Normal	50%	Mod Red	Normal
L.Peroneus longus	Normal	1+	1+	None	-	Mod Incr	Normal	50%	Mod Red	Normal
L. Gastrocnemius (Medial head)	Normal	None	None	None	-	Normal	Normal	None	Normal	Normal
L.Vastus medialis	Normal	None	None	None	-	Normal	Normal	None	Normal	Normal
L. Peroneus tertius	Increased	2+	2+	None	-	Normal	Normal	None	Mod Red	Normal
L. Gluteus medius	Normal	None	None	None	-	Sl Incr	Normal	25%	Normal	Normal
L. Biceps femoris (short head)	Normal	None	None	None	-	Normal	Normal	None	Normal	Normal
L. L5 paraspinal	Normal	None	None	None	-	Normal	Normal	None	Normal	Normal
R. Tibialis anterior	Normal	1+	1+	None	-	Mod Incr	Normal	25%	Mod Red	Normal
R. Gastrocnemius (Medial head)	Normal	None	None	None	-	Normal	Normal	None	Normal	Normal
R. Peroneus tertius	Normal	None	None	None	-	Mod Incr	Normal	25%	Mod Red	Normal
R. Peroneus longus	Normal	None	None	None	-	Mod Incr	Normal	25%	Mod Red	Normal
R. Vastus medialis	Normal	None	None	None	-	Normal	Normal	None	Normal	Normal

Fig. 19.5 Initial electrodiagnostic testing demonstrated bilateral peroneal neuropathies at the fibular head, left worse than right, with a definite conduction block across the left fibular head (arrows in tracing and highlighted in red in data sheet) and a possible conduction block across the right fibular head (green) (**a**, **b**). Bilateral superficial peroneal sensory responses were preserved and within normal limits (red), a slightly atypical finding but compatible with a primary demyelinating process at the fibular heads (**c**). Electromyography showed abnormalities limited to the distribution of the bilateral common peroneal nerves (left = red, right = green) with only equivocal chronic neurogenic changes evident in the left gluteus medius (blue) but no other abnormalities to suggest a proximal lesion of the left sciatic nerve, lumbosacral plexus, or lumbosacral roots (**d**)

sion. He had also lost his left medial hamstring and ankle reflexes, both of which were present 5 months earlier. Given the interval features concerning for a left L5/S1 radiculopathy, repeat electrodiagnostic testing was performed. Relative to the prior study, this study once again showed preserved lower extremity sensory responses and interval resolution of the left peroneal neuropathy at the fibular head but smaller tibial and peroneal motor responses recorded from the left foot. Electromyography showed interval development of active and chronic denervation in additional muscles of the left L5 and S1 myotomes, findings compatible with a left L5/S1 radiculopathy (Fig. 19.6). Computerized tomography myelography confirmed the presence of severe left neu-

MNC

Nerve / Sites	Latency ms	Amplitude mV	Segments	Distance mm	Lat Diff ms	Velocity m/s
L Peroneal - EDB						
Ankle	6.15	0.2	Ankle - EDB	100		
Fib head	14.95	0.3	Fib head - Ankle	320	8.80	36.4
Pop fossa	17.08	0.3	Pop fossa - Fib head	80	2.14	37.5
			Pop fossa - Ankle		10.94	
R Peroneal - EDB						
Ankle	5.73	2.2	Ankle - EDB			
			Pop fossa - Ankle			
L Tibial - AH						
Ankle	5.10	3.0	Ankle - AH	100		
Pop fossa	13.85	2.4	Pop fossa - Ankle	410	8.75	46.9
L Peroneal - Tib Ant						
Fib head	3.39	5.7	Fib head - Tib Ant	140		
Pop fossa	5.73	5.5	Pop fossa - Fib head	100	2.34	42.7
R Peroneal - Tib Ant						
Fib head	4.58	6.4	Fib head - Tib Ant			

SNC

Nerve / Sites	Onset Lat ms	Peak Lat ms	Amplitude µV	Onset Diff ms	Distance mm	Cond Vel m/s
R Sural - Ankle (Calf)						
Calf	2.6	3.5	5	2.6	140	54
L Sural - Ankle (Calf)						
Calf	3.0	3.8	6	3.0	140	47
L Superficial peroneal - Ankle						
Lat leg	2.7	3.3	5	2.7	100	37
R Superficial peroneal - Ankle						
Lat leg	2.4	3.2	7	2.4	100	41

EMG

Summary										
	Insertional	Spontaneous				MUAP				
Muscle	Activity	Fib	PSW	Fase	Other	Dur.	Amp	Poly	Recruit	Activate
L. L5 paraspinal	Increased	1+	1+	None	-					
L. Gluteus medius	Increased	1+	1+	None	-	Sl Incr	Sl Incr	25%	Mild Red	Sub Max
L. Gluteus maximus	Increased	1+	1+	None	-	Sl Incr	Sl Incr	25%	Mild Red	Normal
L. Tibialis anterior	Increased	1+	1+	None	-	Sl Incr	Mod Incr	None	Mod Red	Normal
L. Gastrocnemius (Medial head)	Increased	2+	2+	None	-	Normal	Normal	None	Mild Red	Normal

Fig. 19.6 This repeat study once again showed preserved lower extremity sensory responses (green) and interval resolution of the left peroneal neuropathy at the fibular head (green) but smaller tibial and peroneal motor responses recorded from the left foot (red). Electromyography showed interval development of active and chronic denervation in additional muscles of the left L5 and S1 myotomes (red), findings compatible with a left L5/S1 radiculopathy

roforaminal stenosis at L4–L5 and L5–S1, and cerebrospinal fluid analysis was normal without evidence of malignancy.

The clinical and electrodiagnostic features at the time of initial presentation were compatible with a left peroneal neuropathy at the fibular head. However, the patient's history of low-back pain with radiation down the left lower limb in the setting of a preserved left superficial peroneal sensory response, and subtle chronic neurogenic motor unit action potentials on EMG of the left gluteus, were more suggestive of a left lumbosacral radiculopathy, i.e., raising the possibility of a double crush syndrome. At follow-up, there was progression of pain heightening the concern for a left lumbosacral radiculopathy. Repeat electrodiagnostic testing confirmed the presence of a left L5/S1 radiculopathy accounting for the persistent and new clinical deficits, given the concurrent evidence of interval resolution of the left peroneal mononeuropathy at the fibular head. Fortunately, his pain responded to conservative measures, in this case physical therapy and targeted nerve root injections.

References

1. Wessel LE, et al. Outcomes following peripheral nerve decompression with and without associated double crush syndrome: a case control study. Plast Reconstr Surg. 2017;139(1):119–27.
2. Upton AR, McComas AJ. The double crush in nerve entrapment syndromes. Lancet. 1973;2(7825):359–62.
3. Dahlin LB, Archer DR, McLean WG. Axonal transport and morphological changes following nerve compression. An experimental study in the rabbit vagus nerve. J Hand Surg Br. 1993;18(1):106–10.
4. Kobayashi S, et al. Effect of lumbar nerve root compression on primary sensory neurons and their central branches: changes in the nociceptive neuropeptides substance P and somatostatin. Spine (Phila Pa 1976). 2005;30(3):276–82.
5. Dahlin LB, McLean WG. Effects of graded experimental compression on slow and fast axonal transport in rabbit vagus nerve. J Neurol Sci. 1986;72(1):19–30.
6. Dellon AL, Mackinnon SE. Chronic nerve compression model for the double crush hypothesis. Ann Plast Surg. 1991;26(3):259–64.
7. Schmid AB, Coppieters MW. The double crush syndrome revisited--a Delphi study to reveal current expert views on mechanisms underlying dual nerve disorders. Man Ther. 2011;16(6):557–62.
8. Baba M, et al. Focal conduction delay at the carpal tunnel and the cubital fossa in diabetic polyneuropathy. Electromyogr Clin Neurophysiol. 1987;27(2):119–23.
9. Cohen BH, et al. Multifocal neuropathy: expanding the scope of double crush syndrome. J Hand Surg Am. 2016;41(12):1171–5.
10. Wood VE, Biondi J. Double-crush nerve compression in thoracic-outlet syndrome. J Bone Joint Surg Am. 1990;72(1):85–7.
11. Wilbourn AJ, Gilliatt RW. Double-crush syndrome: a critical analysis. Neurology. 1997;49(1):21–9.
12. Chodoroff B, Ball RD. Lumbosacral radiculopathy, reflex sympathetic dystrophy and tarsal tunnel syndrome: an unusual presentation. Arch Phys Med Rehabil. 1985;66(3):185–7.
13. Augustijn P, Vanneste J. The tarsal tunnel syndrome after a proximal lesion. J Neurol Neurosurg Psychiatry. 1992;55(1):65–7.
14. Golovchinsky V. Double crush syndrome in lower extremities. Electromyogr Clin Neurophysiol. 1998;38(2):115–20.
15. Zheng C, et al. The prevalence of tarsal tunnel syndrome in patients with lumbosacral radiculopathy. Eur Spine J. 2016;25(3):895–905.
16. Iwasaki M, et al. Double crush of L5 spinal nerve root due to L4/5 lateral recess stenosis and bony spur formation of lumbosacral transitional vertebra pseudoarticulation: a case report and review. NMC Case Rep J. 2017;4(4):121–5.
17. Fassler PR, et al. Injury of the sciatic nerve associated with acetabular fracture. J Bone Joint Surg Am. 1993;75(8):1157–66.
18. McSweeney SC, Cichero M. Tarsal tunnel syndrome-A narrative literature review. Foot (Edinb). 2015;25(4):244–50.
19. Morgan G, Wilbourn AJ. Cervical radiculopathy and coexisting distal entrapment neuropathies: double-crush syndromes? Neurology. 1998;50(1):78–83.
20. Boden SD, et al. Abnormal magnetic-resonance scans of the lumbar spine in asymptomatic subjects. A prospective investigation. J Bone Joint Surg Am. 1990;72(3):403–8.
21. Coster S, de Bruijn SF, Tavy DL. Diagnostic value of history, physical examination and needle electromyography in diagnosing lumbosacral radiculopathy. J Neurol. 2010;257(3):332–7.
22. Osterman AL. The double crush syndrome. Orthop Clin North Am. 1988;19(1):147–55.
23. Lo SF, et al. Clinical characteristics and electrodiagnostic features in patients with carpal tunnel syndrome, double crush syndrome, and cervical radiculopathy. Rheumatol Int. 2012;32(5):1257–63.
24. Davidge KM, et al. The "hierarchical" Scratch Collapse Test for identifying multilevel ulnar nerve compression. Hand (N Y). 2015;10(3):388–95.
25. Schwieterman B, et al. Diagnostic accuracy of physical examination tests of the ankle/foot complex: a systematic review. Int J Sports Phys Ther. 2013;8(4):416–26.

26. Kanamoto H, et al. The diagnosis of double-crush lesion in the L5 lumbar nerve using diffusion tensor imaging. Spine J. 2016;16(3):315–21.
27. Chhabra A, et al. Incremental value of magnetic resonance neurography of lumbosacral plexus over non-contributory lumbar spine magnetic resonance imaging in radiculopathy: a prospective study. World J Radiol. 2016;8(1):109–16.
28. Metin Okmen B, Okmen K, Altan L. Investigation of the effect of cervical radiculopathy on peripheral nerves of the upper extremity with high-resolution ultrasonography. Spine (Phila Pa 1976). 2018;43(14):E798–803.
29. Zaidman CM, et al. Detection of peripheral nerve pathology: comparison of ultrasound and MRI. Neurology. 2013;80(18):1634–40.
30. Molinari WJ 3rd, Elfar JC. The double crush syndrome. J Hand Surg Am. 2013;38(4):799–801; quiz 801.
31. Sotaniemi KA. Slimmer's paralysis--peroneal neuropathy during weight reduction. J Neurol Neurosurg Psychiatry. 1984;47(5):564–6.
32. Margulis M, Ben Zvi L, Bernfeld B. Bilateral common peroneal nerve entrapment after excessive weight loss: case report and review of the literature. J Foot Ankle Surg. 2018;57(3):632–4.

Index

C. J. Dy et al. (eds.), *Peripheral Nerve Issues after Orthopedic Surgery*,
https://doi.org/10.1007/978-3-030-84428-8

S

T

V

W

Z

GPSR Compliance

The European Union's (EU) General Product Safety Regulation (GPSR) is a set of rules that requires consumer products to be safe and our obligations to ensure this.

If you have any concerns about our products, you can contact us on ProductSafety@springernature.com

In case Publisher is established outside the EU, the EU authorized representative is:

Springer Nature Customer Service Center GmbH
Europaplatz 3
69115 Heidelberg, Germany

Batch number: 10732807

Printed by Printforce, the Netherlands